BSAVA Manual of Canine and Feline Gastroenterology
third edition

T0203163

Editors:

Edward J. Hall
MA VetMB PhD DipECVIM-CA FRCVS
Langford Vets, Bristol Veterinary School, Langford House, Langford BS40 5DU, UK

David A. Williams
MA VetMB PhD DipACVIM-SAIM DipECVIM-CA
University of Illinois, Department of Veterinary Clinical Medicine,
1008 West Hazelwood Drive, Urbana, IL 61802, USA

Aarti Kathrani
BVetMed(Hons) PhD DipACVIM-SAIM DipACVN FHEA MRCVS
Royal Veterinary College, Hawkshead Lane, Hatfield, Hertfordshire AL9 7TA, UK

Published by:

British Small Animal Veterinary Association
Woodrow House, 1 Telford Way,
Waterwells Business Park, Quedgeley,
Gloucester GL2 2AB

A Company Limited by Guarantee in England
Registered Company No. 2837793
Registered as a Charity

Titles in the BSAVA Manuals series

For further information on these and all BSAVA publications, please visit our website: **www.bsava.com/shop**

Contents

Section 3: Patient management

Section 4: Diseases of specific systems/organs

Contributors

Virginie Barberet
DVM PhD DipECVDI FHEA MRCVS
VetCT specialists,
St John's Innovation Centre, Cowley Road,
Cambridge CB4 0WS, UK

Patrick Barko
MS DVM
University of Illinois,
College of Veterinary Medicine,
2001 South Lincoln Avenue, Urbana, IL 61802, USA

Daniel J. Batchelor
BVSc DSAM PhD DipECVIM-CA MRCVS
Institute of Veterinary Science,
University of Liverpool, Chester High Road,
Neston CH64 7TE, UK

Ian A. Battersby
BVSc DSAM DipECVIM-CA FRCVS
Davies Veterinary Specialists,
Manor Farm Business Park, Higham Gobion,
Hertfordshire SG5 3HR, UK

Andrea Boari
DVM
Small Animal Internal Medicine Service,
Veterinary Teaching Hospital, Faculty of Veterinary
Medicine, University of Teramo, Piano D'accio,
64100 Teramo, Italy

Marcus V. Candido
BVetMed PGBiol MVetSc
Department of Equine and Small Animal Medicine,
Faculty of Veterinary Medicine, University of Helsinki,
PO 57 (Viikintie 49), 00014 Helsinki, Finland

Michael J. Day
BSc BVMS(Hons) PhD DSc Dr(hc) DipECVP FASM FRCPath FRCVS
School of Veterinary and Life Sciences,
Murdoch University, Murdoch 6150,
Western Australia

Clive Elwood
MA VetMB MSc PhD CertSAC DipACVIM-SAIM DipECVIM-CA FRCVS
The Old Schoolhouse, 23 Church Road,
Little Berkhamsted, Hertfordshire SG13 8LY, UK

Maggie Fisher
BVetMed CBiol FRSB DipEVPC MRCVS
Veterinary Research Management,
The Mews Studio, Portland Road, Malvern,
Worcestershire WR14 2TA, UK

Alexander J. German
BVSc PhD CertSAM DipECVIM-CA SFHEA FRCVS
Institute of Ageing & Chronic Disease and Institute of
Veterinary Science, University of Liverpool,
Chester High Road, Neston CH64 7TE, UK

Edward J. Hall
MA VetMB PhD DipECVIM-CA FRCVS
Langford Vets, Bristol Veterinary School,
Langford House, Langford BS40 5DU, UK

Peter Holdsworth
AO BSc(Hons) PhD FRSB FAICD
Veterinary Research Management,
The Mews Studio, Portland Road, Malvern,
Worcestershire WR14 2TA, UK

Aarti Kathrani
BVetMed(Hons) PhD DipACVIM-SAIM DipACVN FHEA MRCVS
Royal Veterinary College,
Hawkshead Lane, Hatfield, Hertfordshire AL9 7TA, UK

Peter Kook
DrMedVet Privatdozent DipACVIM-SAIM DipECVIM-CA
Clinic for Small Animal Internal Medicine,
Vetsuisse Faculty, University of Zurich,
Winterthurerstrasse 260, 8057 Zurich, Switzerland

Rachel Lavoué
DVM PhD DipECVIM-CA
IRSD, INSERM U 1220 UMR INRA – ENVT
Departement of Clinical Sciences,
Ecole Nationale Vétérinaire de Toulouse,
23 Chemin des Capelles, 31076 Toulouse, France

Nicole Luckschander-Zeller
DrMedVet PhD DipACVIM-SAIM DipECVIM-CA
Department IV, Klinik für Kleintiere,
Abteilung für Interne Medizin, Veterinärplatz,
A-1210 Wien, Austria

Alison Ridyard
BVSc DSAM DipECVIM-CA MRCVS
School of Veterinary Medicine,
University of Glasgow, 464 Bearsden Road,
Glasgow, G61 1QH, UK

Marcella Ridgway
VMD MS DipACVIM
University of Illinois,
Veterinary Teaching Hospital,
1008 West Hazelwood Drive,
Urbana, IL 61802, USA

Thomas Spillmann
DipMedVet DrMedVet DipECVIM-CA
Department of Equine and Small Animal Medicine,
Faculty of Veterinary Medicine, University of Helsinki,
PO 57 (Viikintie 49), 00014 Helsinki, Finland

Mickey Tivers
BVSc(Hons) PhD CertSAS DipECVS MRCVS
Paragon Veterinary Referrals,
Paragon Business Village, Red Hall Crescent,
Wakefield WF1 2DF, UK

Penny Watson
MA VetMD CertVR DSAM DipECVIM-CA FRCVS
Department of Veterinary Medicine,
Madingley Road, Cambridge CB3 0ES, UK

Mike Willard
DVM MS DipACVIM-SAIM
College of Veterinary Medicine & Biomedical Sciences,
Texas A&M University,
College Station 77843, USA

David A. Williams
MA VetMB PhD DipACVIM-SAIM DipECVIM-CA
University of Illinois,
Department of Veterinary Clinical Medicine,
1008 West Hazelwood Drive, Urbana, IL 61802, USA

John Williams
MA VetMB LLB CertVR DipECVS FRCVS
Vets Now 24/7 Emergency Hospital,
98 Bury Old Road, Whitefield, Manchester M45 6TQ, UK

Foreword

It is a great pleasure that I have been asked to write the foreword for this new edition of the *BSAVA Manual of Canine and Feline Gastroenterology*. This revised text provides a current, well-structured and authoritative overview of those gastrointestinal diseases challenging both clinician practitioners and academicians alike. A primary aim of this Manual is to provide veterinarians with knowledge to improve the quality of life of dogs and cats living with these disorders; in other words, to effectively diagnose, treat and cure.

I am honoured to know and have collaborated with editors Hall, Williams and Kathrani who, collectively, bring a compendium of advanced gastroenterology knowledge and practical clinical expertise to the reader. They have assembled an expert team of international authors that have skillfully characterized patient problems, diagnostic approach and principles of patient management for each major disease affecting the alimentary tract, liver and pancreas. Chapters contain abundant tables and figures as well as a diagnostic algorithm to aid veterinarians with rapid acquisition of key points for each disease. Noteworthy also is the quality of the colour photographs found throughout the text but especially those of endoscopic and histopathological lesions. I anticipate that this Manual will quickly become an essential 'must have' for all veterinary libraries.

The editors are to be commended for comprising this latest iteration of the *BSAVA Manual of Canine and Feline Gastroenterology*. This excellent publication continues in the tradition of its predecessors by providing the best in scientific quality regarding diagnosis and treatment of gastrointestinal diseases in dogs and cats. I know my desk copy will be used often.

Albert E. Jergens
DVM PhD DipACVIM AGAF

Donn E and Beth M. Bacon Professor in Small Animal Medicine and Surgery and Associate Chair for Research and Graduate Studies
Department of Veterinary Clinical Sciences,
College of Veterinary Medicine,
Iowa State University,
Ames, Iowa USA

Preface

"As a dog returneth to his vomit, so a fool returneth to his folly"
King James Bible, Proverbs 26:11

It has been over a decade since the second edition of the *BSAVA Manual of Canine and Feline Gastroenterology* was published. Thus, this third edition is timely: our knowledge of the digestive and immunological functions of the gastrointestinal (GI) tract has expanded exponentially since then; and we are now beginning to understand the pivotal role of the other two players in this ecosystem, i.e. nutrition and the microbiome, and how their manipulation can improve GI health. However, challenges remain, not least in our understanding of chronic inflammatory enteropathies and whether inflammatory bowel disease (IBD) is a term that should be abandoned in veterinary medicine.

Two of the previous co-editors have returned to editing this 'folly' and welcome a new co-editor, Aarti Kathrani. Her Diplomas in both Internal Medicine and Veterinary Nutrition make her the ideal expert to ensure the content is relevant and correct.

The whole Manual has been rewritten and reorganized to include new knowledge, and make it more accessible and useful for the busy practitioner. We have invited many of the up and coming GI specialists as authors to provide a current perspective and to reflect the growing numbers of specialists working in private (non-academic) referral practices. Whilst the Manual is biased towards diseases seen in the UK, exotic diseases are mentioned, not only because pet travel and climate change may alter their geographical distribution, but also because BSAVA wishes to make its Manuals relevant to practitioners worldwide. There is extensive cross-reference to other relevant BSAVA Manuals (i.e. *BSAVA Manual of Canine and Feline Abdominal Surgery*; *BSAVA Manual of Canine and Feline Dentistry and Oral Surgery*; *BSAVA Manual of Canine and Feline Endoscopy and Endosurgery*; *BSAVA Manual of Canine and Feline Head, Neck and Thoracic Surgery*; *BSAVA Manual of Canine and Feline Oncology*), where some specific diseases or techniques are detailed. All drug dose rates are cross-referenced to the *BSAVA Small Animal Formulary*.

The Manual is divided into four sections. The first section starts with the critical role of history taking and physical examination, and then the generic techniques of clinical pathology, imaging and biopsy are discussed and beautifully illustrated. The second section features twenty succinct chapters on the diagnostic approach to, and differential diagnoses for presenting complaints/problems affecting the GI tract, pancreas and liver, providing the busy practitioner with a practical approach. Although specific treatment regimens are covered in the final section, the third section deals with the rationale behind the treatments available for GI, pancreatic and liver disease. This includes not only antimicrobials, parasiticides and drugs for symptomatically managing vomiting, diarrhoea and constipation, but also a crucial chapter on fluid and nutritional therapy, including non-pharmacological methods of manipulating the microbiome. The final section discusses specific conditions of organs of the GI tract (from mouth to rectum, the pancreas and the hepatobiliary system), describing their pathophysiology and clinical signs, their diagnosis, their treatment and their prognosis.

The busy small animal practitioner is likely to see a dog or cat with GI signs most days and having this Manual as a resource should give them greater insight into the conditions they are treating and hopefully make their job more satisfying. References for each chapter are largely restricted to important papers published since the last edition, with older, seminal papers and key reviews cited for the interested reader. However, given the increasing specialization even within the field of laboratory testing, links to online sources for niche GI tests and other information have been provided when appropriate.

In summary, the Editors believe this third edition of the *BSAVA Manual of Canine and Feline Gastroenterology* presents the most up-to-date information on GI, pancreatic and hepatobiliary disease, in a format that gives the busy practitioner a logical approach to GI problems and their solutions.

To misquote a line from *The Madness of King George*, 'We've always found the stool more eloquent than the pulse'. We hope the reader shares the Editors' interest in gastroenterology.

Ed Hall
David Williams
Aarti Kathrani
October 2019

Chapter 1

Introduction

Edward J. Hall

The gastrointestinal (GI) tract is a complex organ: it is responsible for the coordinated digestion and assimilation of nutrients, simultaneously tolerating dietary antigens and the enteric commensal microbial population (the GI microbiome) whilst excluding pathogens. It is perhaps, therefore, not surprising that it is also the largest immunological organ in the body. Diarrhoea, perhaps the cardinal sign of GI dysfunction in most cases, is common. Yet, thankfully, most cases are mild, transient and self-limiting. Indeed, the majority of episodes never require any veterinary involvement (Hubbard *et al.*, 2007). It is only when signs

are severe or persistent that intervention is needed, and even then, in many acute GI cases, supportive care, in particular fluid therapy, is all that is required.

The main presenting problems related to GI disease are listed in Figure 1.1, which correlates them to the anatomical regions of the GI tract and the associated organs (i.e. liver and pancreas) most likely to be affected. However, it is important to recognize that GI signs can also occur secondary to conditions in other organ systems and, therefore, Figure 1.1 also lists the non-GI diseases that may produce the same clinical signs, mimicking primary GI diseases.

Problem	Primary gastrointestinal disease	Secondary gastrointestinal disease
Abdominal pain	<ul><li>Acute hepatitis</li><li>Cholecystitis</li><li>Enteritis</li><li>Gastritis/ulcer</li><li>Intestinal obstruction</li><li>Pancreatitis</li><li>Peritonitis (GI, pancreas origin)</li><li>Intestinal volvulus</li></ul>	<ul><li>Hypoadrenocorticism</li><li>Lead poisoning</li><li>Peritonitis (non-GI origin)</li><li>Prostatitis</li><li>Pyelonephritis</li><li>Splenic torsion</li><li>Testicular torsion</li><li>Urinary obstruction</li></ul>
Anorexia/hyporexia	<ul><li>All</li></ul>	<ul><li>Many</li></ul>
Ascites	<ul><li>Protein-losing enteropathy</li><li>Portal hypertension<ul><li>Liver fibrosis/cirrhosis</li><li>Portal vein thrombosis</li></ul></li></ul>	<ul><li>Cardiac disease<ul><li>Right-sided heart failure</li></ul></li><li>Pericardial disease</li><li>Peritonitis</li><li>Protein-losing nephropathy</li><li>Uroabdomen</li></ul>
Bloating	<ul><li>Stomach<ul><li>Gastric dilatation-volvulus</li></ul></li><li>Intestinal ileus<ul><li>Chronic intestinal pseudo-obstruction</li></ul></li></ul>	<ul><li>Respiratory disease<ul><li>Dyspnoea and aerophagia</li></ul></li></ul>
Constipation	<ul><li>Large intestinal disease</li><li>Anorectal disease</li><li>Dietary</li><li>Drug-induced</li></ul>	<ul><li>Dehydration</li><li>Endocrine disease<ul><li>Hypothyroidism</li><li>Hypercalcaemia</li></ul></li><li>Hypokalaemia</li><li>Orthopaedic disease</li><li>Neuromuscular disease</li><li>Prostatic disease</li><li>Perineal hernia</li></ul>
Diarrhoea	<ul><li>Dietary</li><li>Intestinal disease</li><li>Liver disease</li><li>Pancreatic disease</li></ul>	<ul><li>Endocrine disease<ul><li>Hypoadrenocorticism</li><li>Hyperthyroidism</li><li>Hypothyroidism (secondary bacterial overgrowth)</li></ul></li><li>Acute/chronic kidney disease</li></ul>

1.1 Classical presenting complaints and the likely (but not consistent) primary gastrointestinal (GI) diseases and potential non-GI (secondary GI) diseases that cause them. CNS = central nervous system. (continues) ▶

Problem	Primary gastrointestinal disease	Secondary gastrointestinal disease
Drooling	• Oropharyngeal disease • Salivary gland disease (sialadenosis) • Oesophageal disease • Gastric ulceration • Hepatoencephalopathy (cats)	• Dental disease • Local irritant • Nausea • Vestibular disease
Dysphagia	• Oropharyngeal disease • Salivary gland disease	• Dental disease
Generalized bleeding	• Liver disease	• Platelet disorders • Coagulopathy

Haematemesis	• Gastric ulceration
	• Small intestinal ulceration
		• Generalized bleeding
		• Swallowed blood
		  • Oral
		  • Nasal
		  • Pulmonary

Haematochezia	• Large intestinal ulceration	• Generalized bleeding disorder
Halitosis	• Dietary • Oropharyngeal disease • Intestinal malabsorption • Pancreatic enzyme supplementation	• Lung disease (e.g. foreign body, tumour)

Melaena	• Gastric ulceration
	• Small intestinal ulceration
		• Generalized bleeding disorder
		• Hypoadrenocorticism
		• Swallowed blood
		  • Oral
		  • Nasal
		  • Pulmonary

Neurological signs	• Liver (hepatoencephalopathy) • Hypocobalaminaemia	• CNS disease • Hyperlipidaemia • Toxins • Thiamine deficiency

Polyphagia	• Exocrine pancreatic insufficiency
	• Small intestinal malabsorption
		• Drugs
		  • Anticonvulsants
		  • Glucocorticoids
		• Endocrine disease
		  • Diabetes mellitus
		  • Hyperadrenocorticism
		  • Hyperthyroidism
		  • Acromegaly
		• Gluttony
		• Physiological (e.g. exercise)

Regurgitation	• Oesophageal disease	• Myasthenia gravis • Psychogenic or limbic epilepsy • Upper airway obstruction (e.g. brachycephalic obstructive airway syndrome, laryngeal obstruction)
Tenesmus	• Anal disease • Rectal disease	• Pelvic obstruction • Perineal hernia • Prostatic disease • Urinary tenesmus

Vomiting	• Salivary gland disease
	(sialadenitis/infarction)
	• Gastric disease
	• Intestinal disease
	• Liver disease
	• Pancreatic disease
		• CNS disease
		  • Inflammation
		  • Space-occupying lesion
		  (e.g. tumour, hydrocephalus)
		  • Vestibular disease
		• Endocrine disease
		  • Hypoadrenocorticism
		  • Hyperthyroidism
		• Metabolic acidosis
		(e.g. diabetic ketoacidosis)
		• Urogenital disease
		  • Prostatitis
		  • Pyometra
		  • Acute/chronic kidney disease
		  • Urinary obstruction or rupture

Weight loss	• Oropharyngeal disease
	• Oesophageal disease
	• Gastric disease
	• Intestinal disease
	• Liver disease
	• Exocrine pancreatic disease
		• Dietary
		• Cardiac cachexia
		• Endocrine disease
		  • Diabetes mellitus
		  • Hypoadrenocorticism
		  • Hyperthyroidism
		• Multicentric lymphoma
		• Neoplasia
		• Physiological (e.g. lactation)
		• Acute/chronic kidney disease

1.1 (continued) Classical presenting complaints and the likely (but not consistent) primary gastrointestinal (GI) diseases and potential non-GI (secondary GI) diseases that cause them. CNS = central nervous system.

Diagnostic approach

A detailed diagnostic approach to each presenting problem is given in Section 2 of the Manual, but it is helpful first to understand how non-GI causes can be ruled out. This process starts with the history and physical examination, and typically includes a laboratory minimum database. Diagnostic imaging and more specialized tests may be needed to confirm the existence of non-GI disease. Thus, initial investigations of GI problems are performed as much to rule out these secondary causes as to define a primary GI problem. The specific findings of these investigations in primary GI disease are covered in the chapters referring to each organ in Section 4.

History

Breed predispositions to specific GI conditions may point the clinician towards a diagnosis (Figure 1.2). It is then appropriate to focus the history on the nature of the GI signs when presented with a case of suspected GI disease, but it is important that the clinician asks about signs that may be related to other organ systems. A series of quick, closed questions should flag up the possibility of non-GI disease(s). For example, dyspnoea, polyuria/polydipsia, seizures and syncope, are unlikely to be caused by primary GI disease. Then, for each presenting GI problem, it is important to ascertain in more detail the severity, duration, frequency and progression, and, in particular, whether there is evidence of bleeding.

Breed	Gastrointestinal disease
Basenji	• Immunoproliferative small intestinal disease
Belgian Shepherd Dog	• Gastric carcinoma
Boxer	• Mastocytoma • Granulomatous (histiocytic ulcerative) colitis
Collies	• Gastric carcinoma • Exocrine pancreatic insufficiency
French Bulldog	• Hiatal hernia • Granulomatous (histiocytic ulcerative) colitis
German Shepherd Dog	• Persistent right aortic arch • Gastric dilatation-volvulus • Exocrine pancreatic insufficiency • Small intestinal dysbiosis (includes antibiotic-responsive diarrhoea) • Lymphoplasmacytic enteritis • Eosinophilic gastroenteritis
Irish Setter	• Persistent right aortic arch • Gastric dilatation-volvulus • Gluten-sensitive enteropathy
Miniature Schnauzer	• Pancreatitis • Haemorrhagic gastroenteritis
Norwegian Lundehund	• Gastric neuroendocrine carcinoma • Lymphangiectasia
Rottweiler	• Parvovirus • Intestinal lymphangiectasia
Shar Pei	• Gastro-oesophageal intussusception • Lymphoplasmacytic enteritis
Staffordshire Bull Terrier	• Gastric carcinoma
Soft Coated Wheaten Terrier	• Protein-losing enteropathy and nephropathy
Yorkshire Terrier	• Intestinal lymphangiectasia

1.2 Breed predispositions for specific gastrointestinal diseases.

Physical examination

Examination of the GI tract in conscious patients is limited to oral and digital rectal examinations and abdominal palpation. However, a full physical examination should be performed to identify potential cardiorespiratory, endocrine and neurological diseases. For example, a head tilt and nystagmus suggest that any vomiting is most likely caused by vestibular disease.

Routine haematology

There are no specific changes on haematological examination that will definitively identify any primary GI disease, and indeed often there are no changes at all in primary GI disease. However, results will indicate if any problem is associated with anaemia and possible GI bleeding, or an inflammatory leucogram or thrombocytopenia. More importantly, results may give clues that there is non-GI disease present; for example, the lack of a stress leucogram in hypoadrenocorticism.

Serum biochemistry

There are no pathognomonic biochemical changes in primary GI disease. Indeed, results are often unremarkable, but this helps rule out the presence of most endocrine and renal diseases. Panhypoproteinaemia helps identify protein-losing enteropathies, and hypocholesterolaemia may indicate malabsorption, but the main value of serum biochemical testing is to identify hepatic and non-GI diseases.

Faecal examination

This is mandatory in cases of chronic diarrhoea and is detailed in Chapter 2.

Imaging

Plain thoracic radiography will identify most oesophageal causes of regurgitation. Plain radiographs are taken before contrast studies, as the diagnosis may be obvious (e.g. oesophageal foreign body, megaoesophagus) and contrast medium either obscures the lesion or risks inhalation. Contrast studies are generally reserved for investigating functional swallowing disorders and oesophageal conditions such as strictures, radiolucent foreign bodies and gastro-oesophageal junction conditions where no abnormalities are seen on plain radiographs, particularly if upper GI endoscopy is not available. Abdominal radiography is most useful in identifying or ruling out conditions that require surgical intervention, but also allows evaluation of other organ systems. Ultrasonography does not replace abdominal radiography but is especially helpful in identifying abnormalities of the internal structure of the liver and the surrounding vasculature, pancreas and GI wall, as well as surgical conditions. Ultrasonography is considered complementary to radiography (see Chapter 3). Although positive findings have good specificity, the sensitivity of abdominal ultrasonography is never 100% due to luminal gas obscuring some areas and the absence of gross morphological changes in some diseases.

Specific tests

Tests of pancreatic and intestinal function (e.g. trypsin-like immunoreactivity (TLI), pancreatic lipase immunoreactivity

(PLI), folate and cobalamin) are discussed in the relevant chapters (see Chapters 18, 34 and 36), but specific tests of thyroid and adrenal function may be needed to rule out endocrine diseases causing GI signs. In particular, an adrenocorticotropic hormone (ACTH) stimulation test (or at least a basal cortisol measurement) should be performed in dogs with chronic vomiting, diarrhoea and/or weight loss to rule out hypoadrenocorticism. Serum thyroxine concentrations should be measured in older cats with polyphagia, diarrhoea or weight loss to rule out hyperthyroidism.

Cytology

Ultrasound-guided fine-needle aspirates of the liver are helpful for the diagnosis of neoplasia and feline hepatic lipidosis, but show poor correlation with histopathological findings for conditions such as chronic hepatitis and cholangitis where the tissue architecture helps define the condition. Fine-needle aspirates of thickened GI wall and enlarged mesenteric lymph nodes are possible to obtain, and a diagnosis of neoplasia may be achieved. However, the identification of inflammatory cells is unhelpful, as they are normally present in these tissues and, without evidence of architectural changes, cannot be interpreted. Cytology of squash endoscopic biopsy samples shows reasonable correlation with specimens obtained by endoscopic biopsy, but the only advantage is the immediacy of the results, and histology should always be performed as well.

Biopsy

GI biopsy inevitably carries a risk of harm due to the need for general anaesthesia and the potential for bleeding, endoscopic perforation or surgical wound dehiscence, and should only be undertaken if the outcome is likely to result in a change in treatment. Therefore, biopsy is rarely indicated in acute GI disease, and it is often considered too risky to anaesthetize a patient with acute pancreatitis.

Biopsy is generally indicated in chronic GI diseases, where a diagnosis cannot be made by laboratory testing and/or imaging, and where empirical treatment trials have failed. Endoscopic biopsy of the oesophagus is difficult because the tissue is very tough, unless very inflamed or neoplastic; however, oesophagitis is generally readily diagnosed by visual inspection, and most tumours yield adequate biopsy samples. Conversely, gastric and intestinal pathology cannot be reliably diagnosed by visual inspection and biopsy is essential. However, if the patient is relatively well, still eating, and has normal serum albumin, cobalamin, folate and imaging findings, intestinal biopsy is usually deferred until empirical anthelmintic, dietary and even antibiotic trials have been attempted and failed. Biopsy in such cases, and especially in young animals, is often unremarkable or shows non-specific inflammation, and empirical trials are still needed to reach a presumptive diagnosis. Cases of GI bleeding, or protein-losing enteropathies with hypoalbuminaemia without hypoglobulinaemia, or cases with abnormalities on palpation/imaging generally need biopsy.

Endoscopic biopsy of the GI tract (see Chapter 4) is preferred unless there is focal disease, identified by palpation and/or imaging, that is either beyond the reach of the endoscope or requires surgical correction. Exploratory laparotomy and full-thickness GI biopsy of various sites provide specimens considered most reliable for a histopathological interpretation, but the risk of surgical dehiscence and septic peritonitis is reported to be between 2 and 12% (Shales *et al.*, 2005; Swinbourne *et al.*, 2017). Except for congenital portosystemic shunts, liver biopsy is always necessary to make a diagnosis in chronic hepatopathies and to determine specific treatment needs, such as copper chelation. Pancreatic biopsy can confirm pancreatitis and identify pancreatic adenocarcinoma.

Summary

In conclusion, investigation of the GI tract is challenging, as it is complex and largely inaccessible and we still have very limited understanding of the aetiopathogenesis of many conditions (Westermarck, 2016). However, through a synthesis of the results of the history, physical examination findings, laboratory testing, imaging, biopsy and empirical trials, a diagnosis can often be reached and logical treatment prescribed.

References and further reading

Hubbard K, Skelly BJ, McKelvie J and Wood JLN (2007) Risk of vomiting and diarrhoea in dogs. *Veterinary Record* **161**, 755–757

Shales CJ, Warren J, Anderson DM *et al.* (2005) Complications following full-thickness small intestinal biopsy in 66 dogs: a retrospective study. *Journal of Small Animal Practice* **46**, 317–321

Swinbourne F, Jeffery N, Tivers MS *et al.* (2017) The incidence of surgical site dehiscence following full-thickness gastrointestinal biopsy in dogs and cats and associated risk factors. *Journal of Small Animal Practice* **46**, 495–503

Westermarck E (2016) Chronic diarrhea in dogs: what do we actually know about it? *Topics in Companion Animal Medicine* **31**, 78–84

Chapter 2

Faecal examination

Edward J. Hall

Laboratory-based faecal examinations, especially microscopy for the identification of intestinal parasites, are important in investigating gastrointestinal (GI) disease, whereas macroscopic faecal examination is of limited value. Gross faecal appearance will confirm diarrhoea, melaena or haematochezia (see Chapters 20 and 21), and allow numerical scoring of faecal consistency. Steatorrhoea is occasionally evident grossly without the need for faecal fat analysis, and colour changes can indicate rapid transit and incomplete bacterial metabolism of faecal bile pigments, but both are non-specific findings. Direct microscopic smear examination with staining for undigested starch granules (Lugol's iodine), fat globules (Sudan stain) and muscle fibres (Wright's or Diff-Quik stains) is also not helpful because results are very non-specific.

Traditionally, laboratory-based faecal examinations have largely been aimed at trying to identify infectious causes, although bacteriological culture results are often hard to interpret as the same, potentially pathogenic organisms may be found in the faeces of healthy animals. Indeed, they are of limited value in patients with acute diarrhoea, although they will identify potential zoonotic risks, and can be very misleading in patients with chronic diarrhoea. Many historical tests, such as quantification of faecal fat and proteolytic activity, are unhelpful or unsuitable for practice. However, an increasing range of faecal biomarkers for intestinal disease is available, although some are not yet commercially available worldwide.

Faecal biomarkers

The quantification in faeces of molecules released into the intestine by diseased patients can act as a marker of GI pathology, although dilution by diarrhoea and poorly digestible dietary components potentially affect the reliability of such tests.

Occult blood

Peroxidase-based guaiac tests are used to search for evidence of GI bleeding that is not grossly visible as melaena or haematochezia. The major indication is when microcytosis and iron deficiency anaemia are detected by haematological examination and biochemical assessment of iron status (see BSAVA Manual of Canine and Feline Clinical Pathology) and gross bleeding has not been observed. The test is sensitive enough to detect 2 ml blood per 30 kg bodyweight, but bleeding could be occurring anywhere within the GI tract. The test merely detects the peroxidase activity of haemoglobin, so false-positives can be caused by meat-based diets, which contain blood, and also by fresh, uncooked vegetables containing peroxidases. In order to obtain a meaningful positive test, the patient must be fed a meat-free diet for at least 72 hours before samples are obtained; a vegetarian or hydrolysed diet is recommended. If bleeding is intermittent, repeat testing may be required.

Immunoglobulin A

Several studies have measured canine faecal immunoglobulin A (IgA), with the aim of identifying IgA deficiency as an underlying cause of chronic enteropathies.

Alpha$_1$-proteinase inhibitor (α_1-PI)

This is a naturally occurring endogenous serum antiprotease resistant to degradation when mucosal damage allows it to leak into the intestinal lumen. Its presence in faeces (faecal α_1-PI) is thus a marker of a protein-losing enteropathy, and is more sensitive than serum albumin as a marker of early disease. Three fresh faecal samples collected after voluntary defecation are tested because of inherent variability and because abrasion of the rectal wall by digital evacuation can produce false-positives. The test cannot be interpreted if there is spontaneous GI bleeding, and the immunoassay is currently only available from a single laboratory in the USA, and only for dogs.

Calgranulin/calprotectin

Calgranulin comprises a range of calcium-binding proteins expressed by the *S100* gene, and is released by activated neutrophils. Calgranulin A (S100A8) and B (S100A9) form a heterodimer called calprotectin. In humans, faecal calprotectin helps distinguish between inflammatory bowel disease (IBD) and irritable bowel syndrome (IBS), a functional disorder with no associated inflammation. Immunoassays for canine calprotectin and calgranulin C (S100A12) have been developed as research tools, but are not currently available to practitioners. Increased faecal calprotectin concentrations in dogs correlate with intestinal inflammation and the degree of histological change, but not necessarily with clinical signs. Increased faecal S100A12 concentrations in canine chronic inflammatory enteropathies have been shown to correlate with a poor response to treatment.

Faecal elastase measurement

Tests to measure faecal elastase are of no clinical value when investigating intestinal disease, and are unreliable for diagnosing exocrine pancreatic insufficiency (EPI) (see Chapter 36). An immunoassay for elastase in canine faeces has been validated, and it is a reasonably sensitive and specific test of EPI, although poorer than serum trypsin-like immunoreactivity (TLI) measurement, and is rarely used clinically.

Lactoferrin

Preliminary studies indicate that faecal lactoferrin may be another useful marker of intestinal inflammation, but assays are not currently available.

Parasites

Microscopic examination of faecal samples can detect intestinal parasitic infections (Dryden *et al.*, 2005). Generally, fresh, non-preserved specimens are examined, but because ova or cysts are shed intermittently, multiple faecal samples may need to be examined. Three-day pooled samples may increase sensitivity for helminth detection, but the vegetative stages of protozoa may be missed because of delays in processing.

Helminths and protozoa are more likely to be associated with chronic GI signs than viruses and bacteria, and investigations in chronic cases may be best restricted to searching for parasites. However, logical interpretation is as important as methodology, and discovery of a parasite may not necessarily prove causation. Indeed, most cestode and roundworm infestations do not cause clinical signs in adult animals, although their ova may be a zoonotic risk and the worms unsightly when expelled.

Direct faecal examination

Wet faecal preparations

Unstained wet mounts can be used to identify motile protozoal trophozoites, such as *Giardia* and *Tritrichomonas*, but a sensitivity of only 14% is reported. A tiny drop of fresh faecal material is put on a slide with a similar volume of warm saline. A cover slip is then placed over the sample and the slide is examined immediately at dry high-power (X400) magnification. The sample must be fresh and kept warm because trophozoites rapidly encyst when cooled: cysts are better identified by faecal concentration methods. Differentiation of *Giardia* and *Tritrichomonas* depends on their characteristic motion under microscopy: *Tritrichomonas* trophozoites progress rapidly across the field of view, while *Giardia* trophozoites tumble slowly like falling leaves. *Trichomonas*, *Pentatrichomonas*, *Balantidium* and *Entamoeba* are occasionally significant findings in cases of colitis (see Chapter 35).

Direct faecal smear

Rapid fixation and staining allows more accurate identification of various protozoa from their characteristic morphology in smears. *Cryptosporidium parvum* can be identified with Ziehl-Neelsen, Heine or safranin stains. Oocysts are extremely small, round, and red or orange bodies when stained, and approximately 1/10 the size of *Cystoisospora* (formerly *Isospora*) oocysts. Immunofluorescent staining improves sensitivity for identifying protozoal infections (see below).

Faecal concentration methods

Faeces can be 'concentrated' either with flotation using sugar or a salt solution, or by sedimentation for examination, or by culture in the case of *Tritrichomonas*, providing greater sensitivity than a direct smear or wet slide preparation. The methodologies are described in Figure 2.1, and their relative advantages and disadvantages are listed in Figure 2.2. The Parasep® faecal filtration and Flotac® systems can be used in practice and are more convenient, mess-free and potentially more sensitive than routine flotation methods (Becker *et al.*, 2011).

Flotation with sugar or salt solutions reveals the majority of parasites, including coccidia and *Cryptosporidium* spp., but the fat content of canine and feline faeces makes the formalin-ether sedimentation technique more suitable for the discovery of roundworm, hookworm and whipworm ova (Figure 2.3). Zinc sulphate flotation is recommended for detecting *Giardia* oocysts because they become deformed by salt flotation. Due to fluctuating excretion of *Giardia*, examination of three separate samples collected over 3 to 5 days is recommended, and has a reported sensitivity of >90%. Identification of *Cryptosporidium* by faecal flotation or centrifugation requires oil immersion microscopy but is insensitive without staining. Sedimentation or the Baermann technique can identify larvae of *Strongyloides* spp., although the latter technique is more commonly used to detect lungworm larvae.

Wet preparation
1. The sample must be fresh (warm).
2. A tiny drop of faecal material is put on a slide with a similar volume of warm saline.
3. A cover slip is immediately placed over the sample.
4. The slide is examined immediately at dry high-power (X400) magnification.

Faecal flotation
1. Place 2–3 g of faeces in 15 ml of saturated sugar or salt solution.
   - Sugar solution = 454 g sugar + 355 ml water (SG 1.27) (+ 6 ml formaldehyde in modified Sheather's solution)
   - Salt solutions (SG 1.18–1.20)
     - Sodium chloride = 350 g per litre of water
     - Sodium nitrate = 338 g per litre of water
     - Zinc sulphate = 330 g per litre of water
2. Mix thoroughly, then strain through a tea strainer or cheesecloth.
3. If there is excess fat after filtration, mix with 2–3 ml of ethyl acetate or ether, centrifuge and discard the supernatant.
4. Place in a 15 ml polypropylene tube.
5. Centrifuge at 1,500 rpm for 5 minutes.
6. Place a cover slip on top, touching the meniscus, for 3–4 minutes (alternatively use a bacteriology loop).
7. Place the cover slip on a microscope slide and examine.
   - Stain with Lugol's iodine for zinc sulphate flotation, if desired.

Faecal sedimentation

Water
1. Mix sample of fresh faeces with water and strain to remove debris.
2. Allow sample to settle for between 30 minutes and 2 hours.
3. Place the sediment on a microscope slide, place a cover slip over the sediment and examine.

Formalin-ether
1. Mix sample of fresh faeces with water and strain to remove debris.
2. Centrifuge strained faeces and re-suspend in 9 ml of 5% formalin solution.
3. Add 3 ml of ethyl acetate and shake vigorously.
4. Re-centrifuge and discard the debris at the formalin-ethyl acetate interface.
5. Examine the sediment as above.

2.1 Methodologies for performing faecal examination for intestinal parasites. SG = specific gravity. (Dryden *et al.*, 2005)

Methodology	Advantages	Disadvantages
Direct wet preparation	• Fast • No distortion of parasites if isotonic saline is used as diluent • Only way to see live trophozoites	• Insensitive, especially if concentration is too low, or if too much debris or fat is present, or sample not fresh
Saturated sucrose or salt flotation	• Inexpensive • Suitable for most common helminth ova and coccidian oocysts	• Ideally requires centrifugation • Unsuitable for: • Fatty stool samples • Tapeworm ova • *Giardia* cysts
Zinc sulphate (ZnSO₄) flotation	• Recommended for most faecal examinations • Floats most helminth eggs • Best for protozoan cysts, especially *Giardia*	• Procedure will not float some trematode ova and some tapeworm ova • Unsuitable for fatty stool samples • ZnSO₄ is relatively expensive
Formalin-ether sedimentation	• Procedure recovers **all** types of helminth ova, larvae, and most protozoan cysts • Best technique for formalin-fixed samples and for faeces with high fat content	• More difficult to perform than other techniques • Ether and ethyl acetate are flammable • More debris remains

2.2 Relative advantages and disadvantages of different methodologies for performing faecal examination for intestinal parasites.

Examples of parasites that can be identified by faecal concentration methods are shown in Figures 2.4–2.9.

Immunodetection

Immunofluorescence

Immunofluorescent antibody (IFA) staining of faecal smears is considered one of the most sensitive methods for detecting *Giardia* and *Cryptosporidium* organisms.

Antigen detection

Copro-antigen tests may be available for parasite infections, including *Giardia*, hookworms, roundworms and whipworms. They can detect parasite infections even if the number of excreted oocysts or ova is low. Enzyme-linked immunosorbent assays (ELISAs) are often used, but the rapid immunochromatographic (SNAP®) method can be used to detect *Giardia* antigen and is suited to in-house use (Figure 2.10). *Giardia* antigen tests are convenient to perform in practice, although, theoretically, they do not have greater sensitivity than zinc sulphate flotation when performed by an experienced technician. However, they do not correlate well with IFA (Rishniw *et al.*, 2010).

Culture

Tritrichomonas can be cultured from feline faeces using a commercially available system, Feline In Pouch™ TF (Biomed Diagnostics). Pouches are inoculated with freshly voided faeces, incubated at 25°C, and then examined under a microscope every couple of days until motile

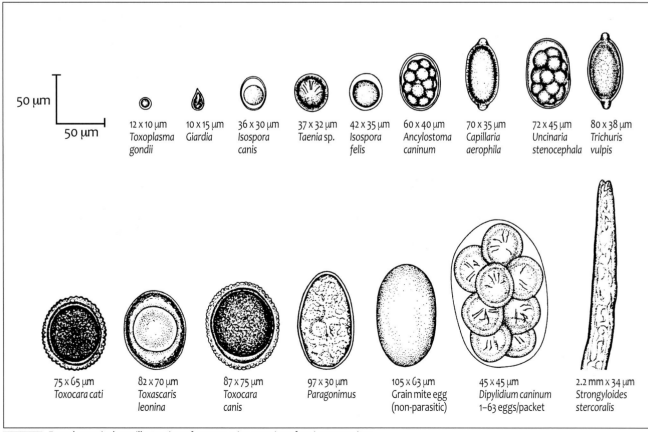

50 µm
50 µm

12 x 10 µm
Toxoplasma gondii

10 x 15 µm
Giardia

36 x 30 µm
Isospora canis

37 x 32 µm
Taenia sp.

42 x 35 µm
Isospora felis

60 x 40 µm
Ancylostoma caninum

70 x 35 µm
Capillaria aerophila

72 x 45 µm
Uncinaria stenocephala

80 x 38 µm
Trichuris vulpis

75 x 65 µm
Toxocara cati

82 x 70 µm
Toxascaris leonina

87 x 75 µm
Toxocara canis

97 x 30 µm
Paragonimus

105 x 63 µm
Grain mite egg (non-parasitic)

45 x 45 µm
Dipylidium caninum
1–63 eggs/packet

2.2 mm x 34 µm
Strongyloides stercoralis

2.3 Faecal parasitology: illustration of comparative egg size of various parasites.
(Courtesy of Hoechst-Roussel-Agri Vet Company, USA; permission requested)

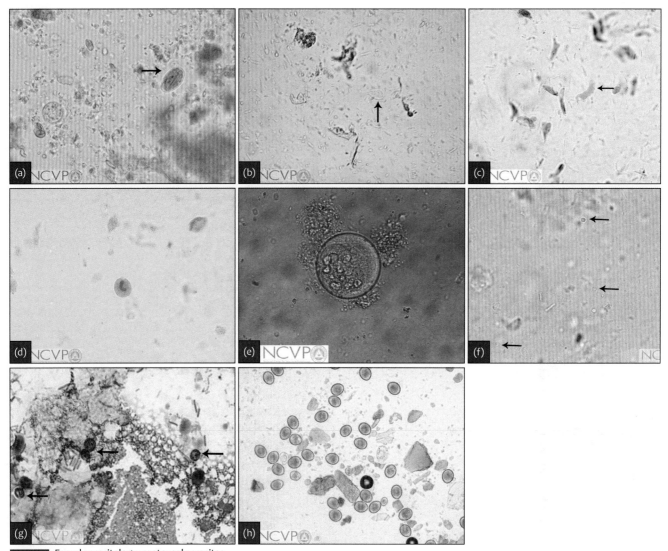

2.4 Faecal parasitology: protozoal parasites.
(a) Cyst of *Giardia* sp. in a faecal preparation stained with iodine. Cysts of *Giardia* sp. are 9–13 x 7–9 µm and typically ovoid. Note the four nuclei, two median bodies and intracytoplasmic flagella within the cyst (arrowed).
(b) Trophozoite of *Giardia* sp. in a direct faecal smear from an infected dog. Trophozoites are 12–17 x 7–10 µm and are tear-drop-shaped with eight flagella, two nuclei and two median bodies (arrowed).
(c) Trichrome-stained *Tritrichomonas foetus* trophozoites. Note the undulating membrane (arrowed).
(d) *Balantidium coli* cyst (stained). Note the large kidney bean-shaped macronucleus.
(e) *Balantidium coli* cyst (not stained). Note the large kidney bean-shaped macronucleus is not easily observed.
(f) Oocysts of *Cryptosporidium* sp. in a sugar faecal floatation (arrowed). Depending on species, oocysts range from 3.5–7 µm in diameter.
(g) Modified Kinyoun's acid-fast stain of *Cryptosporidium* sp. oocysts (arrowed).
(h) Oocysts of *Cystoisospora* spp. in a canine faecal float. Note the two different sizes and that several are sporulated.
(© The National Center of Veterinary Parasitology at Oklahoma State University, www.ncvetp.org/)

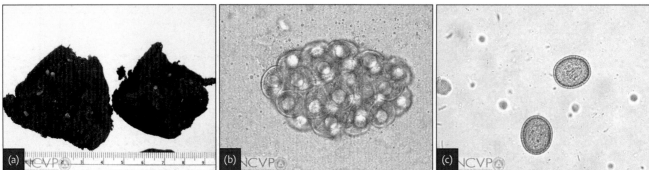

2.5 Faecal parasitology: tapeworms. (a) Proglottids of *Dipylidium caninum* are often readily apparent in canine faeces. (b) *Dipylidium caninum* eggs are found in clusters 120–200 µm in size. Individual eggs measure 35–60 µm in diameter and contain an embryo bearing hooks. (c) Taeniid eggs of *Taenia* spp. and *Echinococcus* spp. are morphologically indistinguishable, measure 25–40 µm, and consist of a thick, striated wall surrounding a hexacanth embryo.
(© The National Center of Veterinary parasitology at Oklahoma State University, www.ncvetp.org/)

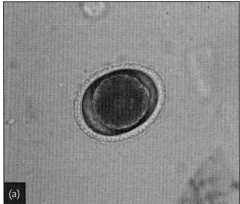

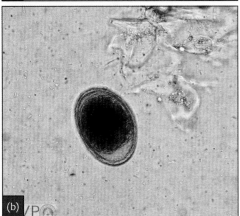

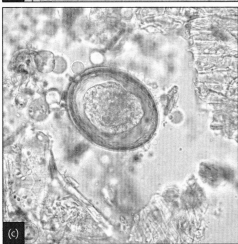

2.6 Faecal parasitology: ascarids. (a) Egg of *Toxocara canis*. The eggs are 85–90 x 75 μm, subspherical and have a thick and pitted shell. (b) Egg of *Toxocara cati*. The eggs are similar to those of *Toxocara canis*, but are 65 x 75 μm and tend to be more elliptical. (c) Egg of *Toxascaris leonina*. The eggs are approximately 70–80 μm and resemble those of *Toxocara* spp., but have a smooth shell and the embryo takes up less space within the egg.

(© The National Center of Veterinary Parasitology at Oklahoma State University, www.ncvetp.org/)

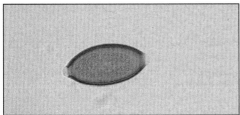

2.7 Faecal parasitology: whipworm. Egg of *Trichuris vulpis* from an infected dog. Eggs are symmetrical, have plugs at both polar ends, and measure approximately 72–90 x 32–40 μm.

(© The National Center of Veterinary Parasitology at Oklahoma State University, www.ncvetp.org/)

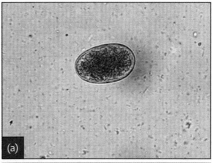

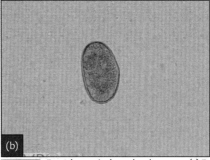

2.8 Faecal parasitology: hookworms. (a) Egg of *Ancylostoma caninum*. Eggs have an elliptical shape, a thin shell and are approximately 52–79 x 28 μm. In fresh faeces, eggs contain morulae, which develop to first-stage larvae within eggs in the environment. (b) Egg of *Uncinaria stenocephala*. This hookworm infects dogs (rarely cats) in cooler temperate regions, including the northern USA, Canada and Europe. The eggs resemble those of *Ancylostoma* spp. in that they are elliptical, thin-shelled and contain morulae in fresh faeces, but *Uncinaria* eggs are slightly larger (71–92 x 35–58 μm).

(© The National Center of Veterinary Parasitology at Oklahoma State University, www.ncvetp.org/)

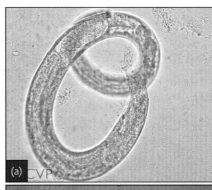

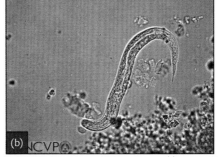

2.9 Faecal parasitology: larvae. (a) Larva of *Ollulanus tricuspis*. Third-stage larvae are approximately 500 μm long and have a tricuspid tail similar to that of the adult female (second- and fourth-stage larvae also have this type of tail). Adults and larvae are found in the stomach of domestic cats and other felids. Diagnosis is based on the identification of larvae or small adults (1 mm) in vomitus using the Baermann test. (b) In fresh faeces, *Strongyloides* spp. larvae rapidly develop to the infective filariform stage, which enters the host via skin or mucosal penetration. 'Filariform' refers to the elongated shape of the oesophagus. In dogs and cats, *Strongyloides* eggs frequently hatch before leaving the body, thus free larvae are most often found in fresh faeces.

(© The National Center of Veterinary Parasitology at Oklahoma State University, www.ncvetp.org/)

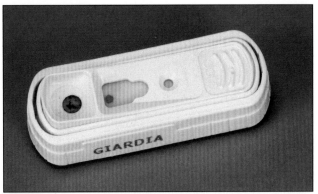

2.10 SNAP® immunochromatographic test for in-house testing for *Giardia* infection.

organisms are seen; this can take from 1 to 12 days from initial inoculation. Although more sensitive than direct smear examination, the method is not as convenient or rapid as polymerase chain reaction (PCR).

Polymerase chain reaction

This is the most sensitive method for detecting *Tritrichomonas*; as few as 10 organisms per gram of faeces can be detected. The faeces can be kept refrigerated for up to a week before testing, but ideally fresh faeces should be tested for better sensitivity, which is improved further by testing mucus and bloody diarrhoea or colonic washings. Samples should not include cat litter, which can contain PCR inhibitors, and patients should not have had antibiotics recently.

Enteropathogenic bacteria

Testing for bacterial pathogens in faeces may be indicated in diarrhoea cases. However, even in acute and definitely in chronic diarrhoea cases, the significance of a positive culture is questionable as pathogenic organisms can be found in the faeces of clinically healthy animals. Furthermore, faecal bacterial isolates do not correlate with the small intestinal bacterial population, and so faecal culture is not suitable for the diagnosis of small intestinal dysbiosis.

Targeted evaluation for potential pathogens, i.e. *Salmonella* spp., *Campylobacter* spp., *Escherichia coli*, *Clostridium perfringens* and *Clostridium difficile*, by culture on selective media is typically performed, but is of questionable significance because of their presence in the faeces of healthy animals. *E. coli* can be cultured from almost all faecal samples, and yet only certain isolates are pathogenic. It is more appropriate to use molecular probes following culture, to detect pathogenicity genes. Similarly, the significance of clostridia in faeces may be more usefully assessed by assays of their toxins or toxin-associated genes, which are probably more sensitive tests and potentially more clinically relevant.

Direct faecal examination

Microscopic examination of a direct smear of fresh faeces may reveal 'seagull'-shaped *Campylobacter* spp. but the sensitivity is poor. Diff-Quik stained faecal smears can be examined for *Clostridium perfringens*

organisms characterized by sub-terminal endospores. If large numbers of spore-forming organisms (>5 per oil field) are detected, *C. perfringens* enterotoxicosis is possible but not necessarily confirmed, i.e. the correlation between sporulation and toxin elaboration is unreliable since endospores and endotoxin can be found in faecal samples from healthy dogs, and toxin can be found in the absence of endospores and *vice versa*. Examination for fungal elements, such as *Histoplasma* and *Pythium*, is important if fungal/oomycete diseases are endemic in the area.

Faecal culture

The interpretation of a positive culture result is problematic because it may not equate with causation, and equally false-negatives are likely with single cultures or rectal swabs: if the sensitivity of the culture method is ≥ 45%, three consecutive negative cultures are needed to be ~90% confident that the sample is truly negative and six cultures would be required to be ~99% confident (Marks *et al.*, 2011). *Campylobacter* is quite labile and may die before postal samples reach the laboratory, so fresh faecal material should be submitted promptly, and placing a swab of the sample in Amies transport medium (containing charcoal) in addition is recommended. Results are most likely to be significant in cases with haemorrhagic diarrhoea, and/or pyrexia, and/or an inflammatory leucogram, and/or if neutrophils are identified on rectal scrape cytology, and/or there has been exposure to a raw food diet.

Salmonella spp.

Most laboratories use a combination of selective enrichment broth followed by subculture on selective agar plates. Presumptive *Salmonella* colonies are then verified using biochemical techniques. Isolates identified as *Salmonella* can be further classified by serotyping performed at reference laboratories.

Campylobacter spp.

Isolation of *Campylobacter* by culture is more likely to be successful from fresh faeces. However, *Campylobacter* isolates are only reliably identified to genus level by standard microbiological culture and biochemical techniques; speciation requires PCR testing of isolates. Thus, an assumption that all *Campylobacter* isolates are the pathogenic *C. jejuni* is false; *C. upsaliensis* isolation is more prevalent in dogs.

Clostridium spp.

Clostridia are ubiquitous isolates from the faeces of healthy cats and dogs, but certain species may be pathogenic under the correct conditions. They can be identified by the presence of the common clostridial antigen (the enzyme glutamate dehydrogenase (GLDH)).

Clostridium difficile: Often considered fastidious to grow, the organism has been isolated by culture from faeces of healthy and diseased dogs at isolation rates varying from zero to 58% depending on the study.

Clostridium perfringens: Unfortunately, isolation by culture has no clinical significance, as *C. perfringens* appears to be a commensal organism, and probably causes disease when triggered to produce toxins.

Toxin assay

The presence of *C. difficile*, and even the identification of potentially toxigenic strains, does not necessarily correlate with the presence of disease. It is the secretion of an enterotoxin (toxin A) with a cytotoxin (toxin B) that is important. An ELISA can be used to detect toxins A and B simultaneously.

Recently, acute haemorrhagic diarrhoea syndrome (AHDS) in dogs, formerly known as haemorrhagic gastro-enteritis (HGE), has been associated with infection by *C. perfringens* type A, producing alpha and netF toxins. One of the other toxins produced is the *C. perfringens* enterotoxin (CPE), encoded by the *cpe* gene. CPE is produced during sporulation and released after bacterial cell lysis, and can induce diarrhoea. As sporulation was assumed to coincide with enterotoxin elaboration, examination of a Diff-Quik stained faecal smear for >5 sporulating organisms per oil field was suggested as a simple screening test. It has subsequently been shown to be unreliable and is no longer recommended. The detection of CPE by reverse passive latex agglutination or by ELISA is more likely indicative of disease, but CPE can be found in the faeces of healthy animals.

Polymerase chain reaction

Although PCR assays are available to identify *Salmonella* and toxigenic strains of *C. difficile*, they are not used routinely. PCR for speciation of *Campylobacter* spp. is now commercially available and aids differentiation of pathogenic *C. jejuni* from the likely commensal *C. upsaliensis*. PCR can be used to identify *Clostridium perfringens* carrying the *cpe* gene but up to one-third of both healthy and diarrhoeic cats and dogs have been shown to carry the gene, and so the test has no discriminatory value.

Molecular fingerprinting

Many bacteria in the intestine cannot be cultured and can only be identified by high throughput gene sequencing of the bacterial 16S rRNA. This method is currently not helpful in individual patients; it is a tool for investigating disturbances of the microbiome in a population.

Viruses

Viral diarrhoea is usually acute and self-limiting, and there is rarely a need to make a positive diagnosis. A variety of tests are available for the identification of viruses, but it must be noted that identification of feline coronavirus in faeces is **not** proof of feline infectious peritonitis (FIP).

Electron microscopy

This can be used to reveal characteristic viral particles of rotavirus, coronavirus, astrovirus, norovirus and parvovirus, but is not generally available.

Polymerase chain reaction

Viruses in faeces can be identified by PCR, and parvo- and coronaviruses are now included in screening panels offered by some laboratories. PCR has been shown overall to be the most sensitive method for the identification of parvovirus in faeces, but may actually be too sensitive, as the virus can also be found in the faeces of dogs with chronic diarrhoea and healthy dogs, and mixed infections may be present (Schmitz *et al.*, 2009). Furthermore, many enteric viruses are only mildly pathogenic and a positive isolation does not confirm causation.

Immunological identification

Immunochromatography, immuno-electron microscopy (IEM) and haemagglutination can all be applied to the identification of enteric viruses. For canine parvovirus, antibody-based tests show poor sensitivities ranging from 15.8 to 26.3% *versus* PCR and 50 to 60% *versus* IEM (Schmitz *et al.*, 2009). However, the faecal immunochromatographic (SNAP®) test to detect parvovirus antigen is still the most applicable to the practice situation (Figure 2.11). The test has a reported sensitivity of 98% and a specificity of 100% for samples collected between days 4 and 7 post infection, when shedding rate is highest and a positive test result is most likely to be clinically relevant. Fresh samples should be tested, ideally taken 24 to 36 hours after the onset of clinical signs. False-negatives can arise if samples are taken too early, before shedding (the test should be repeated after 36 to 48 hours, if clinical signs are consistent with parvovirus), or too late, because shedding decreases after the first week. Weak false-positives occur transiently between 5 and 15 days after vaccination with a modified live vaccine.

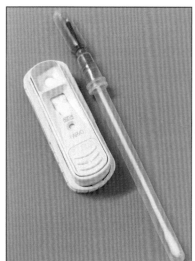

2.11 SNAP® immunochromatographic test for in-house testing for canine parvovirus antigen. After swabbing the sample, the swab tip is placed into the tube. Bending the bulb then breaks the seal and releases conjugate. The bulb is squeezed three times to mix the sample and conjugate, and then squeezed to release five drops into the sample well of the SNAP® device.

References and further reading

Becker SL, Lohourignon LK, Speich B *et al.* (2011) Comparison of the Flotac-400 dual technique and the formalin-ether concentration technique for diagnosis of human intestinal protozoon infection. *Clinical Microbiology* **49**, 2183–2190

Desario C, Decaro N, Campolo M *et al.* (2005) Canine parvovirus infection: which diagnostic test for virus? *Journal of Virological Methods* **126**, 179–185

Dryden MW, Payne PA, Ridley R and Smith V (2005) Comparison of common fecal flotation techniques for the recovery of parasite eggs and oocysts. *Veterinary Therapeutics* **6**, 15–28

Marks SL, Rankin SC, Byrne BA and Weese JS (2011) ACVIM Consensus Statement: Enteropathogenic bacteria in dogs and cats: diagnosis, epidemiology, treatment, and control. *Journal of Veterinary Internal Medicine* **25**, 1195–1208

Rishniw M, Liotta J, Bellosa M *et al.* (2010) Comparison of 4 *Giardia* diagnostic tests in diagnosis of naturally acquired canine chronic subclinical giardiasis. *Journal of Veterinary Internal Medicine* **24**, 293–297

Schmitz S, Coenen C, König M *et al.* (2009) Comparison of three rapid commercial canine parvovirus antigen detection tests with electron microscopy and polymerase chain reaction. *Journal of Veterinary Diagnostic Investigation* **21**, 344–345

Villiers E and Ristić J (2016) *BSAVA Manual of Canine and Feline Clinical Pathology, 3rd edn.* BSAVA Publications, Gloucester

Chapter 3

Imaging of the gastrointestinal tract, liver and pancreas

Virginie Barberet

There are various imaging modalities available for assessing the abdomen and particularly the gastrointestinal (GI) tract, liver and pancreas. Ultrasonography is now more accessible in veterinary practices and is generally the imaging modality of choice. However, despite many limitations, plain radiography can be very helpful in assessing the oesophagus and detecting specific GI diseases, such as gastric dilatation-volvulus (GDV) and mechanical obstructions. The use of computed tomography (CT) is increasing rapidly in veterinary practices and has proven very useful for assessing specific disorders of the liver and pancreas.

Gastrointestinal tract

Pharynx and oesophagus

Plain radiography

In cases of regurgitation or dysphagia, the pharynx and oesophagus can be assessed with lateral radiographic views of the neck and thorax. A dorsoventral view of the thorax can also be useful. Radiography will enable detection of pharyngeal and retropharyngeal masses (e.g. tumour, abscess, lymphadenopathy) and radiopaque foreign bodies (e.g. fish hooks) or stick injuries. In cases of perforation of the pharynx or oesophagus, the presence of free gas in the fascial planes of the neck and/or the mediastinum is common (Figure 3.1) and is often the only radiographic sign, as wooden sticks can be difficult to visualize.

Many oesophageal disorders can be detected on plain thoracic radiographs, such as megaoesophagus and oesophageal diverticulum secondary to vascular ring anomalies, soft tissue masses (tumour, para-oesophageal abscess, *Spirocerca* granuloma), foreign bodies, gastro-oesophageal intussusception and, potentially, hiatal hernia. Aspiration pneumonia (alveolar pattern in the cranioventral lung fields) is also often apparent on plain radiographs of the thorax.

Radiographic signs seen with megaoesophagus may include: dilatation of the oesophagus (with gas or sometimes food), the presence of thin converging soft tissue stripes representing oesophageal walls (Figure 3.2), displacement of the trachea ventrally and to the right, tracheal stripe sign (a thick soft tissue line resulting from summation of the ventral oesophageal wall over the dorsal tracheal wall when there is oesophageal luminal air) and

aspiration pneumonia. As oesophageal dilatation can occur secondary to sedation or general anaesthesia, it is recommended to evaluate megaoesophagus on radiographs of conscious animals only.

An oesophageal diverticulum appears as a focal oesophageal dilatation filled with air or ingesta. In cases of vascular ring anomaly, the secondary diverticulum is

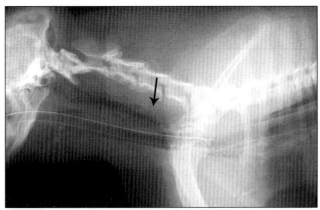

3.1 Lateral view of the neck of a dog with an extensive stick injury. The stick (arrowed) is poorly visible. There is a large amount of gas in the fascial planes of the neck and in the mediastinum outlining the tracheal wall.

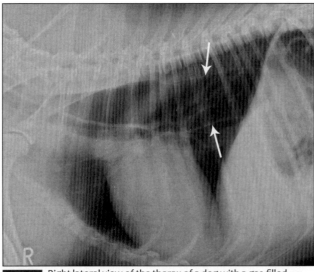

3.2 Right lateral view of the thorax of a dog with a gas-filled megaoesophagus. The dorsal and ventral oesophageal walls (arrowed) appear as thin converging soft tissue stripes.

located cranial to the heart base and induces a focal, ventral deviation of the trachea. Focal leftward curvature of the intrathoracic trachea can also be seen on the dorso-ventral view in cases of persistence of the fourth right aortic arch. An oesophagram is usually not necessary to confirm the diagnosis.

Gastro-oesophageal intussusception appears as a large and well-defined soft tissue opacity within the terminal oesophagus, with possible delineation of gastric rugal folds by intraluminal gas and gas dilatation of the oesophagus cranial to the mass. The gastric silhouette may be absent from the cranial abdomen or decreased in size.

Positive contrast oesophagraphy and swallowing studies

Positive contrast oesophagraphy is performed by oral administration of barium paste or suspension, or preferably food mixed with barium suspension or powder. Plain radiographs should always be obtained first and then views of the neck/thorax can be repeated immediately after the administration of barium. Care should be taken during administration because of the risk of aspiration of barium. This technique will allow the detection and a better assessment of static lesions: megaoesophagus (Figure 3.3) or a diverticulum not seen on plain radiography, oesophageal strictures, marked oesophagitis, oesophageal mass and radiolucent foreign bodies.

Although uncommon in general practice, image-intensified fluoroscopy is available in larger referral practices and academic institutions. Fluoroscopy is necessary for evaluating functional abnormalities of the pharynx and oesophagus, as it enables real-time assessment of the swallowing phases. Studies are usually performed with a liquid phase assessment first (water and barium), followed by a wet food meal (with barium) and eventually a dry food meal (with barium). These techniques are very useful for detecting cricopharyngeal achalasia, decreased or absent motility of the oesophagus, gastro-oesophageal reflux and intermittent hiatal hernia.

Computed tomography

CT can be very useful for assessing perforation of the pharynx or oesophagus (stick injuries, bite wounds), assessing vascular ring anomalies, and detecting and characterizing tumours, abscesses (Figure 3.4) or granulomas in the pharyngeal and oesophageal regions.

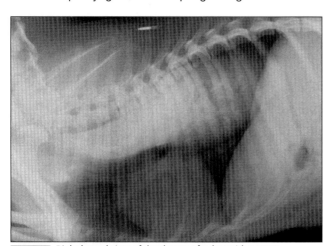

3.3 Right lateral view of the thorax of a dog with a mega-oesophagus after positive contrast oesophagraphy. The oesophagus is severely dilated, inducing a ventral displacement of the trachea.

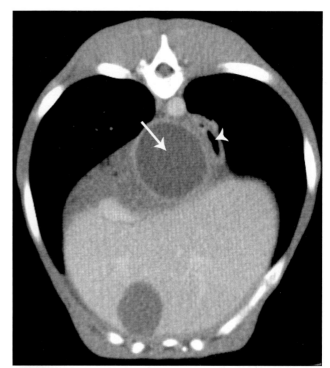

3.4 Transverse CT image (post-contrast soft tissue window) of a dog with a para-oesophageal abscess (arrowed) in the caudal mediastinum. The arrowhead indicates the oesophagus, which contains a small amount of air.

Stomach, small intestine and large intestine
Plain radiography

Abdominal radiography can be useful for detecting some GI disorders, such as GDV, foreign bodies and mechanical obstructions. The contrast in abdominal radiography is inherently low and is dependent on the amount of intra-abdominal fat present. When there is a loss of serosal detail, which can be due to a lack of fat, peritonitis, ascites or carcinomatosis, it can become difficult to distinguish the GI tract margins. Plain radiography is, however, a good modality in cases of GI rupture; in this case, free gas can be present in the peritoneal cavity, most typically seen between the diaphragm and liver and often associated with concurrent peritonitis.

GDV is one of the main indications for GI radiography. The radiographic appearance can vary depending on the content of the stomach, the degree of dilatation and the rotation of the stomach (between 90 and 360 degrees) (Figure 3.5). The radiographic signs can be:

- Dilatation of the stomach with gas/ingesta
- Displacement of the pyloric antrum dorsally and to the left (i.e. gas-filled tubular structure on a right lateral view seen on the craniodorsal aspect of the stomach)
- Compartmentalization of the stomach (i.e. double bubble sign due to a thick soft tissue band separating two gas-filled compartments)
- Gastric wall pneumatosis (i.e. gas lucencies in the wall, indicative of necrosis)
- Paralytic ileus (i.e. diffuse moderate gas dilatation of the small intestinal loops)
- Splenomegaly
- Loss of abdominal serosal detail
- Decreased size of the liver
- Gas-dilated oesophagus.

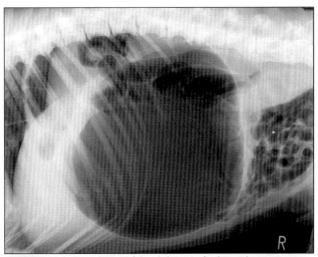

3.5 Right lateral view of the abdomen of a dog with gastric dilatation-volvulus. The stomach is severely gas-dilated and compartmentalized, with the pyloric antrum being located craniodorsally. Paralytic ileus (gas dilatation of the small intestines) and gas dilatation of the oesophagus are also visible.

The stomach can be severely dilated with food, fluid and/or gas without being rotated. In this case, only one compartment is visible. This can be due to aerophagia, over-eating or delayed gastric emptying as a result of functional disturbances or mechanical obstructions at the level of the pylorus or proximal duodenum (e.g. neoplasia, foreign body, pyloric hypertrophy). The cause of obstruction is rarely seen on plain radiography, except in cases of radiopaque foreign material or a mass/foreign body highlighted by luminal gas.

Gastritis cannot be diagnosed with any certainty on plain radiographs, which should always be interpreted with caution, as gastric wall thickening seen radiographically is not always real; it can be due to secretions/debris adhering to the wall mimicking thickening. Thus, gastric wall masses (tumours, polyps) are rarely detected on plain radiography, unless they are large and outlined by luminal gas (Figure 3.6). With uraemic gastritis, thin linear mineralizations may be detected in the gastric mucosa on plain radiography.

Similarly, plain radiography will only detect a limited number of abnormalities at the level of the small and large intestines: radiopaque or linear foreign bodies, mechanical obstructions, paralytic ileus, some intussusceptions, mesenteric or colonic volvulus and megacolon. Only large neoplasms will be detected (often as a tubular soft tissue mass).

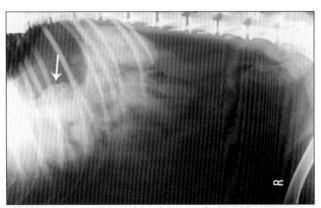

3.6 Right lateral view of the abdomen of a dog with carcinoma in the gastric body and pyloric antrum. The gastric wall is severely thickened and there is a soft tissue mass (arrowed) outlined by luminal gas.

Radiography is very useful for detecting signs of mechanical obstruction of the small intestines. In acute/sub-acute complete obstruction, there is often a segmental gas or fluid dilatation of a few small intestinal loops. Dilatation greater than 12 mm in cats, or thickness of the distended loop greater than 1.6 times the height of the L5 vertebral body in dogs, is suggestive of obstruction, although the use of this ratio does not increase the accuracy of diagnosis significantly. However, the exact cause of the obstruction cannot often be determined with certainty, unless a radiopaque foreign body is clearly visible (Figure 3.7).

In chronic partial obstruction, a gravel sign can be seen (Figure 3.8), but it is also non-specific for the cause of the obstruction (i.e. intussusception, intestinal neoplasia, foreign material). The gravel sign is the accumulation of particulate mineralized material in a small intestinal loop that can mimic colonic content.

Occasionally, signs can be indicative of an intussusception, i.e. an elongated sausage-shaped soft tissue opacity, with luminal gas outlining a convex rounded end on the intussuscepted bowel segment (Figure 3.9) and a linear gas opacity in the lumen of the intussuscepted segment.

Linear foreign bodies are often fixed at their proximal end (often at the pylorus in dogs or under the tongue in cats) with the distal portion being loose in the small intestine, where peristalsis will cause plication of the intestine

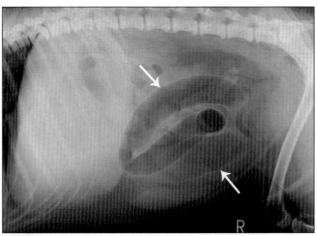

3.7 Right lateral view of the abdomen of a dog with an acute mechanical obstruction by a radiolucent foreign body (not visible). Some small intestinal loops are severely gas-dilated (arrowed) and the stomach is fluid-filled.

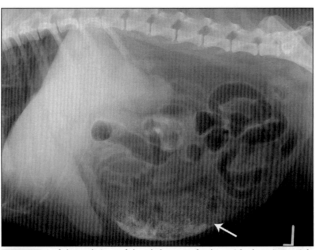

3.8 Left lateral view of the abdomen of a dog with chronic partial obstruction of a small intestinal loop. The affected loop is severely dilated and shows a gravel sign (arrowed).

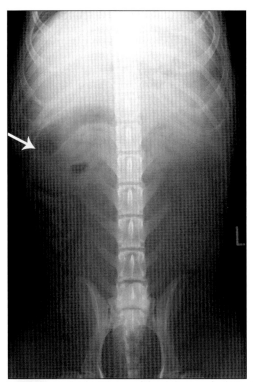

3.9 Ventrodorsal view of the abdomen of a dog with an ileocaecocolic intussusception. The intussuscepted bowel segment is outlined by luminal gas (arrowed).

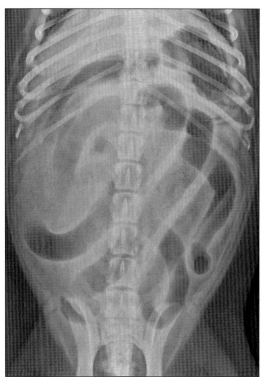

3.11 Ventrodorsal view of the abdomen of a dog with mesenteric volvulus. The small intestinal loops are dilated with gas and show a hairpin aspect.

around the linear foreign body. The radiological signs that can be seen are:

- Bunched and plicated small intestinal loops (Figure 3.10)
- Mild to moderate dilatation of the affected loops
- Abnormally shaped (teardrop, crescent, triangular) gas bubbles in the lumen of the affected loops
- Changes indicative of perforation (presence of free gas, loss of serosal detail due to peritonitis).

A mesenteric or colonic volvulus can be detected on plain radiography, as both will usually induce a severe gas dilatation of the affected segment(s). In the case of mesenteric volvulus (rotation/twisting at the mesenteric root), severe and generalized gas dilatation of all the small intestinal loops is often present and some loops sometimes show a hairpin or fan-shaped aspect (Figure 3.11). In the

case of colonic volvulus, the colon is severely distended with gas and malpositioned and sometimes displaced cranial to the small intestinal loops.

Plain radiography is helpful in assessing the degree of dilatation of the colon in order to differentiate constipation from megacolon. Distension of the colon is suspected when the colonic width is greater than the length of the L7 vertebral body. Megacolon is diagnosed when the colonic width is greater than 1.48 times the length of the L5 vertebral body in cats. The colonic content is usually severely increased in opacity (mineralized opacity) due to desiccation (Figure 3.12). Plain radiography can help rule out mechanical/obstructive causes of megacolon (e.g. perineal hernia, pelvic canal stenosis, prostatomegaly, lymphadenopathy, colonic or intrapelvic mass) and some neurological causes (e.g. cauda equina compression due to sacral fracture, sacrococcygeal luxation).

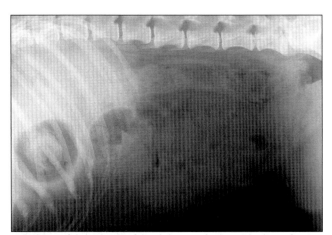

3.10 Left lateral view of the abdomen of a dog with a linear foreign body. The small intestine is severely plicated and some crescent-shaped gas bubbles are visible. Foreign material is also visible in the gas-filled pyloric antrum.

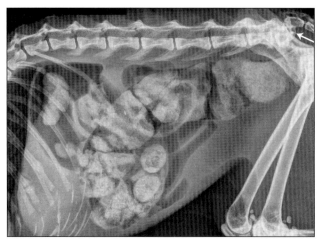

3.12 Lateral view of the abdomen of a cat with megacolon. The faeces are compacted and increased in opacity. There is a chronic sacral fracture (arrowed).

Contrast radiography

Contrast radiography of the GI tract is not commonly used any more, due to the wide availability of other techniques that are better suited to assessing the GI tract (i.e. ultrasonography, endoscopy). Nonetheless, contrast radiography can help diagnose certain conditions that cannot be detected on plain radiography, such as GI wall thickening as a result of inflammation, polyps or neoplasia, ulcers, radiolucent foreign bodies or intussusception.

For performing contrast radiography of the GI tract, it is important to wait for complete emptying of the stomach, if possible, which may require withholding food for 24 hours. Cleansing enemas are necessary before colonography, and plain radiographs should be taken first. GI contrast studies should not be performed (and never with barium) if rupture of the GI tract is suspected. Gastrography or colonography can be positive (barium), negative (air) or double contrast (barium and air). Dosages of contrast agents are detailed in Figure 3.13. Contrast agents can be administered orally or with the help of a nasogastric or orogastric tube for upper GI studies, and per rectum with a balloon-tipped catheter for colonic studies. In the case of gastric tube placement, if sedation is necessary, care should be taken to use drugs that do not have a significant effect on GI motility (e.g. acepromazine or diazepam/ketamine). Lateral (left and/or right) and ventrodorsal views should be taken at regular intervals (for upper GI studies: 0, 5, 15, 30, 60 minutes and then every hour, until the barium reaches the colon). Most of the barium should have left the stomach after 2 hours in cats and 4 hours in dogs. Small intestinal transit time should be approximately 1 hour in cats and 2–4 hours in dogs, but it can vary greatly, particularly when the animal is stressed.

Negative contrast studies have few indications. They are used mostly to look for foreign bodies or large masses in the stomach and to mark the position of the stomach or colon. For a better assessment of the walls, double contrast studies of the stomach and colon are preferred when looking for inflammatory or neoplastic lesions.

Contrast radiographic procedure	Contrast agent	Dose
Negative gastrography	Air	20 ml/kg
Positive gastrography	Liquid barium sulphate suspension (30% w/v)	7–8 ml/kg (large dogs) 10–15 ml/kg (small dogs/cats)
Double contrast gastrography	Liquid barium sulphate suspension (100%) first, then air	3–5 ml/kg barium followed by 10–20 ml/kg air
Upper gastrointestinal study	Liquid barium sulphate suspension (30% w/v)	7–8 ml/kg (large dogs) 10–15 ml/kg (small dogs/cats)
Negative colonography	Air	8 ml/kg
Positive colonography	Liquid barium sulphate suspension (20% w/v)	8 ml/kg
Double contrast colonography	Liquid barium sulphate suspension (20% w/v), then barium removed and air instilled	8 ml/kg barium followed by 8 ml/kg air

3.13 Dosages of contrast agents for contrast radiographic studies of the gastrointestinal tract.

Foreign bodies will typically create intraluminal filling defects within the positive contrast agent, and intestinal dilatation orad to the foreign body will be better appreciated with contrast radiography (Figure 3.14).

Neoplasms of the GI wall may cause mural filling defects, sometimes with an 'apple-core' effect. Conversely, outpouching of contrast agent beyond the limit of the gastric wall usually indicates an ulcerated mucosal surface.

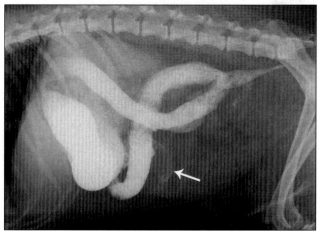

3.14 Right lateral view of the abdomen of a dog with a partial intestinal obstruction due to a peach stone (24 hours after oral administration of barium sulphate). The pyloric antrum and duodenum are moderately dilated; an intraluminal filling defect with an ovoid shape is visible (arrowed). A small amount of barium is visible in the distal part of the small intestine and colon.

Ultrasonography

Ultrasonography is the imaging modality of choice for evaluating the GI tract, as it has very good soft tissue contrast and is a real-time imaging method, which enables the evaluation of GI motility (usually 4–5 contractions per minute for the canine stomach). However, the presence of a large amount of GI gas is a major limitation, as it blocks the progression of the ultrasound waves and, therefore, limits complete evaluation of the GI tract, particularly at the level of the stomach and colon. Ultrasonography is also equipment- and operator-dependent and experience is required to obtain good quality images (e.g. use of intercostal approach for visualizing the stomach, optimizing acoustic windows by changing recumbency) and to interpret them. Typically, it is recommended to withhold food for 12 hours for the stomach to be empty. However, the accumulation of GI gas occurs independently of fasting status.

On ultrasonography, all the walls of the GI tract show a five-layered aspect (Figure 3.15), namely, from internally to externally:

- Hyperechoic mucosal interface
- Hypoechoic mucosa
- Hyperechoic submucosa
- Hypoechoic muscularis
- Hyperechoic serosa.

This layering is usually better assessed with high-frequency linear ultrasound transducers (8–12 MHz). The mucosal layer is usually thicker than the muscularis layer, but they sometimes can have an equal thickness in normal animals. The muscularis layer can be more prominent in the ileum. Measurements of GI wall thickness are detailed in Figure 3.16 but can vary depending on the amount of content, particularly in the stomach and colon.

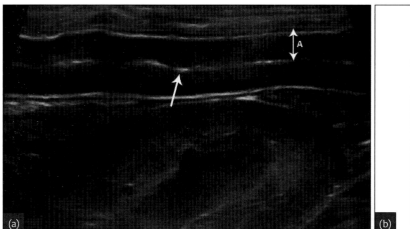

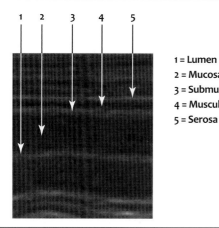

1	= Lumen
2	= Mucosa
3	= Submucosa
4	= Muscularis
5	= Serosa

3.15 (a) Ultrasonographic image of the duodenum of a dog. The wall shows a five-layered appearance (A = whole wall thickness), from internal to external: hyperechoic mucosal-luminal interface (arrowed), hypoechoic mucosa, hyperechoic submucosa, hypoechoic muscularis and hyperechoic serosa. (b) Higher magnification showing the five layers more clearly.

Gastrointestinal segment	Thickness in dogs	Thickness in cats
Stomach (between rugal folds)	3–5 mm	2–3.6 mm
Duodenum	5–6 mm	2.5–4 mm
Jejunum	4–4.5 mm	2.5–3 mm
Ileum	4 mm	3.2 mm
Colon	2–3 mm	1.7–2.5 mm

3.16 Ultrasonographic measurements of gastrointestinal wall thickness.

Mechanical obstructions: Abdominal ultrasonography has a greater accuracy and provides greater diagnostic confidence than radiography for the diagnosis of small intestinal mechanical obstructions. The presence of moderate to severe luminal dilatation of jejunal loops (total width >1.5 cm in dogs) should prompt a thorough search for a cause of mechanical obstruction.

Foreign bodies usually have a characteristic appearance on ultrasonography, with a hyperechoic interface and pronounced acoustic shadowing underneath the interface (Figure 3.17), although the degree of acoustic shadowing depends on the nature of the foreign material. Compact faecal material in the colon and large pieces of food in the stomach can mimic the appearance of a foreign body. Linear foreign bodies usually show a bright linear interface with a variable degree of acoustic shadowing, and often plication of the intestinal wall. A variable degree of luminal dilatation of the affected small intestinal loops can be seen depending on the degree of obstruction by the foreign body. When perforation of the wall occurs, the affected wall can appear thickened and hypoechoic, with a focal loss of layering, and signs of peritonitis (such as hyperechoic mesenteric fat) may be seen in close proximity.

Intussusceptions have a typical multi-layered (concentric rings) appearance on ultrasonography, due to superimposition of wall layers of the intussuscipiens (which can be oedematous, thick and hypoechoic) and intussusceptum (Figure 3.18). Mesenteric fat, blood vessels and lymph nodes may be visible within the intussusception. A lack of blood flow, detected with colour Doppler, in those blood vessels is a good predictive sign that the intussusception will not be manually reducible and that intestinal resection will therefore be necessary. Intussusceptions can occur at any level of the GI tract, but are reported to be more common at the ileocaecocolic junction. They can also be associated with intestinal neoplasia, particularly in older cats.

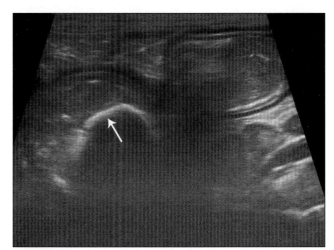

3.17 Ultrasonographic image of a jejunal loop of a cat. The affected loop is severely dilated with fluid/ingesta due to a mechanical obstruction by a foreign body (arrowed) showing a hyperechoic curvilinear surface and strong acoustic shadowing.

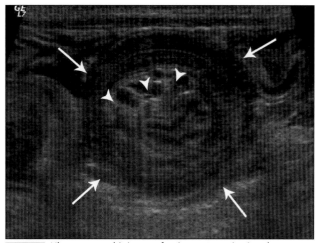

3.18 Ultrasonographic image of an intussusception in a dog (arrowed). The affected loops show a multi-layered appearance (concentric rings) and mesenteric fat and blood vessels (in cross-section; arrowheads) are also present within the intussusception.

Inflammatory diseases: With inflammatory diseases, the GI tract may appear normal or may show diffuse symmetrical wall thickening with preservation of normal wall layering on ultrasonography. However, in severe cases, wall layering may be altered, with changes in the echogenicity of the layers, changes in the relative thickness of the layers or slightly indistinct layers. The ultrasonographic signs of lymphoplasmacytic enteritis are usually:

- Mild to moderate wall thickening affecting the mucosa, submucosa and/or muscularis
- Increased echogenicity of the mucosa (diffuse or showing hyperechoic speckles or striations).

Striations are hyperechoic lines in the mucosa that are perpendicular to the lumen axis and represent dilated lacteals (Figure 3.19). They are usually associated with lymphangiectasia and protein-losing enteropathy. In very severe inflammatory diseases (granulomatous diseases, for example), the wall layering can be completely lost and may mimic neoplastic lesions, due to wall oedema, haemorrhage and fibrosis. In some cats, a mucosal hyperechoic band, parallel to the submucosa, has been described in the small intestine and has been associated with mucosal fibrosis (see Figure 3.22).

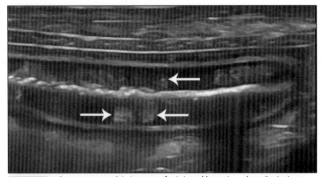

3.19 Ultrasonographic image of a jejunal loop in a dog. Striations are visible within the mucosa as hyperechoic lines perpendicular to the lumen axis (arrowed).

In uraemic gastritis, the gastric wall can appear thickened, with prominent rugal folds and mineralization of the mucosa (hyperechoic lining of the mucosal surface). Gastric wall oedema is sometimes present with severe gastritis and/or gastric ulcers; it appears as an anechoic to hypoechoic layer lining the mucosal surface.

Gastric ulcers may be secondary to severe inflammatory diseases or neoplasia (usually carcinoma). On ultrasonography, they are usually seen as a focal hypoechoic wall thickening with loss of layering (regardless of cause) and a hyperechoic line of gas tracking into the ulcer's crater (Figure 3.20). Fluid accumulation in the gastric lumen is also often present.

Neoplasia: The common ultrasonographic signs seen with GI carcinoma are transmural wall thickening, with altered layering or complete loss of layering. For gastric carcinoma, 'pseudolayering' is sometimes reported (i.e. echogenic line surrounded by outer and inner hypoechoic lines). Intestinal carcinoma tends to be more focal and is more likely to induce mechanical ileus compared with lymphoma.

GI lymphoma can show very variable features:

- It can be diffuse or focal
- It is often associated with regional lymphadenopathy

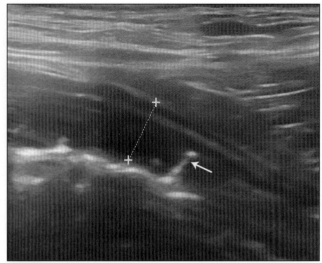

3.20 Ultrasonographic image of a gastric ulcer in a dog previously treated with non-steroidal anti-inflammatory drugs. The gastric wall (in between calipers) is focally thickened (9.7 mm), and there is a thin hyperechoic line of gas tracking into the ulcer's crater in the mucosa (arrowed).

- It can appear as wall thickening with or without loss of wall layering
- It can appear as hypoechoic wall thickening (Figure 3.21)
- It can appear as symmetrical or asymmetrical circumferential wall thickening.

In cats with intestinal lymphoma, significantly increased thickness of the muscularis layer (twice the thickness of the submucosal layer) is sometimes described (Figure 3.22); however, this also can be seen occasionally in patients with chronic inflammatory enteropathies.

Tumours of the muscularis (i.e. GI stromal tumours, leiomyoma, leiomyosarcoma) can present as large, often heterogeneous eccentrically growing mural masses, rarely projecting into the lumen. In cats, intestinal mast cell tumours appear as a hypoechoic non-circumferential eccentric wall thickening or very asymmetric circumferential eccentric wall thickening. Neoplastic mast cells appear to primarily infiltrate the muscularis and submucosa, and altered, rather than complete loss of wall, layering can be seen.

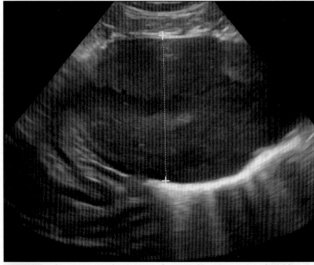

3.21 Ultrasonographic image of gastric lymphoma in a dog. The gastric wall (in between callipers) is focally severely thickened (2.73 cm) and hypoechoic with a complete loss of layering.

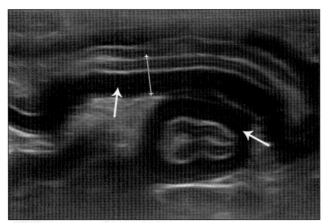

3.22 Ultrasonographic image of intestinal lymphoma in a cat. The jejunal wall (in between calipers) is thickened (4.1 mm) due to a severe thickening of the muscularis layer (arrowed). Mucosal fibrosis is also seen (thin isoechoic line in the mucosa parallel to the submucosa).

Other gastrointestinal diseases

Pyloric stenosis can be due to hypertrophic muscularis or mucosa. This can be difficult to assess on ultrasonography when the stomach is empty and collapsed. It can also be difficult to differentiate from polypoid lesions. Gastric polyps can present as large isoechoic nodules/masses and may also create gastric outflow obstructions.

Interventional procedures

When masses or nodules are detected with ultrasonography in the GI wall, ultrasound-guided fine-needle aspiration can usually be performed. This is particularly helpful when the lesions cannot be accessed with endoscopy, e.g. jejunal or ileal lesions, or eccentric lesions arising from the muscularis. Tru-Cut® biopsies can also be performed, if the mass is large enough and not too mobile. Care should be taken to avoid the GI lumen when performing sampling of the GI wall. Aspiration of the regional lymph nodes is also indicated if they appear abnormal.

Endoscopic ultrasonography

The echo-endoscope is similar to a conventional endoscope, but it has an ultrasound transducer at its tip; they are not currently widely available. Both radial and linear multi-frequency transducers are available. Transducer coupling is either by direct mucosal contact or by inflation of a water-filled balloon surrounding the transducer. Figure 3.23 shows which organs are easy to obtain images of and those which are not as readily visualized.

Structures that are easy to view
• Oesophagus
• Gastric wall
• Liver and associated vessels
• Hepatic lymph nodes
• Left pancreatic limb and body

Structures that are difficult to view
• Distal duodenum and right pancreatic limb
• The entire jejunum
• Ileum
• Caecum

3.23 Organs that are easy and more difficult to visualize by endoscopic ultrasonography.

Computed tomography

In humans, CT is used extensively to evaluate the lumen and walls of the GI tract. It can be helpful for the detection of tumours, obstructions, adhesions and ischaemia. Many GI lesions can be detected with CT but it is still not widely used with small animals (Figure 3.24). Although CT does not identify distinct GI wall layering as precisely as ultrasonography does, distinct mucosal enhancement can be seen on post-contrast images after injection of an iodinated contrast agent. Oral administration of intraluminal contrast agents (e.g. water, milk, barium) has been described, but this is not commonly used in veterinary medicine due to the need for sedation or general anaesthesia to perform CT. Negative gastrography or colonography can also be performed in conjunction with CT.

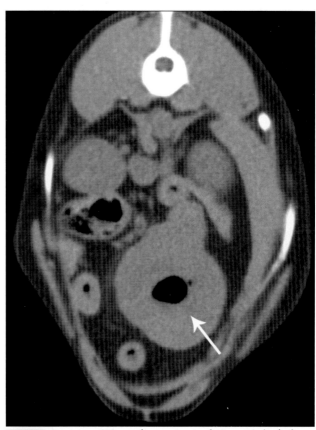

3.24 Transverse CT image (pre-contrast soft tissue window) of a dog with a diffuse colonic wall thickening due to neoplasia (arrowed).

Liver

The imaging modality most commonly used for assessing the liver is ultrasonography, but CT is being used increasingly for that purpose, particularly in larger dogs and when assessing for portosystemic shunts or staging neoplasia.

Radiography

Radiography is mostly used for estimating hepatic size, based on the position of the stomach axis and the margins of the liver lobes relative to the costal arch. The margins of the normal liver should be sharp and triangular, and usually do not extend beyond the costal arch. On lateral abdominal radiographs, the stomach axis (i.e. the line between the fundus and pyloric antrum) should be parallel to the last rib or perpendicular to the cranial lumbar spine in more deep-chested dogs. A cranial displacement of the gastric axis indicates decreased hepatic size (e.g. chronic hepatitis, cirrhosis, portosystemic shunt) or a cranial displacement of the liver (e.g. diaphragmatic rupture, peritoneopericardial diaphragmatic hernia). A caudal displacement of the gastric axis (Figure 3.25) indicates diffuse hepatomegaly (e.g. diffuse or metastatic neoplasia, congestion, nodular hyperplasia, lipidosis, hepatopathies) or the presence of a large hepatic mass (usually neoplasia). In the case of steroid hepatopathy, the liver can be increased in size with rounded margins but usually protrudes markedly caudoventral to the costal arch, rather than displacing the stomach axis.

The biliary tract is usually not visualized by radiography. Rarely, mineralizations can be seen: linear in the bile ducts or more discrete in the gall bladder in cases of cholelithiasis. Gas opacities are rarely seen but may indicate infections with gas-producing bacteria (e.g. emphysematous cholecystitis).

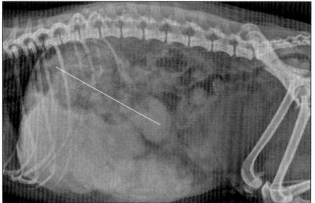

3.25 Right lateral view of the abdomen of a dog with hepatic neoplasia. The stomach axis (indicated by a line) is severely displaced caudally.

Ultrasonography

Ultrasonography is the preferred method for imaging the liver, due to its wide availability and the very good soft tissue detail it provides. It is, however, important to note that whilst ultrasonography is relatively sensitive for detecting parenchymal lesions, it has poor specificity for distinguishing malignant from benign lesions.

The entire liver can often be seen with ultrasonography, but care should be taken to assess the deepest areas by applying enough pressure on the transducer caudal to the costal arch (subcostal approach) or by using an intercostal approach. The lungs and the ribs can sometimes prevent a complete examination of the liver, particularly in deep-chested dogs and in cases of microhepatica. Convex and microconvex probes (frequency range of 5–8 MHz) are usually used.

The diaphragm appears as a hyperechoic line cranial to the liver and a mirror-image artefact is often visible at this level (i.e. a false impression of liver tissue cranial to the diaphragm). The different hepatic lobes cannot be differentiated with ultrasonography unless there is peritoneal effusion and the hepatic size is also sometimes difficult to evaluate objectively. However, some of the criteria used with radiography can be applied (e.g. sharp triangular borders, position of the caudal margin in relation to the

costal arch). The normal hepatic parenchyma is coarse and diffusely hypoechoic compared with the spleen. The gall bladder is usually anechoic with posterior enhancement seen dorsally, although mobile isoechoic sludge is often present, particularly in dogs, and it can be bi-lobed in cats. Gall bladder volume can vary greatly, with the thin, smooth gall bladder wall measuring 1 mm thick in cats and 2–3 mm in dogs. The intra-hepatic biliary ducts are not visible in normal dogs and cats; only the common bile duct can be seen, measuring up to 4 mm wide in cats and 3 mm in dogs. In cats, it can be followed easily to the duodenal papilla.

In normal animals, the main portal vein should be visible at the hepatic hilus; its main branches can be seen within the parenchyma as anechoic tubes with hyperechoic walls (independently of their orientation relative to the ultrasound beam). The hepatic veins also appear as anechoic tubes, but their walls are not hyperechoic, unless the ultrasound beam is perpendicular to the wall. The larger hepatic veins can be followed to the caudal vena cava. The use of colour Doppler can help differentiate portal vessels (red with standard colour-map settings) from hepatic veins (blue). A ratio can be calculated between the maximal diameter of the aorta (AO) and the main portal vein (PV): this PV/AO ratio should be 0.71–1.25 in normal dogs and cats. This measurement can be useful for investigating portosystemic shunts.

Variation in hepatic size

In cases of decreased liver size, the differential diagnoses include chronic hepatitis, cirrhosis, portosystemic shunt, portal vein hypoplasia and hypovolaemia. The liver parenchyma usually appears normal with a portosystemic shunt but it can be diffusely hyperechoic or heterogeneous with chronic hepatitis or cirrhosis.

Diffuse hepatomegaly can reflect hepatitis/cholangiohepatitis, diffuse neoplasia (round-cell neoplasia, extensive carcinoma or metastatic disease), congestion, amyloidosis, steroid hepatopathy, lipidosis and changes secondary to diabetes mellitus. Focal hepatomegaly is usually due to the presence of a mass lesion (e.g. benign or malignant neoplasia, haematoma, abscess, cyst, granuloma or lobar torsion).

Diffuse and focal variations in parenchymal echogenicity

Diffuse hypoechogenicity of the liver can be due to congestion, acute hepatitis (e.g. leptospirosis), lymphoma and other round-cell tumours, and amyloidosis. Diffuse hyperechogenicity of the liver can be the result of lipidosis, steroid hepatopathy, vacuolar hepatopathy, lymphoma, mast cell tumours, fibrosis, chronic hepatitis, cirrhosis or hepatocutaneous syndrome. However, many of these diseases can also be responsible for a diffusely heterogeneous parenchyma with mixed echogenicities (e.g. a combination of diffuse mild hyperechogenicity with ill-defined hypoechoic and/or hyperechoic nodules).

Lymphoma and mast cell tumours can induce diffuse changes in the echogenicity of the hepatic parenchyma, but hypoechoic nodules may also be present (Figure 3.26). It is also important to note that infiltrated hepatic parenchyma can still appear normal on ultrasonography. Therefore, it is recommended to perform fine-needle aspiration of the liver even in the absence of ultrasonographic lesions when neoplastic diseases are suspected. With histiocytic neoplasia, diffuse hypoechogenicity or hypoechoic nodules and masses have been reported.

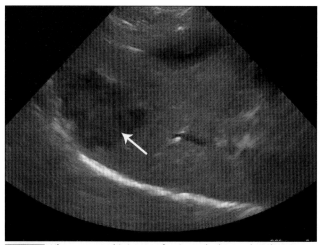

3.26 Ultrasonographic image of an irregular hypoechoic lesion (arrowed) in the liver of a cat affected by lymphoma.

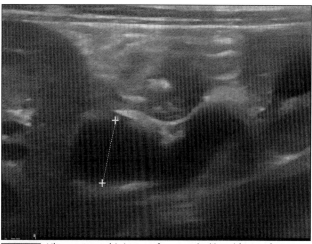

3.28 Ultrasonographic image of a severely dilated (7.7 mm) common bile duct in a cat affected by cholangiohepatitis.

Hepatic and biliary carcinomas can be focal or diffuse and usually appear as mixed lesions (Figure 3.27). However, benign lesions such as haematomas and hepatomas can present the same ultrasonographic appearance.

Biliary tract diseases

In cases of extra-hepatic biliary obstruction (due to plugs, choleliths, neoplasia, cholecystitis, duodenitis or pancreatitis), the common bile duct becomes widened (larger than 4 mm in cats) and tortuous. Retrograde dilatation is then expected to develop at the level of the extra-hepatic and then intra-hepatic bile ducts. The gall bladder is not always dilated in cases of biliary obstruction. Dilatation of the intra-hepatic bile ducts appears as multiple tortuous anechoic tubes with hyperechoic walls and is not associated with colour flow on Doppler.

Gall bladder wall thickening is usually due to cholecystitis (hypoechoic thickening with inner and outer hyperechoic rims if acute or a thick hyperechoic wall if chronic) or oedema (usually hypoechoic thickening with inner and outer hyperechoic rims, secondary to hypoalbuminaemia or portal hypertension), and very less commonly neoplasia. Dilatation of the common bile duct is also sometimes seen in cases of cholecystitis (Figure 3.28) and it can be difficult to differentiate it from obstructive causes.

Polyps and neoplasia originating from the gall bladder wall are rare. Gall bladder mucocoeles have a characteristic appearance on ultrasonography, with the hypoechoic mucus creating a rim around central isoechoic sludge. It will usually show a radiate or kiwi fruit-like pattern with hyperechoic striations (Figure 3.29). The gall bladder wall can be thickened, and rupture may also occur, leading to focal peritonitis.

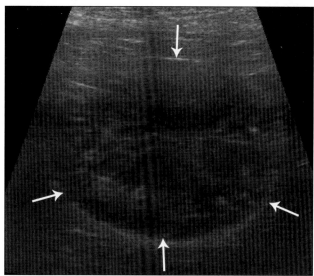

3.29 Ultrasonographic image of a gall bladder mucocoele (arrowed).

Disorders of the hepatic vasculature

Congenital portosystemic shunts can be detected with ultrasonography, but this is highly dependent on the level of experience of the operator, the amount of GI gas and the size of the liver. The right intercostal approach (dorsal aspect of the 11th or 12th intercostal space) is usually preferred, but some less common types of shunts may be missed with this approach. The use of colour Doppler can be useful to follow the vessels and determine the direction of flow. In the case of shunts, the liver is usually small and the kidneys enlarged (mostly in dogs; uroliths may also be detected). Extra-hepatic shunts can be challenging to detect: the shunt leaves one branch of the portal vein before it enters the liver and may join the caudal vena cava, the azygos vein or a phrenic vein. In that case, the portal vein is usually small or undetectable at the level

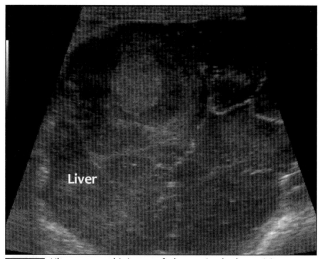

3.27 Ultrasonographic image of a large mixed echogenicity mass lesion (carcinoma) in the liver of a dog.

of the porta hepatis (a PV/AO ratio <0.65 predicts the presence of an extra-hepatic shunt). Intra-hepatic shunts are usually easier to detect. Portal hypertension (secondary to chronic hepatitis, cirrhosis, some hepatic neoplasms, or congenital diseases) is suspected when the portal flow (measured with spectral Doppler) shows a decreased velocity (<10 cm/s) or is hepatofugal. This is, however, sometimes difficult to assess, as ascites and oedema of the pancreas and gall bladder wall can also be seen, together with the presence of acquired shunts, which are often in the region of the left kidney.

Interventional procedures

It is often recommended to sample lesions under ultrasound guidance (fine-needle aspiration or Tru-Cut® biopsy) to further characterize abnormalities. It is also recommended to sample the liver when lymphoma or mast cell tumours are suspected, despite the lack of ultrasonographic abnormalities. As haemorrhage is a potential complication, it is recommended to check the coagulation status of the animal prior to the procedure.

Ultrasound-guided cholecystocentesis can also be performed. It is recommended to use a transhepatic approach (through the parenchyma) and to empty the gall bladder as much as possible. It should not be performed when the gall bladder is too dilated or its wall appears too thin or abnormal, or when there is obstruction of the common bile duct.

Contrast-enhanced ultrasonography

Contrast-enhanced ultrasonography uses a contrast agent composed of microscopic bubbles of inert gas administered intravenously. These bubbles show a non-linear oscillation when subjected to ultrasound waves and enhance the echogenicity of perfused tissue. This technique has proved useful for differentiating benign from malignant hepatic nodules in dogs, with malignant nodules being hypoechoic to the rest of the hepatic parenchyma at peak enhancement whilst benign nodules are isoechoic (O'Brien et al., 2004; O'Brien, 2007). This technique has also proved useful for detecting haemangiosarcoma metastases that were not visible on conventional B-mode ultrasonography of the liver in three dogs.

Computed tomography

CT is a very good technique for assessing the liver, as it overcomes the problems arising from overlying ribs, lung and gas-filled GI structures that could mask lesions on ultrasonography. Intravenous contrast medium is routinely administered during CT to demonstrate focal lesions. Triple-phase CT can sometimes be useful for differentiating malignant lesions (hepatocellular carcinoma, metastatic tumours) from nodular hyperplasia in the canine liver. CT can also be used for evaluating the resectability of liver masses and for performing complete staging. Finally, CT angiography is the preferred imaging modality for diagnosing and characterizing the morphology of portosystemic shunts (Figure 3.30).

Scintigraphy

Scintigraphy is based on the use of radiopharmaceutical agents. It is only available in a few veterinary referral centres, but has proved useful for diagnosing portosystemic shunts.

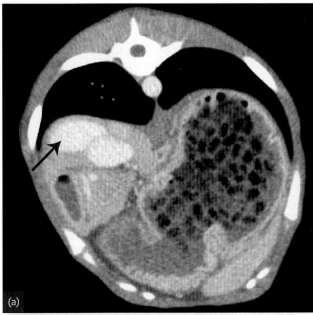
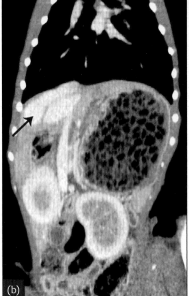

3.30 CT images (post-contrast soft tissue window) in (a) a transverse and (b) a dorsal plane of a dog with a right-divisional intra-hepatic portosystemic shunt (arrowed). The liver is very small.

Pancreas

The pancreas is difficult to view entirely due to its small size and its position in the cranial abdomen. The imaging modality of choice for pancreatitis is ultrasonography, whilst CT with contrast is preferred for detecting insulinomas.

Radiography

The normal pancreas is not visible on radiography, except the left limb, which can sometimes be seen on the ventrodorsal view in obese cats. Therefore, radiography is rarely useful for diagnosing pancreatic disorders. Normal radiographs do not rule out pancreatic diseases, particularly in cases of very acute or chronic pancreatitis or small pancreatic lesions (cysts, insulinomas, other nodules).

In cases of severe pancreatitis, some radiographic signs can be detected: widening of the gastroduodenal angle on ventrodorsal views (descending duodenum displaced laterally and pyloric antrum displaced cranially), caudal displacement of the colon, persistent gas dilatation of the descending duodenum due to focal paralytic ileus, and loss of serosal detail due to focal peritonitis in the right craniodorsal abdomen. Large pancreatic masses (usually carcinomas) can also produce a mass effect inducing a widening of the pyloroduodenal angle and a caudal displacement of the transverse colon (Figure 3.31).

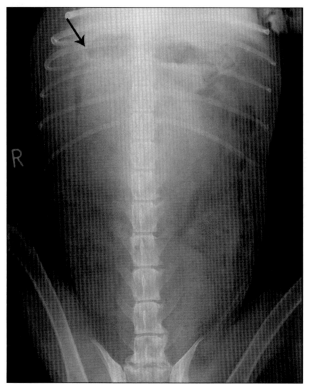

3.31 Ventrodorsal view of the abdomen of a dog with pancreatic neoplasia. The pyloroduodenal angle (arrowed) is widened due to a large pancreatic mass. The colon is also displaced caudally and to the left.

Ultrasonography

Ultrasonography is the current imaging modality of choice to assess the pancreas, but it is operator-dependent. Complete pancreatic visualization is often difficult in dogs, due to the gas present in the stomach and colon and the deep cranial position of the pancreas under the ribs. The right lobe in dogs and the left lobe in cats are easier to detect. The normal pancreas is isoechoic or slightly hyperechoic to the liver and it can sometimes be isoechoic to the surrounding fat; margins can, therefore, be difficult to delineate. The pancreaticoduodenal vein, or pancreatic duct, can sometimes be used to find the pancreas. The maximal thickness of the pancreas is 1 cm in cats and very variable in dogs (1–2.5 cm).

Pancreatitis

In dogs, acute pancreatitis appears as an enlarged hypoechoic pancreas with ill-defined margins (Figure 3.32) surrounded by hyperechoic mesenteric fat (due to saponification). In severe cases, focal peritoneal effusion can be detected as well as duodenitis and paralytic ileus of the descending duodenum, secondary to the peritonitis. A case of intramural haematoma has been reported in the duodenum of a dog affected by pancreatitis. In cats, similar changes can be seen but are usually less obvious,

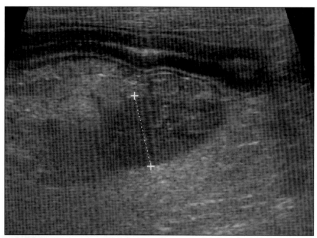

3.32 Ultrasonographic image of pancreatitis in a dog. The pancreas is mildly thickened (1.1 cm), hypoechoic with ill-defined margins and surrounded by hyperechoic fat.

and a normal pancreas on ultrasonography does not exclude the possibility of pancreatitis. In necrotizing pancreatitis, the pancreas may appear very heterogeneous with indistinct borders. Pancreatitis can induce an extrahepatic biliary obstruction with dilatation of the common bile duct.

The diagnosis of chronic pancreatitis is challenging, as the pancreas may appear ultrasonographically normal. Conversely, it can be decreased in size with a heterogeneous parenchyma (due to nodules, fibrosis and mineralization). Pancreatic duct dilatation is not specific, as it can be seen with acute and chronic pancreatitis and in normal older cats. Pancreatic oedema may be associated with pancreatitis or secondary to hypoalbuminaemia or portal hypertension. On ultrasonography, the pancreas is enlarged with hypoechoic stripes separating pancreatic lobulations (Figure 3.33).

Focal pancreatic lesions

These are usually hypoechoic or anechoic. Numerous causes are possible: cysts, pseudocysts (usually a sequel of pancreatitis), retention cysts and abscesses. It is often not possible to distinguish them on ultrasonography.

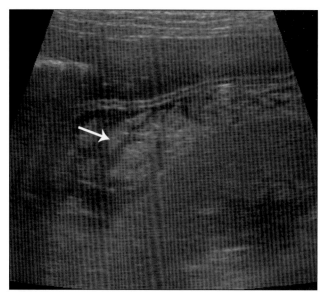

3.33 Ultrasonographic image of pancreatic oedema in a dog. Note the hypoechoic stripes (arrowed) separating pancreatic lobulations.

Pancreatic abscesses may appear large, contain isoechoic cellular fluid and be surrounded by focal peritonitis.

Isoechoic to hypoechoic nodules can also be due to nodular hyperplasia or neoplasia (carcinoma, insulinoma, gastrinoma). A search for potential metastases in the local lymph nodes, liver and mesentery should be conducted. Insulinomas are usually very small nodules (less than 2 cm) and can be very difficult to find on ultrasonography.

Computed tomography

CT angiography is very useful for detecting small pancreatic insulinomas that can be overlooked on ultrasonography. On CT, endocrine pancreatic tumours are usually markedly contrast-enhancing (hyperattenuating to the rest of the parenchyma) in the arterial phase (Figure 3.34) and iso/hyperattenuating in the portal phase. Carcinomas usually remain hypoattenuating to the rest of the pancreas in all phases. CT is also the imaging modality of choice for staging pancreatic tumours, particularly at the level of the regional lymph nodes and liver.

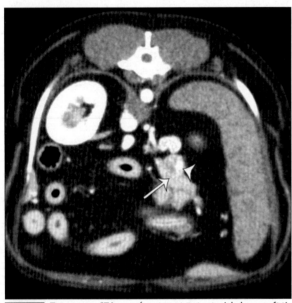

3.34 Transverse CT image (post-contrast arterial phase soft tissue window) of a dog with an insulinoma (arrowhead), which appears hyperattenuating to the rest of the left pancreatic limb (arrowed).

References and further reading

Ciasca TC, David FH and Lamb CR (2013) Does measurement of small intestinal diameter increase diagnostic accuracy of radiography in dogs with suspected intestinal obstruction? *Veterinary Radiology and Ultrasound* **54**, 207–211

Daniaux LA, Laurenson MP, Marks SL *et al.* (2014) Ultrasonographic thickening of the muscularis propria in feline small intestinal small cell T-cell lymphoma and inflammatory bowel disease. *Journal of Feline Medicine and Surgery* **16**, 89–98

Fischetti AJ, Saunders HM and Orobatz KJ (2004) Pneumatosis in canine gastric dilatation-volvulus syndrome. *Veterinary Radiology and Ultrasound* **45**, 205–209

Garcia DAA and Froes TR (2014) Importance of fasting in preparing dogs for abdominal ultrasound examination of specific organs. *Journal of Small Animal Practice* **55**, 630–634

Gaschen L, Kircher P, Wolfram K (2007) Endoscopic ultrasound of the canine abdomen. *Veterinary Radiology and Ultrasound* **48**, 338–349

Heng HG, Huang A, Baird DK *et al.* (2010) Spontaneous intramural canine duodenal hematoma. *Veterinary Radiology and Ultrasound* **51**, 178-181

Hoey S, Drees R and Hetzel S (2013) Evaluation of the gastrointestinal tract in dogs using computed tomography. *Veterinary Radiology and Ultrasound* **54**, 25–30

Kutara K, Seki M, Ishikawa C *et al.* (2014) Triple-phase helical computed tomography in dogs with hepatic masses. *Veterinary Radiology and Ultrasound* **55**, 7–15

Laurenson MP, Skorupski KA, Moore PF *et al.* (2011) Ultrasonography of intestinal mast cell tumors in the cat. *Veterinary Radiology and Ultrasound* **52**, 330–334

Mai W and Cáceres AV (2008) Dual-phase computed tomographic angiography in three dogs with pancreatic insulinoma. *Veterinary Radiology and Ultrasound* **49**, 141–148

O'Brien RT (2007) Improved detection of metastatic hepatic hemangiosarcoma nodules with contrast ultrasound in three dogs. *Veterinary Radiology and Ultrasound* **48**, 146–148

O'Brien RT, Iani M, Matheson J *et al.* (2004) Contrast harmonic ultrasound of spontaneous liver nodules in 32 dogs. *Veterinary Radiology and Ultrasound* **45**, 547–553

O'Brien TR (1981) *Radiographic Diagnosis of Abdominal Disorders in the Dog and Cat*. WB Saunders, Philadelphia

Patsikas MN, Papazoglou LG, Jakovljevic S *et al.* (2005) Color Doppler ultrasonography in prediction of the reducibility of intussuscepted bowel in 15 young dogs. *Veterinary Radiology and Ultrasound* **46**, 313–316

Penninck D and D'Anjou MA (2015) *Atlas of Small Animal Ultrasonography, 2nd edn*. Wiley-Blackwell, Ames

Penninck DG, Webster CR and Keating JH (2010) The sonographic appearance of intestinal mucosal fibrosis in cats. *Veterinary Radiology and Ultrasound* **51**, 458–461

Sharma A, Thompson MS, Scrivani PV *et al.* (2011) Comparison of radiography and ultrasonography for diagnosing small-intestinal mechanical obstruction in vomiting dogs. *Veterinary Radiology and Ultrasound* **52**, 248–255

Sutherland-Smith J, Penninck DG, Keating JH *et al.* (2007) Ultrasonographic intestinal hyperechoic mucosal striations in dogs are associated with lacteal dilation. *Veterinary Radiology and Ultrasound* **48**, 51–57

Trevail T, Gunn-Moore D, Carrera I *et al.* (2011) Radiographic diameter of the colon in normal and constipated cats and in cats with megacolon. *Veterinary Radiology and Ultrasound* **52**, 516–520

Zwingenberger AL, Schwarz T and Saunders HM (2005) Helical CT angiography of canine portosystemic shunts. *Veterinary Radiology and Ultrasound* **46**, 27–37

Chapter 4

Endoscopy

Mike Willard

The role of flexible and rigid endoscopy of the GI tract

The most typical indications for gastrointestinal (GI) endoscopy in small animal practice include:

- Mucosal biopsy looking for infiltrative diseases (either inflammatory or neoplastic)
- Removal of foreign objects
- A search for bleeding lesions.

Endoscopy is rarely useful for diagnosing functional oesophageal diseases (e.g. oesophageal weakness, cricopharyngeal achalasia), functional gastric diseases (e.g. gastroduodenal reflux) or diarrhoea caused by diet or by bacteria, except for granulomatous (histiocytic ulcerative) colitis of Boxers and French Bulldogs. Most GI endoscopic procedures are best done with flexible equipment; however, there are some situations in which rigid equipment is more effective and preferred.

Regardless of the part of the GI tract that is being examined, endoscopy is generally considered 'minimally invasive surgery', but it is only of value if it can be done so well as to avoid the need for more invasive, classic, open surgery. This is especially true with respect to endoscopic biopsies. Endoscopic biopsies are much easier and quicker to perform than surgical biopsies; however, it is very easy to take inadequate, non-diagnostic tissue samples that waste time and resources. If one is not trained in taking high quality tissue samples endoscopically, then it may be best either to refer the patient to a more skillful endoscopist or to obtain the GI tissue samples at surgery.

Oesophageal diseases

Endoscopy is the best way to look for oesophagitis and it is useful in defining oesophageal masses (e.g. malignancies), as well as spirocercosis. Endoscopy is effective in diagnosing and, more importantly, treating benign oesophageal strictures, as well as determining whether an apparent stricture is in fact a vascular ring anomaly. In addition, endoscopy (especially rigid) is the preferred way to remove oesophageal foreign bodies, whenever possible. Sliding hiatal hernias (see Chapter 32) may not always be immediately apparent, but various physical manipulations (e.g. manual compression of the abdomen, occlusion of the endotracheal tube for three consecutive breaths, lifting the rear quarters of the patient) can be performed in order to increase the chance of detection during endoscopy.

Gastric diseases

Flexible endoscopy is the best way to diagnose gastric ulcers and erosions as well as infiltrative mucosal diseases (e.g. neoplasia) and *Helicobacter* infections. It is the preferred way to remove foreign bodies, whenever possible. It is also the best way to remove gastric polyps that are causing outflow obstruction, although that is an uncommon indication. Rarely, flexible endoscopy can be used to cauterize lesions that are causing life-threatening haemorrhage.

Small intestinal diseases

Flexible endoscopy of the small intestine is indicated to look for and biopsy infiltrative diseases (e.g. alimentary lymphoma, fungal infections and other chronic enteropathies). It is the preferred way to remove intestinal foreign bodies, although most are actually beyond the reach of the endoscope.

Large intestinal diseases

Flexible endoscopy is typically used to look for infiltrative and ulcerative diseases, especially of the upper large intestine, caecum and ileum. Rigid endoscopy can readily detect lesions in the descending colon, but it is particularly effective when taking biopsy samples of rectal infiltrates and masses. This is because it is critically important to obtain generous amounts of submucosa in the tissue sample when trying to distinguish benign from malignant anorectal lesions. Occasionally, ileocolic and caecocolic intussusceptions may be diagnosed endoscopically.

Equipment and technique for upper and lower GI endoscopy

It is hard enough to become proficient at flexible endoscopy with good equipment; to try to do so with poor quality equipment is to guarantee frustration. All new flexible GI endoscopes sold today are fully immersible; second-hand, non-immersible endoscopes should be avoided as they cannot be disinfected effectively. Any endoscope designed for GI procedures must have the capability to insufflate with air, wash off the viewing lens and aspirate luminal contents. Four-way deflection is routine, although some paediatric gastroscopes may only have two-way deflection; such endoscopes are not recommended for the novice endoscopist. The light source must provide a very bright light, and it is usually also the source of insufflation. The channel providing insufflation is generally also used to wash off the viewing lens (i.e. a jet of water and/or air is shot at a 90-degree angle across the viewing lens). Some GI endoscopes have an additional feature, whereby a large jet of water is shot straight out of the tip of the endoscope to facilitate washing the mucosa to reveal lesions.

Almost all GI endoscopes now sold are videoscopes as opposed to fibreoptic scopes; hence, a video processor and a monitor are required. The monitor does not need to be extremely expensive, but should be large enough with sufficient resolution to allow easy viewing. A suction pump is essential so that air insufflated into the GI lumen can be removed, as well as unwanted luminal contents (e.g. water, mucus, blood). Some type of image capture system is desirable, but is not critical. Necessary accessories include biopsy forceps and an assortment of foreign body retrieval devices. Optional accessories for the more experienced endoscopist include 'hot' snares, 'hot' probes, 'hot' forceps, balloon catheters, transfer wires and/or injection catheters.

The clinician must carefully consider which species they will be examining most of the time when choosing an endoscope. A 2.8 mm biopsy/aspiration channel is much more desirable than a 2.2 mm channel because it allows many more options regarding accessories, it allows bigger biopsy samples to be obtained and it is much less likely to clog up when aspirating GI contents. Conversely, the smaller the outer diameter of the insertion tube, the easier it will be to pass it through tight spots (e.g. the pylorus, especially in cats) and through winding loops of intestine. An endoscope with an outer diameter of 8.5 mm and a 2.8 mm aspiration/biopsy channel is optimal for the vast majority of canine and feline procedures. A skilled endoscopist can use an endoscope of these dimensions to routinely enter the duodenum of dogs and cats weighing only 2–3 kg.

Almost all GI endoscopes have an insertion tube at least 1 m in length, and this is sufficient for the vast majority of cases. In dogs greater than 30 kg or with very long bodies (e.g. Greyhounds), it is possible for the less experienced endoscopist to 'run out' of insertion tube before reaching the pylorus. Endoscopes with 1.4–1.6 m long insertion tubes are available, and these can reach the pylorus in all but the largest dogs. However, the excessive insertion tube length is cumbersome when performing procedures on smaller animals.

There are numerous foreign body retrieval devices, and the old adage that 'you get what you pay for' is borne out here. Good retrieval devices tend to be expensive; nonetheless, it is advisable to have an assortment of these at hand so one does not waste hours trying to remove a foreign object only to have to finally resort to surgery. The author recommends having a minimum of four devices: a simple snare, a 4- or 6-wire basket, a shark's tooth and an alligator jaw device (Figure 4.1). A W-type coin retrieval device is also very useful if one sees many such foreign bodies. Baskets need to have soft, flexible wires, which open up as widely as possible (at least 2 cm) and will drape and fall over the edges of the foreign object. Baskets with stiff wires (which are often advertised as a less expensive alternative) are often ineffective, as they tend to push the object away.

For more information, see also the *BSAVA Manual of Canine and Feline Endoscopy and Endosurgery*.

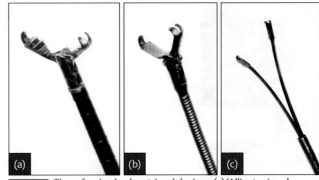

4.1 Three foreign body retrieval devices. (a) 'Alligator jaws'; (b) 'shark's tooth'; (c) W-type coin retrieval device.
(Reproduced from Steiner (2008), with permission from the publisher)

Upper GI endoscopy (oesophago-gastro-enteroscopy)

Animals with GI pathology may have slow gastric emptying times. Therefore, prior to oesophago-gastro-duodenoscopy, the patient should be prepared by withholding all food, ideally for at least 24 or even 36 hours, and withholding water for at least 8 hours, unless this may harm the patient. Prokinetics (e.g. metoclopramide, cisapride, erythromycin, ranitidine), sucralfate and barium sulphate should be avoided for at least 24 hours prior to the procedure. The patient must be anaesthetized to a surgical plane and have a good mouth gag firmly inserted; sedation alone is inadequate. If the stomach is overly distended with air (a common occurrence), there will be decreased ventilation and decreased venous return. If such a patient is being maintained with an anaesthetic agent that is poorly absorbed (e.g. isoflurane, sevoflurane, desflurane), it will be very easy for them to suddenly start waking up during the procedure; therefore, the patient may have to be ventilated to ensure an adequate plane of anaesthesia. Using a mechanical ventilator with the anaesthetic machine is optimal, assuming it can be used safely.

The patient is placed in left lateral recumbency. The tip of the endoscope is advanced through the cricopharyngeal sphincter and insufflation is used as needed to allow thorough examination of the oesophageal mucosa as the endoscope is advanced towards the stomach. Upon entering the stomach, the clinician will typically find a deflated lumen with large rugal folds, making it impossible to do an adequate examination (Figure 4.2). At this point, the clinician should either insufflate the stomach sufficiently to examine it before going into the duodenum, or insufflate the stomach minimally, pass the tip of the endoscope along the parallel rugal folds of the greater curvature, and then enter the antrum and pylorus to examine and biopsy the duodenum before coming back to the stomach. The latter approach is important in larger patients, in order to avoid overly distending the stomach, which would make the distance the endoscope must travel to the pylorus too long to allow entry into the duodenum.

In order to examine the stomach adequately, sufficient air must be instilled to distend the stomach and flatten most of the rugal folds (Figure 4.3). Doing so often causes some degree of gastric dilation, with subsequent hypoventilation and stimulation of gastric peristalsis. Excessive gastric peristalsis can make it more difficult to enter the pylorus. However, it is critical to examine the entire gastric

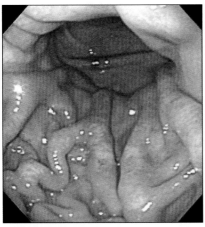

4.2 Endoscopic view of the gastric lumen before it is insufflated. Large rugal folds obscure the majority of the gastric mucosa, preventing thorough examination for gastric mucosal lesions.

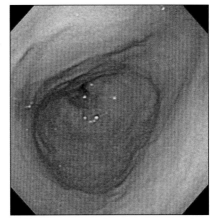

4.4 Endoscopic view of a normal canine antrum with the pylorus seen at the back of the antrum.

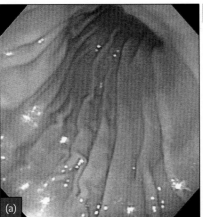

4.3 (a) Endoscopic view of a partially insufflated gastric lumen. Compare this image with Figure 4.2; more of the gastric mucosa can be visualized here. (b) Endoscopic view of a properly insufflated gastric lumen. The gastric lumen can be thoroughly examined now, but this degree of insufflation will soon cause hypoventilation and increased gastric peristalsis.

(a)

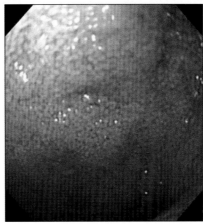

4.5 Endoscopic view of normal duodenal mucosa showing the texture caused by the villi. Compare the mucosal texture seen in this image with that seen in Figures 4.2–4.4.

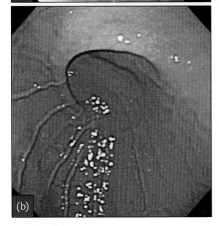

(b)

the duodenal mucosa and cause bleeding, which can obscure subtle lesions or ulcers. If there is pathology near the pylorus, associated inflammation may make it harder to pass the endoscope tip through this area.

The basic principles of endoscopic examination are:

* Only advance the endoscope when you can see where you are going
* If it is difficult to see where you are, then put more air into the lumen and/or pull the tip of the endoscope back and try to get a panoramic view
* It is beneficial to aim the endoscope into the centre of the lumen (i.e. centralize) unless looking at a specific lesion.

mucosal surface carefully because many patients have focal gastric lesions that are easily missed by careless examination. Superficial ulcers in particular, but even deep ulcers, are easily hidden by folds of mucosa, and most are not bleeding at the time of examination.

Enteroscopy begins when the tip of the endoscope passes into the duodenum. The pylorus is visualized as the endoscope enters the antrum (Figure 4.4). When the patient is in left lateral recumbency, the pylorus is at the furthermost aspect of the antrum, typically to the left. The duodenum curves to the right immediately after one enters the pylorus. Normal gastric mucosa is relatively smooth, but normal small intestinal mucosa will be distinctly textured due to the villi (Figure 4.5). A biopsy instrument can be passed through the biopsy channel of the endoscope and into the closed pylorus to act as a guide wire, but this technique is best avoided because it is easy to traumatize

Lower GI endoscopy (rectocolonocaecoileoscopy)

Preparing for colonoscopy begins by withholding all food for at least 24 hours and preferably 48 hours prior to the procedure. This prevents additional faeces from entering the colon. Faeces already in the colon are removed with lavage solutions and/or enemas. Commercial lavage solutions (e.g. polyethylene glycol plus electrolytes or sodium phosphate solutions) are administered the day before the procedure. Commercial polyethylene glycol solutions are usually administered via orogastric tube two or three times the night before the procedure at 25 ml/kg, with each administration 1–2 hours apart. A cleansing enema is typically administered the next morning to further clean out the colon. Alternatively, enemas alone (i.e. three or four the night before the procedure and then one early the morning of the procedure) are often sufficient, especially in patients weighing less than 25 kg. It is easy to administer an enema incorrectly. In dogs, a round-tipped red or silicone rubber enema tube is gently inserted as far into the colon as it will go without resistance or causing pain. Then warm water is allowed to flow into the colon by gravity (using a funnel or enema bucket attached to the tube) until water is coming out of the rectum, around the tube. Faeces are gently loosened by moving the enema tube back and forth, as the fluids are entering the colon. If the patient shows signs of pain or becomes nauseated, the infusion is stopped. In cats, a 50 ml syringe and a soft red latex male dog urinary catheter is used. The colon is slowly filled without trying to get the cat to eliminate water during the procedure. In both dogs and cats, administration of 5 mg of bisacodyl the night before the procedure typically enhances the efficacy of the enemas.

Anaesthesia is typically used, but it is not absolutely necessary for most colonoscopies; it makes the procedure much easier, especially in patients with rectal/anal pain or when being performed by a less than highly experienced endoscopist. The patient is placed in left lateral recumbency for flexible endoscopy and right lateral recumbency for rigid endoscopy. A digital rectal examination should always be performed first to find lesions close to the anus that may be missed or traumatized by the endoscope. The tip of the colonoscope is lubricated and then gently inserted approximately 2.5–7.5 cm into the rectum. If air starts to escape the rectum as insufflation begins (and consequently the colon will not inflate), an assistant is needed to hold the anus tightly around the endoscope to prevent air from escaping.

With flexible colonoscopy, the endoscope should be advanced up to the ileocolic valve. Ileal and colonic biopsies are generally indicated; caecal biopsy samples are less commonly obtained, unless there is an obvious lesion present. Ileal biopsy samples may be obtained by passing the tip of the endoscope into the ileum, or just by passing the biopsy forceps through the ileocolic valve (especially in the cat, which has a very small ileocolic valve) (Figure 4.6). In the dog, it is easy to slide the tip of the endoscope past a normal ileocolic valve and into the caecum without realizing that the caecum has been entered. If this happens, the endoscopist will find that the 'colon' is making turns that the endoscope cannot go past.

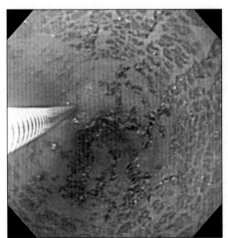

4.6 Endoscopic view of the feline ileocaecal region. Biopsy forceps have been passed into the ileum. The caecum is represented by the blind pouch below the biopsy forceps.

Rigid proctoscopy/colonoscopy

Rigid proctoscopy/colonoscopy is very useful for lesions in the descending colon and especially the rectal area. Hollow, rigid endoscopes with diameters of 19–23 mm can usually be used in dogs. Cats often require rigid endoscopes with diameters of 11–15 mm. There should be an obturator with a smooth surface, which facilitates atraumatic insertion into the rectum. There must be a means to insufflate air, and this usually necessitates a viewing window, which is hinged to allow insertion of rigid biopsy forceps. Proctoscopes are shorter (e.g. 70–130 mm) and are typically 10–25 mm in diameter. Alligator biopsy instruments used with rigid endoscopes need to be of high quality in order to obtain optimal mucosal samples. The author prefers biopsy instruments with tips that cut and shear the mucosa as opposed to clam-shell biopsy cups that pinch off a piece of mucosa (Figure 4.7).

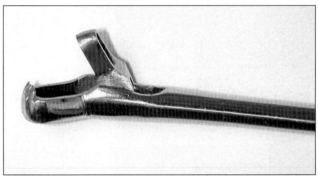

4.7 Rigid biopsy forceps are ideal to obtain submucosal tissue when biopsying infiltrative, anorectal lesions.

Normal appearance

Upper GI endoscopy

The normal canine oesophagus should appear relatively smooth and pink in colour. The diameter of the distended lumen may vary, but it should be relatively uniform except for the expected narrowing at the thoracic inlet. There should be no hyperaemia, blood or obvious roughness, but superficial blood vessels can often be seen in the mucosa. The feline oesophagus will look similar except that the distal segment will have 'ribs' of tissue (where the oesophagus is composed of smooth muscle instead of striated muscle) and blood vessels are more easily seen (Figure 4.8).

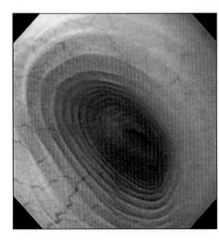

4.8 Endoscopic view of a normal feline oesophagus showing the 'ribbed' appearance where the oesophagus has smooth muscle.

The stomach appears similar in dogs and cats. When collapsed, the gastric lumen will be filled with folds of tissue. When distended, the gastric mucosa is smooth and pink. There may be umbilicated lymphoid follicles, and, occasionally, the cardiac region may have innumerable 'red dots', which are gastric glands. The pylorus is a dynamic structure and may be wide open, partially open or shut appearing like a slit of tissue, and rarely is seen protruding into the lumen like a mushroom.

Videoendoscopes show the duodenal mucosa to have a distinct texture quite different from the oesophagus or stomach. Villi can often be seen as finger-like projections. The duodenal papilla (Figure 4.9) and duodenal lymphoid follicles (Peyer's patches; Figure 4.10) tend to be more obvious in dogs than cats.

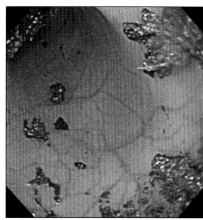

4.11 Endoscopic view of normal canine colonic mucosa showing submucosal blood vessels and residual faecal matter.

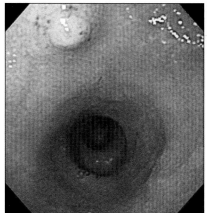

4.9 Endoscopic view of a normal canine duodenum showing the major duodenal papilla.

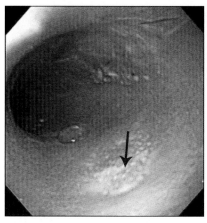

4.10 Endoscopic view of a normal canine duodenum showing a lymphoid follicle (i.e. a so called 'Peyer's patch') (arrowed).

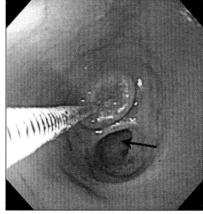

4.12 Endoscopic view of the canine ileocaecal region. The biopsy forceps are being passed into the ileum. The caecocolic orifice is below (arrowed).

Lower GI endoscopy

The colonic mucosa appears similar in dogs and cats. The mucosa is smooth and pink, and careful examination often reveals small 'holes' (i.e. openings of colonic glands). Submucosal blood vessels are visible because the colonic mucosa is thinner than the duodenal or gastric mucosa (Figure 4.11). The canine ileocolic valve is dynamic and may appear as a 'mushroom' or a simple opening, or anything in between (Figure 4.12). The feline ileocolic valve is less dynamic and usually appears as a slit. The feline caecum is a short, blind pouch (see Figure 4.6), whereas in the dog it is a longer, coiled chamber that is easy to enter by mistake without noticing the adjacent ileocolic valve.

Technique for endoscopic biopsy

Gastric and intestinal biopsy is the most commonly performed endoscopic procedure in most practices; biopsy of the normal oesophagus is almost impossible with flexible endoscopes. Good biopsy forceps are critical: most endoscopists prefer biopsy forceps with elongated (ellipsoid) jaws as opposed to round jaws; however, after that, there is almost no consensus. Options include serrated jaws, fenestrated jaws, a needle between the jaws, and reusable or disposable forceps. Each feature has experienced endoscopists who love it and those who hate it. The author recommends new endoscopists try several different types and see which works best for them. It is often wise to consult the pathologists and ask them their opinion about which provides the best tissue samples.

It is good practice to avoid taking biopsy samples while the alimentary tract is maximally distended; 'thicker' bites of mucosa can be obtained if the organ is somewhat deflated. It should always be noted how difficult it is to biopsy a particular lesion; some infiltrative diseases (i.e. scirrhous carcinomas, pythiosis) characteristically produce so much connective tissue that the flexible biopsy forceps cannot 'bite' into the tissue and tear off a piece. Such a finding suggests that a full-thickness biopsy might be required. However, the normal gastric antrum near the pylorus has a mucosa that is much more difficult to biopsy than the rest of the stomach or intestines.

Biopsying is often best performed when the opened biopsy forceps can be pushed against the mucosa at a near 90-degree angle. This is usually relatively easy in the stomach as there is room to manoeuvre the tip of the endoscope. However, in the intestines it is often necessary to deflect the tip of the endoscope by 90 degrees so that the forceps can be pushed directly into the mucosa as opposed to being pushed down the lumen, thereby scraping villus tips off the mucosa. The forceps are pushed into the mucosa so that they indent the mucosa a little, but not so hard that the jaws turn and are not pointed directly into the mucosa. The mucosa is grasped tightly and the forceps withdrawn. It is not necessary to jerk the biopsy forceps hard to remove the tissue, except when taking antral/pyloric samples.

Diagnostic laparoscopy

Laparoscopy allows for superior examination and biopsy of the liver than is possible with ultrasonography and core needle biopsy techniques, as well as pancreatic biopsy. It allows minimally invasive full-thickness biopsy of the intestines, but the value of random biopsies is often not clear (see the *BSAVA Manual of Canine and Feline Endoscopy and Endosurgery* for more discussion of this topic).

Specialized techniques

There are several specific procedures that can be performed with specialized endoscopes or equipment.

Dilation of benign strictures is an important technique. This requires oesophageal dilation balloon catheters or bougies of various diameters. There are many nuances to the procedure and it is strongly recommended that this not be done unless one has had substantial training (i.e. has successfully completed at least 10 procedures under supervision). Excessive trauma often ensures that the stricture will quickly reform. It is also surprisingly easy to rupture the oesophagus, and severe bleeding may occur following the procedure. Adjunctive procedures (i.e. intra-lesional injection of steroids, cutting the stricture prior to ballooning, topical application of mitomycin or sucralfate, insertion of a stent, placement of a percutaneous endoscopic gastrostomy tube, placement of a balloon-oesophagastomy tube) may be required. No technique is consistently effective.

Removal of gastric, duodenal and colonic polyps can be performed with endoscopic electrocautery loops. While these procedures are technically relatively easy, it is important to note that careless use of electrocautery may damage/destroy the camera in the tip of the endoscope and even destroy the circuitry of the videoprocessor. Attention must be paid to the settings on the electrocautery unit: too much current can produce a severe mucosal burn that can perforate the bowel or cause severe signs (e.g. anorexia, vomiting).

Endoscopic mucosal resection is a more advanced technique for removing masses and large biopsy samples from the GI mucosa, in which fluid is injected into the mucosa below the lesion to allow a more complete excision. It requires electrocautery loops and endoscopic injection needles, and appears to be rarely needed in veterinary medicine.

Double-balloon enteroscopy allows the endoscopist to advance the tip of the endoscope far into the jejunum and sometimes even down to the ileum. This technique may require several hours and is primarily indicated when looking for a source of GI bleeding not found in the stomach or duodenum. Alternatively, a gastroduodenoscopy during an exploratory laparotomy may be performed, which involves the surgeon inserting the endoscope through a gastrotomy and manually pushing the small intestine over the tip of the endoscope so that most of the jejunal mucosa is examined. Finally, video-capsule endoscopy can be performed in dogs (>7 kg) using a small device swallowed by the dog. Bleeding lesions can be visualized but tissue samples cannot be obtained.

Endoscopic retrograde cholangiopancreatography is performed to cannulate the bile duct and/or pancreatic duct so as to perform contrast radiographic procedures of the biliary tree or to place stents to allow drainage. It requires a side-viewing (90-degree) duodenoscope specifically designed for this purpose. Considerable experience and skill are required to perform this technique reliably.

References and further reading

Casamian-Sorrosal D, Willard MD, Murray JK *et al.* (2010) Comparison of histopathological findings in biopsies from the duodenum and ileum of dogs with enteropathy. *Journal of Veterinary Internal Medicine* **24**, 80–83

Lhermette P and Sobel D (2008) *BSAVA Manual of Canine and Feline Endoscopy and Endosurgery*. BSAVA Publications, Gloucester

Mansell J and Willard MD (2003) Biopsy of the gastrointestinal tract. *Veterinary Clinics of North America* **33**, 1099–1116

Sarria R, Lopez Albors O, Soria F *et al.* (2013) Characterization of oral double balloon endoscopy in the dog. *Veterinary Journal* **195**, 331–336

Steiner JM (2008) *Small Animal Gastroenterology*. Schlütersche, Hannover, Germany

Tams TR and Rawlings CA (2011) *Small Animal Endoscopy, 3rd edn*, Elsevier Mosby, St. Louis

Willard MD, Mansell J, Fosgate GT *et al.* (2008) Effect of sample quality upon the sensitivity of endoscopic biopsy for detecting gastric and duodenal lesions in dogs and cats. *Journal of Veterinary Internal Medicine* **22**, 1084–1089

Chapter 5

Gastrointestinal surgery

John Williams

Exploratory laparotomy or coeliotomy is the term used to refer to the ventral midline approach to the abdomen. This is the approach that is commonly performed in order to establish or confirm a diagnosis, to determine the extent of involvement of abdominal organs by disease processes, to treat surgically correctable diseases and to ascertain a prognosis.

When performing gastrointestinal (GI) tract surgery, it is all too easy to overlook the need for gentle handling of tissues, and this pertains not only to manual disruption but also to desiccation. Desiccation of peritoneal cells occurs very rapidly under the hot lights in an operating room. This can be readily and cheaply prevented with the use of large sterile swabs soaked in warm sterile saline. Such swabs should also be used under the tines of self-retaining retractors to protect tissues. Swabs, of any size, should be counted at the start and end of an abdominal procedure and must have a radiopaque marker within them to allow for non-invasive detection, should the need arise.

Adequate exposure and a consistent, systematic technique are keys to performing exploratory surgery efficiently and reliably. In order to explore the entire abdomen thoroughly, the incision should extend from the xiphoid to just cranial to the brim of the pelvis. The skin incision needs to be diverted parapreputially in the male dog to avoid the prepuce, and so it is essential to ligate or cauterize the preputial vessels. Shorter incisions may allow for palpation of most of the abdominal structures, but visualization is limited and the risk of missing lesions is greatly increased.

An incision is made through the linea alba to enter the abdominal cavity (see the *BSAVA Manual of Canine and Feline Abdominal Surgery*).

Abdominal exploration

A complete exploratory laparotomy includes visual inspection of all abdominal contents in a systematic manner so that the risk of missing lesions is minimized. If no gross lesions are identified, biopsies of appropriate organs are indicated based on the history, clinical signs and results of preoperative diagnostic tests.

Abdominal closure

The external fascia of the rectus sheath is closed with a simple continuous pattern using absorbable or non-absorbable suture material, taking wide bites in the fascia,

---

Systematic technique for evaluating the abdominal cavity

1. Examine the diaphragm by retracting the liver caudally.
2. Evaluate the liver using a combination of palpation and visual inspection: examine the left, central and right divisions.
3. Retract the proximal duodenum caudomedially to expose the extra-hepatic biliary tree. Unless severe biliary disease is suspected, gently express the gall bladder to help identify the common bile duct and assess patency of the biliary system. If necessary, catheterize the common bile duct through a duodenotomy over the major duodenal papilla.
4. Inspect and thoroughly palpate the stomach, beginning at the oesophageal hiatus and progressing distally to the pylorus.
5. Examine the spleen and left limb of the pancreas.
6. Examine the duodenum and right limb of the pancreas. Retract the duodenum towards the midline and use the mesoduodenum as an 'anatomical retractor' to expose the right abdominal 'gutter'. Cranially, the epiploic foramen, bounded by the hepatic artery, is located between the caudal vena cava dorsally, and the portal vein ventrally.
7. Progressing caudally, the right adrenal gland is located under the caudal vena cava but is difficult to visualize unless the vena cava is retracted medially.
8. Evaluate the kidneys, ureters and (in female patients) genital tract.
9. Evaluate the urinary bladder, terminal ureters, proximal urethra, prostate and sublumbar lymph nodes.
10. Identify and retract the descending colon medially to expose the contents of the left abdominal 'gutter'. The left adrenal gland is readily apparent medial to the kidney, with the phrenico-abdominal vein coursing across its ventral surface.
11. Examine the intestinal tract and mesenteric lymph nodes from one end to the other. The ileum can be identified because it is unique in having an antimesenteric blood supply in addition to vessels in the mesentery. Care must be taken to avoid twisting the root of the mesentery and creating a mesenteric volvulus as the bowel loops are examined. If this does occur, the intestines will become congested very rapidly and the jejunal veins will distend.

Prior to abdominal closure:

1. Check all sites for haemorrhage.
2. Omentalize any biopsy sites.
3. Carry out a swab and 'sharps' count.

---

a minimum of 5 mm from the edge (Figure 5.1). It is important to note that, when closing the laparotomy, suturing the peritoneum is contraindicated, as it will inhibit healing and predispose to adhesion formation. The peritoneum rapidly migrates and seals over a defect such as a closed laparotomy incision. To minimize contamination from visceral contents, the veterinary surgeon (veterinarian) should reglove and use clean instruments to close the laparotomy wound if the gastrointestinal lumen has been entered.

As all fascial tissues heal slowly and extended wound support is required, it is essential to use an appropriate gauge and type of suture material. The choice is between simple interrupted sutures of a non-absorbable monofilament, such as nylon 66 (Ethilon®, Ethicon®), polypropylene (Prolene®, Ethicon®), or a simple continuous pattern of a synthetic absorbable suture material which retains its tensile strength, e.g. polydioxanone (PDS®II, Ethicon®). The gauge depends on the size of the patient but, generally, 3 metric (2/0 USP) or 3.5 metric (0 USP) are suitable. In a giant-breed dog, it is preferable to use a double-looped strand of material of 3 or 3.5 metric rather than a larger gauge, as knot security may become compromised. The external abdominal fascia is no more likely to dehisce with a continuous suture pattern than if simple interrupted sutures are used. The security of a continuous suture is only as good as the two end knots and, therefore, a sufficient number of throws must be used with this pattern. Polydioxanone (PDS®II, Ethicon®) requires five throws for the start knot and seven for the end knot.

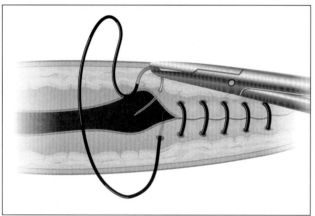

5.1 Simple continuous closure of the external rectus sheath/linea alba.

Gastrointestinal biopsy

Pre-biopsy considerations

The collection of surgical GI biopsy samples involves entering a viscus containing high numbers of bacteria and, as such, needs to be considered as either a clean or clean-contaminated surgical procedure. In most cases, there is no justification for administering any antibiotics when performing GI biopsies. However, if diffuse inflammation is suspected, then the procedure is more likely to be clean-contaminated, and consideration should be given to administering a single perioperative dose of an antibiotic, such as clavulanic acid-potentiated amoxicillin or a second-generation cephalosporin. There is no indication for using postoperative antibiotics in these cases (Brown et al., 1997).

Surgical biopsy

Surgical GI biopsies are full thickness (Mansell and Willard, 2003) and are recommended when endoscopic biopsies are not feasible (e.g. the desired sample site is not accessible by endoscopy) or where further information is required about the deeper layers of the intestinal wall (Evans et al., 2006). It must be remembered that intestinal surgery is not a benign procedure, as there is a risk of dehiscence reported, with the potential development of peritonitis (Shales et al., 2005), although a recent study has shown this risk to be in the order of 2% (Swinbourne et al., 2017). Low serum albumin is associated with an increased risk of dehiscence, and neoplastic infiltration is associated with a higher risk of death (Swinbourne et al., 2017).

When carrying out an intestinal procedure, it is best practice to exteriorize the intestine to be incised and to pack it off from the remainder of the abdominal cavity with saline-soaked swabs. Prior to carrying out an enterotomy, the intestinal contents should be milked away cranially and caudally from the proposed incision site. The author does not routinely use either finger compression or intestinal clamps when taking biopsy samples. A longitudinal perpendicular full-thickness incision is made with a No. 15 scalpel blade in the antimesenteric portion of the intestine and is then converted to an elliptical incision with a blade or fine scissors (Figure 5.2). Prior to closure of the site, any mucosa ballooning out from the wound is trimmed away either with a scalpel or fine Metzenbaum scissors. If routine longitudinal closure is likely to lead to significant narrowing of the intestinal

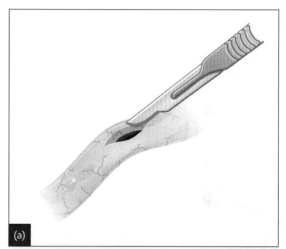

(a)

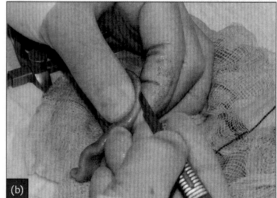

(b)

5.2 (a–b) A full-thickness longitudinal incision is made in the antimesenteric border of the intestine with a No. 15 scalpel blade.
(b, © John Williams)

lumen, a transverse closure is preferred. In cats, transverse closure is always required following elliptical biopsy. The defect is closed with a simple interrupted or simple continuous pattern of 1.5 or 2 metric (4/0 or 3/0 USP) monofilament absorbable sutures (Figure 5.3). The suture line can then be reinforced by overlying with omentum, which should be tacked to the serosa with 1.5 metric (4/0 USP) absorbable suture material.

An alternative to creating an elliptical incision for biopsy is to use a sterile 4 or 6 mm skin punch biopsy instrument which is 'pushed' through from the serosa to the lumen (Figure 5.4). The resulting defect is closed with simple interrupted 1.5 metric (4/0 USP) sutures (Keats *et al.*, 2004), so as to minimize the risk of lumen narrowing. This can be done either longitudinally or transversely, depending on the width of the intestine.

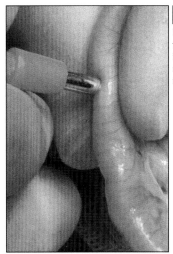

5.4 A 4 mm skin punch biopsy instrument being used to obtain a full-thickness antimesenteric intestinal biopsy sample. Care must be taken to ensure that the mesenteric wall is not damaged.

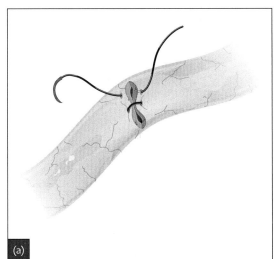

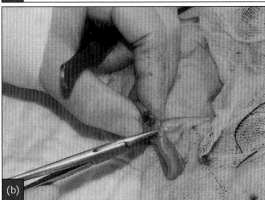

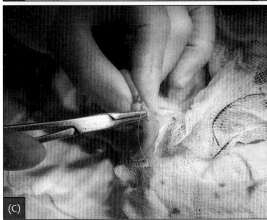

5.3 (a–c) Longitudinal intestinal incisions are closed transversely with 1.5 metric (4/0 USP) absorbable suture material.
(b, c, © John Williams)

Hepatic and pancreatic biopsy

Hepatic biopsy

Pre-biopsy considerations

Biopsy samples may be collected for histopathology, immunohistochemistry, heavy metal (copper, zinc and iron) quantification and bacterial culture. Severe haemorrhage is a potential consequence of hepatic biopsy in dogs and cats, but is rare; it is likely only if there is a significantly prolonged bleeding time or a concurrent thrombocytopenia (usually when the patient has a disseminated intravascular coagulopathy) or thrombocytopathia. In animals with hepatocellular dysfunction, or a suspected complete extra-hepatic bile duct obstruction, a coagulation profile should be obtained preoperatively. It is now recognized that postoperative haemorrhage is rare in patients with only mild coagulation abnormalities. If animals are severely hypoalbuminaemic as a consequence of their liver disease, wound healing may be impaired, and such patients should be given a pre-biopsy plasma transfusion regardless of the technique employed (Vasanjee *et al.*, 2006).

Percutaneous ultrasound-guided liver biopsy

The competent ultrasonographer can identify focal hepatic lesions, such as neoplasia, cysts or abscesses, or identify generalized changes in the hepatic parenchyma. This can allow for accurate guided needle or core biopsy samples to be taken from solid lesions. The advent of spring-loaded 'one-handed' biopsy instruments has made this easier, but they should not be used in cats as they can cause liver rupture. The disadvantage of such a technique is the size of the sample obtained, and it is recommended that the needle size should be larger than 16 G (Cole *et al.*, 2002; Rawlings and Howerth, 2004) and that up to eight samples may be needed for a valid histopathological interpretation. Cysts and abscesses should not be biopsied percutaneously and the procedure is contraindicated if there is bile duct obstruction.

Surgical biopsy

This has the advantages of allowing exploration of the abdomen and biopsy of specific areas of the liver. The disadvantage is that a general anaesthetic and an invasive surgical procedure are required. The other major advantage of surgical biopsies is that a larger and potentially a more representative sample can be obtained (Cole *et al.*, 2002; Rawlings and Howerth, 2004).

Bleeding from the biopsy site can be identified and controlled. If generalized hepatic disease is present, the biopsy sample can be taken from the most accessible site. With focal disease, the entire liver should be palpated carefully for the presence of intraparenchymal nodules or cavities.

Guillotine technique: Marginal biopsy samples are easy to obtain using ligatures. A loop of a synthetic absorbable ligature is passed over an easily accessible edge of liver lobe and the parenchyma is crushed as the ligature is tightened, thereby ligating vessels and biliary ducts (Figure 5.5). The sample is removed by amputating approximately 5 mm distal to the ligature. If there is any haemorrhage, an absorbable haemostatic material can be applied or the omentum placed over the site.

Forceps technique (parenchymal crushing): A pair of haemostatic forceps is placed across the tip of a liver lobe to crush the parenchyma (Figure 5.6). Tissue distal to the

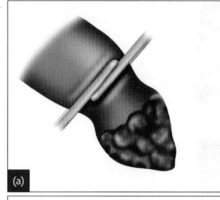
(a)

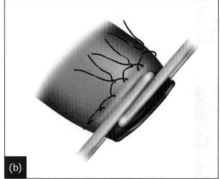
(b)

5.6 Crushing technique for liver biopsy. (a) A pair of haemostatic forceps is placed across the lobe proximal to the lesion. (b) Several overlapping mattress sutures are placed through the liver just proximal to the site of the proposed lobectomy incision. It is important to ensure that the entire width of the hepatic parenchyma is included in the suture and that a stump of crushed tissue is left distal to the ligatures. After tightening the sutures, a sharp scalpel blade is used to remove the hepatic tissue distal to the ligatures, allowing a stump of crushed tissue to remain.
(Reproduced from the *BSAVA Manual of Canine and Feline Abdominal Surgery, 2nd edn*)

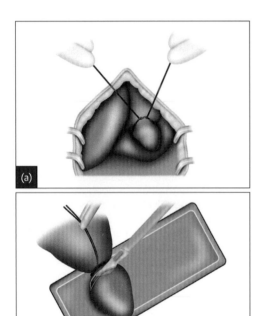
(a)

(b)

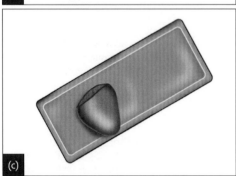
(c)

5.5 Guillotine technique for liver biopsy. (a) A loop of absorbable suture material is placed around a small portion of the tip of a liver lobe. The suture is tied tight to cut through the parenchyma and occlude the blood vessels and bile duct. (b–c) Using a sharp scalpel blade, the hepatic tissue is cut approximately 3–5 mm distal to the ligature. To avoid crushing, the sample should not be handled with tissue forceps.
(Reproduced from the *BSAVA Manual of Canine and Feline Abdominal Surgery, 2nd edn*)

forceps is then excised with a scalpel. Absorbable mattress sutures are placed proximal to the forceps to control haemorrhage if required.

'Skin punch' biopsy: Since the forceps technique is relatively straightforward, a 'skin punch' technique is rarely required. Its use is generally limited to focal lesions on the ventral liver surface, and care must be taken not to penetrate deeper than 50% of the parenchyma (Figure 5.7). The resulting defect can either be sutured with a mattress suture of a synthetic absorbable suture material, or plugged with omentum or an absorbable haemostatic material (e.g. Gelfoam®).

Laparoscopic biopsy

This is a minimally invasive technique that is being used increasingly, as it allows visualization of 85% of the liver surface and permits focal biopsies to obtain samples of an adequate size. The author uses a two-port technique, placing the camera port and a single instrument port slightly caudal and lateral to the umbilicus, one port being placed either side. Occasionally, a third port is placed so that a blunt probe or retractor can be used to manipulate the liver lobes. A 6 mm trocar cannula assembly can be placed to accommodate 5 mm cup biopsy forceps. These biopsy forceps are used to harvest pieces of liver from the edge of a lobe. The tissue is grasped and the instrument then twisted until the tissue comes away from the liver lobe. There is minimal bleeding in healthy dogs and the quality and yield of the tissue samples are excellent. It is

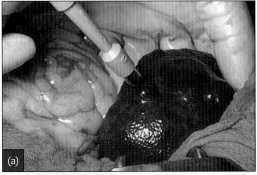
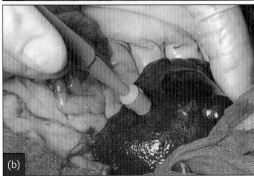
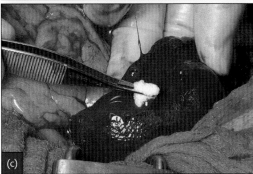
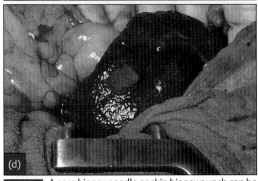

understand the blood supply to the pancreas. It is essential that neither the duct system nor the vascular system are damaged as part of the biopsy procedure, and that pancreatic perfusion is maintained. Pancreatic ischaemia is a very reproducible method by which to induce pancreatitis experimentally!

Pre-biopsy considerations

Anatomy: The pancreas is divided into the right and left lobes and the body (Figure 5.8). The right lobe is adjacent to the duodenum, and is easily exposed by retracting the duodenum ventrally into the abdominal incision. The left lobe of the pancreas is caudodorsal to the greater curvature of the stomach. Retracting the stomach and greater omentum cranially, while retracting the transverse colon caudally, exposes it best. The body of the pancreas is at the confluence of the right and left lobes and is located adjacent to the pylorus (see Chapter 36).

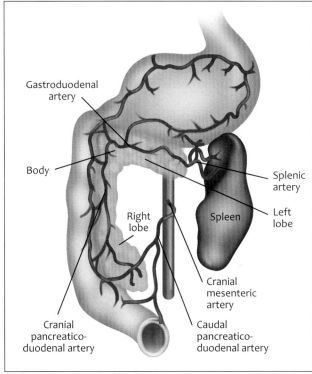

5.8 Anatomy of and blood supply to the pancreas and adjacent structures.
(Reproduced from the BSAVA Manual of Canine and Feline Abdominal Surgery, 2nd edn)

5.7 A core biopsy needle or skin biopsy punch can be used to obtain small pieces of liver tissue. This technique is useful for hepatic lesions located away from the periphery of the lobe. (a) The focal lesion is identified. (b) The skin biopsy punch is pushed into the parenchyma to cut a core sample. (c–d) The biopsy site can be packed with a small piece of Gelfoam® or omentum following removal of the hepatic tissue, to facilitate haemostasis.
(Reproduced from the BSAVA Manual of Canine and Feline Abdominal Surgery, 2nd edn)

also possible to coagulate the periphery of the biopsy site with a vessel-sealing device, and this may help to reduce haemorrhage (Vasanjee *et al.*, 2006). Several biopsy samples should be taken from multiple lobes, unless specific lesions are identified.

Pancreatic biopsy

If pancreatic biopsy is to be carried out, the veterinary surgeon must know the location of the pancreatic ducts and

Pancreatic duct anatomy is variable. In the dog, the pancreatic duct enters the major duodenal papilla immediately adjacent to the common bile duct (Figure 5.9). An accessory pancreatic duct is present in most but not all dogs and is usually the larger of the two entering the duodenum, at the minor duodenal papilla. The minor papilla is more distal in the duodenum than the major papilla. In the cat, a single pancreatic duct is frequently the only pathway for pancreatic secretions to enter the duodenum. Also, in cats, the pancreatic duct and the common bile duct may join before entering the major duodenal papilla.

The blood supply to the pancreas varies according to the lobe (Figure 5.8). The right lobe is supplied by the cranial and caudal pancreaticoduodenal artery and vein, which run parallel to the long axis of the pancreas and duodenum. Blood supply to the left lobe is via branches of the gastroduodenal, common hepatic and splenic arteries.

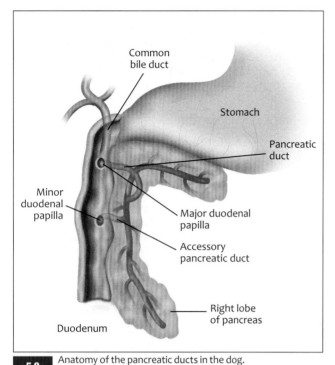

5.9 Anatomy of the pancreatic ducts in the dog.
(Reproduced from the *BSAVA Manual of Canine and Feline Abdominal Surgery, 2nd edn*)

Animals with signs of pancreatic disease coupled with finding a mass or fluid-filled structure (abscess, pseudo-cyst) on abdominal ultrasonography or radiographs would probably indicate the need for abdominal exploratory surgery and biopsy. This is particularly true if serial ultrasound examinations reveal persistence or enlargement of such a structure. Additionally, if during an exploratory laparotomy gross lesions of the pancreas are identified, biopsy of the tissue should be considered.

Surgical technique

In cases where there is diffuse disease, the tip of the right (duodenal) limb is chosen for biopsy; due to its accessibility and given its peripheral position, the risk to ducts and vessels is small. Either a suture fracture or surgical dissection and ligation can be used. Whichever technique is used, it is essential to suture the mesoduodenum closed and to cover the area with omentum. This will help minimize the risk of pancreatic enzyme leakage.

Suture fracture technique: The least traumatic method for procuring a sample of pancreatic tissue (when there is diffuse disease of the pancreas) is the suture fracture technique (Figure 5.10). This involves removing a small piece of tissue from the tip of either the right or left limb of the pancreas.

1. Grasp the descending duodenum and place it into the surgical field to expose the right limb of the pancreas. Alternatively, retract the transverse colon caudally and the stomach cranially to expose the left limb of the pancreas.
2. Isolate the area to be biopsied with laparotomy swabs (sponges).
3. Handle the pancreatic tissue as little as possible and lavage the tissue frequently with warm, sterile, isotonic saline. ▶

4. Dissect the mesenteric attachments from the desired area and then ligate a small (2–3 mm) section of pancreas at the tip with absorbable suture material (1.5 metric (4/0 USP) PDS). Avoid the use of chromic catgut, polyglactin 910 or poliglecaprone 25, as they are rapidly digested by pancreatic enzymes.
5. Sharply resect the ligated segment with a scalpel or fine scissors.
6. Place the tissue sample in formalin and submit for histopathology.
7. If minor bleeding persists at the biopsy site, place sterile absorbable gelatine or cellulose sponge material on the area.

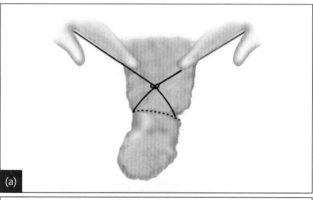
(a)

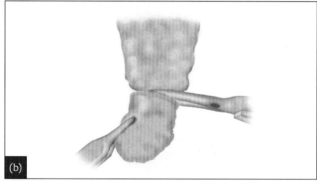
(b)

5.10 Suture fracture technique. (a) Tightening of the ligature crushes the pancreatic parenchyma. (b) Pancreatic tissue distal to the ligature is transected.
(Reproduced from the *BSAVA Manual of Canine and Feline Abdominal Surgery, 2nd edn*)

Electrocautery has been regarded historically as being damaging to the pancreas, as it is more likely to lead to necrosis and pancreatitis. Recent studies have shown that both vessel-sealing devices and harmonic scalpels can be used safely to obtain biopsy samples with minimal clinical effect on the patient (Harmoinen *et al.*, 2002; Barnes *et al.*, 2006). This has opened up the possibility of carrying out laparoscopic biopsies in both the dog and the cat (Webb and Trott, 2008; Cosford *et al.*, 2010) with minimal trauma to the pancreas. However, access to the left limb with laparoscopy is often limited due to its anatomical location adjacent to the greater curvature of the stomach.

Postoperative considerations

A balanced electrolyte solution should be administered intravenously until oral intake of food and water resumes. A commercial therapeutic low-fat diet should be fed for several days to reduce the chance of postoperative pancreatitis.

Partial pancreatectomy

Pancreatic surgery can be challenging and may be associated with serious potential complications. A thorough understanding of the anatomy, physiology and surgical diseases of the organ and the optimum measures for patient care are necessary before considering undertaking pancreatic surgery.

Indications

Partial pancreatectomy is indicated for the removal of insulin-secreting tumours (insulinomas), gastrin-secreting tumours (gastrinomas) (see Chapter 33) and pancreatic adenocarcinomas. Up to 80% of the pancreas can be removed without affecting either exocrine or endocrine function, as long as the duct to the remaining portion is left intact and the remainder of the pancreas is healthy.

Surgical technique

1. Carefully examine and palpate the entire pancreas to detect masses (if the tumour cannot be identified, do not use intravenous methylene blue to facilitate localization of neoplastic tissue due to its limited efficacy and potential for severe hypotensive complications).
2. Determine the section of the pancreas to be removed and isolate the segment from the surrounding structures with moistened laparotomy sponges.
3. Incise the mesentery adjacent to the affected pancreas and ligate blood vessels as needed. When dissecting the right limb, be careful to preserve the pancreaticoduodenal artery and vein. Ligate only the small branches of those vessels that supply the segment to be removed.
4. Place a stay suture (1.5 metric (4/0 USP)) at the end of the lobe to be removed to facilitate manipulation.
5. Prior to sharp transection, either bluntly separate the pancreatic tissue using mosquito haemostatic forceps and ligate the blood vessels (Figure 5.11), or simply ligate the tissue without prior dissection (guillotine style) with absorbable suture material (1.5 or 2 metric (4/0 or 3/0 USP) PDS) to occlude the vessels and pancreatic ducts.
6. Remove the pancreatic tissue at least 1–2 cm proximal to the tumour.
7. Thoroughly explore the abdomen, paying particular attention to the rest of the pancreas, liver and regional lymph nodes to check for metastasis.

If the neoplasm is located at the confluence of the right and left limbs, an enucleation of the mass is necessary, since total pancreatectomy should be avoided. When performing dissection in this area of the pancreas, trauma to the common bile duct and pancreatic ducts should be avoided. Enucleation of the mass is performed by gentle blunt and sharp dissection to separate the tumour from the surrounding pancreatic tissue. Blood vessels should be ligated as necessary.

Insulinoma

An insulinoma is a tumour of the beta-cells of the pancreas and can range in size from 2–3 mm nodules to much larger masses that invade the surrounding structures. They tend to be located with equal frequency in the body and the right and left lobes of the pancreas. An insulinoma is usually malignant in dogs and, therefore, is classified as a carcinoma. It is a functional tumour that secretes excessive amounts of insulin, causing hypoglycaemia. Dogs with insulinoma can be treated medically or surgically. However, a clinical study found significantly longer survival times for dogs treated by partial pancreatectomy (median survival 785 days) compared with those treated medically (median survival 196 days) (Polton *et al.*, 2007) (see the *BSAVA Manual of Canine and Feline Endocrinology*).

Preoperative considerations

Thoracic radiographs should be obtained preoperatively to evaluate for metastasis. Intravenous fluids with glucose (balanced electrolyte solution plus 5% dextrose) should be initiated the day before and continued during surgery to prevent hypoglycaemia. Blood glucose concentration should be measured immediately before surgery and additional glucose given if the concentration is less than 2 mmol/l.

WARNING

Total pancreatectomy is extremely difficult and should not be attempted. It usually requires resection and anastomosis of the proximal duodenum together with cholecystoenterostomy. The patient will also need intensive medical therapy post-surgery not only for diabetes mellitus and exocrine pancreatic insufficiency, but probably also for recurrent ascending infection in the biliary tree, as persistent ascending infection is likely

---

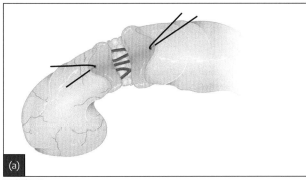
(a)

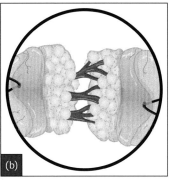
(b)

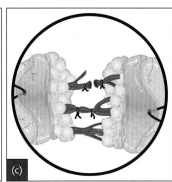
(c)

5.11 Partial pancreatectomy using the (a) dissection and (b–c) ligation techniques.

After removal of the primary pancreatic mass, metastatic nodules in the liver should be removed, if possible, by partial or complete liver lobectomy. In addition, affected lymph nodes should be resected if invaded by the neoplasm or they are palpably enlarged. Prior to closure, the abdomen is lavaged with warm, sterile saline.

Postoperative management

Pancreatitis is a potential complication of insulinoma resection and can be severe (see Chapter 36). However, a recent paper concluded that 'there is no significant risk to surgical pancreatic biopsy *per se* provided good surgical technique and tissue handling are employed' (Pratschke *et al.*, 2015).

A balanced electrolyte solution with 5% dextrose should be administered intravenously until oral intake of food and water resumes. Blood glucose concentrations should be monitored at least twice daily. Intravenous glucose should be discontinued if the animal is hyperglycaemic or has a normal, stable glucose concentration.

After surgery, oral intake of water should be instigated first and then food, if no vomiting has occurred after 48 hours. A highly digestible, low-fat diet should be provided. Oral intake of food should be discontinued if vomiting occurs. Periodic monitoring of serum glucose should be continued.

Persistent hypoglycaemia indicates residual tumour is present. Continued medical management of hypoglycaemia will be necessary (i.e. frequent feedings, dietary management and corticosteroids or other drugs (such as diazoxide or somatostatin analogues)) to increase serum glucose concentrations as needed.

Hyperglycaemia may occur due to atrophy of the normal beta-cells by feedback inhibition; this may resolve with time, and normal pancreatic endocrine function should eventually resume, although insulin therapy may be needed for weeks to months.

Prognosis

Postoperative survival depends upon the stage of disease. One study found that dogs with tumours confined to the pancreas had significantly longer survival time than those with metastasis to regional lymph nodes or distant sites. This study also found that approximately 50% of dogs with tumours confined to the pancreas were free of hypoglycaemia 14 months postoperatively (Tobin *et al.*, 1999).

Surgical treatment of pancreatitis

Medical treatment of pancreatitis is preferred for most animals with pancreatitis (see Chapter 36). However, surgical intervention may be appropriate in certain patients. Surgery should be considered if repeated ultrasound examinations reveal persistence or enlargement of a pancreatic abscess or other mass and if the patient's condition dictates aggressive action. Although pancreatic abscesses or pseudocysts may resolve with conservative management, surgical exploration is frequently necessary.

Indications

The indications for surgery include:

- Failure to respond to appropriate medical therapy
- Presence of a pancreatic mass (abscess, pseudocyst, neoplasia)
- Severe icterus due to extra-hepatic biliary obstruction that is non-responsive to medical management
- Pancreatitis associated with septic peritonitis.

Preoperative considerations

The animal should be thoroughly assessed and the history and clinical course of events reviewed. Patient factors that may increase the likelihood of complications, such as age, debilitation, sepsis, hypoproteinaemia, disseminated intravascular coagulation (DIC), diabetes mellitus, acute kidney injury and disorders of other organ systems, should be considered. The coagulation status in animals with severe pancreatitis and possible DIC should be determined, and any fluid and electrolyte imbalances corrected prior to surgery. Antibiotic therapy should be started and continued during the perioperative period.

The objectives of surgery are to:

- Surgically expose the pancreas and determine the type and extent of disease
- Remove devitalized tissue
- Flush and drain cysts or abscesses; consider bacteriological culture to rule out infection (rare)
- Thoroughly explore the abdominal cavity for evidence of associated lesions or other problems.

Lavage of the peritoneal cavity to remove necrotic tissue debris, toxins, enzymes and exudates is also an important part of the surgery. In animals with severe septic peritonitis, providing postoperative drainage of the peritoneal cavity may be necessary.

Surgical technique

Omentalization of pancreatic abscesses or pseudocysts should be considered, as omentum provides increased blood flow, lymphatic drainage and fills dead space.

1. Expose the left limb of the pancreas by retracting the transverse colon caudally.
2. Carefully and gently examine the pancreas for masses, abscesses, inflammation and necrosis. Gently break down adhesions and abscesses digitally to establish ventral drainage. Obtain samples of fluid or tissue for bacterial culture and sensitivity testing as needed.
3. Carefully and judiciously debride necrotic pancreatic tissue and fat. Do not disrupt the pancreatic blood supply during dissection. Minimize trauma to normal or non-necrotic pancreatic tissue. Flush affected areas with warm, sterile saline.
4. Submit all tissue for histopathology.
5. Grasp the caudal edge of the greater omentum and place it into the abscess cavity.
6. Place several tacking sutures (synthetic, non-absorbable material) from the omentum to the edges of the abscess cavity.
7. Carefully examine the gall bladder and biliary ducts for evidence of obstruction. Gently squeeze the gall bladder to determine whether bile is expressible through the common bile duct. Consider retrograde catheterization of the common bile duct if complete obstruction is suspected.

Postoperative care

Medical therapy for pancreatitis should be continued (see Chapter 36). The administration of plasma for hypoproteinaemia and whole blood transfusions for postoperative anaemia (packed cell volume <20%) should be considered. Potential complications include septic shock, hypoproteinaemia, worsening of pancreatitis and peritonitis, thromboembolism and abdominal pain.

Although most patients recover, pancreatitis is a life-threatening disease that frequently has a prolonged and unpredictable clinical course; thus, a guarded prognosis is warranted if surgical intervention is required. The prognosis is poor when pancreatitis is complicated by septic shock, DIC, acute kidney injury or intestinal infarction.

References and further reading

Allen SW (1989) A comparison of two methods of partial pancreatectomy in the dog. *Veterinary Surgery* **18**, 274–278

Barnes RF, Greenfield CL, Shaeffer DJ *et al.* (2006) Comparison of biopsy samples obtained using standard endoscopic instruments and the harmonic scalpel during laparoscopic and laparoscopic-assisted surgery in normal dogs. *Veterinary Surgery* **35**, 243–251

Brown DC, Conzemius M, Shofer FS and Swann H (1997) Epidemiologic evaluation of postoperative wound infections in dogs and cats. *Journal of the American Veterinary Medical Association* **210**, 1302–1306

Caywood DD, Klausner JS, O'Leary TP *et al.* (1987) Pancreatic insulin-secreting neoplasms: clinical, diagnostic, and prognostic features in 73 dogs. *Journal of the American Animal Hospital Association* **24**, 577–584

Cole TL, Center SA, Flood SN *et al.* (2002) Diagnostic comparison of needle and wedge biopsy specimens of the liver in dogs and cats. *Journal of the American Veterinary Medical Association* **220**, 1483–1490

Cosford KL, Shmon CL, Myers SL *et al.* (2010) Prospective evaluation of laparoscopic pancreatic biopsies in 11 healthy cats. *Journal of Veterinary Internal Medicine* **24**, 104–113

Evans SE, Bonczynski JJ, Broussard JD *et al.* (2006) Comparison of endoscopic and full-thickness biopsy specimens for diagnosis of inflammatory bowel disease and alimentary tract lymphoma in cats. *Journal of the American Veterinary Medical Association* **229**, 1447–1450

Harmoinen J, Saari S, Rinkinen M and Westermarck E (2002) Evaluation of pancreatic forceps biopsy by laparoscopy in healthy beagles. *Veterinary Therapeutics* **3**, 31–36

Keats MM, Weeren R, Greemlee P *et al.* (2004) Investigation of Keyes skin biopsy instrument for intestinal biopsy versus a standard biopsy technique. *Journal of the American Animal Hospital Association* **40**, 405–410

Mansell J and Willard MD (2003) Biopsy of the gastrointestinal tract. *Veterinary Clinics of North America: Small Animal Practice* **33**, 1099–1116

Mizumoto R, Yano T, Sekoguchi T and Kawarada Y (1986) Resectability of the pancreas without producing diabetes, with special reference to pancreatic regeneration. *International Journal of Pancreatology* **185**, 1986

Mooney C and Peterson M (2012) *BSAVA Manual of Canine and Feline Endocrinology, 4th edn.* BSAVA Publications, Gloucester

Nelson RW and Salisbury SK (2000) Pancreatic beta cell neoplasia. In: *Saunders Manual of Small Animal Practice, 2nd ed*, eds. S Birchard and R Sherding, pp 288–294. WB Saunders, Philadelphia

Polton GA, White RN, Brearley MJ and Eastwood JM (2007) Improved survival in a retrospective cohort of 28 dogs with insulinoma. *Journal of Small Animal Practice* **48**, 151–156

Pratschke KM Ryan J, McAlinden A and McLauchlan G (2015) Pancreatic surgical biopsy in 24 dogs and 19 cats: postoperative complications and clinical relevance of histological findings. *The Journal of Small Animal Practice* **56**, 60–66

Rawlings CA and Howerth EW (2004) Obtaining quality biopsies of the liver and kidney. *Journal of the American Animal Hospital Association* **40**, 352–358

Shales CJ, Warren J, Anderson DM *et al.* (2005) Complications following full-thickness small intestinal biopsy in 66 dogs: a retrospective study. *Journal of Small Animal Practice* **46**, 317–321

Swinbourne F, Jeffery N, Tivers MS *et al.* (2017) The incidence of surgical site dehiscence following full-thickness gastrointestinal biopsy in dogs and cats and associated risk factors. *The Journal of Small Animal Practice* **58**, 495–503

Tobin RL, Nelson RW, Lucroy MD *et al.* (1999) Outcome of surgical *versus* medical treatment of dogs with beta cell neoplasia: 39 cases (1990–1997) *Journal of the American Veterinary Medical Association* **215**, 226–230

Vasanjee SC, Bubenik LJ, Hosgood G and Bauer RW (2006) Evaluation of hemorrhage, sample size, and collateral damage for five hepatic biopsy methods in dogs. *Veterinary Surgery* **35**, 86–93

Webb CB and Trott C (2008) Laparoscopic diagnosis of pancreatic disease in dogs and cats. *Journal of Veterinary Internal Medicine* **22**, 1263–1266

Williams JM and Niles JD (2015) *BSAVA Manual of Canine and Feline Abdominal Surgery, 2nd edn.* BSAVA Publications, Gloucester

Chapter 6

Biopsy and cytology

Michael J. Day

Sample collection

Cytological samples

A range of cytological samples may be collected from the gastrointestinal (GI) tract, but most diagnoses will be made, or subsequently confirmed, by histopathological examination of tissue biopsy samples. Oropharyngeal lesions may be sampled by fine-needle aspiration (FNA), surface scraping or impression smear. The technique of rectal mucosal scraping may yield cytological samples relevant to the diagnosis of disease of the terminal alimentary tract. Thickened intestinal loops, mesenteric lymph nodes, the liver and pancreas may be sampled by ultrasound-guided FNA (Crain *et al.*, 2014; Cordner *et al.*, 2015). However, Cohen *et al.* (2003) reported that cytological examination is least reliable for diagnosis of liver lesions compared with samples taken from other anatomical locations. Impression smears may be made from the surface of biopsy samples of liver, pancreas or GI tract before the tissues are placed into fixative. Cytology has the advantages of speed, low cost and in-house availability, but does not always guarantee a definitive diagnosis.

Biopsy samples

Oropharyngeal or salivary gland lesions will generally be sampled by excisional or incisional biopsy. Evaluation of regional lymph nodes may also be indicated, particularly for suspected neoplastic disease. Oesophageal lesions are most often sampled by endoscopy (see Chapters 4 and 32).

The GI tract may be sampled by the collection of endoscopic biopsy samples of the mucosa or by the collection of full-thickness biopsy samples of the wall of the stomach or intestine at laparotomy. Endoscopy is minimally invasive and permits visualization of the mucosal surface of the GI tract, but allows only superficial (mucosal) biopsy and cannot access the mid-small intestine. The superficial nature of the samples means that it is not possible to rule out deeper underlying pathology (Figure 6.1). For example, the mucosa overlying an alimentary tract neoplasm might be ulcerated and inflamed – an endoscopic biopsy might only sample this reactive tissue and miss the underlying tumour. Optimally, endoscopic biopsy samples should be routinely collected from gastric mucosa (fundic and antral), small intestine and colon. Several studies have shown that both the duodenum and ileum should be sampled wherever possible, as in some cases the disease process

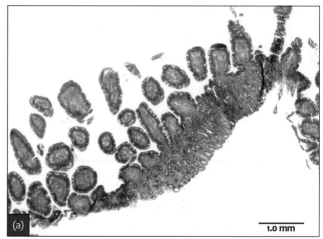

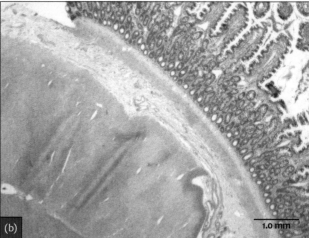

6.1 Sections from (a) endoscopic and (b) full-thickness biopsy samples of small intestine showing the relative levels of tissue sampled by these procedures. The endoscopic samples do not include tissue beneath the level of the mucosa. (Haematoxylin and eosin stain.)

is restricted to one level of the small intestine (Casamian-Sorrosal *et al.*, 2010; Scott *et al.*, 2011; Procoli *et al.*, 2013). Even if there is no apparent indication for sampling these sites, evaluation of the entire GI tract is useful as subclinical lesions may be detected. If endoscopic biopsy samples are taken, a minimum of six good quality samples should be collected from each site (Willard *et al.*, 2008). This will maximize the chance of making a diagnosis and will allow for the variability in quality of tissue and variation in tissue orientation during embedding. Endoscopic biopsy samples may be placed directly into an excess of 10% neutral buffered formalin for submission to the laboratory (Ruiz *et al.*, 2016). Where samples are to be transported over a long distance, the tissues may be placed carefully between purpose-designed 'sponges' within a histology cassette, which is then placed into formalin. It is essential to pre-wet the sponges in formalin before placing the tissues on to their surface because samples placed on to dry sponges will be damaged as they are removed for processing. All samples should be submitted with a thorough clinical history, including relevant serum biochemical data and a summary of major endoscopic or ultrasonographic findings.

Laparotomy permits the collection of full-thickness samples from multiple levels of the GI tract and the additional collection of samples from the liver, pancreas or mesenteric lymph nodes. A pathologist is always more likely to be able to make a more meaningful diagnosis with a full-thickness biopsy sample of intestine taken at laparotomy, particularly in the case of neoplastic disease (Kleinschmidt *et al.*, 2010). Biopsy samples should be taken even if the gut appears grossly normal, as there may still be histological abnormalities. If there is a suggestion of liver or pancreas abnormality, these tissues should also be sampled whilst the opportunity presents – rather than regretting the absence of a key sample later. This is particularly the case in cats, where there may be concurrent intestinal, hepatic and pancreatic inflammatory disease ('triaditis'). Where intestinal neoplasia is suspected, biopsy of the draining mesenteric lymph node to check for metastatic spread is indicated. Full-thickness biopsy samples of intestinal mucosa will tend to curl when placed into formalin, which will make preparation of a well-orientated section difficult. This effect may be prevented if the sample is first placed, serosal side down, on to a small piece of card before immersing the card and sample in formalin.

The liver may be sampled by percutaneous needle core biopsy or by collection of a wedge biopsy sample at laparotomy. Needle core biopsy samples obtained by blind percutaneous sampling are less valuable than percutaneous ultrasound-guided or laparoscopic samples that may target specific focal lesions and provide a larger tissue sample (Figure 6.2). Even if core biopsies include predominantly liver tissue (and percutaneous core biopsies may sometimes comprise chiefly muscle or fat), they do not always permit assessment of the entire hepatic unit. Commonly, a liver core biopsy would include few portal areas that are often the focus of hepatic disease. It has been suggested that a minimum of 15 portal triads should be assessed to determine whether there is portal or periportal pathology. Therefore, ideally, at least two or three core biopsy samples should be taken to increase the likelihood of achieving a histopathological diagnosis. One study has shown that pathological changes are not uniform throughout the liver lobes and that at least two lobes should be sampled in order to increase diagnostic success (Kemp *et al.*, 2015).

Pancreatic tissue may be sampled at laparotomy and excision of an entire mesenteric lymph node is an appropriate sample, if lymphadenomegaly is noted.

Greater scope for sample collection arises at post-mortem examination. When conducting a post-mortem examination of a case with GI disease, samples of grossly affected and unaffected tissue (or samples containing the junction of these types of tissue) should be collected. Sample collection should not be restricted to a single site that may be indicated by ante-mortem diagnostic procedures, and samples should be collected from multiple

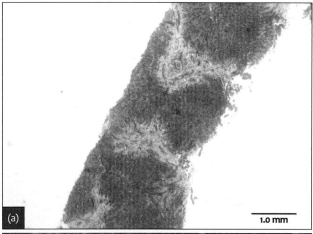

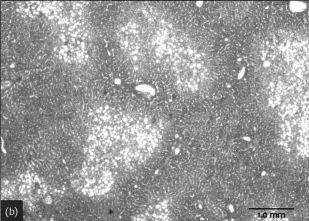

6.2 Sections from (a) a needle core and (b) a wedge biopsy sample of liver showing the relative amount of tissue sampled by these procedures. The wedge biopsy sample includes many more complete hepatic units for assessment. (Haematoxylin and eosin stain.)

locations to check for subclinical pathology. For example, during a post-mortem examination of a dog with colitis, samples might be collected from the stomach, duodenum, jejunum, ileum, mesenteric lymph node, liver and pancreas in addition to affected colonic tissue. For intestinal samples taken at post-mortem examination, an intact 4 cm section of the entire intestine should be sampled. It is best to fix this sample unopened, as a flat portion of intestine will curl during processing as described above for full-thickness biopsy samples.

All samples for routine histopathological examination should be placed, immediately after collection, into an excess (minimum volume 10 times the tissue size) of 10% neutral buffered formalin. Rapid fixation is essential for gut tissue, particularly for samples collected *post mortem*, as autolytic change can be pronounced within 20 minutes after death. Where multiple intestinal sites are sampled, the tissues should be submitted in separate pots that are clearly labelled with the origin of the sample.

Sample processing
Routine cytology and histopathology
Cytological samples from the alimentary tract are generally submitted as multiple, freshly prepared, air-dried smears that are then stained for microscopic examination. Biopsy samples of tissue undergo a more complex procedure that involves movement through a series of graded alcohols in

an automatic tissue processor until they are finally embedded in paraffin wax blocks. Larger tissue samples will be examined, and 'trimmed' by the pathologist to a size optimum for preparation of a standard microscope slide, and sometimes multiple areas of a larger tissue sample will be selected for examination. Endoscopic pinch biopsies provide a particular challenge to the histology technician. The uniformly small size of these samples often necessitates that they are processed within a purpose-designed fine-mesh container within the standard histological 'cassette', and after processing they are difficult, if not impossible, to orientate correctly within the wax block. Where multiple endoscopic biopsy samples are taken from a particular site, these will generally be blocked together to prepare a single microscopic section. Needle core biopsy samples can also be fragile, particularly when the tissue of origin is friable, and these may also fragment during transit. Following embedding in paraffin wax, a standard 4 μm section will be prepared and stained with haematoxylin and eosin (HE) for standard histopathological examination. Processing tissue samples generally takes a minimum of 24 hours, but newer tissue processors are able to run a 'rapid cycle' for small samples (i.e. endoscopic or core biopsy samples) that can reduce this time to several hours.

Special histochemical stains

The examination of an HE-stained section is the first line of the histopathological examination, and, in the majority of cases, no further assessment is required. However, most histopathology laboratories will be able to perform a panel of 'special stains' to assess particular features of a biopsy sample. These will generally be selected by the pathologist on the basis of the examination of the HE-stained section.

In the case of a granulomatous or pyogranulomatous inflammatory lesion, it would be routine to perform a panel of special stains that included Gram stain (for bacteria), periodic acid–Schiff (PAS, for fungi or algae) and Ziehl-Neelsen (ZN, for acid-fast bacteria) to attempt to identify an infectious aetiology. Other special stains used to identify pathogens include:

- Warthin-Starry silver stain, which may be used for the detection of spirochaetal bacteria
- Giemsa stain, which may be used to identify protozoa (e.g. *Leishmania*).

The clinician should be aware that these special stains are relatively insensitive and may be negative where culture or polymerase chain reaction (PCR) may yield a positive result. Where eosinophils may be difficult to appreciate in some HE-stained sections, special stains, such as Sirius Red, can highlight these cells for assessment of their role in an inflammatory enteropathy. In the case of neoplastic disease, the most widely used example of the application of special stains is the use of toluidine blue staining in mast cell neoplasia.

Special stains should be performed routinely in the assessment of liver biopsy samples. The presence of intra-hepatocyte granular pigment is a common finding, and a distinction should be made between iron (haemosiderin, stained by Perls' Prussian blue) and copper (stained by rubeanic acid) (Figure 6.3). Fouchet's stain can be used to highlight bile pigment accumulation in cases of biliary obstruction. Hepatic fibrosis can be assessed by use of the haematoxylin Van-Gieson (HVG) stain for collagen, and silver-based staining, such as the Gordon and Sweet

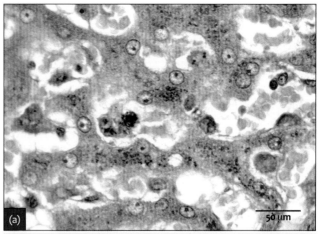

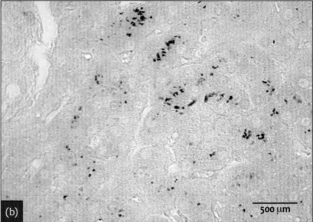

6.3 Sections of liver stained by (a) Perls' Prussian blue for haemosiderin and (b) rubeanic acid for copper, to investigate the nature of the cytoplasmic, brown, granular pigment observed within hepatocytes on a routine haematoxylin and eosin stain.

method for reticulin fibres. Hepatic lipid vacuoles and vacuoles left by glycogen accumulation may be distinguishable on HE-stained tissues: lipid vacuoles are well defined with the nucleus displaced to the periphery, whilst glycogen vacuoles are small, poorly defined and do not displace the nucleus. However, glycogen vacuoles can be confused with hydropic changes. Therefore, frozen tissue sections are required to stain for hepatic lipid by oil red O and for glycogen by PAS to confirm their nature. Amyloid deposition can be detected by Congo red staining and examination of the section by polarized light for birefringence. The same range of special stains for infectious agents described above can be applied to liver or lymph node tissue with evidence of inflammatory change suggestive of microbial involvement.

Electron microscopy

Transmission electron microscopy (TEM) is rarely indicated, or available, in a routine diagnostic pathology setting. However, TEM can sometimes be useful in characterizing microbial agents that might not be easily identified by routine light microscopy (e.g. enteropathogenic *Escherichia coli* or *Cryptosporidium*) or characterizing ultrastructural lesions (e.g. lysosomal storage diseases). TEM can be performed retrospectively by removing a sample of tissue from the paraffin wax block for further processing. For prospective TEM examination, tissue fixed in glutaraldehyde is optimal, and the laboratory should be consulted for specific requirements.

Immunohistochemistry

Immunohistochemistry utilizes an antiserum (a polyclonal antiserum or monoclonal antibody) to detect a specific antigenic molecule within a tissue sample. Some antibodies may be applied to formalin-fixed tissue, making it possible to perform retrospective studies using the same biopsy sample that was processed for routine histopathological evaluation. In contrast, other antibodies may only be used with snap-frozen fresh tissue that has been sectioned with a cryostat. There is a specific protocol for snap-freezing tissue samples for immunohistochemistry, and this is usually not possible to perform in a general practice setting.

The binding of antibody to the target molecule in the tissue is detected via labelling of the primary antibody, or a secondary antibody, with either a fluorochrome (immunofluorescence) or enzyme (immunoperoxidase). Various enhancement procedures (e.g. avidin–biotin immunohistochemistry or polymer detection systems) have been applied to the methodology. Immunohistochemistry is now widely available, as many commercial laboratories have the capacity to perform automated immunolabelling.

Immunohistochemistry may be used to detect specific infectious agents in tissue, and is more sensitive than the special stains described above. For example, detection of coronavirus antigen in the serosal lesions of feline infectious peritonitis would be a useful adjunct to diagnosis. Immunohistochemistry may also be used to detect amyloid and to distinguish between AA and AL forms of the protein.

At the experimental level, immunohistochemistry has been used to characterize the inflammatory cell types in intestinal biopsy samples from dogs and cats with chronic inflammatory enteropathies. The relative proportions of lamina propria and intraepithelial T-cells (CD4+, CD8+, $\gamma\delta$TCR+), plasma cells (IgG, IgM, IgA) and antigen-presenting cells (MHC class II+, MAC387+) have been examined, but at this time such immunohistochemical methods are not routinely applied to the diagnosis of chronic inflammatory enteropathies.

The diagnosis of alimentary tract neoplasia also benefits from the application of immunohistochemistry. The most common indications for this method are to make the distinction between idiopathic lymphocytic inflammation and early-stage alimentary tract lymphoma, and to phenotype the neoplastic lymphoid population. In lymphoma, a lymphocytic infiltrate is clonal, so virtually all of the lymphocytes in the sample will be of one phenotype (e.g. T- or B-cell), whereas in an inflammatory process, a mixture might be expected (Figure 6.4). Immunophenotyping alimentary lymphoma is particularly relevant in the cat in order to distinguish between low-grade alimentary lymphoma (generally T-cell), intermediate to high-grade alimentary lymphoma (T- or B-cell) and large granular lymphocyte lymphoma (generally T-cell) (Barrs and Beatty, 2012; Moore et al., 2012).

Other epithelial or stromal tumour markers may be evaluated immunohistochemically. For example, the neuroendocrine markers synaptophysin and chromogranin are used to identify intestinal carcinoid, and the marker c-kit (CD117) helps differentiate a gastrointestinal stromal tumour (GIST) from a tumour of smooth muscle. A monoclonal antibody against eosinophil peroxidase allows indentification of both intact and degranulated eosinophils. The pathologist will usually advise on the selection of appropriate immunohistochemical markers on the basis of the histopathological findings seen on the HE-stained section and the number of markers chosen may often be determined by cost. Immunohistochemistry is generally batched and so results may take several days to 2 weeks to become available.

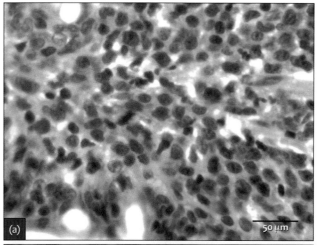
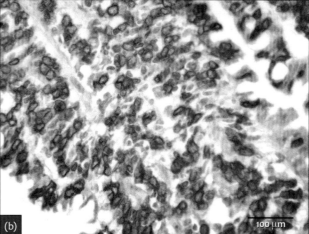

6.4 Section of small intestinal villus from a dog with alimentary lymphoma. (a) The haematoxylin and eosin-stained section shows replacement of normal mucosal structure by a diffuse sheet of neoplastic round cells with mitotic activity. (b) These are identified as T lymphocytes by immunohistochemical expression of CD3.

Molecular analysis

Molecular techniques may now be applied to formalin-fixed and paraffin wax-embedded tissue samples after appropriate extraction of genetic material from 'shavings' of tissue taken from the wax blocks. One such application is in determining the clonality of a lymphoid population within a biopsy sample in order to distinguish lymphoma from inflammation on the basis of restricted genotype. PCR for antigen receptor rearrangements is now available routinely and can improve the diagnostic sensitivity in cases of lymphoma when coupled with immunohistochemistry (Kiupel et al., 2011); however, clonality can also occur in cases of chronic inflammatory enteropathy (Hiyoshi et al., 2015).

The technique of fluorescence in situ hybridization utilizes labelled molecular probes to detect and localize molecular targets in tissue samples. Some laboratories now offer this technique for the detection of bacterial translocation (i.e. from the intestinal lumen through the epithelial barrier into the lamina propria), the identification of E. coli in dogs with granulomatous colitis, detection of gastric Helicobacter spp., the association of Campylobacter coli with neutrophilic enteritis in cats or for the identification of bacteria in liver biopsy samples (Jergens et al., 2009; Mansfield et al., 2009; Twedt et al., 2014; Maunder et al., 2016).

Biopsy sample interpretation

Histopathological interpretation of liver biopsy samples has been greatly improved through the work of the WSAVA Liver Standardization Group (Rothuizen *et al.*, 2006). The nomenclature and definitions of liver pathology given by this group are now used by most diagnostic pathologists when describing hepatic lesions. There is no consensus grading scheme for pancreatic pathology.

The greatest challenge to pathologists still comes from the interpretation of inflammatory change in endoscopic biopsy samples of the GI mucosa. The WSAVA Gastro-intestinal Standardization Group produced a pictorial mono-graph that defines the normal histopathological appearance of the gastric, duodenal and colonic mucosa and defines and grades (as mild, moderate or severe) key architectural (e.g. villus stunting, crypt distortion or abscessation, ulceration or fibrosis) and inflammatory (e.g. lymphoplasmacytic, eosinophilic, neutrophilic or granulomatous) changes in these tissues (Day *et al.*, 2008; Washabau *et al.*, 2010). However, even when the specialist pathologists who were members of the group tested the scoring system in a large blinded study, there was poor correlation between the scores assigned by different pathologists to the same tissue section (Jergens *et al.*, 2014). Correlation was improved when the scoring system was adapted to include only two severity grades or was refined to include fewer parameters (Jergens *et al.*, 2014). Such studies are also likely to yield higher quality data when the tissue sections are prepared and stained by a single laboratory to avoid inevitable inter-institutional variation in methodology (Willard *et al.*, 2010). The parameters assessed in the simplified model are shown in Figure 6.5. Despite these studies, interpretation of endo-scopic biopsy tissues still provides a source of frustration to clinicians and pathologists, particularly when a mucosa with gross endoscopic change is reported to have normal histological structure.

The pathology report should include a gross descrip-tion of the sample submitted (most relevant for biopsy samples taken at laparotomy or post-mortem samples, but for endoscopic biopsy samples, including the number of samples from each site), which can provide a useful cross-check for the clinician that what was submitted to the laboratory has actually been sectioned. A microscopic description of each site sampled should be given, together with an interpretative comment and diagnosis. In the case of endoscopic or core biopsies, the pathologist may seek to provide an overview of the multiple samples, but highlight any specific localized abnormality (e.g. 'The

overall appearance of the samples is normal, but in one of the biopsy samples of fundic mucosa there is a focus of ulceration and neutrophilic inflammation'). Particular problems faced by the pathologist when interpreting endoscopic pinch biopsies (which may be mentioned in the report) include:

- Poor orientation of the biopsy specimen for sectioning, such that a cross-section of individual villi is presented, rather than a longitudinal section through the villus–crypt unit
- Fragmentation of the biopsy specimen with separation of the epithelial layer
- Crush artefact at the base of the biopsy specimen that obliterates fine cellular detail (Figure 6.6).

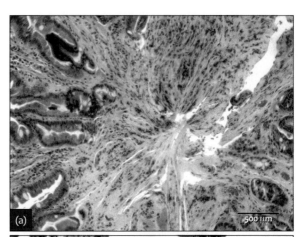

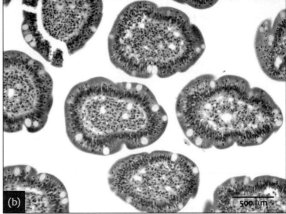

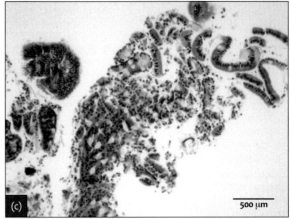

Organ	Microscopic feature scored
Stomach	• Intraepithelial lymphocytes • Lamina propria inflammation • Fibrosis (glandular nesting) • Mucosal atrophy
Small intestine	• Villus atrophy • Epithelial injury • Crypt dilatation or distortion • Intraepithelial lymphocytes • Lamina propria inflammation
Colon	• Epithelial injury • Crypt dilatation • Fibrosis or atrophy • Lamina propria inflammation • Number of goblet cells

6.5 Key microscopic features examined in scoring the severity of chronic inflammatory enteropathy.
(Adapted from Jergens *et al.*, 2014)

6.6 Sections of endoscopic biopsy samples demonstrating common artefacts seen with this procedure. (a) Crush artefact with loss of discernible tissue and cellular structure. (b) Cross-sections of isolated villi when tissue is not oriented in a perpendicular fashion. (c) Fragmentation of a small intestinal tissue biopsy. (Haematoxylin and eosin stain.)

Some pathologists will also score the severity of each architectural and inflammatory change according to the WSAVA guidelines as normal (0), mild (1), moderate (2) or severe (3), but there is no evidence that the cumulative score is of diagnostic or prognostic importance. There is no consensus grading scheme for neoplastic lesions of the alimentary tract. The nature of the neoplastic population (e.g. epithelial, spindle or round cell), the histological arrangement (e.g. sheet, acinar, whorled) and cytological features (e.g. pleomorphism, nuclear:cytoplasmic ratio, nucleoli, chromatin, mitoses) should be described. Other basic parameters, such as the extent of tissue destruction, infiltration of deep margins (difficult to assess with endoscopic pinch biopsies) and invasion of blood or lymphatic vessels or nodal metastasis, should also be reported.

Future possibilities

One study has examined the utility of the technique of confocal endomicroscopy, which allows direct real-time microscopic examination of the mucosa ('virtual biopsy') by local or intravenous application of fluorescent dyes and use of a specialized endoscope (Sharman *et al.*, 2013; 2014). In human medicine, this technique is valuable for assessment of inflammatory or neoplastic change in the intestinal mucosa.

References and further reading

Barrs V and Beatty J (2012) Feline Alimentory Lymphome. Classification, risk factors, clinical signs and non-invasive diagnostics. *Journal of Feline Medicine and Surgery* 14, 182–190

Casamian-Sorrosal D, Willard MD, Murray JK, Hall EJ, Taylor SS and Day MJ (2010) Comparison of histopathological findings in endoscopic biopsies from the duodenum and ileum of dogs with enteropathy. *Journal of Veterinary Internal Medicine* 24, 80–83

Cohen M, Bohling MW, Wright JC, Welles EA and Spano JS (2003) Evaluation of sensitivity and specificity of cytological examination: 269 cases (1999–2000). *Journal of the American Veterinary Medical Association* 222, 964–967

Cordner AP, Sharkey LC and Armstrong PJ (2015) Cytologic findings and diagnostic yield in 92 dogs undergoing fine-needle aspiration of the pancreas. *Journal of Veterinary Diagnostic Investigation* 27, 236–240

Crain SK, Sharkey LC and Cordner AP (2014) Safety of ultrasound-guided fine-needle aspiration of the feline pancreas: a case-control study. *Journal of Feline Medicine and Surgery* 17, 858–863

Day MJ, Bilzer T, Mansell J et al. (2008) Histopathological standards for the diagnosis of gastrointestinal inflammation in endoscopic biopsy samples from the dog and cat: a report from the World Small Animal Veterinary Association Gastrointestinal Standardization Group. *Journal of Comparative Pathology* 138, S1–S43

Hiyoshi S, Ohno K, Uchida K et al. (2015) Association between lymphocyte antigen receptor gene rearrangements and histopathological evaluation in canine chronic enteropathy. *Veterinary Immunology and Immunopathology* 165, 138–144

Jergens AE, Evans RB, Ackermann M et al. (2014) Design of a simplified histopathologic model for gastrointestinal inflammation in dogs. *Veterinary Pathology* 51, 946–950

Jergens AE, Pressel M, Crandell J et al. (2009) Fluorescence in situ hybridization confirms clearance of visible *Helicobacter* spp. associated with gastritis in dogs and cats. *Journal of Veterinary Internal Medicine* 23, 16–23

Kemp SD, Zimmerman KL, Panciera DL, Monroe WE and Leib MS (2015) Histopathologic variation between liver lobes in dogs. *Journal of Veterinary Internal Medicine* 29, 58–62

Kiupel M, Smedley RC, Pfent C et al. (2011) Diagnostic algorithm to differentiate lymphoma from inflammation in feline small intestinal biopsy samples. *Veterinary Pathology* 48, 212–222

Kleinschmidt S, Harder J, Nolte I, Marsilio S and Hewicker-Trautwein M (2010) Chronic inflammatory and non-inflammatory diseases of the gastrointestinal tract in cats: diagnostic advantages of full-thickness intestinal and extraintestinal biopsies. *Journal of Feline Medicine and Surgery* 12, 97–103

Mansfield CS, James FE, Craven M et al. (2009) Remission of histiocytic ulcerative colitis in boxer dogs correlates with eradication of invasive intramucosal *Escherichia coli*. *Journal of Veterinary Internal Medicine* 23, 964–969

Maunder CL, Reynolds ZT, Peacock L et al. (2016) Campylobacter species and neutrophilic inflammatory bowel disease in cats. *Journal of Veterinary Internal Medicine* 30, 996–1001

Moore PF, Rodriguez-Bertos A and Kass PH (2012) Feline gastrointestinal lymphoma: mucosal architecture, immunophenotype, and molecular clonality. *Veterinary Pathology* 49, 658–668

Procoli F, Motskula PF, Keyte SV, Priestnall S and Allenspach K (2013) Comparison of histopathologic findings in duodenal and ileal endoscopic biopsies in dogs with chronic small intestinal enteropathies. *Journal of Veterinary Internal Medicine* 27, 268–274

Rothuizen J, Bunch SE, Charles JA et al. (2006) *WSAVA Standards for Histological and Clinical Diagnosis of Canine and Feline Liver Disease*. Elsevier, Philadelphia

Ruiz GC, Reyes-Gomez E, Hall EJ and Freiche V (2016) Comparison of 3 handling techniques for endoscopically obtained gastric and duodenal biopsy specimens: A prospective study in dogs and cats. *Journal of Veterinary Internal Medicine* 30, 1014–1021

Scott KD, Zoran DL, Mansell J, Norby B and Willard MD (2011) Utility of endoscopic biopsies of the duodenum and ileum for diagnosis of inflammatory bowel disease and small cell lymphoma in cats. *Journal of Veterinary Internal Medicine* 25, 1253–1257

Sharman MJ, Bacci B, Whittem T and Mansfield CS (2013) In vivo confocal endomicroscopy of small intestinal mucosal morphology in dogs. *Journal of Veterinary Internal Medicine* 27, 1372–1378

Sharman MJ, Bacci B, Whittem T and Mansfield CS (2014) In vivo histologically equivalent evaluation of gastric mucosal topologic morphology in dogs by using confocal endomicroscopy. *Journal of Veterinary Internal Medicine* 28, 799–808

Twedt DC, Cullen J, McCord K, Janeczko S, Dudak J and Simpson K (2014) Evaluation of fluorescence in situ hybridization for the detection of bacteria in feline inflammatory liver disease. *Journal of Feline Medicine and Surgery* 16, 109–117

Washabau RJ, Day MJ, Willard MD, et al. (2010) Endoscopic, biopsy, and histopathologic guidelines for the evaluation of gastrointestinal inflammation in companion animals. *Journal of Veterinary Internal Medicine* 24, 10–26

Willard M, Mansell J, Fosgate G et al. (2008) Effect of sample quality upon the sensitivity of endoscopic biopsy for detecting gastric and duodenal lesions in dogs and cats. *Journal of Veterinary Internal Medicine* 22, 1084–1089

Willard MD, Moore GE, Denton BD et al. (2010) Effect of tissue processing on assessment of endoscopic intestinal biopsies in dogs and cats. *Journal of Veterinary Internal Medicine* 24, 84–89

Chapter 7

Polyphagia

Daniel J. Batchelor and Alexander J. German

Definition of the problem

Polyphagia is excessive eating or appetite.

Relevant history

It is important to determine whether the animal is gaining or losing weight, as this will help differentiate between the various causes of polyphagia (Figures 7.1 and 7.2).

Causes of polyphagia associated with weight loss include poor quality diets, chronic regurgitation, maldigestion, malabsorption, diabetes mellitus, exposure to a cold environment, hyperthyroidism and increased exercise. Causes of polyphagia associated with weight gain include primary polyphagia, hypersomatotropism, hyperadrenocorticism, insulinoma, pregnancy, sudden acquired retinal degeneration syndrome (SARDS) and drug-induced polyphagia. Obesity is a common consequence of polyphagia in otherwise healthy dogs or cats that consume food in

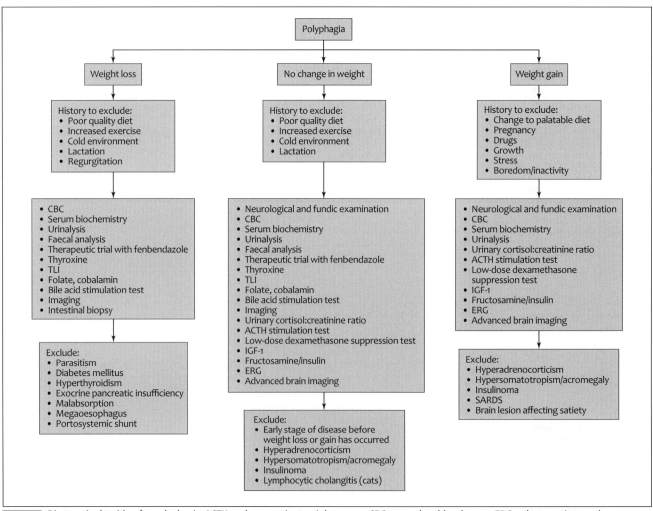

7.1 Diagnostic algorithm for polyphagia. ACTH = adrenocorticotropic hormone; CBC = complete blood count; ERG = electroretinography; IGF-1 = insulin-like growth factor-1; SARDS = sudden acquired retinal degeneration syndrome; TLI = trypsin-like immunoreactivity.

Primary polyphagia

- Lesion affecting brain areas controlling satiety (hypothalamus/brainstem)
- Palatable diet
- Recent stressful event
- Boredom
- Genetic predisposition to excessive appetite (e.g. Labrador Retriever, Beagle, others)
- Other factors causing increased appetite (e.g. neutering)

Secondary polyphagia

- Poor quality diet
- Chronic regurgitation
- Malabsorption
  - Exocrine pancreatic insufficiency
  - Inflammatory/infiltrative intestinal diseases
  - Intestinal lymphangiectasia
  - Intestinal parasites
- Diabetes mellitus
- Hypersomatotropism/acromegaly
- Hyperadrenocorticism
- Sudden acquired retinal degeneration syndrome (SARDS)
- Insulinoma
- Increased metabolic rate
  - Growth
  - Late-stage pregnancy
  - Lactation
  - Cold environment
  - Increased exercise
  - Hyperthyroidism (hyperplasia, adenoma or carcinoma of thyroid gland or ingestion of uncooked (raw) diet containing thyroid gland tissue)
- Drugs
  - Glucocorticoids
  - Progestagens
  - Thyroxine excess
  - Phenobarbital
  - Benzodiazepines
  - Cyproheptadine
  - Mirtazapine
  - Capromorelin
- Portosystemic shunt (reported, but reduced appetite more common)
- Lymphocytic cholangitis (cats)

7.2 Differential diagnoses for polyphagia.

excess of their caloric requirement, and can be associated with genetic and/or behavioural factors that drive appetite in some individuals and breeds. Uncommonly, thyrotoxicosis in dogs and cats can also occur following the ingestion of an uncooked diet containing thyroid gland tissue.

The clinical history enables the clinician to exclude:

- Poor quality diet
- Recent change to a highly palatable diet
- Increased exercise
- A cold environment
- Pregnancy/lactation
- Regurgitation
- Administration of drugs (glucocorticoids, anticonvulsants, thyroxine, others)
- Recent stressful events, such as the introduction of a new pet.

Apart from weight changes, other clinical signs may be present depending on the underlying cause of the polyphagia. Concurrent polyuria/polydipsia (PU/PD) is expected in diabetes mellitus, hyperadrenocorticism (dogs), hyperthyroidism (mainly cats), SARDS and hypothalamic lesions. Hyperadrenocorticism in dogs is also associated with panting, abdominal enlargement, skin and hair coat changes, weakness, exercise intolerance

and lethargy. Hyperthyroidism can be associated with gastrointestinal signs (e.g. vomiting or diarrhoea) and also behavioural changes such as increased activity and irritability. Sudden-onset blindness suggests SARDS, but PU/PD and polyphagia can occur before the blindness. When polyphagia is due to malabsorption, signs such as small intestinal diarrhoea and vomiting are usually (but not always) present. Insulinoma may be associated with ataxia, weakness, trembling, collapse and, possibly, seizures. Animals with primary polyphagia may have a history of head trauma, or may be showing other neurological signs or behavioural changes compatible with a hypothalamic or multifocal central nervous system (CNS) lesion.

Physical examination

For polyphagic animals, examination should include a general physical examination along with neurological and fundic examinations. Late-stage pregnancy or lactation should be obvious at this stage. Cats with hyperthyroidism usually have a detectable goitre, and often show restlessness and an unkempt hair coat. They may also have tachycardia, arrhythmia, gallop sounds or a cardiac murmur. Hyperthyroidism is rare in dogs but can occur with a functional thyroid carcinoma, which is usually palpable as a cervical mass. Hyperadrenocorticism is associated with a range of possible abnormalities on examination, including hair coat changes (symmetrical alopecia, hyperpigmentation, thinning of skin, calcinosis cutis, poor regrowth of clipped areas), loss of muscle mass, abdominal enlargement and hepatomegaly. Acromegaly may be associated with changes in body conformation (enlargement of the head and paws, widened interdental spaces, prognathism) or inspiratory stridor. Physical examination can be normal in SARDS because the retinas may be normal in the early stages.

In cases with malabsorption, physical examination may be normal. In conditions that lead to loss of protein (e.g. protein-losing enteropathy, protein-losing nephropathy), there may also be weight loss, ascites and subcutaneous oedema. Identifying 'turgid' intestinal loops is usually a non-specific finding, but firm or irregular thickening of the intestines can indicate infiltrative disease. Abdominal pain may be present in some conditions including pancreatitis and gastric ulceration.

Animals with primary polyphagia may show other neurological signs compatible with a hypothalamic or midbrain lesion (e.g. incessant pacing, circling, central blindness, ataxia, proprioceptive deficits, upper motor neuron signs in the limbs, or signs associated with disturbances of adrenal, thyroid or reproductive function depending on the exact site of the lesion). Other neurological abnormalities may be present in multifocal CNS diseases.

Diagnostic tests

After the initial basic tests (complete blood count), serum biochemistry panel, urinalysis, and serum thyroxine assay in patients with possible hyperthyroidism), faecal examination for parasites may be performed (three-pooled samples is recommended) (Figure 7.3). Trial therapy with parasiticides should be considered as false-negative faecal results are possible. Serum folate and cobalamin

- CBC
- Serum biochemistry
- Urinalysis
- Total thyroxine assay ± free thyroxine
- Faecal examination
- Serum folate and cobalamin assays
- Serum trypsin-like immunoreactivity
- Bile acid stimulation test
- Faecal alpha$_1$- proteinase inhibitor if available (currently USA only)
- Thoracic radiography
- Abdominal ultrasonography
- Adrenal function tests to investigate or exclude hyperadrenocorticism
  - Urinary cortisol:creatinine ratio
  - ACTH stimulation test
  - Low-dose dexamethasone suppression test
- Growth hormone assay (if available) or IGF-1 assay
- Blood glucose ± fructosamine ± serum insulin
- Electroretinography
- Endoscopy or coeliotomy and intestinal biopsy
- Advanced brain imaging (CT or MRI) ± CSF analysis

7.3 Diagnostic tests for the investigation of polyphagia. ACTH = adrenocorticotropic hormone; CBC = complete blood count; CSF = cerebrospinal fluid; CT = computed tomography; IGF-1 = insulin-like growth factor-1; MRI = magnetic resonance imaging.

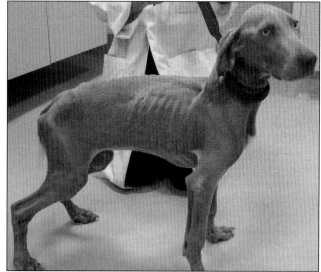

7.4 Patient presented with polyphagia and weight loss. The dog was diagnosed with exocrine pancreatic insufficiency (see Chapter 36).

assays may provide evidence for malabsorption. Serum trypsin-like immunoreactivity is a sensitive and specific test for exocrine pancreatic insufficiency (Figure 7.4). A bile acid stimulation test may support a diagnosis of portosystemic shunt. Faecal alpha$_1$-proteinase inhibitor may detect protein-losing intestinal diseases before serum albumin starts to decrease, but the test is not currently available outside the USA.

Imaging studies can be helpful: thoracic radiography may demonstrate megaoesophagus, and abdominal ultrasonography may be useful in the investigation of intestinal diseases or portosystemic shunts (see Chapter 3). Adrenal function tests can be used to investigate or exclude hyperadrenocorticism. Assays of growth hormone (if available) or insulin-like growth factor-1 in serum can be used to investigate the possibility of hypersomatotropism/acromegaly. The diagnosis is supported in cats by demonstration of a pituitary mass on computed tomography (CT) or magnetic resonance imaging (MRI).

Insulinoma is supported by finding low blood glucose and/or serum fructosamine. If insulinoma is suspected, a sample for serum insulin assay should be taken when the blood glucose concentration is <3 mmol/l. SARDS can be diagnosed on appropriate history and physical examination findings, and confirmed by electroretinography. Intestinal biopsy may be part of the investigation of intestinal diseases. Advanced brain imaging (CT or MRI), along with cerebrospinal fluid analysis, may be performed to investigate central causes of polyphagia if the neurological examination is abnormal.

Chapter 8

Anorexia and hyporexia

Daniel J. Batchelor and Alexander J. German

Definition of the problem

Anorexia is defined as a lack of appetite for food. Hyporexia means a reduction in appetite, and is sometimes referred to as partial anorexia. Prolonged anorexia is harmful and leads to villus atrophy and reduced epithelial barrier and immune functions.

Relevant history

Anorexia and hyporexia are non-specific clinical signs with numerous causes. For animals with anorexia or hyporexia caused by a medical condition, a detailed clinical history may help to direct subsequent investigations (Figure 8.1). The owner should be asked if there has been any recent change in the animal's circumstances that could lead to anorexia or hyporexia, such as the introduction of a new pet into the household, addition or absence of a family member, change to a more unpalatable diet, change in feeding pattern or location, or stress.

Anorexia and hyporexia should be distinguished from situations where the animal seems interested in food but then is unwilling or unable to eat it, suggesting a disorder of the oral cavity, nose or skull that causes difficulty or pain during eating (Figures 8.2 and 8.3).

The history should include both medical and environmental aspects, including whether the animal is receiving any drugs. Many drugs can cause a reduction in appetite, including non-steroidal anti-inflammatory drugs, chemotherapeutic agents, opioid analgesics, some antibiotics (including amoxicillin, cefalexin, chloramphenicol, erythromycin and sulphonamides), cardiac glycosides, penicillamine, omeprazole and ferrous sulphate.

- Vomiting/signs of nausea
- Regurgitation
- Dysphagia
- Halitosis
- Diarrhoea or constipation
- Coughing or other respiratory signs
- Collapsing
- Lameness
- Behavioural changes
- Neurological signs
- Changes in weight or body conformation
- Appearance of new masses or swelling
- Presence of any ocular, nasal, otic, vulval or preputial discharge
- Polyuria/polydipsia

8.1 Important aspects of the history in cases of anorexia or hyporexia: useful areas of questioning for the owner.

Potential causes

- Inflammatory disease
  - Bacterial infection
  - Viral infection
  - Fungal infection
  - Protozoal infection
  - Immune-mediated disease
  - Tissue necrosis
  - Pancreatitis
- Pyrexia
- Cancer
- Chronic pain
- Disease causing pain in oral cavity, nose, skull, oesophagus or stomach
  - Fracture
  - Mass
  - Foreign body
  - Stomatitis
  - Dental/periodontal disease
  - Masticatory myositis
  - Retrobulbar abscess
  - Trigeminal neuritis
  - Temporomandibular joint problem
  - Sinonasal aspergillosis
  - Osteomyelitis
  - Neoplasia
- Alimentary tract disease
- Pancreatic disease
  - Small intestinal disease
  - Large intestinal disease
- Respiratory disease
- Heart disease
- Metabolic disease
  - Kidney disease
  - Liver disease
  - Adrenal dysfunction
  - Diabetic ketosis/ketoacidosis
  - Hypercalcaemia
- Anaemia
- Nausea
- Central nervous system disease
- Loss of sense of smell (anosmia)
- Psychological cause
  - Bereavement
  - New pet in household
  - Altered environment
  - Stress
  - Hospitalization
- Unpalatable diet
- Drug affecting appetite
  - Non-steroidal anti-inflammatory drug
  - Chemotherapeutic agent
  - Opioid analgesic
  - Antibiotic (beta lactams, chloramphenicol, erythromycin, sulphonamides)
  - Cardiac glycosides
  - Other (e.g. penicillamine, omeprazole, ferrous sulphate)

8.2 Differential diagnoses for anorexia or hyporexia.

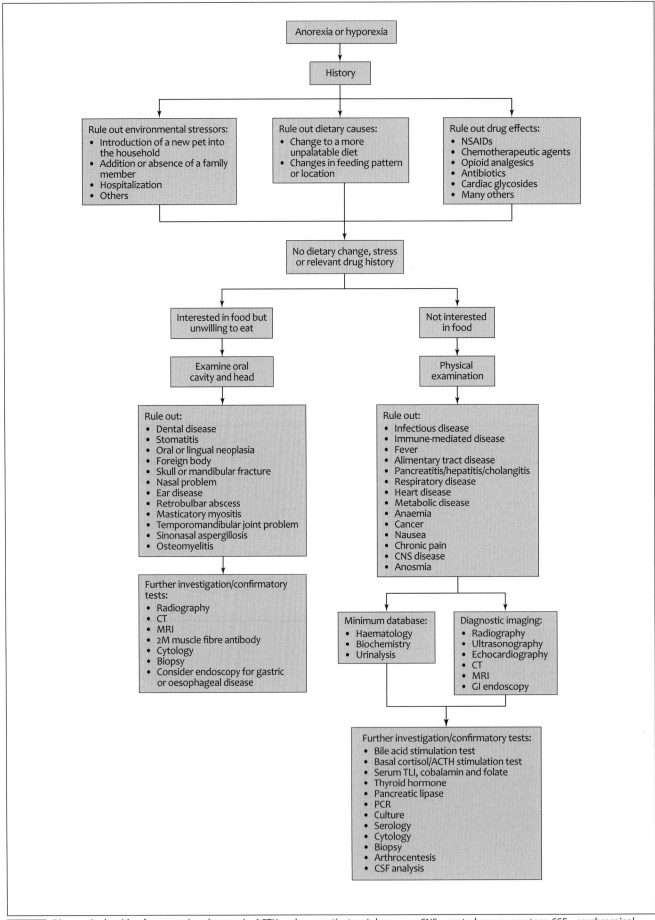

8.3 Diagnostic algorithm for anorexia or hyporexia. ACTH = adrenocorticotropic hormone; CNS = central nervous system; CSF = cerebrospinal fluid; CT = computed tomography; GI = gastrointestinal; MRI= magnetic resonance imaging; NSAIDs = non-steroidal anti-inflammatory drugs; PCR = polymerase chain reaction; TLI = trypsin-like immunoreactivity.

Physical examination

A careful, complete physical examination is essential in cases presenting with anorexia or hyporexia because causes are many and varied. For animals that are keen to eat and can smell food but are then unable to eat it, detailed examination of the oral cavity and head is required. In some cases, sedation or anaesthesia might be required in order to examine these regions properly. Particular attention should be paid to inflammation or structural abnormalities of the teeth, lips, gums, tongue and oropharynx, noting the presence of any ulcers, fractures, masses, foreign bodies or anatomical abnormalities. Difficulty or pain on opening the mouth can suggest a temporomandibular joint abnormality, masticatory myositis, retrobulbar abscess or ear disease. The nose should be examined for discharge, depigmentation, pain and the presence of normal airflow through the nostrils using a wisp of cotton wool. The ears should be examined for pain, redness, discharge and abnormal odours. The temporal muscles should be examined for swelling, pain and atrophy. Any abnormalities of cranial nerve function should be noted.

Since a range of systemic diseases can cause anorexia or hyporexia, it is essential that the clinician examines all body systems, looking for evidence of abnormalities. For example:

- The cardiovascular system should be evaluated by determining the heart rate and assessing pulse quality and peripheral perfusion, as well as examining for the presence of a murmur, gallop sound or arrhythmia
- The respiratory system should be evaluated by determining the respiratory rate and effort, as well as auscultating the lung fields
- The abdomen should be evaluated by palpation, including rectal examination, assessing for:
  - Areas of pain
  - Masses
  - Enlargement of the liver, spleen, mesenteric lymph nodes, urinary bladder, kidneys, uterus or prostate
  - Gas- or fluid-filled distension of the gastrointestinal tract
  - Intussusception
  - Foreign body
  - The presence of firm faeces in the colon that may suggest constipation/obstipation
  - Urinary bladder abnormalities
- Peripheral lymph nodes should be palpated to determine if lymphadenopathy is present and the location
- Ocular examination should be performed
- The spinal column should be palpated for areas of pain and manipulation of the neck should be performed to detect cervical pain
- Orthopaedic examination should be performed to assess for pain or joint swelling that may suggest a painful orthopaedic condition or polyarthritis
- Neurological examination should be performed

- Rectal temperature should be measured to detect fever
- Skin/hair coat should be assessed.

Rarely, an animal may lose its sense of smell, which may cause it to appear to be interested in food but then not eat. Gastric carcinoma should also be considered in older dogs that go to the food bowl to eat, but then do not subsequently ingest anything.

Diagnostic tests

A variety of tests may be required for investigating cases of anorexia or hyporexia, depending on the information obtained from the history and physical examination (Figure 8.4). Useful screening tests in nearly every case include haematology, serum biochemistry and urinalysis. Depending on findings from the history and physical examination, more specific tests could include faecal analysis, radiography, ultrasonography, echocardiography and gastrointestinal endoscopy. Specific blood tests could include a bile acid stimulation test and assays for cortisol/adrenocorticotropic hormone stimulation test, serum trypsin-like immunoreactivity, cobalamin and folate, thyroxine, pancreatic lipase or 2M muscle fibre antibody. Microbial infection may be diagnosed by direct observation of the organism, polymerase chain reaction, culture or serology.Inflammatory or neoplastic disease can be investigated by cytology or biopsy of masses, enlarged lymph nodes or abnormal areas, or by analysis of synovial or cerebrospinal fluid. Some disorders require advanced imaging, such as computed tomography or magnetic resonance imaging, for investigation.

Required in most cases
• Haematology
• Biochemistry
• Urinalysis
• Radiography
• Ultrasonography
Employed when indicated by specific signs or initial test results
• Faecal analysis
• Bile acid stimulation test
• Serum cortisol/ACTH stimulation test
• Serum TLI, cobalamin and folate
• Thyroxine assay
• Pancreatic lipase
• 2M muscle fibre antibody
• Cytology
• Polymerase chain reaction
• Culture
• Serology
• Biopsy
• Arthrocentesis
• Cerebrospinal fluid analysis
• Echocardiography
• Gastrointestinal endoscopy
• Computed tomography
• Magnetic resonance imaging

8.4 List of possible diagnostic tests for cases of anorexia or hyporexia. ACTH = adrenocorticotropic hormone; TLI = trypsin-like immunoreactivity.

Chapter 9

Weight loss

Alexander J. German and Daniel J. Batchelor

Definition of the problem

Weight loss occurs when energy expenditure exceeds dietary energy intake. Normal animals are able to offset any deficiency of intake by decreasing energy expenditure, slowing the rate of weight loss. The predominant body tissue lost is adipose tissue, with lean tissue loss (from muscle and organs) being limited initially. However, lean tissue loss is inevitable if the energy deficit is severe.

Cachexia refers to a syndrome of severe weight loss resulting from metabolic derangements, and this often cannot be corrected by increasing dietary energy intake alone. Furthermore, the mechanisms that normally preserve lean tissue mass during negative energy balance are circumvented, resulting in severe lean tissue loss. Examples of diseases that lead to cachexia include chronic kidney disease, cancer, cardiac disease and chronic inflammatory disease. In humans, cachexia is known to be a significant predictor of mortality and a similar effect is likely in cats and dogs, given that suboptimal body condition is often a negative prognostic indicator.

Relevant history

In some cases, the owner will recognize weight loss and present their animal for veterinary attention (Figures 9.1 and 9.2). Alternatively, they might be concerned about other clinical signs, or the weight loss might go unnoticed until the time of presentation. Even when weight loss is

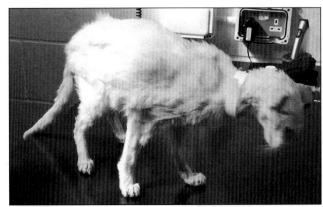

9.2 A 7-year-old neutered female Domestic Shorthaired cat is in extremely poor body condition (BCS 2/9) and there is evidence of muscle wasting.

present, it can be difficult for owners to be precise about the magnitude. Therefore, the clinician should aim to quantify the severity of the weight loss accurately, by comparing current weight to previous weight measurements. Change in weight can be a sensitive indicator for impending health problems. In the authors' opinion, a loss of >5% bodyweight within a 3-month period, or >10% overall loss whatever the time frame, should be investigated.

Given the range of possible causes (Figures 9.3 and 9.4), a complete medical history is important. Dietary history should include all food currently fed and consumed (together with the amounts, including treats and supplements), how the portions are measured out, how the food is

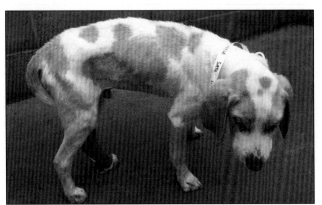

9.1 A 9-month-old entire male Beagle with a portosystemic shunt. The dog has a poor body condition (BCS 3/9) and there is some loss of muscle mass.

Inadequate nutrient intake

• Nutritionally incomplete or unbalanced diet
• Inadequate food intake of a nutritionally complete diet
  • Deliberate starvation
  • Errors when calculating energy requirements
  • Controlled weight loss programmes
• Decreased voluntary food intake
  • Pain
  • Reduced appetite (e.g. pyrexia, nausea)
  • Altered sense of smell (e.g. nasal cavity disease)
• Problems with prehension, chewing and swallowing
  • Head trauma
  • Dental disease
  • Temporal myositis cricopharyngeal achalasia, etc.
• Severe regurgitation
• Excessive vomiting or nausea

9.3 Differential diagnoses for weight loss. (continues) ▶

Malabsorption

- Small intestinal malabsorption
- Exocrine pancreatic insufficiency
- Liver disease
- Short bowel syndrome

Excessive energy demand

- Excessive protein or calorie loss
  - Diabetes mellitus
  - Protein-losing enteropathy
  - Protein-losing nephropathy
  - Exudative skin diseases
- Increased metabolic rate
  - Hyperthyroidism
  - Extreme exercise
  - Decreased ambient temperature
  - Pregnancy and lactation
  - Growth
- Metabolic derangements leading to cachexia
  - Neoplasia
  - Cardiac disease
  - Chronic kidney disease
  - Chronic inflammatory diseases
  - Hypoadrenocorticism

9.3 (continued) Differential diagnoses for weight loss.

fed (number of meals/day, use of a bowl or puzzle feeder, individual *versus* group feeding) and any recent dietary changes. If necessary, the owner should be asked to provide label information. For home-prepared food, it might be necessary to contact a specialist (board-certified) veterinary nutritionist for further analysis or use a food-testing laboratory to determine nutrient content. The WSAVA Global Nutrition Committee provides guidance on nutritional assessment in dogs and cats.

It is important to determine whether appetite is increased, decreased or unchanged. This can help refine the list of differential diagnoses. In some conditions, increased appetite would be expected (e.g. increased energy demand from exercise or lactation, many diseases causing malabsorption, diseases leading to regurgitation). In other cases, appetite is reduced (e.g. diseases causing pain, azotaemia and/or other metabolic derangements). In some circumstances, the appetite is increased, but the animal is subsequently unwilling to swallow food after prehension occurs. This can suggest painful disorders of the head or oral cavity. The clinician should also question the owner about whether any changes have occurred in the animal's environment, for instance, changes in housing, weather conditions and activity levels.

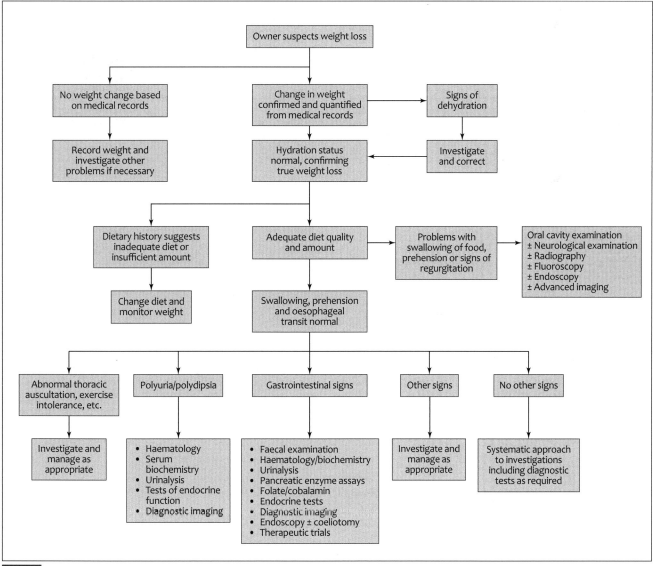

9.4 Diagnostic algorithm for weight loss.

Other signs identified in the history can help to direct the diagnostic approach, for example, gastrointestinal signs (prehension of food, swallowing, vomiting, regurgitation and changes in faecal consistency). Small intestinal diarrhoea can be associated with malabsorption, but is not invariably present. Constipation in older animals, especially cats, can be a sign of dehydration caused by diseases such as chronic kidney disease. Other useful signs include polyuria/polydipsia, coughing and exercise intolerance.

Physical examination

During the oral cavity inspection, mucous membrane colour can be assessed to identify possible icterus or anaemia, and capillary refill time is determined. Dental arcades and gingival surfaces should be examined and this may determine whether weight loss is the result of anorexia due to dental disease. Swallowing is usually best assessed visually by using the external gag reflex, where the clinician applies gentle external pressure to the pharynx, which normally stimulates swallowing. Cardiac auscultation coupled with assessment of pulse quality and rate is important to determine whether cardiac disease is present, as well as inspecting the rest of the body for other signs of cardiovascular disease, such as ascites, subcutaneous oedema, jugular distension, and temperature of the extremities. Thoracic auscultation is indicated to detect evidence of pulmonary or pleural disease. The abdomen should be palpated to determine whether there is any pain, abdominal masses, solid faecal matter (suggesting constipation), or fluid. Finally, rectal examination can be useful, enabling palpation of the prostate and inspection of faeces if necessary.

Bodyweight should be measured and body condition assessed. Electronic scales should be regularly calibrated to ensure precision and accuracy. The WSAVA Global Nutrition Committee recommends use of the nine-point body condition score (BCS) system.

These assessments mainly detect changes in peripheral body fat mass, rather than lean tissue, and also lack sensitivity: it typically takes approximately 10% change in bodyweight before a change in BCS is noted. That said, muscle mass loss of varying severity is usually seen in dogs and cats with BCS 1–2 out of 9. To identify more subtle changes and/or muscle mass loss in otherwise overweight cats and dogs, muscle condition scoring (MCS) is recommended. A 4-category MCS has been validated and it involves inspecting and palpating specific areas of the body (spine, scapulae, skull, and the wings of the ilia).

Although subjective and not validated, a subjective system for muscle scoring can help identify diseases that might lead to cachexia in animals that are overweight. Hydration status should be assessed to ensure that rapid changes in bodyweight are not the result of global fluid shifts. Finally, neurological examination can be considered as an extension of the physical examination.

Diagnostic tests

Given the extensive differential diagnosis list for weight loss, an array of diagnostic tests may be needed (Figure 9.5). Some tests are used in most cases, such as routine clinicopathological tests (e.g. haematology, serum biochemistry, thyroxine measurement (cats), urinalysis, faecal analysis and serology (cats)) and diagnostic imaging procedures (e.g. radiography and ultrasonography). Some tests are

Required in most cases
- Routine clinicopathological tests
  - Haematology
  - Serum biochemistry (± thyroxine in cats)
  - Urinalysis
- Faecal analysis
  - Parasitology
  - Bacteriology
- Serology (cats especially)
  - Feline leukaemia virus
  - Feline immunodeficiency virus
  - Feline enteric coronavirus
- Diagnostic imaging
  - Radiography
  - Abdominal ultrasonography

Employed when indicated by specific signs or initial test results
- Serum tests to assess calcium status
  - Ionized calcium
  - Parathyroid hormone
  - Parathyroid hormone-related protein
  - Vitamin D
- Serum pancreatic enzyme testing
  - Pancreatic lipase
  - Trypsin-like immunoreactivity
  - DGGR lipase (NB not pancreas-specific)
- Serum vitamin concentrations
  - Folate
  - Cobalamin
- Endocrine testing
  - Serum cortisol ± ACTH stimulation testing
  - Total thyroxine ± free thyroxine (free T4)
  - Fructosamine
  - Other
- Serology
  - Acetylcholine receptor antibodies
  - *Toxoplasma*
  - *Neospora*
  - Other
- Microbiological testing of faeces
  - Bacterial culture
  - Fungal culture
  - Other
- Diagnostic imaging
  - Ultrasound-guided biopsy
  - Contrast studies
- Therapeutic trials
  - Exclusion diet
  - Antiparasitic medication
  - Increased food intake

Occasionally employed (in a minority of cases, when signs or initial test results dictate)
- Endoscopy and sample collection
  - Oesophagoscopy
  - Gastroduodenoscopy
  - Colonoscopy (± ileoscopy)
  - Bronchoscopy
  - Other
- Exploratory surgery and biopsy
  - Coeliotomy
- Advanced imaging
  - Fluoroscopy (barium swallow)
  - Computed tomography
  - Magnetic resonance imaging
- Neurological evaluation
  - Cerebrospinal fluid analysis
  - Muscle and nerve biopsy
- Cardiac evaluation
  - Cardiac biomarkers
  - Electrocardiography
  - Echocardiography
  - Holter monitoring
- Glomerular filtration rate
  - SDMA
  - Iohexol clearance
  - Exogenous creatinine clearance
- Nutritional evaluation of the diet

9.5 Diagnostic tests for weight loss. ACTH = adrenocorticotropic hormone; DGGR = 1,2-0-dilauryl-rac-glycero glutaric acid-(6'-methylresorufin) ester; SDMA = symmetric dimethylarginine.

employed only when there are particular clinical signs or clinicopathological abnormalities, including tests of endocrine function, dynamic bile acid measurement, and assay of serum trypsin-like immunoreactivity or pancreatic lipase, folate and cobalamin concentrations. All other tests are used only in occasional cases, and where specific clinical signs or other test results require it.

Differential diagnoses

Pathophysiological mechanisms that can lead to weight loss as a clinical sign include inadequate nutrient intake, malabsorption and excessive energy demand (see Figure 9.3).

Useful websites

WSAVA Global Nutrition Committee – Nutritional Guidance:
http://www.wsava.org/nutrition-toolkit

WSAVA Global Nutrition Committee – Muscle Condition Score (cats):
https://www.wsava.org/WSAVA/media/Documents/Committee%20Resources/Global%20Nutrition%20Committee/Muscle-condition-score-chart-Cats-1.pdf

WSAVA Global Nutrition Committee – Muscle Condition Score (dogs):
http://www.wsava.org/WSAVA/media/Documents/Committee%20Resources/Global%20Nutrition%20Committee/Muscle-condition-score-chart-2013-1.pdf

Chapter 10

Drooling

Patrick Barko

Definition of the problem

Saliva secreted into the oral cavity comes from the parotid, mandibular, sublingual and zygomatic salivary glands. Between meals, salivation occurs at a constant rate but is increased in anticipation of feeding and by the presence of food or bitter substances in the oral cavity. The composition and volume of salivary secretions are regulated by the autonomic nervous system, and parasympathetic stimulation from the central nervous system (CNS) is the most potent stimulus for salivation. Saliva has several important functions including lubrication, binding, solubilization of food, maintenance of oral hygiene and evaporative cooling.

Drooling is a general term describing two different clinical signs: ptyalism and pseudoptyalism. Ptyalism (also known as sialorrhoea) refers specifically to a physiological or pathological increase in the production and secretion of saliva (also known as hypersalivation), whereas pseudoptyalism describes any condition in which salivary secretion is normal but saliva accumulates in the oral cavity and may then leak from the mouth, leading to the problem of drooling (Figure 10.1). This is due to either an inability to retain saliva within the mouth or to swallow. Ptyalism and pseudoptyalism often overlap, and thus the clinical distinction between them is not possible without further investigation.

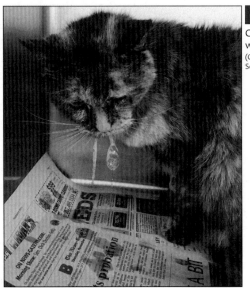

10.1
Cat presenting with drooling. (Courtesy of Amy Somrak)

Aetiology and pathogenesis

The aetiopathogeneses of ptyalism and pseudoptyalism are varied, encompassing disorders of the salivary glands, oropharynx and nervous system, in addition to congenital/conformational anomalies, metabolic syndromes, immune-mediated disease, infectious agents and toxin/drug exposures. Note that for many conditions there are overlapping mechanisms for drooling. For instance, neurological conditions may increase salivary secretion at the same time as affecting the ability to swallow, causing ptyalism and pseudoptyalism, respectively. Similarly, exposure to certain toxins can cause ptyalism by local irritation in the oral cavity and by their effects on the gastrointestinal and neurological systems; for example, *Bufo* toads can secrete a venom on to the skin which can contain a variety of toxins, depending on their species, which causes hypersalivation if an animal tries to pick it up or licks it.

Differential diagnoses

The most common causes of drooling are those originating from within the oropharyngeal cavity. See Figure 10.2 for a comprehensive overview of differential diagnoses for drooling in dogs and cats.

Signalment, history and physical examination

Signalment

Young patients presenting for evaluation of excessive drooling are more likely to have congenital/conformational anomalies. In large-breed dogs (e.g. Bloodhound, St Bernard, Mastiff), brachygnathism and/or excessive lip fold tissue can be associated with pseudoptyalism. Hepatoencephalopathy caused by congenital portosystemic shunts should be considered an important differential diagnosis in cats presenting with ptyalism. Dogs and cats of any age can present with drooling caused by toxin/drug exposure, oropharyngeal foreign bodies or acute viral infections, which can occur in any age group, but should be considered more likely in young animals.

Affected body system or disease process	Specific disease
Conformational	• Brachygnathism • Excessive lip fold tissue
Neurological	• Cranial nerve lesions affecting swallowing function (glossopharyngeal, hypoglossal and vagus nerves) • Cranial nerve lesions affecting jaw, lip or facial tone (trigeminal neuropraxia, trigeminal neuritis, facial nerve paralysis, nerve sheath tumours) • Dysautonomia • Vestibular dysfunction • Seizure disorders • Focal myasthenia gravis causing dysphagia and/or megaoesophagus
Oropharyngeal	• Periodontal disease (gingivitis, stomatitis) • Foreign body/obstruction • Neoplasia • Glossitis • Local irritants: plants containing insoluble calcium oxalate (e.g. *Philodendron* sp., *Dieffenbachia*, *Calladium* sp.), other houseplants (e.g. *Poinsettia*, Kentucky coffee tree), household cleaners • Bitter substances: metronidazole, trimethoprim-sulfamethoxazole, tylosin, tramadol • Candidiasis
Oesophageal	• Obstruction (foreign body, stricture) • Megaoesophagus • Oesophagitis • Spirocercosis
Salivary	• Sialolith • Sialocoele • Neoplasia • Sialadenitis • Sialadenosis • Idiopathic
Gastrointestinal	• Nausea (variety of causes) • Hiatal hernia • Gastric ulceration • Foreign body • Gastric dilatation-volvulus • Gastric adenocarcinoma
Metabolic	• Uraemia • Hepatic encephalopathy (portosystemic shunt, hepatic insufficiency) (more common in cats)
Infectious	• Viral: calicivirus (cats), herpesvirus (cats), rabies, pseudorabies (Aujeszky's disease) • Bacterial (tetanus, botulism) • Fungal (candidiasis)
Immune-mediated	• Lymphoplasmacytic gingivostomatitis (cats) • Chronic ulcerative paradental stomatitis (dogs) • Toxic epidermal necrolysis • Pemphigus vulgaris • Bullous pemphigoid • Masticatory myositis • Polymyositis
Toxins/drugs	• Drugs: opiates, caffeine, zolpidem, tricyclic antidepressants, 5-hydroxytryptophan • Toxins: organophosphates, cholinergics, pyrethrin, pyrethroids, boric acid, zinc phosphide, aldicarb, metaldehyde, *Amanita* mushrooms • Illicit drugs: cocaine, amphetamines • Animal venoms and toxins: black widow spider, coral snake, *Bufo* toad toxin
Behavioural	• Pavlovian: anticipation of food • Emotional: contentment (especially in cats) • Pain response
Trauma	• Temporomandibular dislocation or dyspraxia • Mandibular or maxillary fracture

10.2 Differential diagnoses for ptyalism and pseudoptyalism.

History

An acute onset of drooling is most often associated with oropharyngeal foreign bodies, viral infections, toxin/drug exposure or trauma. In patients with chronic drooling, metabolic, neoplastic and periodontal conditions are more likely. The presence of signs of oesophageal or gastrointestinal dysfunction (regurgitation, vomiting, diarrhoea) or weight loss, reduced appetite, coughing, sneezing, difficulty eating or drinking, behavioural changes, neurological dysfunction, or some combination thereof, may reflect systemic disorders and conditions originating outside of the oropharyngeal cavity.

Physical examination

Patients presenting for evaluation of drooling may not have evidence of active drooling during physical examination. In these instances, the hair around the mouth and forepaws should be examined for pink-brown discolouration caused by porphyrin, a pigmented substance abundant in salivary secretions (Figure 10.3). Additionally, evidence of moist dermatitis can be identified in facial skin folds of dogs with excessive drooling. Sanguinous or purulent salivary secretions are indicative of a condition primarily affecting the oropharyngeal cavity.

In all patients presenting for drooling, complete examination of the oropharyngeal cavity and maxillofacial structures is essential. When an oropharyngeal cause of drooling is suspected, procedural sedation or general anaesthesia is typically required to perform a comprehensive examination, including the teeth, gingiva, palate and sublingual area. Patients requiring anaesthesia for oropharyngeal examination should receive a full neurological assessment (including the gag reflex) and a minimum database (complete blood count, serum biochemistry panel, urinalysis) should be obtained prior to sedation or anaesthetic induction. Neurological assessment of patients with drooling should focus on cranial nerve function, behaviour, level of consciousness, the likelihood of CNS involvement and localization of any neurological lesion. Patients with drooling and signs of neurological dysfunction with an unknown vaccination history, either residing in or imported from countries where rabies is endemic, should be treated with extreme caution due to the risk of human rabies exposure.

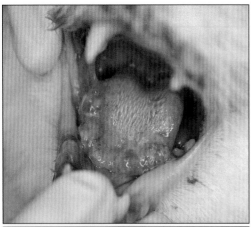

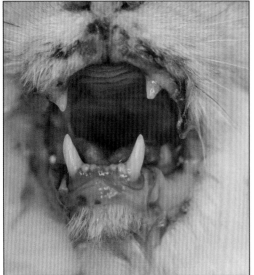

10.3 Ptyalism in a 9-year-old Domestic Shorthaired cat with glossitis. Note the red-brown discolouration of the fur surrounding the mouth caused by salivary porphyrin staining.
(Courtesy of Amy Somrak)

Diagnostic tests

In many cases, a thorough physical examination, emphasizing the oropharyngeal cavity, maxillofacial structures and assessment of neurological function, is sufficient to identify the cause of excessive drooling. Additional diagnostic tests should be utilized on a case-by-case basis to exclude less common differential diagnoses.

Clinical pathology

A minimum clinicopathological database should be assessed in patients presenting for evaluation of drooling, especially when there is no visually identifiable evidence of oropharyngeal disease. The minimum database should include a complete blood count, serum biochemistry panel and urinalysis. In many cases, the results of clinicopathological assessment are unrewarding; however, the benefits of these diagnostics are two-fold:

- They can aid in the exclusion of metabolic causes of ptyalism
- They provide necessary information to gauge the risk of general anaesthesia in patients requiring a full oropharyngeal and periodontal examination.

Patients with uraemia will have increases in serum urea and creatinine concentrations, with or without electrolyte disturbances, and isosthenuria. Hepatic insufficiency and hepatic encephalopathy are often associated with microcytic anaemia, decreased serum concentrations of albumin, glucose, cholesterol and urea, and ammonium biurate crystalluria. Measurement of pre- and postprandial serum bile acids can aid in the assessment of hepatic function. Patients with inflammatory or infectious disease may have inflammatory changes on their leucograms, although a normal leucogram does not exclude such disorders. If a neuromuscular condition is suspected, serum titres of antibodies to the acetylcholine receptor should be measured to rule out myasthenia gravis.

Diagnostic imaging

Patients with regurgitation or clinical signs referable to the respiratory tract benefit from thoracic imaging. In those with signs of gastrointestinal dysfunction, abdominal radiography, ultrasonography or both should be recommended. If the cause of excessive drooling can be localized to the oropharyngeal cavity, salivary glands or maxillofacial structures, advanced imaging of the head may be required. Dental radiographs can aid in the detection of periodontal disorders, while computed tomography of the skull or focused ultrasonographic examination of specific structures (e.g. salivary glands, tongue, lymph nodes) may be required. These advanced imaging modalities may require consultation with or referral to a veterinary diagnostic imaging specialist.

Infectious disease testing

Feline patients should be tested for feline leukaemia and feline immunodeficiency viruses, as they may be associated with secondary infections, neoplasia, ulcerative lesions or gingivostomatitis that can cause drooling. Several laboratories offer diagnostic panels to screen for viruses that can cause lesions in the oral cavity and upper respiratory tract. Rabies can only be excluded as a differential diagnosis by post-mortem analysis of brain tissue. Contact the appropriate local or national health authority if rabies is a differential diagnosis.

Diagnostic procedures

Cytology and histopathology can be useful in the diagnosis of inflammatory, infectious and neoplastic disorders causing drooling. If, during the course of oropharyngeal examination, a mass is identified, cytological analysis of a fine-needle aspirate or tissue impression sample can provide a rapid and inexpensive diagnosis. Brush cytology and scrape samples can also aid in the diagnosis of oral candidiasis. Tissue samples should be collected and preserved in formalin in case cytology does not yield a definitive diagnosis. Histopathology is the diagnostic test of choice for neoplastic and ulcerative lesions identified in the oral cavity and mucocutaneous junctions.

Treatment

Therapeutic management of drooling will depend on its specific cause. Information regarding the treatment of these conditions can be found in their corresponding chapters in this and other veterinary medical texts. A full review of these diverse therapies is beyond the scope of this chapter.

If a lesion affecting a single salivary gland is identified, surgical excision may be a challenging but effective therapeutic option. In cases of idiopathic ptyalism, or those that do not respond to treatment of the underlying disorder causing ptyalism, a variety of symptomatic therapies have been proposed. Anticholinergic drugs (atropine, glycopyrrolate) are effective in reducing the volume of salivary secretions. Some dogs with idiopathic salivary gland enlargement (sialadenosis) and ptyalism often respond to phenobarbital. In humans, injection of botulinum toxin into the salivary gland, radiation therapy, transdermal scopolamine, and acupuncture have been described as adjunct treatments for refractory ptyalism. The use of drug or adjunct therapies for ptyalism should be carefully weighed against the potential for inducing xerostomia and other drug-specific adverse effects. It is prudent to consider these therapies only after a thorough diagnostic evaluation and if ptyalism is significantly impacting quality of life or risk of mortality.

Several non-specific supportive care measures can promote comfort and quality of life in animals with ptyalism. Appropriate analgesic therapy should be provided to any patient with drooling caused by a painful condition. Dogs and cats with lesions causing pain may also benefit from a soft or liquefied diet to reduce pain associated with prehension and chewing. Patients with swallowing dysfunction or other lesions that prevent normal feeding are candidates for assisted enteral nutrition. In those with normal oesophageal function, placement of an oesophagostomy tube offers a minimally invasive and simple method of enteral feeding. Gastrostomy tubes should be placed in patients with oesophageal dysmotility. Petroleum jelly can be applied to skin around the mouth to prevent moist dermatitis.

Zoonotic and public health considerations

Rabies is a universally fatal, zoonotic disease that can cause excessive drooling in affected animals. Any mammal from an endemic country presenting with excessive drooling that has not been vaccinated for rabies, or whose vaccination status is unknown, should be treated with extreme caution, especially when concurrent neurological or behavioural changes are identified. Contact the appropriate health officials before handling or evaluating patients when rabies is suspected.

References and further reading

Boyce WH and Bakheet MR (2005) Sialorrhea: a review of a vexing, often unrecognized sign of oropharyngeal and esophageal disease. *Journal of Clinical Gastroenterology* **39**, 89–97

Niemiec BA (2013) Local and regional consequences of periodontal disease. In: *Veterinary Periodontology*, ed. BA Niemiec, pp. 69–80. Wiley and Sons, Hoboken

Niemiec BA (2016) Halitosis and ptyalism. In: *Textbook of Veterinary Internal Medicine: Diseases of the Dog and Cat, 8th edn*, ed. SJ Ettinger and EC Feldman. WB Saunders, Philadelphia

Chapter 11

Halitosis

Patrick Barko

Definition of the problem

Halitosis is defined as a noticeably unpleasant odour emitted from the mouth during breathing. Clinically, halitosis can be subdivided into two categories: physiological and pathological. Physiological halitosis is characterized by malodour originating from normal putrefactive processes in the oral cavity in the absence of an identifiable pathological lesion. Physiological halitosis is typically transient and associated with the consumption of odoriferous foods, inadequate oral hygiene, or both. Pathological halitosis is associated with any disease process that can alter the chemical composition of the breath. Pathological halitosis is further designated as oral or extra-oral, depending on its aetiological origin. Halitosis is common in dogs and cats and is a significant cause for concern among pet owners. Persistent or severe halitosis is not normal and warrants diagnostic investigation to determine its cause and implement effective treatment.

Pathophysiology

Halitosis is most likely associated with conditions affecting the oral cavity. The true prevalence of oral halitosis is unknown in dogs, but in humans approximately 87% of halitosis is associated with lesions in the oropharyngeal cavity. Thus, bacterial putrefaction in the oral cavity is considered the most common mechanism of halitosis in small animals. Bacterial metabolism of food debris, saliva, mucus, desquamated epithelial cells and blood substances by anaerobic, Gram-negative bacteria generates malodorous chemicals, including volatile sulphur compounds (VSCs), short-chain fatty acids and diamines (cadaverine and putrescine). Saliva has several properties that inhibit bacterial metabolism and conditions that decrease saliva production (xerostomia) or dry the oral mucous membranes and can promote the generation of malodorous compounds. Transient physiological halitosis results from bacterial metabolism, of food debris after a meal. Pathological conditions causing halitosis are associated with necrosis, infection, inflammation, ulceration and haemorrhage in the oropharyngeal cavity. These conditions cause halitosis by altering the composition of the oral microbiome, increasing the quantity and quality of substrate available for microbial putrefaction, and changing the quantity or chemical composition of salivary secretions.

Extra-oral diseases associated with halitosis result from exhalation of volatile compounds from the respiratory tract or their emission from the gastrointestinal tract. Transient, physiological halitosis can follow the ingestion of certain foods (e.g. garlic) whose volatile metabolites circulate in the blood and are transported across the alveolar capillaries into the breath. Pathological halitosis can originate from volatile compounds generated as a consequence of malabsorption or metabolic disorders, including uraemia, ketosis and hepatic insufficiency. Diseases of the respiratory and digestive tract cause halitosis due to the generation of malodorous compounds within their respective lumens. Upper respiratory diseases resulting in post-nasal drip and nasopharyngeal obstruction cause halitosis due to the accumulation of respiratory secretions and mucus in the caudal oropharynx and dehydration of the oropharyngeal mucosa due to open-mouthed breathing, respectively. Lower respiratory tract diseases, including bronchitis, asthma, bronchiectasis, pneumonia, bronchial foreign bodies, abscesses and neoplasia, can cause halitosis as a result of the accumulation of respiratory secretions, tissue necrosis, haemorrhage and ulceration, as well as putrefaction of inhaled plant material or food.

Differential diagnoses

Diseases listed in Figure 11.1 have been associated with halitosis in small animals and/or humans. Due to a paucity of studies in small animals, some of these have not been described in dogs and cats. However, the likelihood that they could contribute to halitosis in small animals warrants their consideration in its diagnostic investigation.

Affected body system	Specific disease
Oropharyngeal cavity	• Physiological 　• Poor oral hygiene 　• Consumption of malodorous foods 　• Mouth breathing 　• Coprophagia 　• Anal licking • Pathological 　• Periodontitis 　• Gingivitis 　• Tonsillitis 　• Pharyngitis 　• Dental abscessation 　• Oronasal fistulae 　• Neoplasia 　• Xerostomia

11.1 Differential diagnoses for halitosis. (continues) ▶

BSAVA Manual of Canine and Feline Gastroenterology, third edition. Edited by Edward J. Hall, David A. Williams and Aarti Kathrani. ©BSAVA 2020

Affected body system	Specific disease
Metabolic	• Uraemia • Ketosis • Hepatic insufficiency
Upper respiratory	• Rhinitis • Nasal obstruction (foreign body, neoplasia) • Neoplasia
Lower respiratory	• Inflammatory airway disease (bronchitis, asthma) • Pneumonia • Neoplasia • Foreign body • Bronchiectasis • Abscessation • Broncho-oesophageal fistula
Gastrointestinal	• Oesophageal foreign body • Gastroesophageal reflux disease • Gastric ulceration • Gastritis associated with *Helicobacter* infection • Proximal gastrointestinal obstruction (pylorus, duodenum) • Malabsorption

11.1 (continued) Differential diagnoses for halitosis.

Signalment, history and physical examination

Signalment

Small-breed dogs have an increased risk of halitosis due to their predisposition for periodontal disease, because of their small mouths with teeth that are closer together than larger dogs. These factors promote the development of tartar and plaque, which favours bacterial putrefaction of food debris. The likelihood of periodontitis, oral neoplasia and metabolic disorders increases with age.

History

Dog and cat owners commonly observe halitosis in a home environment because of their frequent and often intimate contact with their pet. An owner's ability to detect halitosis is likely to be associated with their willingness to allow their pet to lick them. Owners who are willing and able to examine and brush their pet's teeth at home are also more likely to notice halitosis. As halitosis is often associated with other diseases of the oral cavity, affected animals may also present for examination of pain or difficulty while eating, ptyalism, haemorrhage or purulent oronasal discharge, reduced appetite, or some combination thereof. Animals with metabolic causes of halitosis may present with lethargy, anorexia and vomiting. Respiratory disorders associated with halitosis can manifest as coughing, sneezing, nasal discharge, open-mouth breathing and increased respiratory rate. Patients with gastrointestinal conditions can be presented for evaluation of abdominal pain, vomiting, diarrhoea and anorexia.

Physical examination

In all patients presenting for halitosis, complete examination of the oropharyngeal cavity is essential. When an oropharyngeal cause of halitosis is suspected, procedural sedation or general anaesthesia is typically required to perform a comprehensive examination including the teeth, gingiva, palate and sublingual area. Figures 11.2–11.4 represent gross findings of various oral lesions associated

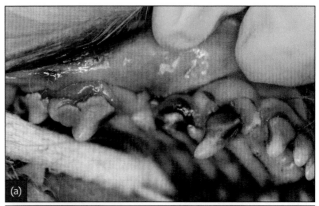
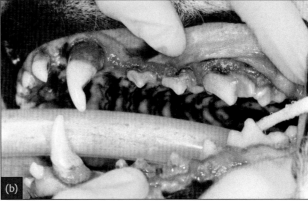

11.2 Periodontitis is a common cause of halitosis. (a) A 5-year-old Maltese dog with severe periodontitis, dental calculus and gingival haemorrhage. (b) A 6.5-year-old mixed-breed dog with severe periodontitis, gingivitis and dental calculus.
(Courtesy of Amy Somrak)

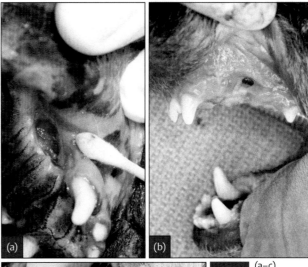

11.3 (a–c) Oronasal fistulae in three dogs.
(Courtesy of Amy Somrak)

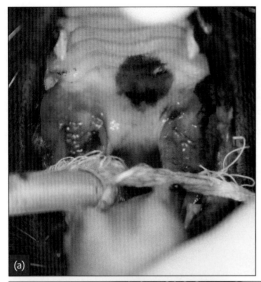

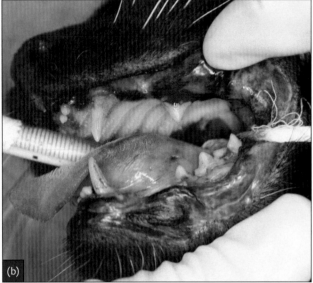

11.4 (a, b) Gingivostomatitis in a 7.5-year-old castrated male Domestic Shorthaired cat.
(Courtesy of Amy Somrak)

with halitosis. Patients requiring anaesthesia for oropharyngeal examination should receive a full minimum database (complete blood count, serum biochemistry panel, urinalysis) prior to sedation or anaesthetic induction to screen for metabolic causes of halitosis.

Diagnostic tests

Assessment of volatile and odoriferous compounds in the breath

In humans, halitosis was traditionally diagnosed via organoleptic assessment. Applied in a formal and clinical setting, this method requires an affected individual to exhale into a tube through a privacy barrier and an observer trained in scent detection and characterization to smell their breath and determine the severity of halitosis on a numerical scale. Informal versions of this method, where a pet owner or veterinary surgeon (veterinarian) detects halitosis by smelling an animal's breath, are the most common methods used to detect halitosis in small animals. The subjective nature of the organoleptic method has led to the development of quantitative techniques for measuring volatile compounds in the breath. The most sensitive of these is gas chromatography (GC). The technical complexity of GC typically precludes its clinical practicality; however, a portable GC device has recently been used to assess the efficacy of dietary intervention in dogs with halitosis (DiCerbo et al., 2015). Portable electrochemical sensors that measure VSCs in the breath can provide rapid, quantitative assessment of halitosis. This method has been used to demonstrate a correlation between VSC concentrations in the breath and organoleptic severity of halitosis in dogs (Rawlings and Culham, 1998). Although GC and electrochemical instruments provide an objective, quantitative assessment of halitosis, these methods are not widely available or practical in a clinical setting. Modifications or informal versions of the organoleptic method are likely to remain the most practical screening methods for halitosis in small animals.

Clinical pathology

Clinicopathological assessment of halitosis is useful in detecting metabolic disorders that can affect the chemical composition of the breath. Assessment of a serum biochemistry panel and urinalysis are the most useful means of screening for metabolic syndromes implicated in the development of halitosis. Measurement of fasting hyperglycaemia, glucosuria and ketonuria is consistent with diabetic ketosis and should prompt a more thorough evaluation for diabetes mellitus. Patients with uraemia will have increases in serum urea and creatinine concentrations, with or without electrolyte disturbances, and isosthenuria. Hepatic insufficiency is often associated with microcytic anaemia, decreased serum concentrations of albumin, glucose, cholesterol and urea, and ammonium biurate crystalluria. Measurement of pre- and postprandial serum bile acids can aid in the assessment of hepatic function.

Diagnostic imaging

If the cause of halitosis is localized to the oropharyngeal cavity, advanced diagnostic imaging may be required. Dental radiographs are a sensitive means of detecting pathology involving the tooth roots and surrounding bone. A gross examination lacking dental radiography will fail to identify approximately 50% of dental lesions. In addition to their diagnostic utility, dental radiographs are essential in ensuring that no tooth root fragments remain following dental extraction. In patients with clinical signs of nasal cavity disease and in those where oral examination and dental radiography are unrewarding, computed tomography (CT) scans of the skull may be required. Patients with clinical signs referable to the lower respiratory tract benefit from thoracic radiography or CT. In those with signs of gastrointestinal obstruction or dysfunction, abdominal radiography, ultrasonography or both should be recommended.

Diagnostic procedures

The most useful procedure for the diagnosis of halitosis is a comprehensive oral examination under general anaesthesia. For ulcerative lesions and masses, cytological analysis can provide a rapid and inexpensive diagnosis. Tissue samples should be collected and preserved in formalin in case cytology does not yield a definitive diagnosis. Histopathology is the diagnostic test of choice for neoplastic and ulcerative lesions identified in the oral cavity and mucocutaneous junctions.

Treatment

Therapeutic management of halitosis will depend on the specific cause. Information regarding treatment of these conditions can be found in their corresponding chapters in this and other veterinary medical texts. A full review of these diverse therapies is beyond the scope of this chapter. In cases of periodontitis, a comprehensive dental cleaning should include subgingival scaling and polishing. Dental extractions may be required to treat infected tooth roots or otherwise non-viable teeth. Routine dental prophylaxis, daily brushing of teeth and the use of chlorhexidine rinses and medicated chew toys can reduce halitosis associated with oral cavity disease. Oronasal fistulae should be treated surgically and closure of the defect may require mucoperiosteal, buccal or palatal flap grafts (see the *BSAVA Manual of Canine and Feline Dentistry and Oral Surgery* and *BSAVA Manual of Canine and Feline Head, Neck and Thoracic Surgery*). The majority of oronasal infections are caused by opportunistic commensal microbes and resolve after correction of the underlying disorder. However, antibiotic therapy may be required in some cases to manage severe infections or in patients with infectious respiratory or gastrointestinal disease.

Selection of an appropriate antimicrobial agent should be based on the results of culture and sensitivity testing whenever possible.

References and further reading

Brockman D, Holt D and ter Haar G (2018) *BSAVA Manual of Canine and Feline Head, Neck and Thoracic Surgery, 2nd edn.* BSAVA Publications, Gloucester

Di Cerbo A, Pezzuto F, Canello S, Guidetti G and Palmieri B (2015) Therapeutic effectiveness of a dietary supplement for management of halitosis in dogs. *Journal of Visualized Experiments* **101**, e52717

Eubanks DL (2009) Doggy breath: what causes it, how do I evaluate it, and what can I do about it? *Journal of Veterinary Dentistry* **26**, 192–193

Madhushankari GS, Yamunadevi A, Selvamani M, Mohan Kumar KP and Basandi PS (2015) Halitosis – an overview: Part–I–Classification, etiology, and pathophysiology of halitosis. *Journal of Pharmacy and Bioallied Sciences* **7**, 339–343

Murata T, Yamaga T, Iida T, Miyazaki H and Yaegaki K (2002) Classification and examination of halitosis. *International Dental Journal* **52**, 181–186

Niemiec BA (2013) Local and regional consequences of periodontal disease. In: *Veterinary Periodontology*, ed. BA Niemiec, pp. 69–80. J Wiley and Sons, Hoboken

Niemiec BA (2016) Halitosis and ptyalism. In: *Textbook of Veterinary Internal Medicine: Diseases of the Dog and Cat, 8th edn.* ed. SJ Ettinger and EC Feldman. WB Saunders, Philadelphia

Rawlings JM and Culham N (1998) Halitosis in dogs and the effect of periodontal therapy. *Journal of Nutrition* **128**, 2715–2716

Reiter AM and Gracis M (2018) *BSAVA Manual of Canine and Feline Dentistry and Oral Surgery, 4th edn.* BSAVA Publications, Gloucester

Chapter 12

Dysphagia

Aarti Kathrani

Definition of the problem

Dysphagia is the medical term for difficulty swallowing. The causes of dysphagia can be subdivided into functional (e.g. secondary to a neurological or muscular abnormality of the swallowing reflex) or structural (e.g. secondary to a stricture, traumatic injury, foreign body or neoplasia involving the oropharynx or oesophagus). Dysphagia can also be further subdivided into oral dysphagia, pharyngeal dysphagia and oesophageal dysphagia, depending on the localization of the structural or functional abnormality. The various causes of dysphagia in dogs and cats are illustrated in Figure 12.1.

Pathogenesis, clinical signs and possible causes

Oral dysphagia

Oral dysphagia occurs when there are abnormalities of prehension, mastication, lubrication or transportation of food from the tongue to the pharynx. Clinically, oral dysphagia may manifest as difficulty prehending or masticating food or an inability for food to pass to the base of the tongue. Possible aetiologies include:

- Dental disease
- Lingual disease
- Oral neoplasia
- Oral ulceration
- Masticatory myopathy
- Difficulty opening the jaw resulting from mandibular or maxillary fracture
- Retrobulbar abscess
- Craniomandibular osteopathy
- Temporomandibular joint disease or trigeminal neuritis.

Pharyngeal dysphagia

Pharyngeal dysphagia occurs when the food bolus cannot be advanced from the oropharynx, through the hypopharynx and into the proximal oesophagus. Cricopharyngeal dysphagia is difficulty in passage of the food bolus through the upper oesophageal sphincter. It is either due to a partial or complete lack of opening or relaxation of the

Cause	Oral dysphagia	Pharyngeal dysphagia	Oesophageal dysphagia
Functional	Rabies Masticatory myositis Peripheral neuropathy CNS disease	Rabies Botulism Tetanus Cricopharyngeal asynchrony Polyradiculoneuritis Peripheral neuropathy CNS disease Polymyositis Myasthenia gravis	Botulism Tetanus Distemper Polyradiculoneuritis Peripheral neuropathy CNS disease Polymyositis Myasthenia gravis Megaoesophagus Hiatal hernia
Structural	Dental disease Oronasal fistula Stomatitis Ulcer Foreign body Mass Neoplasia Retrobulbar abscess Lingual frenulum disorder Cleft palate Temporomandibular joint disease Trauma (fracture, luxation) Glossitis Craniomandibular osteopathy	Foreign body Neoplasia Abscess Polyp Granuloma Cricopharyngeal achalasia Pharyngitis	Foreign body Neoplasia Oesophagitis Diverticulum Stricture Spirocercosis Vascular ring anomaly

12.1 Differential diagnoses for dysphagia in dogs and cats, separated into functional and structural causes with localization. CNS = central nervous system.

upper oesophageal sphincter (structural; cricopharyngeal achalasia), or from inappropriate timing of its opening or relaxation (functional; cricopharyngeal asynchrony). Clinically, pharyngeal dysphagia may present with repetitive swallowing attempts, gagging or retching, nasal regurgitation of food, coughing related to swallowing, excessive head movements and dropping of food from the mouth during swallowing. Possible aetiologies include:

- Pharyngeal foreign body
- Neoplasia
- Ulceration or neuromuscular disease
- Cricopharyngeal dysphagia.

Oesophageal dysphagia

Oesophageal dysphagia is difficulty in passage of the food bolus down the oesophagus. Regurgitation is associated with oesophageal dysphagia (see Chapter 32). Possible aetiologies include:

- Oesophageal foreign body
- Neoplasia
- Stricture or diverticulum
- Oesophagitis
- Megaoesophagus
- Hiatal hernia
- Vascular ring anomaly.

Signalment, history and physical examination

Signalment

Young dogs are more likely to be presented with congenital abnormalities, such as vascular ring anomaly or cricopharyngeal achalasia, which may be first apparent at weaning. Ingestion of a foreign body or caustic agent is more likely in young to middle-aged animals. Geriatric large-breed dogs can exhibit a progressive neuropathy with associated pharyngeal weakness, pharyngeal dysphagia and oesophageal dysfunction (Stanley *et al.*, 2010). Cats with dysphagia are more likely to have a structural disorder, such as an oral tumour, ulcer or stomatitis. Dog breeds that have a predisposition to pharyngeal dysphagia include:

- Golden Retriever for pharyngeal weakness
- Cocker Spaniel and Springer Spaniel for cricopharyngeal dysphagia
- Bouvier des Flandres and Cavalier King Charles Spaniel for muscular dystrophy
- English Bulldog and French Bulldog for redundant oesophagus
- German Shepherd Dog for vascular ring anomaly
- Boxer for inflammatory myopathy
- Boston Terriers and Pugs for hiatal hernia.

History

Determining the exact clinical signs an animal with dysphagia is exhibiting may help to localize the dysphagia as oral, pharyngeal or oesophageal (see above). It is also important to ascertain whether the animal is coughing or has a high respiratory rate or difficulty breathing, as animals with dysphagia can present with concurrent aspiration pneumonia, which is a complication that may occur with any form of dysphagia. Dehydration and/or weight loss may also be noted due to decreased water or caloric intake, respectively.

Collection of a detailed medication history is important to rule out oesophagitis or stricture caused by oral doxycycline or clindamycin administration. Similarly, enquiring about any recent general anaesthesia is important, as general anaesthesia can result in oesophagitis or stricture due to gastro-oesophageal reflux. Access to foreign bodies and caustic agents should be ruled out, and travel history to countries with endemic rabies should be excluded in all animals with dysphagia.

Physical examination

Physical examination of the dysphagic animal must include careful palpation of the pharynx and neck to assess for masses, asymmetry or pain. The thorax should be auscultated thoroughly to assess for any abnormalities associated with aspiration pneumonia. A thorough neurological examination, including evaluation of cranial nerves, should be performed, together with assessment of the tongue, jaw tone and gag reflex. If neurological deficits are present with dysphagia, a nervous system disorder, such as a neuropathy, neuromuscular junction disorder or myopathy, is more likely. A complete oral and laryngeal examination under sedation or general anaesthesia is essential to rule out obstructions (e.g. foreign body, mass), inflammatory processes (e.g. stomatitis, dental disease), anatomical abnormalities (e.g. cleft palate, lingual abnormalities) or laryngeal paralysis (e.g. polyneuropathy).

Diagnostic tests

It is essential to observe the animal eating and drinking to help localize the dysphagia to oral, pharyngeal or oesophageal. Oral dysphagia can often be diagnosed by watching the animal eat or by physical or neurological examination. Unfortunately, animals with pharyngeal dysphagia can be more challenging to diagnose, as they often present with non-specific signs, such as gagging, retching or repetitive swallowing. The presence of regurgitation helps to localize the dysphagia to the oesophagus. The various diagnostic tests that may be considered or performed in animals with dysphagia are listed and explained below. An algorithm for diagnostic testing of a dog or cat with dysphagia is illustrated in Figure 12.2.

Clinical pathology

A complete blood count, biochemistry panel with creatine kinase and electrolytes, and urinalysis should be performed in animals with dysphagia where the underlying cause is not readily apparent after the collection of a history, performance of a physical and neurological examination, and visual assessment of the animal eating and drinking. Collection of a minimum database will allow for assessment of systemic disease as well as general health prior to sedation or general anaesthesia for more advanced diagnostic testing. Measurement of creatine kinase activity may help in the assessment of neuromuscular disease, although a value within the reference range does not rule this out.

A thyroid panel to rule out hypothyroidism as a cause of neuromuscular weakness or megaoesophagus (tentative association), and an acetylcholine receptor antibody titre to rule out myasthenia gravis, which could present as a focal disease in cases of acquired megaoesophagus,

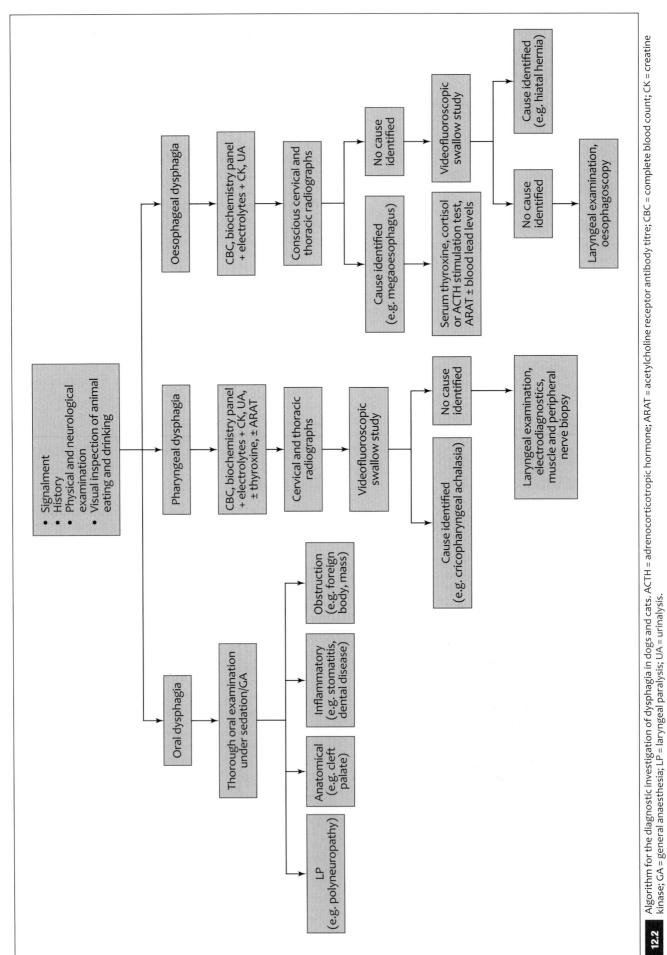

12.2 Algorithm for the diagnostic investigation of dysphagia in dogs and cats. ACTH = adrenocorticotropic hormone; ARAT = acetylcholine receptor antibody titre; CBC = complete blood count; CK = creatine kinase; GA = general anaesthesia; LP = laryngeal paralysis; UA = urinalysis.

should be considered in relevant cases. Also, for cases of acquired megaoesophagus, a basal cortisol or adrenocorticotropic hormone stimulation test and measurement of blood lead levels, if an applicable history of exposure is present, should be considered.

Diagnostic imaging

Radiography

Cervical and thoracic radiographs allow for the assessment of any pharyngeal abnormalities, such as a mass or foreign body, oesophageal abnormalities, such as megaoesophagus, or signs consistent with aspiration pneumonia.

Videofluoroscopic swallow study

This imaging modality is normally only available in a referral setting. It involves real-time capture of images while the conscious animal swallows liquid barium or dry or tinned food mixed with barium. This imaging modality is one of the most important procedures for assessing the functional integrity of the swallow reflex, particularly the function of the pharyngeal and oesophageal phases of swallowing.

Laryngeal examination

A thorough examination of the function of the larynx under a light plane of anaesthesia should be considered in animals with pharyngeal and oesophageal dysphagia to rule out laryngeal paralysis associated with polyneuropathies.

Oesophagoscopy

Performed under general anaesthesia, oesophagoscopy allows for a structural assessment of the oesophagus and is helpful in the diagnosis of oesophagitis, oesophageal stricture, diverticulum, mass or foreign body and hiatal hernia.

Electrodiagnostics

Electrodiagnostics, available in a referral setting, includes electromyography and measurement of motor and sensory nerve conduction velocities. Although this diagnostic modality does not provide a specific diagnosis in most cases, it can provide important information on the severity, distribution and character of a myopathic or neuropathic disease process, and can also indicate the best site for biopsy. As this diagnostic modality can take some time under general anaesthesia, the animal's health status should be considered before embarking on this test.

Muscle and peripheral nerve biopsy

In an animal with dysphagia suspected to be caused by a neuromuscular disorder, muscle and nerve biopsies may provide a definitive diagnosis and help with prognosis of the disease. However, they should be collected early in the diagnostic investigation process and evaluated by a laboratory with expertise in neuromuscular disease.

Treatment

Treatment should focus on the underlying disease and an accurate diagnosis is therefore important. Dietary management focusing on food consistency and the frequency and position of feeding is important as an adjunctive treatment and for those disorders where the underlying disease cannot be treated. An assisted enteral feeding tube is necessary if the animal cannot meet its daily caloric requirement. Complications, such as aspiration pneumonia, should also be addressed when present.

References and further reading

Lopez J (2016) Dysphagia. In: *Textbook of Veterinary Internal Medicine: Diseases of the Dog and Cat, 8th edn*, ed. SJ Ettinger and EC Feldman, pp. 154–158. WB Saunders, Philadelphia

Marks SL (2014) Oropharyngeal dysphagia. In: *Kirk's Current Veterinary Therapy XV*, ed. JD Bonagura and DC Twedt, pp. 495–500. Elsevier Saunders, St Louis

Stanley BJ, Hauptman JG, Fritz MC, Rosenstein DS and Kinns J (2010) Esophageal dysfunction in dogs with idiopathic laryngeal paralysis: a controlled cohort study. *Veterinary Surgery* **39**, 139–149

Chapter 13

Regurgitation

Aarti Kathrani

Definition of the problem

Regurgitation is defined as the passive expulsion of food or fluid from the oesophagus. Diseases that cause inflammation, obstruction or dysmotility of the oesophagus can disrupt its function, resulting in regurgitation (see Chapter 32). Owners may confuse regurgitation with vomiting, which is a centrally mediated reflex, where gastric or proximal duodenal contents are forcefully expelled. Therefore, careful questioning of the owner is important to help differentiate between the two and to enable formulation of an accurate problem and differential diagnosis list, as well as to help guide diagnostic investigations in the regurgitating animal.

Differential diagnoses

The differential diagnoses for a dog or cat with regurgitation are presented in Figure 13.1. Megaoesophagus is the most common cause of repeated regurgitation in the dog.

Signalment, history and physical examination

Signalment

Young dogs are more likely to be presented for congenital abnormalities, such as vascular ring anomaly or congenital megaoesophagus, which may be first apparent at weaning. Ingestion of foreign bodies or a caustic agent is more likely in young to middle-aged animals. Geriatric large-breed dogs can exhibit a progressive neuropathy with associated pharyngeal weakness, pharyngeal dysphagia and oesophageal dysfunction (Stanley *et al.*, 2010). Labrador Retrievers, Newfoundlands and Chinese Shar Peis have an increased prevalence of congenital megaoesophagus, whereas Great Danes, German Shepherd Dogs and Irish Setters have an increased prevalence of both congenital and idiopathic acquired forms of megaoesophagus. Clinical spirocercosis occurs more often in young adult, large-breed dogs in endemic countries (Mylonakis *et al.*, 2006). As regurgitation is relatively uncommon in cats, vomiting can be anticipated rather than regurgitation in this species.

Category of cause of regurgitation		Cause
Megaoesophagus	Focal	Vascular ring anomaly Stricture
	Generalized	Congenital Idiopathic acquired Hypoadrenocorticism Myasthenia gravis Lead poisoning Botulism Tetanus Hypothyroidism Polyradiculoneuritis Thallium toxicity Gastroesophageal reflux-induced oesophagitis Dermatomyositis
Structural		Foreign body Neoplasia (extra- and intramural oesophageal) Diverticulum Granuloma Stricture
Infectious		Distemper *Spirocerca lupi* *Neospora caninum* *Pythium insidiosum*
Neurological disease		Polyneuropathy Polyneuritis Dysautonomia Organophosphate toxicity
Inflammatory disease		Oesophagitis

13.1 Differential diagnoses for regurgitation in dogs and cats.

History

The history should initially focus on confirming whether the animal is truly regurgitating rather than vomiting. Asking owners to describe the episodes is useful, since with vomiting owners will generally describe abdominal contractions, retching, bile in the vomitus or prodromal signs of nausea, such as salivation or lip smacking. Conversely, with regurgitation owners will generally describe that the animal simply lowers its head and material is expelled with no active effort and, typically, with no associated noise. However, it should be noted that on rare occasions, bile might be seen in regurgitation due to reflux of bile from the stomach into the oesophagus prior to regurgitation. Unfortunately, measuring the pH of the material is not useful in helping to differentiate between vomiting and regurgitation, as in some cases the animal may regurgitate stomach contents, and in some they may vomit bicarbonate-rich fluid from the proximal duodenum. Similarly, the timing of the episode in relation to feeding, or the amount of material produced, does not help to differentiate between regurgitation and vomiting. Whether the material is digested or undigested also does not help in differentiating between the two, as animals may vomit undigested food or regurgitate digested food. If the history is unable to distinguish between regurgitation and vomiting, asking the owner to video record an episode might be helpful.

Enquiring about any recent general anaesthesia and oral administration of doxycycline or clindamycin is important, as these are the most common causes of oesophageal stricture (Davies *et al.*, 2015). Laryngeal paralysis has been associated with oesophageal dysfunction (Stanley *et al.*, 2010). Travel to countries with endemic *Spirocerca lupi* should be included in the history. Additional clinical signs reported by owners may include polyphagia, weight loss, odynophagia, ptyalism, weakness and other neurological abnormalities. If aspiration pneumonia is present, the animal may present with dyspnoea, pyrexia and cough.

Physical examination

Physical examination may reveal a thin body condition score due to decreased caloric intake. The neck should be assessed for any bulging, which could reflect oesophageal dilatation. The thorax should be auscultated thoroughly to assess for potential aspiration pneumonia. A complete neurological examination should be performed to rule out any abnormalities that may occur with myasthenia gravis, neuropathies or myopathies.

Diagnostic testing

An algorithm for diagnostic testing of a dog or cat with regurgitation is presented in Figure 13.2.

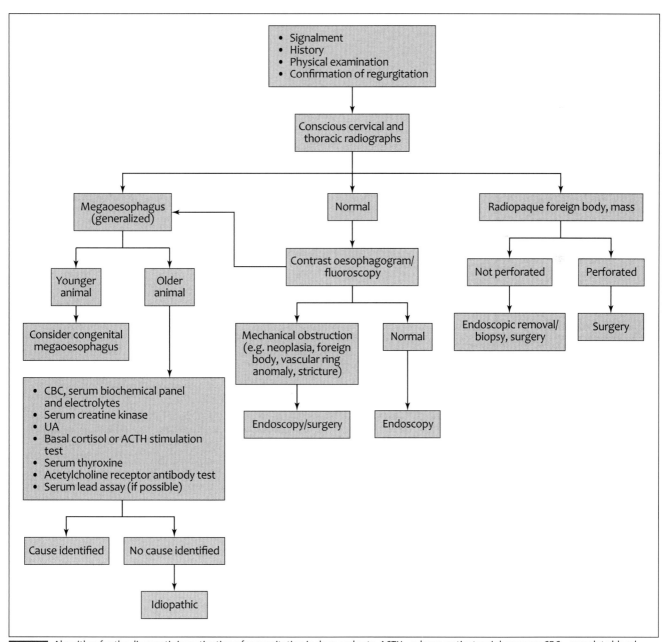

13.2 Algorithm for the diagnostic investigation of regurgitation in dogs and cats. ACTH = adrenocorticotropic hormone; CBC = complete blood count; UA = urinalysis.

Clinical pathology

A minimum database consisting of a complete blood count, serum biochemistry panel with electrolytes and creatine kinase, and urinalysis should be performed if the animal is systemically unwell or megaoesophagus has been diagnosed. Additional testing for confirmed acquired mega-oesophagus cases include a basal cortisol or adrenocorticotropic hormone stimulation test for hypoadrenocorticism, a thyroid panel for hypothyroidism, acetylcholine receptor antibody titre for myasthenia gravis and blood lead concentrations if there is a compatible history of exposure. Faecal analysis should be performed in those cases that have travelled to a *Spirocerca lupi*-endemic country.

Diagnostic imaging

Cervical and thoracic radiographs are recommended to assess for oesophageal dilatation (generalized due to megaoesophagus or focal due to stricture or vascular ring anomaly), radiopaque foreign body, intra- or extraluminal masses, widening of the mediastinum and changes indicative of aspiration pneumonia. Conscious radiographs are necessary for the diagnosis of oesophageal dilatation, as sedation or general anaesthesia may be associated with iatrogenic oesophageal dilatation.

Contrast oesophagogram or videofluoroscopic study

If plain cervical and thoracic radiographs are non-diagnostic, then a contrast oesophagogram or a videofluoroscopic study may be considered. Contrast oesophagograms provide further structural assessment, whereas a videofluoroscopic study is used to better define oesophageal motility.

Laryngeal examination

A thorough examination of laryngeal function under a light plane of anaesthesia should be considered in animals with regurgitation, as laryngeal paralysis has been associated with oesophageal dysfunction (Stanley *et al.*, 2010).

Oesophagoscopy

Endoscopy is a valuable diagnostic tool as it can allow retrieval of foreign bodies, biopsy of masses, treatment of strictures, identification of oesophagitis or hiatal hernia, and placement of a percutaneous gastrostomy tube.

Treatment

Treatment should focus on the underlying disease if possible. Dietary management focusing on food consistency, frequency of feeding and position of feeding is important as an adjunctive treatment and for those disorders where the underlying disease cannot be treated (e.g. congenital or idiopathic acquired megaoesophagus). Trial and error is needed to help determine the right consistency and texture of food for each animal, as this may vary from meatballs to a liquefied diet. For cases of megaoesophagus or oesophageal dysmotility, ensuring the animal is kept upright during and after feeding, either manually or with the aid of a Bailey chair, is recommended to help with the passage of food down the oesophagus (see Chapter 32). A gastrostomy feeding tube may be necessary to ensure adequate caloric intake, as well as to reduce regurgitation episodes. Complications, such as aspiration pneumonia, should also be addressed when present.

Prokinetic drugs, such as cisapride and metoclopramide, should be avoided in dogs with megaoesophagus, as they may make it harder for food to pass into the stomach as they increase lower oesophageal sphincter tone. However, bethanechol may be beneficial in some dogs with oesophageal dysmotility, and sildenafil in dogs with megaoesophagus (Washabau, 2003; Quintavalla *et al.*, 2017). Cisapride may be a more effective prokinetic agent in cats, as it targets cholinergic neurons of the oesophagus (Moses *et al.*, 2000). Animals with primary oesophagitis or gastro-oesophageal reflux disease should be treated with sucralfate and a proton pump inhibitor or H_2-receptor antagonist to reduce gastric acid, together with a prokinetic agent to increase lower oesophageal sphincter tone and a low-fat diet to reduce gastric retention.

References and further reading

Davies JA, Fransson BA, Davis AM, Gilbertsen AM and Gay LM (2015) Incidence of and risk factors for postoperative regurgitation and vomiting in dogs: 244 cases (2000–2012). *Journal of the American Veterinary Medical Association* **246**, 327–335

Gallagher A (2016) Vomiting and regurgitation. In: *Textbook of Veterinary Internal Medicine: Diseases of the Dog and Cat, 8th edn*, ed. SJ Ettinger and EC Feldman, pp. 158–164. WB Saunders, Philadelphia

Hillsman S and Tolbert K (2018) Differential diagnosis: regurgitation. *Clinician's Brief* **16**, 21

Johnson BM, DeNovo RC and Mears EA (2009) Canine megaesophagus. In: *Kirk's Current Veterinary Therapy XIV*, ed. JD Bonagura and DC Twedt, pp. 486–492. Elsevier Saunders, St Louis

Lopez J (2016). Dysphagia. In: *Textbook of Veterinary Internal Medicine: Diseases of the Dog and Cat, 8th edn*, ed. SJ Ettinger and EC Feldman, pp. 154–158. WB Saunders, Philadelphia

Moses L, Harpster NK, Beck KA and Hartzband L (2000) Esophageal motility dysfunction in cats: a study of 44 cases. *Journal of the American Animal Hospital Association* **36**, 309–312

Mylonakis ME, Rallis T, Koutinas AF *et al.* (2006) Clinical signs and clinicopathologic abnormalities in dogs with clinical spirocercosis: 39 cases (1996–2004). *Journal of the American Veterinary Medical Association* **228**, 1063–1067

Quintavalla F, Menozzi A, Pozzoli C *et al.* (2017) Sildenafil improves clinical signs and radiographic features in dogs with congenital idiopathic megaoesophagus: a randomised controlled trial. *Veterinary Record* **180**, 404

Stanley BJ, Hauptman JG, Fritz MC, Rosenstein DS and Kinns J (2010) Esophageal dysfunction in dogs with idiopathic laryngeal paralysis: a controlled cohort study. *Veterinary Surgery* **39**, 139–149

Washabau RJ (2003) Gastrointestinal motility disorders and gastrointestinal prokinetic therapy. *Veterinary Clinics of North America: Small Animal Practice* **33**, 1007–1028

Chapter 14

Acute vomiting

Clive Elwood

Definition of the problem

Vomiting is a reflex, facilitated by a sequence of programmed, overlapping events coordinated centrally in the brainstem, which reduce the risks of adverse consequences (such as aspiration of acidic stomach contents) whilst achieving elimination of noxious substances.

Vomiting comprises 'prodromal' (often accompanied by signs of nausea), 'retching' and 'expulsion' phases. The reflex is controlled within the brainstem in the 'vomiting centre', which receives inputs from peripheral receptors in the abdomen and pharynx via the vagus nerve and glossopharyngeal nerves, respectively, the 'chemoreceptor trigger zone' of the brainstem, the vestibular system and, possibly, higher centres of the brain. The activities associated with the events include:

- Hypersalivation
- Increased swallowing and relaxation of the lower oesophageal sphincter
- Retrograde duodenal peristalsis
- Relaxation of the cardia
- Increased abdominal pressure
- Closure of the glottis.

The reflex action of vomiting should be distinguished from regurgitation (see Chapter 13).

The majority (up to 85%) of acute gastrointestinal upsets (vomiting and/or diarrhoea, with or without haemorrhage) are self-limiting and require variable amounts of supportive and symptomatic treatment without extensive investigation. Careful application of history taking and physical examination skills, combined with a logical and proportionate approach, should determine the severity of the disease process and differentiate those patients in which outpatient or no treatment is necessary, those which need to be supported (e.g. with intravenous fluids or enteral nutrition) and treated symptomatically (e.g. with antiemetics) and those which need further diagnostic testing and/or specific treatment. In addition, this initial assessment may give clear indications of the underlying cause of the vomiting.

'Acute' vomiting is vomiting that has been evident for less than 3–4 weeks. The distinction between acute and chronic vomiting (see Chapter 15 for a discussion of the approach to chronic vomiting) is not of critical importance excepting that most self-limiting causes of acute vomiting will have resolved within 3 weeks and, if they have not, alternatives should be considered. The differential diagnoses for acute vomiting are shown in Figure 14.1.

Gastrointestinal (GI) conditions

- Acute self-limiting vomiting/diarrhoea (with or without haemorrhage)
- Sialadenitis/salivary gland infarction (not truly GI)
- Gastric ulceration
  - Non-steroidal anti-inflammatory drugs (NSAIDs)
  - Metabolic
  - Irritant
  - Endocrine
- Gastric/intestinal entrapment
  - Ruptured diaphragm
  - Adhesions
- Gastric dilatation-volvulus
- Feline acute haemorrhagic vomiting syndrome
- Foreign body (gastric or intestinal)
- Infection/infestation
  - Canine parvovirus
  - Canine distemper virus
  - Feline parvovirus
  - Salmonellosis
  - Helminthiosis
  - Toxoplasmosis (cat)
  - Leptospirosis
  - Coronavirus (canine and feline)
- Intussusception
- Intestinal volvulus
- Intestinal infarction

Abdominal conditions

- Peritonitis
  - Septic
  - Bile
  - Urine
  - Idiopathic
- Hepatobiliary disease
  - Hepatitis
  - Infectious
  - Immune
  - Toxic
  - Metabolic
  - Cholangiohepatitis
  - Gall bladder mucocoele
  - Cholangitis
  - Cholelithiasis
  - Lobe torsion
  - Abscess
- Splenic
  - Torsion
  - Abscess
  - Infarction
- Pancreatic
  - Pancreatitis
- Renal
  - Pyelonephritis
  - Nephrolithiasis

14.1 Differential diagnoses for acute vomiting in dogs and cats. (continues) ▶

Abdominal conditions *continued*

- Urogenital
  - Pyometritis
  - Metritis
  - Prostatitis/prostatic abscess
  - Uterine rupture
  - Ureterolithiasis

Systemic conditions

- Metabolic
  - Uraemia
  - Ketoacidosis
  - Hepatic encephalopathy
  - Hypoadrenocorticism
  - Hypercalcaemia
  - Hypokalaemia
  - Hyper/hyponatraemia
  - Septicaemia
  - Hyperviscosity syndrome
- Endocrine
  - Hypoadrenocorticism
  - Hyperthyroidism
- Toxic
  - Lead
  - Ethylene glycol
  - Ethanol
  - Theobromine
  - Many others
- Drugs
  - Chemotherapeutics
  - Digoxin
  - Erythromycin
  - Many others

Neurological diseases

- Trauma
- Meningitis
- Encephalitis
- Motion sickness
- Vestibular disease
  - Idiopathic peripheral vestibular syndrome
  - Otitis interna
- Cerebellar disease
  - Infarction
- Visceral epilepsy
- Sialadenosis (retching)

14.1 (continued) Differential diagnoses for acute vomiting in dogs and cats.

- Persistent non-productive retching
- Peracute onset
- Sudden abdominal distension
- Abnormal behaviours (e.g. hiding, circling, aggression)
- Marked malaise
- Marked abdominal pain (e.g. withdrawal, relief postures)
- Haematemesis
- Inability to retain food in the stomach
- Fever
- Polyuria/polydipsia
- Stranguria
- Severe dehydration/hypovolaemia/shock
- Bradycardia

14.2 Clinical signs potentially indicative of more severe disease in dogs and cats with acute vomiting.

contain fresh or digested blood, or fragments of a foreign body, may be of note. Voluminous, frequent, green liquid vomitus, which may be refluxed passively as well as vomited, can be seen with upper small intestinal obstruction.

The patient's general management and living environment may be relevant. An indoor-only cat, for example, will be at reduced risk of infectious disease, whereas a relatively free-roaming dog may be at increased risk of dietary indiscretion and toxin exposure. Exposure to potential infections, such as viral enteritis, should be considered. The travel history and vaccination and worming status of any patient, but particularly puppies and kittens, is important, as is their provenance. In some circumstances, accurate records cannot be assumed, and certification may not be proof of effective vaccination. In vulnerable puppies and kittens, caution might dictate a more proactive approach to diagnosis and management if the clinical suspicion of infectious disease is high.

Clients should be questioned about access to, and disappearance of, toys or other objects (e.g. indigestible foodstuffs) that could act as foreign bodies. Similarly, the potential for exposure to toxins, such as ethylene glycol, or any ongoing drug therapy, should be explored.

Recent changes of diet or known dietary indiscretion might be relevant and be considered as triggers of acute vomiting.

In entire bitches, an oestrus in the previous few weeks, polydipsia and resolving or persistent vaginal discharge should alert to the possibility of a pyometra.

Owners should also be questioned about other signs that might accompany vomiting, such as abdominal enlargement, diarrhoea, weakness, anorexia or inappetence, ptyalism (an indicator of nausea, but can also accompany swallowing problems and feline hepatic encephalopathy) (see Chapter 10), neurological signs (particularly loss of balance, gait abnormalities and head tilt that can accompany vestibular disease) and abnormal urination, all of which might point the clinician in a particular direction for investigation and management.

Signalment and history

The initial history should attempt to clarify whether the presenting signs represent regurgitation or vomiting. Vomiting is an active reflex process with a predictable sequence of events, whereas regurgitation is a passive event in which (typically) undigested food and/or saliva is returned under the influence of gravity, often unexpectedly. Owners should be questioned about the presence of the prodromal signs nausea, retching and abdominal contraction, which typically accompany vomiting. The distinction between vomiting and regurgitation can be less clear in cats than in dogs and, in cats, megaoesophagus, oesophagitis or hiatal hernia are often reported as 'vomiting'.

The signalment of the patient presenting with acute vomiting is important. Infectious disease and foreign bodies may be more likely in kittens and puppies. Certain breeds of dog, such as Bearded Collies and Nova Scotia Duck Tolling Retrievers, have increased incidence of hypoadrenocorticism, and older entire female dogs are at risk of pyometra.

Historical features that indicate potentially more severe or complex disease than an acute self-limiting condition are shown in Figure 14.2. A vomitus which is reported to

Physical examination

As with history taking, physical examination skills in the acutely vomiting dog or cat should primarily be applied to the question 'Is there any reason not to manage this as a probable acute self-limiting condition?'. General demeanour should be assessed by observation during history taking and demonstration of signs such as relief postures (Figure 14.3) noted.

Body temperature may be elevated with viral and bacterial enteritis or other sources of pyrogens, such as

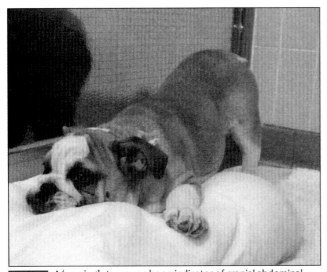

14.3 A 'praying' stance can be an indicator of cranial abdominal pain.

(Reproduced from the BSAVA Manual of Canine and Feline Anaesthesia and Analgesia)

inflammation (e.g. pancreatitis) or focal infections of specific organs of the abdominal cavity. Subnormal body temperature may accompany shock and dehydration and, in cats, can be seen in severe sepsis.

Heart and pulse rate should be assessed and related to each other as well as other indicators of circulatory status, such as pulse strength, mucous membrane colour, mucous membrane hydration and capillary refill time. Tachycardia, particularly with dry mucous membranes and weak pulse strength, may be an indicator of hypovolaemia/hypotension. Tachycardia with a dysrhythmia in a vomiting patient could be due to systemic inflammatory disease, such as pancreatitis, splenic disease, metabolic disease (e.g. electrolyte disturbances) or, potentially, toxicities. Bradycardia (absolute or relative) in the face of other signs suggestive or anticipatory of shock should be recognized because it can be seen with serious electrolyte disturbances, for example, hyperkalaemia in hypoadrenocorticism.

Mucous membrane colour should be assessed for pallor (anaemia, hypovolaemia), icterus (most likely indicating hepatobiliary or post-hepatic disease in the vomiting patient) and increased redness or injection of capillaries (systemic inflammatory responses). Capillary refill time can be increased with hypovolaemia and decreased with sepsis. Decreased skin turgor can be indicative of dehydration and the need for hydration support.

The mouth should be opened and the oral cavity thoroughly examined, including elevation of the tongue. In cats particularly, linear foreign bodies may be seen fixed under or cutting into the base of the tongue.

Halitosis can be an indicator for the presence of necrosis in the oral cavity, pharynx or oesophagus, for example, due to a foreign body or necrosis of the salivary glands. In acute uraemic syndrome, uraemic breath may be detected and in ketotic syndrome some people can smell the ketones.

The submandibular area should be palpated for salivary gland enlargement/discomfort, which can be indicative of sialadenosis in dogs. Peripheral lymph nodes should be palpated for enlargement, which could accompany, for example, haematological malignancies such as lymphoma.

Respiratory signs (tachypnoea, hyperpnoea, dyspnoea, coughing) should be noted and could indicate a more generalized systemic illness or complications of vomiting such as aspiration pneumonia.

Abdominal palpation is a key clinical skill and can be used to suggest and locate abdominal pain, organ enlargement, focal thickenings, masses and abdominal fluid. Palpation of the cranial abdomen may be facilitated by having the patient in an upright stance with the head elevated (Figure 14.4). When there is marked abdominal pain, complete boarding or splinting (i.e. rigidity) of the abdominal musculature may prevent localization but, more typically, careful gentle pressure can be applied with the fingers or fingertips to indicate possible sources of pain and discomfort. Although not definitive, localizing the pain can be possible and can suggest which organs may be involved (Figure 14.5). Often, particularly in cats and smaller (or less deep-chested) dogs, intestinal foreign bodies do not cause generalized pain and may be readily identified sitting within a loop of intestine. A swollen abdomen with tympani and pain may indicate gaseous distension ('bloat'), which may need immediate relief, and, if accompanied by gastric or intestinal volvulus, can be a true life-threatening emergency.

The presence of peritoneal fluid may be suspected by perceiving a round, distended abdomen and a 'fluid thrill/wave' palpable across the abdominal cavity when the opposite side is tapped. These signs can also be present when loops of intestine are fluid filled. In the presence of significant amounts of abdominal fluid, organ enlargements may still be perceived by ballottement. Abdominal fluid can be apparent with protein-losing enteropathy, protein-losing nephropathy, acute hepatic disease, acute pancreatitis, neoplasia, bile peritonitis, a ruptured urinary bladder, acute septic peritonitis and intra-abdominal bleeding, amongst other possibilities (see Chapter 24).

The anus and perianal region should be examined for signs of faecal staining that might indicate diarrhoea, or sometimes the presence of linear foreign bodies. Similarly, where possible, a rectal examination should be performed to include prostatic or vaginal palpation per rectum. Faeces should be visually inspected for consistency and the presence of melaena, haematochezia or worms.

Vaginal discharge should be identified. Purulent and mucopurulent vaginal discharge can be seen in bitches with pyometritis and metritis.

Neurological examination may be appropriate to confirm deficits that can accompany neurogenic sources of vomiting such as a head tilt, nystagmus and/or gait abnormalities, which can be seen with acute vestibular events (e.g. idiopathic peripheral vestibular syndrome or cerebellar infarction).

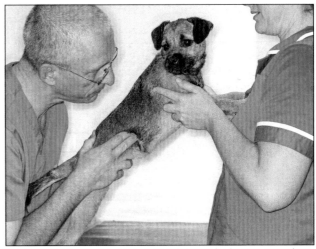

14.4 Raising the front legs during abdominal palpation can make it easier to identify cranial abdominal organs.

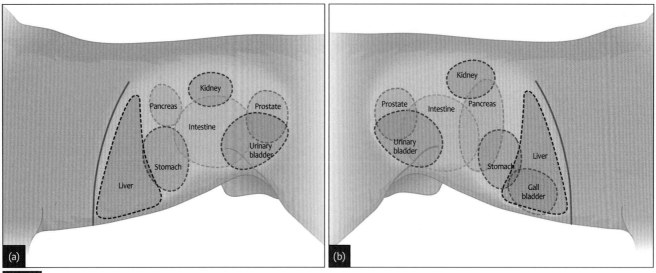

14.5 Approximate location of abdominal organs and associated pain on abdominal palpation in dogs and cats. (a) Left side. (b) Right side.

Diagnostic tests

Clinical decision making in acute vomiting is initially aimed at determining whether or not supportive and symptomatic treatment is sufficient (Figure 14.6). Otherwise, depending on historical and physical findings, certain diagnostic tests (Figure 14.7) may be appropriate.

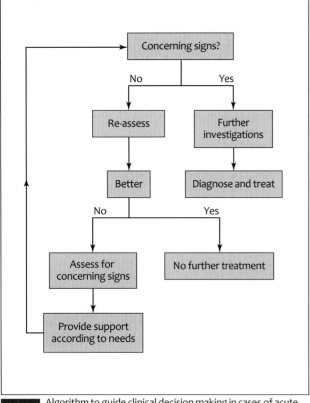

14.6 Algorithm to guide clinical decision making in cases of acute vomiting in dogs and cats.

- Packed cell volume/total protein
- Haematology (red and white cell indices)
- Serum electrolytes
- Blood lactate
- Serum total and ionized calcium
- Plasma urea, creatinine, SDMA
- Liver enzymes (ALT, ALP, AST, GGT)
- Urinalysis (specific gravity, bilirubin, blood cells, ketones, glucose, protein)
- Faecal analysis (microscopy, parasitology, culture, ELISA, e.g. for parvovirus)
- Serology for infectious disease (e.g. leptospirosis, toxoplasmosis)
- Canine or feline pancreatic lipase immunoreactivity
- Serum cobalamin and folate
- Bile acid stimulation test
- ACTH stimulation test
- Serum thyroxine/free thyroxine (free T4)
- Serum toxin screens
- Abdominal radiography
- Contrast fluoroscopic examination
- Abdominal ultrasound scan
- Abdominal CT scan
- Abdominocentesis/diagnostic peritoneal lavage
- Upper gastrointestinal endoscopy
- Exploratory laparotomy
- Tissue biopsy and histopathology

14.7 Appropriate diagnostic tests when investigating acute vomiting in dogs and cats. ACTH = adrenocorticotropic hormone; ALP= alkaline phosphatase; ALT = alanine aminotransferase; AST = aspartate aminotransferase; CT = computed tomography; ELISA = enzyme-linked immunosorbent assay; GGT = gamma-glutamyl transferase; SDMA = symmetric dimethylarginine.

References and further reading

Batchelor DJ, Devauchelle P, Elliott J et al. (2013) Mechanisms, causes, investigation and management of vomiting disorders in cats: a literature review. Journal of Feline Medicine and Surgery **15**, 237–242

Duke-Novekovski, de Vries M and Seymour C (2016) BSAVA Manual of Canine and Feline Anaesthesia and Analgesia, 3rd edn. BSAVA Publications, Gloucester

Elwood CM (2003) Investigation and differential diagnosis of vomiting in the dog. In Practice **25**, 374–386

Elwood CM, Devauchelle P, Elliott J et al. (2010) Emesis in dogs: a review. Journal of Small Animal Practice **51**, 4–22

Chapter 15

Chronic vomiting

Clive Elwood

Definition of the problem

A presentation of vomiting becomes 'chronic' after 3–4 weeks and, even if there are no other concerning signs, it should be considered worthy of investigation to rule out serious underlying disease and for welfare reasons. The differential diagnoses for chronic vomiting are shown in Figure 15.1. For a definition of vomiting and a description of the vomiting reflex, as well as how to distinguish vomiting from regurgitation, see Chapters 13 and 14.

Intra-abdominal, non-gastrointestinal conditions

- Peritoneal neoplasia
- Steatitis
- Peritonitis
  - Septic
  - Bile
  - Urine
  - Idiopathic
- Hepatobiliary disease
  - Neoplasia
  - Hepatitis
  - Infectious
  - Immune
  - Toxic
  - Metabolic
  - Cholangitis
  - Cholelithiasis
  - Cyst
  - Lobe torsion
  - Abscess
  - Portosystemic shunt
- Splenic
  - Torsion
  - Abscess
  - Infarction
  - Neoplasia
- Pancreatic
  - Pancreatitis
  - Neoplasia
- Adrenal tumour
- Renal
  - Chronic kidney disease
  - Pyelonephritis
  - Nephrolithiasis
  - Neoplasia
- Urogenital
  - Uterine rupture
  - Ureterolithiasis
  - Pyometra
  - Metritis
  - Prostatitis
  - Prostatic abscess

Gastrointestinal conditions

- Chronic gastritis
  - Eosinophilic
  - Lymphoplasmacytic
  - Granulomatous
  - Induced by spiral bacteria (unproven)
- Gastric neoplasia
  - Lymphoma
  - Carcinoma
  - Leiomyoma/sarcoma
  - Gastric mast cell tumour
- Gastric ulceration
  - Non-steroidal anti inflammatory drugs (NSAIDs)
  - Neoplasia
  - Metabolic
  - Hypergastrinaemia (pancreatic gastrinoma)
  - Hyperhistaminaemia (cutaneous mast cell tumour)
  - Irritant
- Gastric/intestinal entrapment
  - Ruptured diaphragm
  - Adhesions
  - Peritoneopericardial diaphragmatic hernia
  - Inguinal or umbilical hernia
  - Internal (mesenteric) hernia
- Gastric dilatation-volvulus
- Hiatal hernia
- Pyloric stenosis
- Chronic hypertrophic pyloric gastropathy
- Dietary intolerance
- Foreign body
  - Gastric
  - Intestinal
- Infection/infestation
  - Salmonellosis
  - Campylobacterosis
  - Fungal infection
  - Helminthiasis
  - Feline infectious peritonitis
- Chronic inflammatory enteropathies
  - Eosinophilic
  - Lymphoplasmacytic
  - Granulomatous
- Intestinal neoplasia
- Intussusception
- Intestinal volvulus
- Motility disorders
  - Dysautonomia
  - Localized autonomic dysfunction

Systemic conditions

- Metabolic
  - Uraemia
  - Ketoacidosis
  - Hepatic encephalopathy

15.1 Differential diagnoses for chronic vomiting in dogs and cats. (continues)

▶

Systemic conditions *continued*

- Metabolic *continued*
  - Hypoadrenocorticism
  - Hypercalcaemia
  - Hypokalaemia
  - Hyper/hyponatraemia
  - Septicaemia
  - Hyperviscosity syndrome
- Endocrine
  - Hyperthyroidism
  - Hypoadrenocorticism
  - Hypothyroidism
  - Vitamin D deficiency
- Neoplastic
  - Leukaemia
  - Histiocytic disease
  - Hypereosinophilic syndrome
  - Lymphoma
  - Systemic mastocytosis
- Toxicity
  - Lead
  - Radiation
  - Many others
- Drugs
  - Chemotherapeutics
  - Digoxin
  - Erythromycin
  - Many others
- Other
  - *Dirofilaria immitis* (cats)
  - Cardiomyopathy (cats)
  - Pyothorax
  - Thoracic tumours
  - Bronchial disease

Neurological diseases

- Hydrocephalus
- Space-occupying lesion
- Motion sickness
- Vestibular disease
- Cerebellar disease
- Visceral epilepsy
- Sialadenosis (retching)

15.1 (continued) Differential diagnoses for chronic vomiting in dogs and cats.

Signalment and history

Initial history taking for a patient showing chronic vomiting should attempt to establish whether there is true vomiting or regurgitation (see Chapters 13 and 14).

The signalment of the patient may be important. Regarding breed, for example, juvenile renal disease and subsequent uraemia is noted in Boxers, Shar Peis and Soft Coated Wheaten Terriers (amongst others), whereas pyloric stenosis is most common in brachycephalic dogs; Persian cats appear predisposed to peritoneopericardial diaphragmatic hernia (PPDH); chronic hypertrophic pyloric gastropathy is seen more commonly in toy breeds of dog; Siamese cats have increased incidence of gastrointestinal (GI) adenocarcinoma; and Cocker Spaniels appear predisposed to chronic pancreatitis. Hypoadrenocorticism has a greater incidence in female *versus* male dogs, and reproductive conditions, such as pyometra, are obviously sex dependent. The age of the patient is relevant, with congenital disease more likely in younger patients and degenerative or neoplastic conditions more likely in adult or older patients.

The provenance of the patient, including the genetic background and any family history of problems, as well as any potential exposure to atypical agents, should be considered. The general management of the patient (indoors *versus* outdoors, contact with other animals, potential exposure to infections and toxins) should also be established. The travel, vaccination and antiparasitic prophylactic treatment history should be made clear.

Any disease in animals or people in contact with the patient should be questioned. In multi-cat households, the provenance and viral status of other cats should be considered.

A good dietary history should be obtained, including, where possible, diets, treats, supplements and ingredients fed currently and previously, and the clinical signs associated with these. Potential access to non-standard food or recurrent dietary indiscretion should be considered.

Potential access to foreign bodies should be questioned. This should include toys and, particularly in cats, linear foreign bodies, as well as recent events such as parties and barbeques where dogs, in particular, might gain access to bones, corn cobs, cocktail and kebab sticks, etc.

A patient's previous clinical history may well be relevant. A history of trauma, for example, might be associated with conditions, such as a diaphragmatic rupture or bile peritonitis from damage to the biliary system. A history of musculoskeletal pain, treated with non-steroidal anti-inflammatory drugs, might point to gastric ulceration. Prior and ongoing medication should always be considered.

In entire females, the reproductive history, including timing of oestrus and any parturition, might indicate the possibility of pyometra or metritis.

Owners should be questioned about the nature, timing and frequency of vomiting. Vomiting of bile-stained fluid on an empty stomach (i.e. some hours after eating) is more typical of conditions associated with gastric mucosal irritation, such as gastritis and gastric foreign bodies. Vomiting of food soon after eating may indicate a real or functional gastric outflow or upper small intestinal obstruction, such as a foreign body or pyloric ulcers or pancreatitis. Vomiting of food after a number of hours may indicate a component of gastric motility disorder, which could be primary or secondary (e.g. from pancreatitis).

As well as the presence of food, other aspects of the vomitus are important; the presence of digested blood ('coffee grounds') suggests loss of mucosal integrity (Figure 15.2; see Chapter 19). Occasionally fresh blood is seen in vomitus as an apparent result of the increased venous pressures associated with the vomiting reflex and may not be a true indicator of mucosal disease. In cats with trichobezoars, these may be readily apparent in the vomitus.

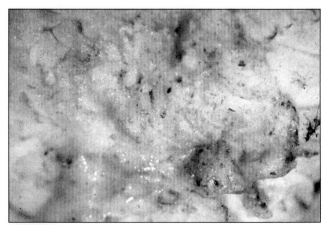

15.2 The 'coffee grounds' appearance of digested blood in vomitus.

The patient's appetite should be considered and related to bodyweight changes and condition scores (see Chapters 8 and 9). Decreased appetite may be seen where there is associated pain and nausea or where vomiting is a component of a systemic illness, such as neoplasia. Severe weight loss (with or without increased appetite) may be noted where there is cancer cachexia, maldigestion/malabsorption, protein-losing enteropathy or nephropathy, and with endocrine diseases such as hyperthyroidism or diabetes mellitus. Appetite may be increased in some conditions, such as hyperthyroidism in cats, with maldigestion/malabsorption and, on occasion, with gastric irritation, for example, gastritis. However, a normal appetite does not rule out the presence of a serious condition. In dogs with gastric carcinoma, for example, a normal appetite may be preserved until very late in the disease course, despite marked ulceration, thickening and distortion of the stomach wall.

Signs of pain and discomfort should be ascertained and may manifest as aggressive or withdrawn behaviour, difficulty or inability to find a comfortable resting position and adoption of relief postures. Patients that show interest in eating but subsequently refuse to do so might be experiencing pain or nausea in association with eating or the sensory perception of food; in some cases this may be associative or learned behaviour and should be considered in future management.

Occasionally owners will report obvious abnormal sounds arising from the patient's abdomen, such as borborygmi with increased GI motility, or musical sounds, with a distended or obstructed viscus.

The pattern of progression of chronic vomiting and associated signs is helpful (Figure 15.3). A slow unremitting worsening of signs could indicate a degenerative or neoplastic condition; a low-grade steady state of signs might be seen with 'static' conditions such as congenital pyloric stenosis; waxing and waning signs can be seen in conditions such as idiopathic chronic enteropathies and chronic pancreatitis; severe persistent signs might be seen with sustained 'acute' illnesses such as a splenic torsion; and remitting signs might be seen with conditions that are transient but recurrent, such as ureterolithiasis.

It is not unusual for chronic vomiting patients to have been treated non-specifically or symptomatically prior to in-depth investigation, and a response or a lack of response to prior treatment can provide useful information. Antacids may provide some relief to conditions associated with gastric irritation, such as gastritis and ulcerative disease. Antiemetics can provide symptomatic relief in many patients but may be much less effective with severe conditions. Antibiotics can effectively suppress causes of chronic vomiting associated with bacterial infection, such as cholecystitis or foreign body penetration. Corticosteroids can suppress inflammation and rectify deficiency in hypoadrenocorticism.

Responses to dietary management are also relevant. Owners and clinicians may have tried various formulations and consistencies of food, and the variation in clinical signs associated with these can indicate whether an underlying dietary sensitivity is more likely or if certain formulations or consistencies of food are better tolerated.

Beyond obtaining history about the vomiting *per se*, associated signs should be explored. These should include: information about the respiratory system (e.g. coughing and sneezing, in case there is associated disease such as aspiration pneumonia); whether or not there is diarrhoea and, if so, its nature (small intestinal *versus* large intestinal *versus* mixed); whether there is increased drinking and the duration thereof; and abnormalities in the willingness or ability to exercise, including weakness or

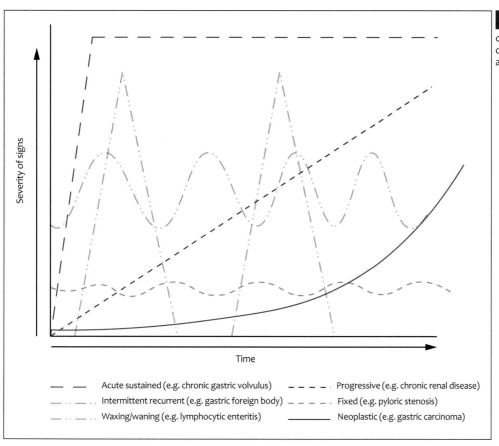

15.3 The pattern of change in severity and frequency of clinical signs can aid differential diagnosis of chronic vomiting in dogs and cats.

— — Acute sustained (e.g. chronic gastric volvulus) — — — — Progressive (e.g. chronic renal disease)

— ·· — Intermittent recurrent (e.g. gastric foreign body) — — — — Fixed (e.g. pyloric stenosis)

— · — ·· Waxing/waning (e.g. lymphocytic enteritis) ———— Neoplastic (e.g. gastric carcinoma)

collapsing episodes. Signs of neurological dysfunction may be relevant, and any skin disease might indicate metabolic disease (e.g. chronic hepatopathy) or an allergic predisposition.

Physical examination

A primary objective of physical examination in patients with chronic vomiting is to assess their immediate needs for supportive and symptomatic therapy whilst investigation is pursued (Figure 15.4); the criteria are the same as for acute vomiting (see Chapter 14).

- **Body condition** – The patient's overall body condition should be assessed as an indicator of general debility and potential cachexia, malassimilation and metabolic disease. Muscle, coat and skin condition should be similarly assessed.

- **Mucous membranes** – The colour of the mucous membranes is important. Pale mucous membranes in a patient that shows no signs of hypovolaemia and has, for example, strong to hyperdynamic regular pulses might indicate chronic GI blood loss and a well-compensated anaemia. Icterus may be noted with hepatic and extra-hepatic causes of vomiting (Figure 15.5; see Chapter 25).
- **Mouth** – The mouth should be examined for foreign material and ulceration, and the smell of the breath assessed for halitosis, a uraemic odour or ketones.
- **Pharynx/larynx** – The pharynx/larynx and salivary glands should be palpated for swelling and pain and, particularly in elderly cats, a careful palpation of the cervical region should be performed to check for goitre.
- **Peripheral lymph nodes** – The peripheral lymph nodes should be assessed for enlargement and pain.
- **Heart and lungs** – The heart and lungs should be carefully auscultated, in particular noting dullness, which could be associated with the presence of intervening tissue (PPDH, diaphragmatic rupture) or adventitious lung sounds (squeaks and rasps) associated with, for example, complicating aspiration pneumonia.
- **Thorax** – Palpation of the surface of the thorax should be performed to look for evidence of historical trauma (e.g. rib fractures) and evidence of mass lesions.
- **Abdomen** – Abdominal palpation should proceed as described in Chapter 14.
- **Anal and perineal examination** – This should include examination for evidence of diarrhoea and vaginal discharge.
- **Rectal examination** – This should assess for faecal consistency and the presence of melaena and allow palpation of the anal sacs, prostate or vagina and, occasionally, urethra and urinary bladder.

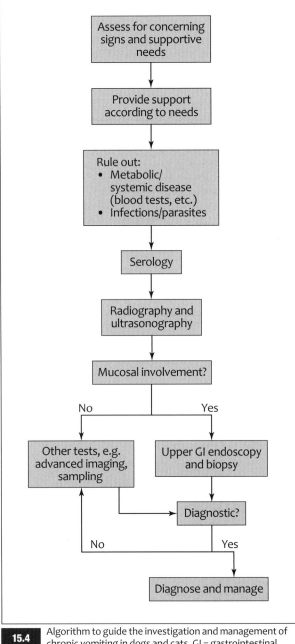

15.4 Algorithm to guide the investigation and management of chronic vomiting in dogs and cats. GI = gastrointestinal.

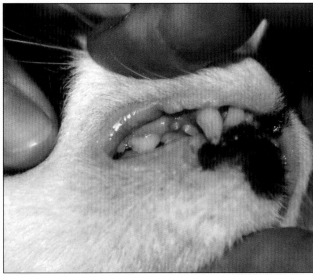

15.5 Icterus in chronically vomiting patients may direct investigations to the liver or causes of extra-hepatic biliary obstruction.

Diagnostic tests

Diagnostic tests should be chosen and prioritized after history taking and physical examination, with an appropriate differential diagnosis list in mind (Figure 15.6).

- Packed cell volume/total protein
- Haematology (red and white cell indices)
- Serum electrolytes
- Serum total and ionized calcium
- Plasma urea, creatinine and SDMA
- Liver enzymes (ALT, ALP, AST, GGT)
- Urinalysis (specific gravity, blood cells, ketones, glucose, bilirubin, protein)
- Faecal analysis (microscopy, parasitology, culture, ELISA, FeLV and FIV, e.g. for parvovirus)
- Serology for infectious disease (e.g. leptospirosis, toxoplasmosis)
- Canine or feline pancreatic lipase
- Serum TLI, cobalamin and folate
- Exclusion diet trial
- Bile acid stimulation test
- ACTH stimulation test
- Thyroid hormone profiles
- Other hormone profiles (APUDoma)
- Autonomic function testing (pilocarpine response tests)
- Serum toxin screens
- Abdominal radiography
- Contrast fluoroscopic examination
- Abdominal ultrasonography
- Abdominal CT scan
- Needle aspirate cytology and culture
- Cholecystocentesis
- Abdominocentesis/diagnostic peritoneal lavage
- Upper gastrointestinal endoscopy
- Exploratory laparotomy
- Tissue biopsy and histopathology

15.6 Diagnostic tests to consider when investigating chronic vomiting in dogs and cats. ACTH = adrenocorticotropic hormone; ALP = alkaline phosphatase; ALT = alanine aminotransferase; APUDoma = amine precursor uptake and decarboxylation tumour; AST = aspartate aminotransferase; CT = computed tomography; ELISA= enzyme-linked immunosorbent assay; FeLV = feline leukemia virus; FIV = feline immunodeficiency virus; GGT = gamma-glutamyl transferase; SDMA = symmetric dimethylarginine; TLI = trypsin-like immunoreactivity.

References and further reading

Batchelor DJ, Devauchelle P, Elliott J *et al.* (2013) Mechanisms, causes, investigation and management of vomiting disorders in cats: a literature review. *Journal of Feline Medicine and Surgery* **15**, 237–242

Elwood CM (2003) Investigation and differential diagnosis of vomiting in the dog. *In Practice* **25**, 374–386

Elwood CM, Devauchelle P, Elliott J *et al.* (2010) Emesis in dogs: a review. *Journal of Small Animal Practice* **51**, 4–22

Chapter 16

Bloating

Rachel Lavoué

Definition of the problem

There are a variety of mechanisms and differential diagnoses that can cause abdominal distension (Figure 16.1). Abdominal bloating refers to a condition in which the abdomen feels swollen and is uncomfortable because of distension of the gastrointestinal (GI) tract. It is a non-specific and subjective sign that may or may not be associated with other more objective physical signs (e.g. distended, tensed or painful abdomen (Figure 16.2); presence of belching and flatulence or diarrhoea). Bloating is rarely the primary reason for consultation in veterinary practice, while it is a frequent symptom in humans, with a prevalence ranging from 16 to 21% of cases. Despite its low apparent prevalence in small animals, this problem should not be overlooked too quickly. Indeed, if it is not usually a life-threatening condition, bloating can orientate the clinician toward a more chronic digestive or respiratory disorder, and is likely to be underdiagnosed in small animals.

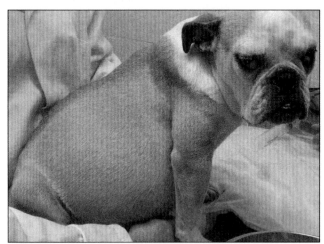

16.2 Marked abdominal distension secondary to ascites in an English Bulldog.

Gas accumulation:
- Gastric dilatation-volvulus
- Aerophagia in dyspnoeic animals
- Bacterial fermentation
  - Dietary
  - Dysbiosis
- Ileus (functional or mechanical)
- Mesenteric torsion
- Pneumoperitoneum

Increased gastrointestinal content:
- Heavy roundworm burden (puppies and kittens)
- Constipation/obstipation/idiopathic megacolon
- Over-eating
- Gastric outflow obstruction
- Mesenteric torsion
- Ileus (functional or mechanical)

Fluid accumulation:
- Effusion (transudate, modified transudate, exudate, neoplastic; see Chapter 24)
- Pyometra
- Urinary obstruction (bladder, hydronephrosis)
- Ileus (functional or mechanical)
- Cyst
- Abscess

Increase in size of intra-abdominal structures:
- Organomegaly
- Fat deposition
- Neoplasia
- Granuloma
- Pregnancy

Abdominal wall abnormalities:
- Muscle weakness in hyperadrenocorticism (with hepatomegaly)
- Abdominal wall or prepubic tendon rupture

16.1 Differential diagnoses for abdominal distension.

Pathophysiology and aetiology

Different causes have been postulated to explain bloating, which may involve more than one of the following in the same animal:

- Increased luminal contents (i.e. gas, ingesta, liquid)
- Impaired gastric or intestinal emptying
- Altered intra-abdominal volume displacement
- Individual variability in perception of intestinal stimuli.

With organomegaly and an increased amount of liquid or ingesta within the digestive tract, the primary complaint is likely to be more specific and may be associated with diarrhoea, tenesmus or constipation (see Chapters 17, 18 and 23 for additional details). In most cases, the sensation of bloating is a direct consequence of the presence of gases within the digestive tract.

Increased luminal content of gas

Gases are physiologically present within the intestines and result from swallowed air, chemical luminal reactions and diffusion from the bloodstream. In the upper GI tract, the reaction of neutralizing acids and alkalis is responsible for endogenous gas formation, while bacterial fermentation is the primary endogenous source in the lower digestive tract. Gas output is achieved by belching, absorption into the blood, bacterial consumption and perianal evacuation.

Aerophagia may be amplified with excitement, competitive or increased rate of food consumption, brachycephalic obstructive airway syndrome or with any respiratory disorder (Figure 16.3).

Endogenous production of gas may increase concomitantly with bacterial fermentation. In dogs, the intestinal microbiome may partly be breed-dependent (Simpson *et al.*, 2002; Cutrignelli *et al.*, 2009; Hand *et al.*, 2013), which indirectly affects gas production and fermentation kinetics. Some breeds of dog might, therefore, be predisposed to abdominal bloating, as well as animals that develop intestinal dysbiosis. The composition of ingested food is also directly related to endogenous gas production. In humans, flatulogenic diets have been demonstrated to be associated with abdominal distension episodes in susceptible patients, and high-fibre foods, fatty meals and dairy products are frequently reported as offending causes. In dogs fed once daily, the peak production of gases is approximately 2 hours after a meal. Diets with a high content of fermentable fibre, such as fructo-oligosaccharides, increase the volume of gas produced by fermentation in both dogs and humans.

Impaired gas emptying

Although intestinal gas may lead to significant discomfort when it is present in excessive quantity and/or cannot be eliminated properly, various studies indicate that bloating in human patients is rather a consequence of abnormal distribution of gases and individual susceptibility. Indeed, only a minimal increase in the total volume of gas is demonstrated in humans suffering from chronic bloating because of irritable bowel syndrome (IBS). In veterinary medicine, some similarities have been found in dogs suffering from idiopathic large intestinal diarrhoea and presumed IBS.

Ineffective eructation and defective gas transit promote abnormal gas repartitioning and can induce abdominal bloating. Failure to eructate, a sedentary lifestyle and ingestion of fermentable fibres have all been associated with increased frequency of flatulence and have the ability to slow intestinal transit. The composition of digestive gases may also alter motility. In human patients with inflammatory bowel disease (IBD) or IBS, physiological concentrations of methane slow transit and induce constipation and abdominal discomfort. All dogs and cats with chronic digestive disorders might, therefore, be at risk of abdominal bloating.

Gastric dilatation, with or without volvulus, is a common cause of abdominal bloating in large- and giant-breed dogs. Although not fully understood, many factors have been reported to cause gastric dilatation, including genetic predisposition, bacterial fermentation and abnormal motility (Van Kruiningen *et al.*, 2013; Gazzola and Nelson, 2014).

See Chapter 33 for more information on gastric dilatation-volvulus (GDV) and the *BSAVA Manual of Canine and Feline Abdominal Surgery* for its surgical treatment.

History and physical examination

Abdominal bloating is rarely the primary reason for veterinary consultation and it is difficult to objectively evaluate and diagnose. Animals with episodes of standing with an arched back, temporarily distended abdomen or painful cramping may be suffering from bloating. Abdominal discomfort may also present as a stiff gait or the prayer position (see Chapter 14).

Given its pathophysiology, bloating should also be suspected in patients that are suffering from dyspnoea, chronic eructation and flatulence. With these patients, an exhaustive questionnaire regarding any other signs indicative of an underlying digestive disorder should be completed. Indeed, bloating and gas-related symptoms are reported by most human patients with GI disorders, such as IBS, IBD and functional constipation.

The presence of a tense abdomen on palpation, intestinal gaseous distension and abdominal tympanism are the most specific findings in affected animals. The absence of these findings, however, does not exclude abdominal bloating, as signs may fluctuate. Although transient, signs associated with gas-related disorders should not be dismissed too rapidly, as they can be the first signs of GDV or be indicative of more chronic, but nonetheless serious, abdominal diseases.

An extensive review of the animal's history, and associated respiratory and digestive signs, is mandatory. Prior medical disorders (e.g. GDV) or medical treatments (e.g. antimicrobials) that could be associated with intestinal transit alteration or microbiome modification should be assessed. Obtaining specific and detailed information regarding dietary habits is crucial, as abdominal bloating mostly develops after meals in humans, especially because specific foods (e.g. beans, cabbage, lentils, Brussel sprouts) promote fermentation. The level of exercise and activity should also be recorded.

Diagnostic tests

In the presence of gas-related signs, thoracic and abdominal radiographs may be useful to characterize the severity and location of gas accumulation (Figure 16.3). In cases of overt signs of GDV, megaoesophagus, generalized ileus and hiatal hernia, specific management is essential. Investigations should be carried out when dysmotility and malassimilation-malabsorption syndrome are suspected (see Chapter 34 for more details).

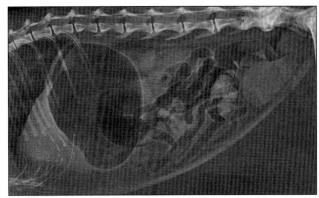

16.3 Lateral abdominal radiograph showing bloating secondary to marked aerophagia in a dyspnoeic cat.

Treatment

Specific treatment should be based on a specific diagnosis, when possible. Some treatments may improve the gas-related signs of the patient. However, given the multifactorial pathophysiology implicated in bloating, its management remains empirical and focuses on decreasing gas production and modulating digestive transit. To date, no treatment has been reported as universally effective in human medicine.

Changes in feeding habits, with a highly digestible and novel protein source fed twice daily, may decrease bacterial fermentation and the number of flatulence episodes in dogs (see Chapter 27). Supplementation with fermentable fibre may help to treat a subset of dogs suffering from idiopathic large intestinal diarrhoea. Additionally, promoting physical exercise is an easy approach to improve flatulence in dogs and digestive transit time in humans.

Although there is a lack of clear evidence for probiotic administration in dogs, specific probiotics lead to relief of bloating in humans suffering from IBS. The effect of prokinetic drugs on bloating in small animals remains largely unknown, while the clinical use of 5-HT$_4$ receptor agonists (e.g. cisapride) in humans is limited because of their cardiovascular side effects (see Chapter 27). Myorelaxant drugs are commonly used in human patients suffering from IBS and are superior to placebo in the treatment of bloat. No specific data are available in veterinary medicine, although antispasmodic drugs were not helpful in the management of a few patients with canine idiopathic large bowel diarrhoea. Finally, adsorbing agents (simethicone and charcoal) have been shown to decrease bloating in humans. In veterinary medicine, administration of charcoal, *Yucca schidigera* and zinc acetate diminished the percentage of odoriferous gases in dogs, supposedly because of decreased production of hydrogen sulphites (Giffard *et al.*, 2001). However, it did not decrease the total gas production and its efficacy in abdominal bloating is unknown.

Summary

Although abdominal bloating remains an ill-defined syndrome in veterinary medicine, attention should be given to patients suffering from vague abdominal signs, as it could be an indication of a more serious condition. The diagnostic investigation should focus on the possible underlying disorder, while management of abdominal bloating relies on specific treatment of the underlying cause, when possible. Despite the lack of data on bloating in veterinary medicine, symptomatic treatment can provide relief to animals suspected of having this condition.

References and further reading

Bendezu RA, Barba E, Burri E *et al.* (2015) Intestinal gas content and distribution in health and in patients with functional gut symptoms. *Neurogastroenterology and Motility* **27**, 1249–1257

Byron JK, Shadwick SR and Bennett AR (2010) Megaesophagus in a 6-month-old cat secondary to a nasopharyngeal polyp. *Journal of Feline Medicine and Surgery* **12**, 322–324

Chassany O, Marquis P, Scherrer B *et al.* (1999) Validation of a specific quality of life questionnaire for functional digestive disorders. *Gut* **44**, 527–533

Coffin B, Bortolloti C, Bourgeois O and Denicourt L (2011) Efficacy of a simethicone, activated charcoal and magnesium oxide combination (Carbosymag®) in functional dyspepsia: results of a general practice-based randomized trial. *Clinics and Research in Hepatology and Gastroenterology* **35**, 494–499

Collins SB, Perez-Camargo G, Gettinby G *et al.* (2001) Development of a technique for the in vivo assessment of flatulence in dogs. *American Journal of Veterinary Research* **62**, 1014–1019

Cutrignelli MI, Bovera F, Tudisco R and D'Urso S (2009) In vitro fermentation characteristics of different carbohydrate sources in two dog breeds (German shepherd and Neapolitan mastiff). *Journal of Animal Physiology and Animal Nutrition* **93**, 305–312

Gazzola KM and Nelson LL (2014) The relationship between gastrointestinal motility and gastric dilatation-volvulus in dogs. *Topics in Companion Animal Medicine* **29**, 64–66

Giffard CJ, Collins SB, Stoodley NC *et al.* (2001) Administration of charcoal, *Yucca schidigera*, and zinc acetate to reduce malodorous flatulence in dogs. *Journal of the American Veterinary Medical Association* **218**, 892–896

Gonlachanvit S, Coleski R, Owyang C and Hasler WL (2006) Nutrient modulation of intestinal gas dynamics in healthy humans: dependence on caloric content and meal consistency. *American Journal of Physiology-Gastrointestinal and Liver Physiology* **291**, 389–395

Hand D, Wallis C, Colyer A and Penn CW (2013) Pyrosequencing the canine faecal microbiota: breadth and depth of biodiversity. *PLoS One* **8**, 53115

Hungin AP, Mulligan C, Pot B *et al.* (2013) Systematic review: probiotics in the management of lower gastrointestinal symptoms in clinical practice – an evidence-based international guide. *Alimentary Pharmacology and Therapeutics* **38**, 864–886

Jiang X, Locke GR, III, Choung RS *et al.* (2008) Prevalence and risk factors for abdominal bloating and visible distention: a population-based study. *Gut* **57**, 756–763

Lecoindre P and Gaschen FP (2011) Chronic idiopathic large bowel diarrhea in the dog. *Veterinary Clinics of North America: Small Animal Practice* **41**, 447–456

Nandi R and Sengupta S (1998) Microbial production of hydrogen: an overview. *Critical Reviews in Microbiology* **24**, 61–84

Pimentel M, Lin HC, Enayati P *et al.* (2006) Methane, a gas produced by enteric bacteria, slows intestinal transit and augments small intestinal contractile activity. *American Journal of Physiology-Gastrointestinal and Liver Physiology* **290**, 1089–1095

Poncet CM, Dupre GP, Freiche VG *et al.* (2006) Prevalence of gastrointestinal tract lesions in 73 brachycephalic dogs with upper respiratory syndrome. *Journal of Small Animal Practice* **46**, 273–279

Poynard T, Regimbeau C and Benhamou Y (2001) Meta-analysis of smooth muscle relaxants in the treatment of irritable bowel syndrome. *Alimentary Pharmacology and Therapeutics* **15**, 355–361

Schmitz S, Glanemann B, Garden OA *et al.* (2015) A prospective, randomized, blinded, placebo-controlled pilot study on the effect of *Enterococcus faecium* on clinical activity and intestinal gene expression in canine food-responsive chronic enteropathy. *Journal of Veterinary Internal Medicine* **29**, 533–543

Serra J, Azpiroz F and Malagelada J (2001) Impaired transit and tolerance of intestinal gas in the irritable bowel syndrome. *Gut* **48**, 14–19

Simpson JM, Martineau B, Jones WE, Ballam JM and Mackie RI (2002) Characterization of fecal bacterial populations in canines: effects of age, breed and dietary fiber. *Microbial Ecology* **44**, 186–197

Williams J and Niles J (2015) *BSAVA Manual of Canine and Feline Abdominal Surgery, 2nd edn.* BSAVA Publications, Gloucester

Van Kruiningen HJ, Gargamelli C, Havier J *et al.* (2013) Stomach gas analyses in canine acute gastric dilatation with volvulus. *Journal of Veterinary Internal Medicine* **27**, 1260–1261

Yamka RM, Harmon DL, Schoenherr WD *et al.* (2006) *In vivo* measurement of flatulence and nutrient digestibility in dogs fed poultry by-product meal, conventional soybean meal, and low-oligosaccharide low-phytate soybean meal. *American Journal of Veterinary Research* **67**, 88–94

Chapter 17

Acute diarrhoea

Ian A. Battersby

Definition of the problem

Acute diarrhoea is defined as an abnormally frequent passage of semi-solid or fluid faecal matter, lasting less than 14 days. Diarrhoea is a primary sign of intestinal disease; however, it may also be a manifestation of other systemic diseases. Diarrhoea can occur as a consequence of small or large intestinal disease, although it is not uncommon for both regions to be affected by diffuse disease. During diarrhoea there is an increased loss of water and electrolytes (sodium, chloride, potassium and bicarbonate) in the liquid faeces. Dehydration and blood electrolyte abnormalities occur when these losses are not replaced adequately.

History and physical examination

A good clinical history and thorough physical examination are the first steps to determine what diagnostic investigations and level of treatment are required (Figure 17.1). It is important to determine any occurrence of scavenging, the animal's worming/vaccination status and the presence of similar clinical signs in any in-contact animals or people.

Clinical findings can also help determine whether the diarrhoea is large intestinal or small intestinal in origin (see Chapter 18), although most cases of acute diarrhoea involve both regions.

Examples of physical examination abnormalities that warrant further investigation and hospitalization for treatment include:

- Tachycardia, bradycardia or arrhythmias
- Dehydration and hypovolaemia
- Melaena or significant fresh blood in the faeces (see Chapters 20 and 21)
- Abdominal pain or palpable abnormalities (e.g. mass/foreign body).

Formulation of a problem list and development of diagnostic and treatment plans

The majority of animals presenting with acute diarrhoea will be cases of simple dietary indiscretion and will not require

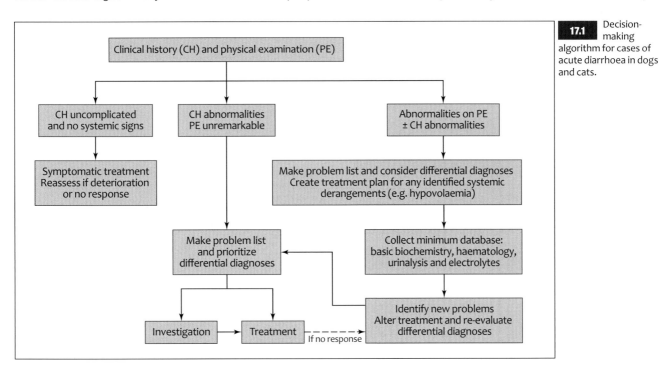

17.1 Decision-making algorithm for cases of acute diarrhoea in dogs and cats.

extensive investigations and/or treatment. However, if any abnormalities are evident in the clinical history or on physical examination, a list of the main findings should be made and the differential diagnoses for each problem considered and prioritized to optimize diagnostic testing.

Differential diagnoses

Figure 17.2 outlines the differential diagnoses for acute diarrhoea and the text below expands on some of the causes identified.

Dietary causes

Dietary-related problems are probably the most common cause of acute diarrhoea, and may be the result of dietary indiscretion (e.g. scavenging), intolerance, food poisoning (e.g. spoiled food) or hypersensitivity (allergy).

Dietary
• Hypersensitivity (allergy) • Intolerance • Rapid dietary change (especially in puppies and kittens) • Poor-quality and/or spoiled foods
Infectious

• Parasitic:
  • Helminths/ascarids: *Toxocara, Uncinaria* spp., *Trichuris*
  • Protozoa: *Cystoisospora, Cryptosporidium, Giardia, Tritrichomonas* (C)
• Viral:
  • Parvovirus (D, C)
  • Coronavirus (D, C)
  • Related to feline leukaemia virus and/or feline immunodeficiency virus
  • ? Rotavirus (D, C)
  • Distemper virus
  • ? Feline astrovirus
  • Canine adenovirus
  • ? Reovirus (D, C)
  • ? Feline torovirus
  • ? Enteroviruses
• Bacterial:
  • *Salmonella*
  • *Clostridium perfringens*
  • Pathogenic *Escherichia coli*
  • *Campylobacter jejuni*
  • *Yersinia*
  • Other bacteria
• Algal:
  • *Prototheca*[a]
• Fungal[a]

Neoplastic
• Lymphoma • Adenocarcinoma
Anatomical
• Intussusception
Toxin ingestion
• Heavy metals (e.g. lead) • Drugs (e.g. antibiotics, cytotoxics, non-steroidal anti-inflammatory drugs)
Metabolic
• Hypoadrenocorticism
Miscellaneous
• Haemorrhagic gastroenteritis/acute haemorrhagic diarrhoea syndrome • Acute pancreatitis

17.2 Potential causes of acute diarrhoea in dogs and cats. Note: causes of chronic diarrhoea that may initially present acutely are not listed. [a] Rare in the UK. C = cat; D = dog; ? = uncertain whether clinically significant.

Infectious causes

Endoparasites: Endoparasites can cause acute and/or chronic diarrhoea when heavy infestations are present. *Trichuris vulpis*, which infects the caecum and colon of the dog, can in severe infestations cause abdominal pain, weight loss, hyponatraemia and hyperkalaemia.

Protozoa:
Coccidia: Heavy infestations with *Cystoisospora* (formerly *Isospora*) spp. can occur in puppies and kittens kept in unsanitary conditions, and may result in diarrhoea. *Cryptosporidium parvum* has also been associated with diarrhoea in dogs and cats, predominantly in those animals that are immunocompromised.

Giardia: *Giardia* species can affect both dogs and cats. The majority of infections are subclinical, but clinical signs can vary from acute to chronic small or large intestinal diarrhoea.

Tritrichomonas: *T. foetus* has been identified as an intestinal pathogen in cats, resulting in large intestinal diarrhoea, which is more commonly chronic in nature.

Bacteria: Gastrointestinal infection with a number of potentially pathogenic bacteria (*Campylobacter jejuni, Campylobacter upsaliensis, Salmonella, Clostridium, Escherichia coli*) may result in acute or chronic diarrhoea. However, since these bacteria can also be found in the faeces of healthy dogs and cats, the significance of a positive faecal test result should be interpreted with caution (see Chapter 2).

Viruses:
Parvovirus: Canine parvovirus is a highly contagious and life-threatening cause of acute enteritis in young unvaccinated dogs. The virus is very stable in the environment and infection occurs via faecal–oral transmission. Clinical signs develop 4–7 days following infection, but viral shedding can occur before the onset of signs. Disease occurs in tissues where cells are undergoing rapid multiplication (i.e. lymphoid tissues, bone marrow and intestinal crypt cells), resulting in leucopenia, intestinal crypt necrosis and severe haemorrhagic diarrhoea. When severe mucosal damage occurs, bacterial translocation can result in septicaemia, endotoxaemia and disseminated intravascular coagulation. Puppies infected *in utero*, or shortly after birth, may develop myocarditis, although this is rare due to the high prevalence of maternally derived antibody protection.
Feline parvovirus is very similar to canine parvovirus in terms of its pathogenicity and gastrointestinal signs, but *in utero* infection can also result in cerebellar hypoplasia.

Coronavirus: Canine coronavirus has been associated with diarrhoea of varying severity, but its significance as a primary pathogen is uncertain. Feline coronavirus is an ubiquitous virus, which may cause mild self-limiting diarrhoea; however, in some patients, coronavirus can result in the development of feline infectious peritonitis.

Torovirus: Torovirus has been linked with a syndrome of diarrhoea and protruding nictitating membranes in cats, but a causative association has never been proven.

Distemper virus: Animals presenting with clinical signs are usually young dogs. Gastrointestinal signs are normally preceded by a cough, rhinitis and pyrexia.

Neoplastic causes

Diarrhoea can occur in association with neoplasia, due to a number of mechanisms, although typically the diarrhoea becomes chronic. The most commonly recognized gastrointestinal tumours are lymphoma (solitary or diffuse) and adenocarcinoma (solitary mass or large ulcerated area).

Intussusception

An intussusception may occur at any location along the intestinal tract but the ileocolic region is most common. They occur spontaneously more frequently in young animals and are often associated with concurrent enteritis. In older animals, intussusception is often associated with a small lesion acting as a nidus.

Toxin ingestion

Various toxins (e.g. insecticides) can result in both vomiting and diarrhoea (see the BSAVA/VPIS Guide to Common Canine and Feline Poisons). However, often the exact cause remains undetermined unless the animal was witnessed ingesting the toxin, and most of the time the animal will respond favourably to symptomatic treatment as for dietary intolerance.

Heavy metals: Ingestion of heavy metals can result in diarrhoea; for example, gastrointestinal signs are the most common clinical signs associated with chronic low-level lead poisoning.

Drugs: When an animal receiving any medication develops diarrhoea, consideration should be given as to whether the medication itself might be the cause. Non-steroidal anti-inflammatory drugs are a common cause of drug-induced diarrhoea. Although commonly used, antibiotics are rarely indicated in the treatment of acute diarrhoea and can themselves cause diarrhoea.

Hypoadrenocorticism

Hypoadrenocorticism (Addison's disease) is more commonly diagnosed in dogs, but also rarely in cats. Clinical signs include anorexia, vomiting and diarrhoea; other reported signs include lethargy, weakness and collapse. Abnormalities on bloodwork that should raise suspicion of hypoadrenocorticism include hyperkalaemia, hyponatraemia, absence of a stress leucogram and eosinophilia. An atypical form of hypoadrenocorticism is infrequently reported in the dog. In these cases, the animal is deficient in glucocorticoids only; hence, the electrolyte changes discussed above are absent.

Acute haemorrhagic diarrhoea syndrome

Acute haemorrhagic diarrhoea syndrome (AHDS) (Unterer et al., 2014), formerly known as haemorrhagic gastroenteritis (HGE), is a clinical syndrome characterized by acute profuse bloody diarrhoea and haemoconcentration, with packed cell volume (PCV) often exceeding 60%, but usually with total protein within the reference range. This feature, together with the absence of leucopenia, helps differentiate AHDS from parvovirus infection. The aetiology of AHDS is unknown but an association has been made with infection by a Clostridium perfringens organism secreting netE and netF toxin (Sindern et al., 2018). The prognosis for most dogs is good if treated appropriately (see Chapter 34).

Pancreatitis

In the dog, the most common clinical signs of pancreatitis reported are anorexia and vomiting, but concurrent diarrhoea is reported in some cases. In cats, while anorexia is the most frequent clinical sign, a wide spectrum of additional signs can occur, and a concurrent enteropathy is often present and may contribute to or cause clinical signs.

Diagnostic tests

When performing a diagnostic test, the clinician must consider how the results should be interpreted based on an understanding of the test's limitations and performance (i.e. sensitivity and specificity) (see the BSAVA Manual of Canine and Feline Clinical Pathology).

Minimum database

In all patients hospitalized for the treatment of acute diarrhoea, a minimum database including basic biochemistry, haematology and urinalysis should be performed. The minimum database and electrolyte levels allow assessment of hydration status, electrolyte abnormalities (which may indicate primary endocrine disease or arise secondary to gastrointestinal losses) and haematological abnormalities that may be indicative of an underlying disease (e.g. elevated PCV in AHDS/HGE).

Faecal testing

There are a number of faecal tests (see below) that can be used in cases of acute diarrhoea (also see Chapter 2). Interpretation of the results can be clouded by the presence of some enteropathogens in the faeces of healthy cats and dogs. The author does not perform faecal analysis routinely in acute diarrhoea cases, unless there are signs of systemic involvement or there is evidence to suggest the diarrhoea is infectious in nature (e.g. multiple animals affected, poor vaccination history suggesting parvovirus). In cases in which worming history is poor or there is a known geographical parasite burden, analysis should be considered or, alternatively, a trial anthelmintic therapy could be prescribed.

- Culture – for Salmonella, Campylobacter and pathogenic Escherichia coli.
- Parasitology microscopy to identify endoparasites, protozoa and to perform an egg count.
- Faecal antigen enzyme-linked immunosorbent assay (ELISA) – for Giardia, parvovirus, hookworms, whipworms, roundworms and Cryptosporidium.
- Faecal ELISA – for Clostridium perfringens enterotoxin and Clostridium difficile toxin A and B.
- Faecal polymerase chain reaction – for Tritrichomonas, Clostridium toxins and genes, Salmonella, Campylobacter, coronavirus, distemper virus and Cryptosporidium.

Blood testing

The following blood tests may be useful to investigate cases of acute diarrhoea:

- Retroviral serology – for feline leukaemia virus/feline immunodeficiency virus

- Basal cortisol or adrenocorticotropic hormone stimulation test
- Canine/feline pancreatic lipase – for suspected pancreatitis cases.

Imaging

The following diagnostic imaging techniques may be helpful for the investigation of acute diarrhoea:

- Abdominal radiography (see Chapter 3)
    - Plain radiographs
    - Barium-impregnated spheres/liquid barium studies
- Abdominal ultrasonography.

Endoscopy and exploratory laparotomy

These should only be considered when non-invasive tests have been exhausted, or clinical findings indicate laparotomy to be necessary (e.g. a foreign body).

References and further reading

Battersby I and Harvey A (2006) Differential diagnosis and treatment of acute diarrhoea in the dog and cat. *In Practice* **28**, 480–488

BSAVA/VPIS Guide to Common Canine and Feline Poisons (2012) BSAVA Publications, Gloucester

Greene C and Marks SL (2011) Gastrointestinal and intra-abdominal infections. In: *Infectious Diseases of the Dog and Cat, 4th edn*, ed. C Greene, pp. 950–980. Elsevier Saunders, St. Louis

Marks SL, Rankin SC, Byrne BA and Weese JS (2011) Enteropathogenic bacteria in dogs and cats: diagnosis, epidemiology, treatment, and control. *Journal of Veterinary Internal Medicine* **25**, 1195–1208

Sindern N, Suchodolski JS, Leutenegger CM *et al.* (2018) Prevalence of *Clostridium perfringens* net*E* and net*F* toxin genes in the feces of dogs with acute hemorrhagic diarrhea syndrome. *Journal of Veterinary Internal Medicine* **33**, 100–105

Unterer S, Busch K, Leipig M *et al.* (2014) Endoscopically visualized lesions, histologic findings, and bacterial invasion in the gastrointestinal mucosa of dogs with acute hemorrhagic diarrhea syndrome. *Journal of Veterinary Internal Medicine* **28**, 52–58

Villiers E and Ristić J (2016) *BSAVA Manual of Canine and Feline Clinical Pathology, 3rd edn*. BSAVA Publications, Gloucester

Willard MD (2013) Diarrhea. In: *Canine and Feline Gastroenterology*, ed. RJ Washabau and MJ Day, pp. 99–105. Elsevier Saunders, St. Louis

Chapter 18

Chronic diarrhoea

Nicole Luckschander-Zeller

Definition of the problem

Diarrhoea is an increase in volume or fluidity of the faeces and, often, a consequent increase in the frequency of defecation (Marks, 2012). The general mechanisms, which may overlap, are increased osmotic drag, increased secretion or permeability, or altered motility (Battersby and Harvey, 2006). If the signs persist or are intermittently present for more than 14 days, the diarrhoea is classified as being chronic. Therefore, the disease is not self-limiting and every patient with chronic diarrhoea needs a thorough diagnostic investigation. Although breed predisposition and local disease prevalence influence the investigation of chronic diarrhoea, there are general guidelines that should be applied.

Relevant history

Before taking the history, it is essential to pay attention to the signalment of the patient as certain breeds are predisposed to specific gastrointestinal diseases (see Chapter 1). The priority of underlying diseases varies with age; for example, infectious diseases in young animals *versus* neoplastic diseases in older animals.

It is also essential to take a thorough history for all patients with chronic diarrhoea. A diet history is always important, including any dietary changes (Figure 18.1). As many pet owners change the food provided very often, it is important to document every food fed in order to select an appropriate elimination diet. Response to any previous treatment and association with any stressful events are important in the history.

The history of the patient and the description of the faeces are helpful to distinguish between acute and chronic diarrhoea, to estimate the severity of the disease and sometimes to characterize the most obvious localization (small intestinal *versus* large intestinal) (Figure 18.2). Nevertheless, it should be kept in mind, that fresh blood can also be a sign of fast intestinal transit time, and so it does not exclude small intestinal disease. In addition, animals with evident large intestinal signs can have generalized intestinal diseases (e.g. lymphoma or histoplasmosis), so it is useful to run tests for both small and large intestinal diseases in all affected patients.

Diarrhoea often is not the only clinical sign present and might be accompanied by anorexia, hyporexia, vomiting, weight loss, pruritus, polyuria/polydipsia, or changes in the respiratory system (Figure 18.1). These details might help identify the underlying aetiology of the diarrhoea, including extra-intestinal causes. It is important to recognize that the absence of diarrhoea does not exclude the presence of even severe gastrointestinal disease.

It is helpful to have a standardized approach when taking the history to ensure that all necessary information is asked about and recorded (Figure 18.1).

Dietary history
• What does the patient eat, including treats and supplements?   • Food changes?   • Time point(s)?   • Scavenging?   • Foreign bodies?
Medical history

• Any treatment before?
   • What medication?
   • How long?
   • Did it help?
 • Any examinations before?
   • Blood?
   • Faeces?
   • Imaging?
 • Vaccination?
 • Deworming?
   • What and when?

Stressful events
• Especially important for patients with chronic diarrhoea. For example, dog shows, house move, etc.
Diarrhoea

• Description of diarrhoea
 • How long has the dog/cat suffered from diarrhoea?
 • Intermittent/continuous?
 • What does the diarrhoea look like?
   • Mucus?
   • Blood (fresh or digested)?
 • Any tenesmus?
 • Collectable – is it possible to grade?

Other signs
• Vomiting?   • Weight loss?   • Polyuria/polydipsia?   • Anorexia/hyporexia?   • Pruritus?   • Coughing?   • Increased respiratory rate?
Travel history
• Has the dog/cat recently travelled abroad?

18.1 Standardized approach to taking a history in dogs and cats with chronic diarrhoea.

Clinical sign	Small intestine	Large intestine
Mucus	–	++
Fresh blood	–	±
Digested blood (melaena)	±	±
Tenesmus	–	++
Weight loss	++	(+)
Vomiting	+	+
Quantity	Large	Small
Consistency	Soft-formed, watery	Stringy (due to increased mucus)
Frequency	+	++
Influence on general condition	+	(+)
Abnormal folate and/or cobalamin	±	–
Borborygmi	+	–
Faecal urgency	–	+

18.2 Differences in clinical signs in dogs and cats with small intestinal *versus* large intestinal diarrhoea. However, it should be noted that many dogs and cats with large intestinal signs will have evidence of small intestinal involvement too and, therefore, the investigation should also evaluate the small intestine (e.g. serum cobalamin and folate, abdominal ultrasound examination, and duodenal and ileal endoscopic biopsy).

Physical examination

A thorough physical examination is important to define the severity and the possible origin (intestinal *versus* extra-intestinal) of the underlying disease.

The physical examination should start with observation of the unrestrained animal. This is necessary in order to observe characteristics such as mentation, body condition, posture and breathing pattern. The behaviour of the patient can also be evaluated in order to assess signs of nervousness.

Even though abdominal examination is one of the most important parts of the physical examination in cases of chronic diarrhoea, the physical examination should include all organ systems.

The examination should start with body condition scoring (see Chapter 9), followed by evaluation of the hair coat, skin surface, muscle condition, skin turgor, body temperature, pulse and mucous membranes. A detailed examination of the oral cavity is required; the clinician should look under the tongue to detect string foreign bodies. Thyroid palpation should always be performed, especially in adult cats, in order to detect thyroid nodules. The cardiorespiratory system should be assessed in detail, to avoid missing pleural effusion possibly due to hypoalbuminaemia, perhaps secondary to gastrointestinal loss, and the peripheral lymph nodes should be palpated.

The examination of the abdomen should start with observation. The animal should be observed from behind as well as from the left and right sides to assess changes in abdominal girth. An increase in abdominal size can be due to ascites but may also be due to an increase in size of organs or bloating (see Chapter 16).

Palpation of the abdomen should assess the tension of the abdominal wall, the size and shape of intra-abdominal organs, and areas of pain. A decrease in apparent abdominal size, or increased tension of the abdominal wall, can be a sign of abdominal pain. It is important to take time for abdominal palpation in order to avoid muscle tensing. Both hands are laid flat on both sides of the animal's abdomen and while slowly increasing pressure the abdomen should be palpated systematically from cranial to caudal (Figure 18.3a) The intestines should move freely between the fingers of the examiner and should feel soft and smooth.

A digital rectal examination is an important part of the physical examination in dogs (Figure 18.3b). This provides not only a faecal sample but also allows assessment of the faecal consistency, colour and odour as well as for the presence of mucus, fresh blood, melaena or foreign material. Furthermore, rectal masses, strictures or irregular thickening of the rectal wall can be detected. Digital palpation of the rectum in cats is usually performed under general anaesthesia or deep sedation (Marks, 2012).

It might be helpful to use a clinical scoring system, such as the canine inflammatory bowel disease activity index (CIBDAI) (Jergens *et al.*, 2003) or canine chronic enteropathy clinical activity index (CCECAI) (Allenspach *et al.*, 2007) or, in feline patients, the feline chronic enteropathy activity index (FCEAI) (Jergens *et al.*, 2010) to objectively record the patient's signs (see Chapter 34c).

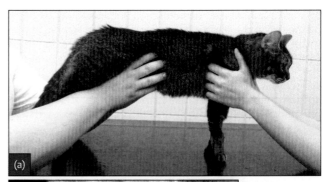
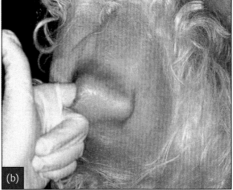

18.3 (a) Abdominal palpation of a cat. (b) Digital rectal examination of a dog.
(b, Courtesy of J Williams)

Differential diagnoses

The diagnostic approach to the causes of chronic diarrhoea in dogs and cats is shown in Figure 18.4.

Intestinal disorders

Figure 18.5 lists the potential causes for intestinal disorders that can cause chronic diarrhoea in cats and dogs.

Extra-intestinal disorders

Figure 18.6 details the potential causes for extra-intestinal disorders in cats and dogs.

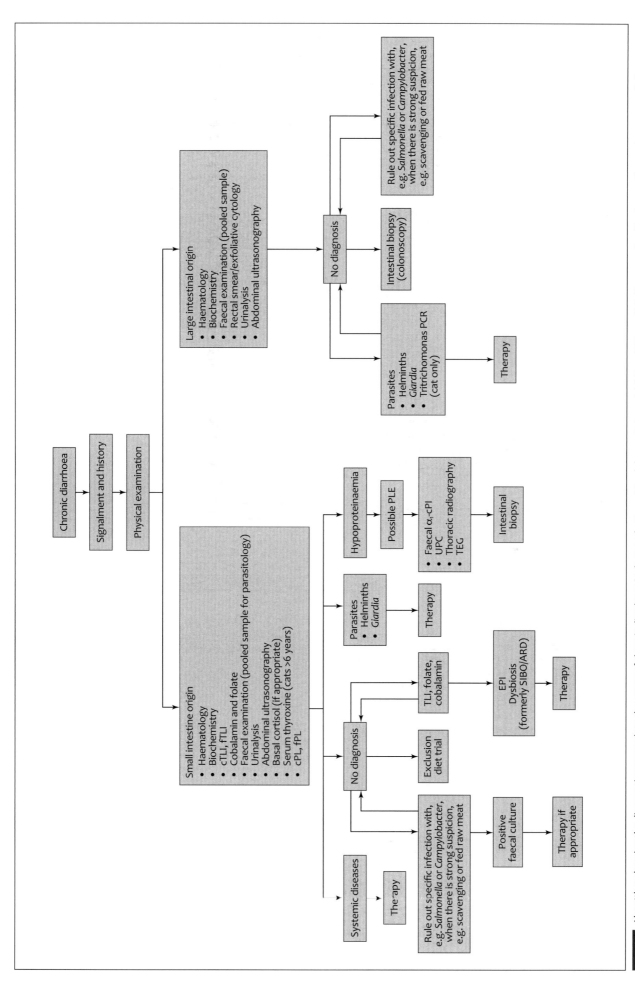

18.4 Algorithm showing the diagnostic approach to the cause of chronic diarrhoea in dogs and cats. α₁-PI = alpha₁-proteinase inhibitor; ARD = antibiotic-responsive diarrhoea; cPL = canine pancreatic lipase; cTLI = canine trypsin-like immunoreactivity; EPI = exocrine pancreatic insufficiency; fPL = feline pancreatic lipase; fTLI = feline trypsin-like immunoreactivity; PCR= polymerase chain reaction; PLE = protein-losing enteropathy; SIBO = small intestinal bacterial overgrowth; TEG = thromboelastography; TLI = trypsin-like immunoreactivity; UPC = urine protein:creatinine ratio.

Dietary

- Dietary intolerance
- Food allergy

Inflammatory

- Chronic enteropathies (eosinophilic, lymphoplasmacytic, other)
  - Food responsive
  - Antibiotic responsive
  - Idiopathic chronic enteropathy (with inflammation and/or villous atrophy)
  - Lymphangiectasia

Infectious

- Fungal
  - *Pythium insidiosum* (dogs)
  - Histoplasmosis (primarily dogs)
  - Cryptococcosis (rare)
- Algal
  - *Prototheca zopfii* (large intestinal signs)
- Parasitic
  - Whipworms
  - Roundworms
  - Hookworms
  - Tapeworms
- Protozoal
  - *Tritrichomonas* (cats)
  - *Giardia* spp.
  - *Coccidia*
  - *Cryptosporidium*
- Rickettsial
  - *Neorickettsia helminthoeca*
- Bacterial
  - *Clostridium perfringens*
  - *Clostridium difficile*
  - *Salmonella* spp. (typically acute diarrhoea or asymptomatic)
  - *Escherichia coli* (adherent invasive *E. coli*, granulomatous colitis, large bowel signs)
- Viral
  - Parvovirus (typically acute)
  - Distemper (typically acute)
  - Feline infectious peritonitis
  - Feline leukaemia virus
  - Feline immunodeficiency virus
    - Chronic intussusception
    - Annular neoplasm
    - Stricture (rare)
    - Foreign body

Infiltrative

- Infiltrative neoplasia (lymphoma, carcinoma, mast cell tumour, histiocytic disease)
- Other infiltrative diseases (amyloidosis)

Mechanical/motility

- Irritable bowel syndrome (IBS) (extrapolated from human IBS)
- Partial intraluminal obstruction

18.5 Causes of intestinal disorders associated with chronic diarrhoea in dogs and cats.

Pancreatic diseases

- Pancreatitis
- Exocrine pancreatic insufficiency
- Pancreatic neoplasia

Liver diseases

- Liver failure
- Intra-hepatic cholestasis
- Bile duct obstruction

Kidney diseases

- Uraemia
- Nephrotic syndrome

Metabolic disorders

- Hypoadrenocorticism
- Hyperthyroidism
- Hypokalaemia

18.6 Causes of extra-intestinal disorders associated with chronic diarrhoea in dogs and cats. APUDoma = amine precursor uptake and decarboxylation tumour. (continues) ▶

Metabolic disorders *continued*

- Hypoalbuminaemia
- Hypocobalaminaemia
- APUDoma (e.g. gastrinoma)

Various drugs and toxins

- Non-steroidal anti-inflammatory drugs
- Antibiotics
- Digoxin
- Cancer chemotherapeutics
- Others

18.6 (continued) Causes of extra-intestinal disorders associated with chronic diarrhoea in dogs and cats. APUDoma = amine precursor uptake and decarboxylation tumour.

Diagnostic tests

Figure 18.7 details the diagnostic tests that can be employed to investigate chronic diarrhoea.

Blood tests

- Haematology
- Serum electrolytes, including ionized calcium
- Serum biochemistry panel
- Serum thyroxine assay, in cats >6 years old
- Serum folate (decreased folate is compatible with proximal small intestinal disease)
- Serum cobalamin (there is a high prevalence of decreased serum concentrations in chronic small intestinal disease; also a negative prognostic factor)
- 12-hour fasted serum trypsin-like immunoreactivity is a sensitive and specific test for exocrine pancreatic insufficiency
- Canine and feline pancreatic lipase can be negative prognostic factors with a likely poor response to glucocorticoid treatment
- Serum basal cortisol >55 nmol/l to exclude hypoadrenocorticism (Lennon *et al.*, 2007)
- Adrenal function tests if necessary, e.g. an ACTH stimulation test if basal cortisol <55 nmol/l to confirm hypoadrenocorticism
- Feline leukaemia virus, feline immunodeficiency virus status
- C-reactive protein
- Pre- and postprandial bile acids

Urinalysis

- Urine specific gravity
- Sediment evaluation
- Urine protein:creatinine ratio

Faecal tests (see Chapter 2)

- Faecal cytology (dry and wet mount)
- Faecal flotation for parasites – three pooled samples are recommended due to intermittent shedding
- *Giardia* antigen test
- Trial therapy with antiparasitic agent should be considered as false-negative faecal results are possible
- *Tritrichomonas foetus* polymerase chain reaction (cats)
- Faecal alpha$_1$-proteinase inhibitor may detect protein-losing intestinal diseases before the serum albumin starts to decrease (assay only available in the USA and currently only for dogs)
- For suspected bacterial-associated diarrhoea: faecal culture and *Clostridium* toxin measurement are not helpful

Imaging

- Thoracic radiography may demonstrate pleural effusion
- Abdominal ultrasonography may be useful
  - Characterize extra-intestinal diseases
  - Describe intestinal wall layering and thickening

Gastroduodeno-colonoscopy

- It is recommended to perform endoscopy of the ileum after duodenal endoscopy in every patient with chronic diarrhoea (both small intestinal and large intestinal) in order to increase the diagnostic yield

18.7 Specific diagnostic tests for dogs and cats with chronic diarrhoea. ACTH = adrenocorticotropic hormone.

References and further reading

Allenspach K (2013) Diagnosis of small intestinal disorders in dogs and cats. *Veterinary Clinics of North America: Small Animal Practice* **43**, 1227–1240

Allenspach K, Wieland B, Gröne A and Gaschen F (2007) Chronic enteropathies in dogs: evaluation of risk factors for negative outcome. *Journal of Veterinary Internal Medicine* **21**, 700–708

Battersby I and Harvey A (2006) Differential diagnosis and treatment of acute diarrhoea in the dog and the cat. *In Practice* **28**, 480–488

Berghoff N, Parnell NK, Hill SL, Suchodolski JS and Steiner JM (2013) Serum cobalamin and methylmalonic acid concentrations in dogs with chronic gastrointestinal disease. *American Journal of Veterinary Research* **74**, 84–89

Di Donato P, Penninck D, Pietra M, Cipone M and Diana A (2013) Ultra-sonographic measurement of the relative thickness of intestinal wall layers in clinically healthy cats. *Journal of Feline Medicine and Surgery* **16**, 333–339

Elwood C, Devauchekke P, Elliott J *et al.* (2010) Emesis in dogs: a review. *Journal of Small Animal Practice* **51**, 4–22

Goodwin LV, Goggs R, Chan DL and Allenspach K (2011) Hypercoagulability in dogs with protein-losing enteropathy. *Journal of Veterinary Internal Medicine* **25**, 273–277

Jergens AE, Crandell JM, Evans R, Ackermann M, Miles KG and Wang C (2010) A clinical index for disease activity in cats with chronic enteropathy. *Journal of Veterinary Internal Medicine* **24**, 1027–1033

Jergens AE, Schreiner CA, Frank DE *et al.* (2003) A scoring index for disease activity in canine inflammatory bowel disease. *Journal of Veterinary Internal Medicine* **17**, 291–297

Lennon EM, Boyle TE, Hutchins RG *et al.* (2007) Use of basal serum or plasma cortisol concentrations to rule out a diagnosis of hypoadrenocorticism in dogs: 123 cases (2000–2005). *Journal of the American Veterinary Medical Association* **231**, 4163–4166

Marion M, Lecoindre P, Marlois N *et al.* (2017) Link between chronic gastric disease and anxiety in dogs. *Proceedings of the 11th International Veterinary Behaviour Meeting* 14–16 September 2017, Samorin, Slovakia

Marks SL (2012) Diarrhoea. In: *Canine and Feline Gastroenterology*, ed. RJ Washabau and MJ Day, pp. 99–107. Saunders, St. Louis

Marks SL, Rankin SC, Byrne BA and Weese JS (2011) Enteropathogenic bacteria in dogs and cats: diagnosis, epidemiology, treatment and control. *Journal of Veterinary Internal Medicine* **25**, 1195–1208

Reed N, Gunn-Moore D and Simpson K (2007) Cobalamin, folate and inorganic phosphate abnormalities in ill cats. *Journal of Feline Medicine and Surgery* **9**, 278–288

Scott KD, Zoran DL, Mansell J, Norby B and Willard MD (2011) Utility of endoscopic biopsies of the duodenum and ileum for diagnosis of inflammatory bowel disease and small cell lymphoma in cats. *Journal of Veterinary Internal Medicine* **25**, 1523–1527

Chapter 19

Haematemesis

Mike Willard

Definition of the problem

Haematemesis is defined as the vomiting of blood (*Dorland's Illustrated Medical Dictionary*).

Relevant history

Obtaining an accurate history is crucial, and the client must be carefully questioned regarding the exact appearance of the vomitus. The blood may be undigested and have the typical red colour associated with blood (Figure 19.1), or it may be partially to completely digested and resemble 'coffee grounds' or 'dregs' from a tea bag or even 'dirt' (Figure 19.2). While most clients recognize undigested blood because it is red, very few clients recognize digested or semi-digested blood in the vomitus.

It is important to try to distinguish vomiting from regurgitation based upon the history, especially if the blood is undigested. If the patient has signs consistent with vomiting (i.e. prodromal signs, active retching, dry heaving and/or bile), then it is almost certainly vomiting. However, if the patient does not have any of these signs, one cannot assume that the patient is regurgitating. While most of these patients are regurgitating, some are vomiting and show signs identical to patients that are regurgitating. If the patient is producing digested blood, then it is almost

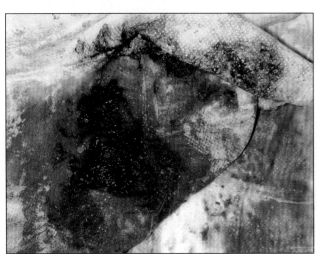

19.1 Typical red appearance of blood which has been vomited. There is dark material in the centre, which represents blood being digested. More completely digested blood is shown in Figure 19.2.

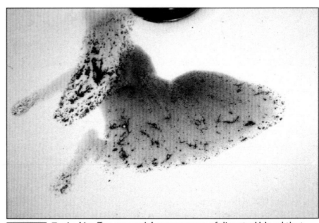

19.2 Typical 'coffee grounds' appearance of digested blood that has been vomited.

certainly vomiting. If the patient is producing red blood, then it becomes important to determine whether the blood is coming from the oesophagus or is swallowed blood originating from the respiratory tract, as opposed to coming from the stomach or intestines.

If haematemesis is chronic, then acute haemorrhagic diarrhoea syndrome (AHDS), formerly called haemorrhagic gastroenteritis (HGE), which is a frequent cause of acute haematemesis, typically with simultaneous haematochezia (see also Chapter 21), can be ruled out. Acute haematemesis can be due to almost any cause of acute vomiting (see Chapter 14).

The amount of blood in the vomited material can be informative. If there are only a few small spots of blood (typically red or reddish brown) interspersed in the vomited material (Figure 19.3), then it is not likely to be clinically important: any animal which is vomiting vigorously may have a few small spots of blood caused by mechanical trauma to the gastric mucosa during vomiting, as the gastric mucosa is forcibly thrust into the oesophagus. Larger amounts of blood, either spread throughout the material or in 'pools', are much more likely to be due to a clinically important lesion.

It is important to understand that, although there may be other signs of gastrointestinal (GI) disease (e.g. anorexia, abdominal pain, diarrhoea, weight loss), some patients with serious disease have haematemesis as their only clinical sign. If large volumes of blood (i.e. tablespoon-sized amounts) are being produced, then it is important to check for evidence of weakness, pale mucous membranes and/or heavy breathing that might suggest hypovolaemia

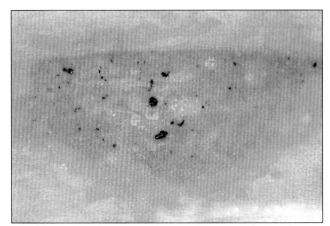

19.3 Small specks of blood in vomited bile-stained fluid. Such specks can be due to various causes, but especially mucosal trauma secondary to vigorous vomiting of any cause.

or anaemia. However, one must realize that most patients vomiting blood do not have signs consistent with anaemia.

When haematemesis is present or suspected, the clinician should specifically question the owner regarding potential causes of upper GI ulceration (GU), as well as toxins that cause coagulopathies. All non-steroidal anti-inflammatory drugs (NSAIDs), including COX-2 NSAIDs as well as topical NSAIDs applied to the eyes, ears or skin, and dexamethasone are particularly ulcerogenic. It is especially easy for owners to forget to mention administration of NSAIDs, since they are over-the-counter medications found in most households; hence, this area should be revisited a couple of times during the anamnesis. Ingestion of vitamin K antagonists, while a rare cause, is important to check for because missing it can be catastrophic. Anything which could cause severe hypoperfusion (e.g. an episode of shock due to trauma or surgery; severe physiological stress due to hard work associated with very hot or very cold temperatures) must be identified. It is important to ask if anything that might be a gastric foreign body is missing from the environment. In addition, it should be remembered that mast cell tumours could cause haematemesis as even the remote release of histamine leads to gastric hyperacidity.

Physical examination

Physical examination is seldom revealing in patients with haematemesis. Anaemia is infrequently found, and hypovolaemia/shock is rare. Abdominal pain is relatively uncommon in patients with bleeding gastric lesions, except when there is deep ulceration near to the point of perforation. Rectal examination rarely reveals melaena because it only occurs when a large amount of blood is lost into the GI tract in a relatively short period of time (see Chapter 20). A thorough dermatological examination is very important to rule out masses that could be mast cell tumours. Despite these findings being uncommon, finding any of them typically mandates a more aggressive diagnostic and therapeutic approach.

Diagnostic tests

A logical diagnostic approach is to rule out bleeding disorders, systemic diseases and NSAID administration before investigating the GI tract (Figure 19.4). Platelet

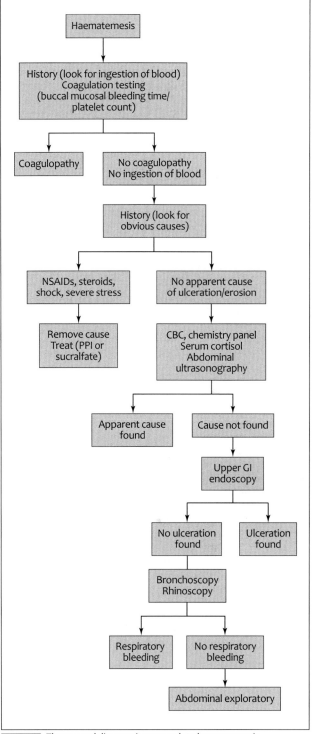

19.4 The general diagnostic approach to haematemesis. CBC = complete blood count; GI = gastrointestinal; NSAIDs = non-steroidal anti-inflammatory drugs; PPI = proton pump inhibitor.

count, buccal mucosal bleeding times and coagulation testing are good screening tests to look for the presence of bleeding disorders. Coagulopathies need to be eliminated early on despite being uncommon causes of haematemesis. If the history and physical examination are not very suggestive of the cause (e.g. NSAID ingestion, shock, mast cell tumour), then the next step is usually abdominal imaging.

Ultrasonography is superior to radiography when looking for GU. Looking for GU radiographically requires a barium contrast procedure, but this is notoriously insensitive and it also makes later endoscopic examination difficult or impossible. Abdominal ultrasonography is more sensitive than abdominal radiography, but it must be understood that ultrasonography is inherently a relatively insensitive test for most gastric disorders; it can miss major gastric infiltrates and ulcers, and it can never be assumed that a major lesion is not present because it was not found by ultrasound examination. If an infiltrate is noted, performing fine-needle aspiration is reasonable as it may diagnose malignancy, an important cause of ulceration.

A complete blood count (CBC) and serum biochemistry panel are typically undertaken simultaneously with or after imaging. The CBC seldom diagnoses the presence or the cause of GU, but might indicate the severity and/or chronicity of the bleeding. The serum biochemistry panel sometimes finds evidence of hepatic failure, an important cause of GU. Hypoalbuminaemia and hypocholesterolaemia, which are often found in severe hepatic insufficiency, can also be caused by GI blood loss; therefore, their presence does not help diagnose hepatic failure. Likewise, many dogs with hepatic failure are not hyperbilirubinaemic. Serum bile acid concentrations and blood ammonia concentrations are typically most helpful in diagnosing hepatic failure.

Some dogs with severe GI bleeding have atypical hypoadrenocorticism with normal serum electrolytes, but hyponatraemia and hyperkalaemia are the classic findings suggestive of hypoadrenocorticism. However, non-adrenal diseases can also cause these electrolyte aberrations. A resting serum cortisol measurement is a good screening test for hypoadrenocorticism, which can closely mimic GI disease and even cause major haematemesis. Hypercalcaemia is an uncommon finding, but, when present, is usually due to hypercalcaemia of malignancy in dogs (although some hypoadrenal dogs are also hypercalcaemic). Lymphoma is perhaps the most common cause of hypercalcaemia of malignancy in dogs; hence, hypercalcaemia may suggest GI lymphoma.

Chronic kidney disease, although often mentioned as a cause of GU, is infrequently responsible for haematemesis in the dog or cat. Sometimes the blood urea is increased due to GI haemorrhage, because the blood acts as a source of protein for intestinal bacteria. However, it requires a lot of GI bleeding in a relatively short time to raise the urea enough to be noticeable. Furthermore, unless a chemistry panel was obtained shortly before the GI bleeding episode, it can be difficult to determine that there has been an increase.

If the cause is still unknown after extensive biochemical testing and imaging, then the clinician must choose between therapeutic trials for GU or further testing, which usually means gastroduodenoscopy. Likewise, if a lesion is found by ultrasonography but cannot be diagnosed by examination of a fine-needle aspirate, then it must be decided whether to perform endoscopy or surgery.

If no lesion is found during ultrasonography, then gastroduodenoscopy is the best next step. If the lesion is in the oesophagus, stomach or proximal duodenum, then endoscopy is the most sensitive and specific investigation for GU. Upper GI endoscopy requires special equipment and anaesthesia. It can be surprisingly easy to miss gastric lesions if the clinician has less than excellent equipment or does not perform a thorough examination (see Chapter 4). If endoscopy is unavailable, an exploratory laparotomy may be performed, but it is quite easy to miss focal gastric or intestinal mucosal lesions when performing surgery. Most gastric lesions are not visible from the serosal surface, and it is very easy to miss GU when looking into the stomach via a gastrotomy incision. Complicating the situation, lesions may only bleed intermittently. Therefore, flexible endoscopy, performed by a competent endoscopist, is preferred, even if it requires referral. Capsule endoscopy can be performed instead of gastroduodenoscopy, and it will examine the entire GI tract.

If a therapeutic trial is elected in place of further diagnostics, a proton pump inhibitor (e.g. omeprazole, pantoprazole) is an excellent choice. While it takes proton pump inhibitors 3–5 days to achieve their maximum efficacy, their initial efficacy is probably better than that of H_2-receptor antagonists. There are no data suggesting that combining a proton pump inhibitor with H_2-receptor antagonists, misoprostol or sucralfate is beneficial. Sucralfate in particular can make endoscopy very difficult to perform adequately later. If a therapeutic trial is going to work, there should be clear evidence of improvement (not necessarily complete resolution) in 5–7 days. If there is not clear, unequivocal evidence of improvement by that time, diagnostics become imperative.

Differential diagnoses

AHDS is a common disease of middle-aged, small-breed dogs; terriers seem to be commonly affected. These patients often have acute haematemesis coupled with haematochezia and hyporexia. A suggestive history coupled with an increased haematocrit and normal serum proteins is most suggestive.

Any dog with vigorous vomiting of any cause may have a few specks of blood in the vomitus. This is usually insignificant. Likewise, any dog with acute gastritis may have minimal erosive disease and have a minimal amount of blood in the vomitus.

GU is the most important cause of haematemesis. GU is commonly iatrogenic and caused by drugs, especially NSAIDs. Dexamethasone is probably the most ulcerogenic of the steroids. Prednisolone does not cause ulceration as reliably as dexamethasone, but using high doses and/or the presence of other stress factors (e.g. poor perfusion) can be associated with substantial gastric haemorrhage. Other causes of GU include various gastric malignancies (i.e. carcinoma (especially scirrhous), leiomyoma, leiomyosarcoma, lymphoma), paraneoplastic hyperacidity (i.e. gastrinoma, mast cell tumour), hepatic failure, and severe physiological stress causing poor visceral perfusion. Hypoadrenocorticism can cause gastric bleeding that appears to be due to GU. While an uncommon cause, it can be very important. Gastric foreign objects are an uncommon cause of GU, unless of sharp metallic or plastic nature. However, a foreign object in the stomach can prevent GU from any other cause from healing, despite treatment with medications. Coagulopathies and benign polyps rarely cause clinically detectable gastric haemorrhage. Blood may reflux into the stomach from duodenal lesions (e.g. duodenal ulceration, bleeding from the gall bladder). Rarely, oesophageal lesions (usually due to foreign bodies or occasionally as an iatrogenic complication from ballooning a stricture) will bleed, and the blood will pass into the stomach and subsequently be vomited. Still less commonly, patients with bleeding lesions in the lungs or nasopharynx may cough up and swallow blood and then subsequently vomit it. Finally, some patients will ingest blood (e.g. by scavenging on waste food or the remains of slaughtered animals) and later vomit it, mimicking GU.

References and further reading

Boston SE, Moens NMM, Kruth SA *et al.* (2003) Endoscopic evaluation of the gastroduodenal mucosa to determine the safety of short-term concurrent administration of meloxicam and dexamethasone in healthy dogs. *American Journal of Veterinary Research* **64**, 1369–1375

Boysen SR (2015) Gastrointestinal hemorrhage. In: *Small Animal Critical Care Medicine, 2nd edn*, ed. D Silverstein and K Hopper, pp. 630–634. Elsevier Saunders, St. Louis

Dorland's Illustrated Medical Dictionary, 32nd edn (2011) Elsevier Saunders, Philadelphia

Monnig AA and Prittie JE (2011) A review of stress-related mucosal disease. *Journal of Veterinary Emergency and Critical Care* **21**, 484–495

Myers M, Scrivani PV and Simpson KW (2018) Presumptive non-cirrhotic bleeding esophageal varices in a dog. *Journal of Veterinary Internal Medicine* **32**, 1703–1707

Peters RM, Goldstein RE, Erb HN *et al.* (2005) Histopathologic features of canine uremic gastropathy: a retrospective study. *Journal of Veterinary Internal Medicine* **19**, 315–320

Webb C and Twedt DC (2003) Canine gastritis. *Veterinary Clinics of North America: Small Animal Practice* **33**, 969–985

Willard MD (2013) Hemorrhage (gastrointestinal). In: *Canine and Feline Gastroenterology*, ed. RJ Washabau and MJ Day, pp. 129–134. Elsevier, St. Louis

Chapter 20

Melaena

Mike Willard

Definition of the problem

Melaena is defined as the passage of dark-coloured faeces stained with blood pigments or with altered blood (*Dorland's Illustrated Medical Dictionary*). Melaena usually indicates upper gastrointestinal (GI) disease, as opposed to haematochezia, which generally indicates lower GI haemorrhage (i.e. colonic/rectal) (see Chapter 21 for a discussion of haematochezia).

Relevant history

An accurate history is essential. Having a client volunteer that their animal's faeces are 'dark' in colour is essentially meaningless. Unless the faeces are black (Figure 20.1) and tarry, the clinician has no assurance that the dark faecal colour represents melaena. It is important to determine if a history of melaena meets these criteria or, if doubt remains, whether melaena is actually present. Furthermore, the entire faeces may be melaenic, or there may be digested blood smeared over and partially covering otherwise normally coloured faeces. The clinician should ask if substances that can mimic melaena (i.e. bismuth-containing products, activated charcoal) could have been ingested. Determining that haematemesis is present (i.e. 'coffee grounds' or 'tea dregs' in the vomitus; see Chapter 19) is consistent with melaena, but its absence does not help to discern whether melaena is present or absent.

The clinician should note things in the history that may promote GI ulceration (e.g. administration of non-steroidal anti-inflammatory drugs or dexamethasone, severe hypoperfusion such as shock, severe physiological stress) and are consistent with melaena. However, many patients with gastric lesions do not vomit; hyporexia may be the major and/or only sign of gastric disease. Hence, many patients with upper GI haemorrhage (e.g. due to GI neoplasia) causing melaena have little or nothing else in their history besides hyporexia to suggest that a GI lesion is present.

Physical examination

Physical examination may be consistent with substantial gastric or duodenal haemorrhage (i.e. pale oral mucous membranes, weak or hyperdynamic pulses). However, this is uncommon. Abdominal palpation infrequently elicits pain in patients with GI ulcers. Digital rectal examination may be the first time that melaenic faeces are noted.

Diagnostic tests

The clinician must, first, be sure that 'dark' faeces in fact represent melaena and not other pigments. Sometimes, simply putting fresh faeces with suspected melaena on white, absorbent paper reveals a red colour diffusing away from the faecal mass, confirming melaena (Figure 20.2).

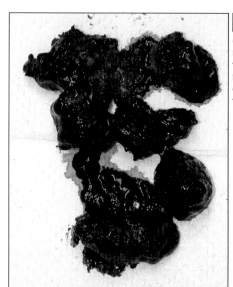

20.2 Brown faeces covered with melaena (black faeces). Note the reddish colour diffusing out from the faeces.

20.1 Typical appearance of melaena from a dog. Note the coal black appearance.

BSAVA Manual of Canine and Feline Gastroenterology, third edition. Edited by Edward J. Hall, David A. Williams and Aarti Kathrani. ©BSAVA 2020

If blood loss has been peracute, there may be no changes on the complete blood count. If there has been upper GI haemorrhage sufficient to cause melaena, then the packed cell volume and serum albumin concentration will typically decrease within a day. A one-time event causing melaena will probably result in a regenerative anaemia within 3–5 days of the event. Chronic blood loss may produce iron deficiency anaemia (i.e. decreased mean cell volume (MCV), hypochromia increased red blood cell distribution width (RDW)). RDW is more sensitive than MCV for detecting microcytosis, and an increased RDW may be seen in patients with a normal MCV. In such cases, examination of the red blood cell histogram may reveal microcytosis that is not apparent from considering the MCV.

Mild to moderate hypoalbuminaemia is classically found in patients with GI blood loss but is not guaranteed; it depends upon what the serum albumin concentration was before the blood loss began. Even serum albumin concentrations at the very low end of the reference range, while technically 'normal', may not be 'normal enough'. Hypocholesterolaemia may reflect intestinal malabsorption but can also be secondary to GI loss of blood, depending upon what the serum cholesterol concentration was prior to the bleeding.

Upper GI haemorrhage (especially from gastric ulcers) is a common cause of melaena; hence, the diagnostic approach (Figure 20.3) is similar to that described for haematemesis (see Chapter 19). Coagulopathies, hepatic disease and hypoadrenocorticism should be excluded by clinical pathology testing early in the course of the investigation. Increased alanine transaminase activity, serum bile acid concentrations and/or blood ammonia concentrations suggest hepatic disease, which may be the cause or the effect of whatever is causing GI bleeding. A resting serum cortisol concentration is useful to screen for hypoadrenocorticism. Hypercalcaemia can be due to hypercalcaemia of malignancy, which itself is most often due to lymphoma (although some hypoadrenal dogs are also hypercalcaemic). The clinician may rarely see erthrocytosis or hypoglycaemia due to intestinal leiomyoma.

Abdominal ultrasonography is typically performed along with clinicopathological testing. If an infiltrative lesion or a mass is noted, fine-needle aspiration may allow a diagnosis. If the nature of the infiltrate cannot be identified with fine-needle aspiration, then abdominal exploratory surgery for biopsy (typically excisional) is usually the next step (since the clinician can have reasonable confidence that there is a lesion that can be visually discerned or palpated at surgery). Gastroduodenoscopy can be performed instead if the lesion appears to be within the reach of the insertion tube.

If abdominal ultrasonography does not reveal any meaningful lesions, then gastroduodenoscopy is typically the next step. Gastroduodenoscopy is much more sensitive for finding mucosal lesions (especially of the stomach) than is surgery. If gastroduodenoscopy is not helpful, then bronchoscopy and examination of the choanae can assess for occult respiratory bleeding in which blood is coughed up and swallowed. However, in some cases, the bleeding lesion may be in the GI tract but beyond the reach of the typical 1 m or even 1.6 m gastroscope (i.e. mid-jejunum). In such a patient, the clinician must perform either 'push enteroscopy' (which involves specialized endoscopic equipment that is seldom available to veterinary surgeons (veterinarians)), capsule endoscopy or an exploratory laparotomy.

If the cause of haemorrhage is not apparent at exploratory surgery, then surgery can be combined with

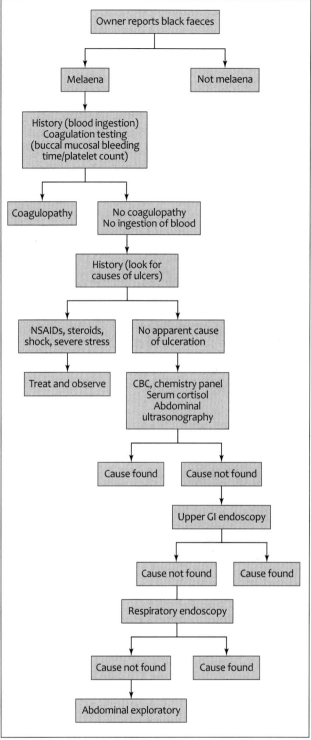

20.3 Overview of the basic diagnostic approach to the patient with melaena. CBC = complete blood count; GI = gastrointestinal; NSAIDs = non-steroidal anti-inflammatory drugs.

endoscopy. A flexible endoscope is advanced as far as possible into the duodenum/jejunum, and then the surgeon manually pushes the intestines over the tip of the endoscope, thus allowing the endoscopist to visualize most of the jejunal mucosa. Alternatively, the clinician may insert a needle into the small intestinal lumen and aspirate at multiple levels during laparotomy, to help localize where the haemorrhage is occurring. Once the level of haemorrhage is identified, an enterotomy can be performed to examine the mucosal surface and locate the source of haemorrhage.

Chapter 21

Haematochezia

Mike Willard

Definition of the problem

Haematochezia is defined as the 'presence of blood in the faeces' *(Dorland's Illustrated Medical Dictionary)*. While this technically includes melaena, it is generally understood that haematochezia refers to red, undigested blood in the faeces (Figure 21.1), while melaena refers to black, tarry, digested blood in the faeces (see Chapter 20).

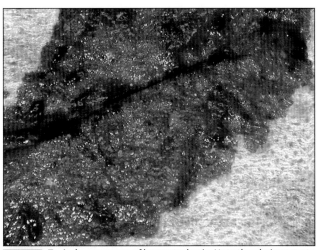

21.1 Typical appearance of haematochezia. Note the obvious spots and streaks of red blood in the dark, diarrhoeic faeces.

Relevant history

Patients with haematochezia may have nothing else in the history to suggest disease, or they may have obvious signs of colonic/rectal disease (e.g. tenesmus, dyschezia, diarrhoea) or systemic illness (e.g. depression, lethargy, hyporexia). It is important to ascertain the degree of haematochezia and the distribution of the blood on the faeces, which is not always easy. Many clients are somewhat 'put off' by their pets' abnormal faeces and have difficulty giving an accurate description. Others are so alarmed by the presence of red blood that they initially make it sound like there is much more blood present than is the case. Determining stressful events can be helpful (understanding that 'stress' is referring to physiological stress, i.e. hypovolaemia, poor perfusion, severe inflammation, etc., more than psychological stress).

Physical examination

A complete physical examination should be performed because signs of systemic disease may be occasionally seen (e.g. pale mucous membranes, injected sclera, abdominal pain). Patients with haematochezia are rarely anaemic (except young puppies with large burdens of *Ancylostoma* spp.), regardless of how severe the haematochezia is. The most important abnormalities (and often the only abnormalities) at physical examination in patients with haematochezia are typically found during digital rectal examination. This examination is the single most important diagnostic test undertaken, so much so that the patient should be sedated/anaesthetized, if that is necessary, to do a careful, complete examination. Rectal/anal lesions can be surprisingly easy to miss during digital rectal examination in conscious patients. All expected structures (i.e. pelvis, wings of ilium, sacrum, anal sacs, prostate/urethra in male dogs, and sometimes the vagina in female dogs) should first be methodically identified and then all the mucosa within reach of the finger carefully palpated. The tip of the finger is used because it is more sensitive than the body of the finger. Masses (especially adenomatous polyps, but also malignancies), strictures (especially adenocarcinoma) and mucosal thickening/irregularity (especially from inflammatory or neoplastic infiltrative diseases) are the most common abnormalities causing haematochezia found on digital rectal examination. Anal sac disease is common but infrequently causes haematochezia, while perineal hernia rarely produces haematochezia.

Smaller polyps often feel like a fold of mucosa or a bit of faeces stuck on the mucosa; most of the time they are not particularly hard or firm. Only by repeatedly feeling the same area over and over will one recognize that it must be a lesion because it is always present in the same place. It rarely feels obviously pedunculated. Partial strictures can be easy to miss in larger animals. This is because their colonic diameter is large enough that, even if the lumen is decreased by 50% in diameter, a finger may still slip in and out without any apparent resistance. Rectal prolapse is occasionally found (especially in young patients with substantial diarrhoea). Rarely, ileocolic intussusceptions will resemble a rectal prolapse. These two lesions are relatively easy to confuse during digital examination; the presence of a fornix should be checked when performing a rectal examination of a dog with intestinal tissue protruding from the anus. Both anal sacs should be repeatedly expressed to ensure that the blood is not coming from them. The correct approach is that, if the history strongly suggests an anorectal lesion, a finger is inserted into the rectum and left there until the lesion is found!

Diagnostic tests

Faecal examination for trichuriasis is important in areas where the parasite is found. The ova are heavy, and the flotation solution must be dense enough to make them float. More than one faecal examination may be needed, as these parasites can shed ova sporadically.

After faecal examination has been performed, digital rectal examination is the single most important diagnostic procedure in patients with haematochezia. If digital rectal examination and faecal examination are non-revealing or if there is an infiltrative lesion in the rectal area, then the next step is generally endoscopy, although imaging is reasonable. Abdominal ultrasonography is possible, but there is not always a window that will allow imaging of rectal/anal lesions. However, even if the primary lesion itself cannot be seen, imaging may reveal evidence of malignant metastasis to the lumbar spine, sublumbar lymph nodes, or abdominal viscera.

Infiltrative lesions require biopsy, and rigid proctoscopy tends to be much more rewarding than flexible endoscopy for lesions near the anus. It is hard to insufflate the anorectal area with a flexible endoscope, and rigid biopsy forceps (see Chapter 4) are preferred because they can reliably obtain relatively generous amounts of submucosa. Obtaining submucosa is critically important when distinguishing benign from malignant anorectal lesions. If the lesion is out of reach of a rigid endoscope, then flexible endoscopy is necessary. Abdominal ultrasonography or flexible colonoscopy will document the rare sliding ileocolic intussusception or a caecocolic intussusception or an infiltrative lesion orad to the anorectal area. Exploratory surgery is generally avoided because of the relatively high incidence of dehiscence with full-thickness incisions into the colon.

Differential diagnoses

If there are simply a few specks of red blood on otherwise relatively normal or somewhat soft faeces, trichuriasis or other relatively mild diseases (mild colitis) are the first concerns. If haematochezia is associated with acute diarrhoea, then acute enterocolitis or trichuriasis are major concerns, although a 'stress colitis', such as is sometimes associated with kennelling or other major changes in environment, must be considered. In such cases, the patient is treated symptomatically and observed. If the patient has acute bloody vomiting and diarrhoea with haematochezia, then acute haemorrhagic diarrhoea syndrome (AHDS; formerly known as haemorrhagic gastroenteritis, HGE) is a common differential diagnosis. Parvoviral diarrhoea can produce haematochezia, but systemic signs usually predominate. If the faeces are relatively normal and the blood is isolated on one side of the faecal mass, then the lesion is suspected to be very close to the anus (e.g. rectal polyp, rectal tumour). If tissue protrudes (even intermittently) from the anus, then ileocolic intussusception is an important consideration. If the blood is haphazardly smeared across the faeces, then the lesion can be almost anywhere in the

distal colonic/anorectal area. If blood is seen on the floor when the animal gets up from lying down or sitting and is not associated with faeces, then an anal sac, perineal or a rectal lesion is suspected.

Chronic haematochezia associated with diarrhoea might be due to many causes, but severe colonic diseases that are more diffuse (e.g. granulomatous (histiocytic ulcerative) colitis, histoplasmosis, pythiosis, protothecosis, lymphosarcoma and *Heterobilharzia Americana* infection) are the most common underlying causes. Dogs with colitis causing haematochezia almost invariably have diarrhoea with mucus, while affected cats sometimes have haematochezia associated with normal faecal consistency. The more common dietary-responsive, fibre-responsive and tylosin-responsive colitides can produce haematochezia, but this association is uncommon. Colonic vascular ectasia is a particularly rare cause but can produce severe haematochezia. These associations between history, physical examination and location are not absolute, but they give the clinician a reasonable idea of the most likely place to find a lesion (Figure 21.2).

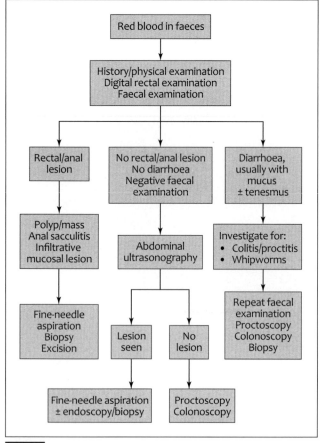

21.2 General diagnostic approach to haematochezia in the dog.

References and further reading

Boysen SR (2015) Gastrointestinal hemorrhage. In: *Small Animal Critical Care Medicine, 2nd edn*, ed. D Silverstein and K Hopper, pp. 630–634. Elsevier Saunders, St. Louis

Daugherty MA, Leib MS, Lanz OI *et al.* (2006) Diagnosis and surgical management of vascular ectasia in a dog. *Journal of the American Veterinary Medical Association* **229**, 975–979

Dorland's Illustrated Medical Dictionary, 32nd edn (2011) Elsevier Saunders, Philadelphia

Hayashi K, Okanishi H, Kagawa Y *et al.* (2012) The role of endoscopic ultrasound in the evaluation of rectal polypoid lesions in 25 dogs. *Japanese Journal of Veterinary Research* **60**, 185–189

Igarashi H, Ohno K, Fujiwara-Igarashi A *et al.* (2015) Inflammatory colorectal polyps in miniature Dachshunds frequently develop ventrally in the colorectal mucosa. *Veterinary Journal* **203**, 256–258

Nucci DJ, Liptak JM, Slemic LE *et al.* (2014) Complications and outcomes following rectal pull-through surgery in dogs with rectal masses: 74 cases (2000–2013). *Journal of the American Veterinary Medical Association* **245**, 684–695

Tefft KM (2017) Melena and hematochezia. In: *Textbook of Veterinary Internal Medicine, 8th edn*, ed. SJ Ettinger, EC Feldman, E Côté, pp. 167–171. Elsevier Saunders, St. Louis

Unterer S, Busch D, Leipig M *et al.* (2014) Endoscopically visualized lesions, histologic findings, and bacterial invasion in the gastrointestinal mucosa of dogs with acute hemorrhagic diarrhea syndrome. *Journal of Veterinary Internal Medicine* **28**, 52–58

Willard MD (2013) Hemorrhage (gastrointestinal). In: *Canine and Feline Gastroenterology,* ed. RJ Washabau and MJ Day, pp. 129–134. Elsevier Saunders, St. Louis

Chapter 22

Dyschezia

Mike Willard

Definition of the problem

Dyschezia refers to difficult or painful elimination of faeces during defecation. Primarily indicative of anorectal disease or perianorectal disorders, it often, but not invariably, coexists with tenesmus. Most animals with dyschezia have tenesmus, but many animals with tenesmus do not have dyschezia. The reader is referred to Chapter 23 for a description of tenesmus. The general diagnostic approach to dyschezia is given in Figure 22.1.

Clinical features

Patients with dyschezia often show evidence of pain by vocalizing when defecating. This is especially common in cats, which may growl loudly or even 'scream' when at or near the litter tray. In dogs, vocalization is usually rather subdued by comparison. A dog may do nothing more than whine or whimper. In more subtle cases, the patient (especially dogs) will repeatedly look back at its rectal area as if searching for something that is hurting it.

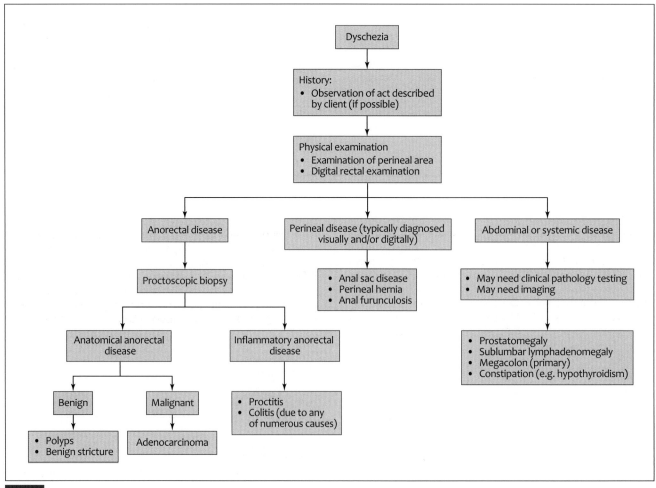

22.1 Algorithm showing an approach to the patient with dyschezia.

Relevant history

A meticulous history is very helpful when trying to differentiate dyschezia from tenesmus. It can be especially confusing because most animals with dyschezia also have tenesmus. It is important to ascertain whether the signs only occur when the patient defecates as opposed to also happening when the patient is urinating. Pain noted before defecating suggests anorectal obstructive disease, while pain noted after defecating is more suggestive of an inflammatory lesion (e.g. proctitis). Sometimes, both obstruction and inflammation coexist in anorectal lesions (e.g. anal furunculosis causing so much swelling that there is also obstruction).

Physical examination

Careful physical examination is sufficient for the diagnosis of many of the causes of dyschezia (Figure 22.2).

- Constipation (can be the cause of dyschezia, the effect of dyschezia, or both)
- Proctitis/colitis (numerous causes)
- Anorectal mass
  - Benign (polyps)
  - Malignant (adenocarcinoma, lymphoma)
  - Foreign body
- Anorectal stricture/obstruction
  - Benign stricture (rare, primarily due to trauma or congenital)
  - Malignant stricture (especially adenocarcinomas)
  - Large anorectal mass (usually neoplastic but may be a very large polyp)
  - Pelvic fracture
  - Inflammatory strictures (cats)
- Perianal/perineal disease
  - Perineal hernia
  - Anal furunculosis
  - Anal sacculitis or abscess
- Caudal abdominal disorders
  - Pelvic fracture

22.2   Causes of dyschezia.

The perineal region

The perineal region must be carefully examined for perineal hernias, anal furunculosis, abnormalities of the anal sacs (i.e. inflammation, rupture, tumour) and perianal masses. Anal furunculosis can be relatively easy to miss in the early stages (Figure 22.3). It is imperative that the clinician is able to perform a very thorough and careful examination of the perianal area, which at times includes washing the area. Anal sac disease is often only detected when the contents are expressed and inspected (i.e. pus or blood is expressed). While many perineal hernias are immediately obvious (i.e. there is a large bulge to the side of the anus), digital examination is necessary to reveal those in which an obvious perineal bulge is not present.

Abdominal palpation

Abdominal palpation may reveal an impacted colon (i.e. a dilated colon filled with hard faeces that does not allow digital pitting during palpation) indicative of constipation or obstipation. If constipation is found, the next step is to determine whether the constipation is the cause of the dyschezia or if it was caused by the dyschezia (i.e. the patient refuses to defecate due to the rectal pain and

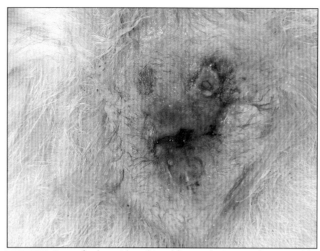

22.3   Anus of a dog with early anal furunculosis. Note that it would be very easy to miss these draining tracts if the patient was conscious and the clinician was not able to perform a careful physical examination.

subsequently becomes constipated). Occasionally, the clinician may find that the colon or the prostate is painful during abdominal palpation. Palpating a very large, firm colon may sometimes be an indication of a long ileocolic intussusception that is extending the length of the colon.

Digital rectal examination

Digital rectal examination is especially important in these patients. It is desirable to initially attempt to perform the digital rectal examination without sedation/anaesthesia to help localize the source of the pain/discomfort. Care must be taken to ensure the patient does not bite the veterinary surgeon (veterinarian), nurses or clients involved. If it is not possible to perform the rectal examination without undue stress to the patient, then sedation or even anaesthesia is indicated. In particular, the clinician needs to look for anorectal strictures, mucosal thickening in the anorectal area, intraluminal masses (e.g. benign polyps or malignant tumours), rectal foreign bodies, prostatic enlargement plus pain, and/or caudal abdominal cavity abnormalities (e.g. painful organs, masses, pelvic fractures). Finding blood on the finger after a careful examination in which the patient did not struggle strongly suggests either inflammatory disease or a friable lesion (e.g. rectal polyp). Sometimes painful anal sac disease, perineal hernias and anal furunculosis will only be appreciated during digital rectal examination. If mucosa is protruding from the rectum, it is important to distinguish rectal prolapse (which has a fornix) from an ileocolic intussusception that is protruding from the anus (in which case there will be no fornix) or a rectal polyp. In larger animals (e.g. >45 kg), it may be necessary to use two fingers during digital rectal examination to find partial strictures.

Diagnostic tests

Additional diagnostic procedures are based upon localization of the pain during digital rectal examination.

Faecal analysis

Performing multiple faecal examinations looking for parasites, ova and cysts is recommended. It is rare for nematodes to cause dyschezia, but *Tritrichomonas* in cats is renowned for producing severe dyschezia that occasionally causes vocalization during defecation. In some cases, the anus will be obviously reddened and protruding. It can be very difficult to find *Tritrichomonas* on direct faecal examination; polymerase chain reaction on faeces is a much more sensitive test (see Chapter 2). Evaluation of direct smears of rectal muscosal scrapings or fresh faeces mixed with physiological saline may reveal *Histoplasma* organisms, *Prototheca* organisms and/or neoplastic inflammatory cells, all indicative of colitis. Cytological examination of a rectal scraping is more likely to be helpful for diagnosing these disorders than faecal cytology.

Diagnostic imaging

Diagnostic imaging (e.g. plain radiographs, contrast radiographs and/or ultrasonography) is occasionally helpful. While most anorectal obstructions are best found by digital rectal examination, occasionally they require imaging (especially in larger animals in which digital examination can only explore a portion of the rectal lumen). Imaging may also reveal rectal foreign bodies, faecal impaction, intraluminal masses, and/or mesenteric or sublumbar lymphadenopathy associated with benign or malignant (e.g. lymphoma, adenocarcinoma) infiltrative diseases.

Proctoscopy

Proctoscopy utilizing a rigid endoscope is typically the most useful procedure for patients with dyschezia. It is difficult to perform a good anorectal examination with a flexible endoscope because it is hard to adequately distend the area with air insufflation. Furthermore, when biopsy is indicated (especially for mass lesions), rigid proctoscopy allows the use of rigid biopsy forceps, which typically produce far superior tissue samples compared with those obtained with biopsy forceps used through flexible endoscopes. With anorectal lesions (e.g. a mass or a mucosal or submucosal stricture), it is critically important to obtain a relatively generous amount of submucosa because it is this area that must often be evaluated to accurately distinguish benign from malignant lesions. In properly obtained tissue samples, typically the submucosa appears as a pale section below the darker mucosa. Animals that are suspected of having a more diffuse proctitis or colitis (i.e. those in which a focal lesion is not found) do not need such a deep biopsy; however, proper use of rigid forceps will still produce a far superior tissue sample. It is always advisable to take at least three or four tissue samples, even when there is an 'obvious lesion'.

Cytology of fine-needle aspiration samples from rectal and perineal masses may allow rapid identification of neoplasms and/or abscesses. However, it is important to note that while aspirate cytology can be very specific, it is notoriously insensitive (i.e. the clinician should almost never eliminate a diagnosis simply because evidence was not found on aspirate cytology).

Clinical pathology laboratory tests

Clinical pathology testing is seldom helpful in patients with dyschezia. Such testing (i.e. haematology and serum biochemistry panel) is primarily indicated to evaluate the patient prior to anaesthesia.

References and further reading

Lamoureux A, Maurey C and Freiche V (2017) Treatment of inflammatory rectal strictures by digital bougienage: a retrospective study of nine cases. *Journal of Small Animal Practice* **58**, 293–297

Chapter 23

Tenesmus

Mike Willard

Definition of the problem

Tenesmus is ineffectual and/or painful straining to urinate or defecate. It is easy to confuse tenesmus with dyschezia, but the latter is only due to anorectal disease, while the former can be due to lower urinary tract disease as well as lower gastrointestinal tract disorders. Many animals with tenesmus do not have dyschezia, but it is uncommon to have dyschezia without tenesmus. The reader is referred to Chapter 22 for a discussion of dyschezia.

One of the main reasons for tenesmus is large intestinal disease, particularly anorectal conditions. Straining is seen as the patient remains postured to defecate for an extended period of time with little faeces being produced. Tenesmus may also be evidenced by repeated, unsuccessful attempts to defecate. Tenesmus is often (but not invariably) associated with other signs of colonic disease, such as large intestinal diarrhoea (i.e. either chronic diarrhoea without weight loss, or diarrhoea with obvious haematochezia (see Chapter 21)) or mucus, or both. However, tenesmus can occur when a patient (especially a cat) has a blocked urethra and is repeatedly attempting to urinate. The general diagnostic approach to tenesmus is outlined in Figure 23.1.

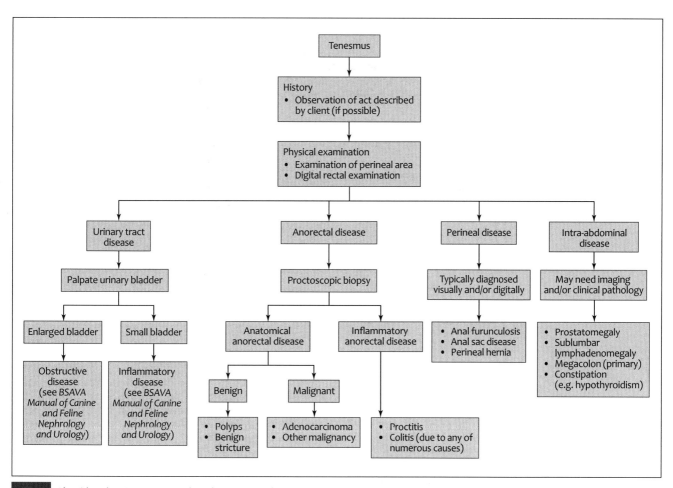

23.1 Algorithm showing an approach to the patient with tenesmus.

Relevant history

A thorough, precise history is the essential starting point for the diagnosis of almost every problem. In the case of tenesmus, it is important to consider both the lower urinary system and the lower gastrointestinal tract. Lower urinary tract disorders producing tenesmus (e.g. cystitis, urethritis, urethral obstruction) can result in protracted, unsuccessful attempts to urinate, a weak or intermittent stream of urine (or even an absent stream despite posturing) and/or urine with haematuria.

It is important to distinguish stranguria/pollakiuria producing tenesmus from polyuria/polydipsia and urinary incontinence. Most clients confuse these problems when they describe the issues to the veterinary surgeon (veterinarian). Dysuria (and tenesmus) is typically confirmed by documenting either very small amounts of urine being produced despite repeated efforts (and this can be very difficult for some clients to perceive, especially in female dogs squatting and urinating in the grass), or seeing the patient position itself to urinate but not producing urine (again, hard for some clients to accurately discern in a female squatting in the grass). Noting the position of the tail during straining can sometimes be helpful, particularly in cats. Straining to defecate is often associated with the tail being held up, while straining to urinate may result in the tail being held down. Haematochezia or faecal mucus (which some clients describe as a 'grey coating' on the faeces) strongly suggests anorectal and/or colonic disease. Finally, a lack of any evidence of abnormalities in urination is suggestive of anorectal disease.

If tenesmus is determined to be due to anorectal disease, then the question is whether the tenesmus is due to an obstruction or an inflammatory process. Tenesmus prior to the production of faeces is usually due to obstruction of the lower colon or the anorectal area. Tenesmus persisting after the production of faeces is suggestive of an inflammatory lesion of the distal colon or anorectal area. Tenesmus associated with the patient squatting tends to suggest inflammatory disease such as colitis, while tenesmus that occurs as the animal is semi-walking or partially squatting is more suggestive of constipation. Excessive grooming of the anal area may be seen in patients with perineal/perianal disease.

The characteristics of the faeces are important to note. Faeces that are normal in consistency but much thinner in diameter than normal (Figure 23.2) (i.e. so-called 'ribbon-like' faeces) strongly suggest an anorectal stricture. Faeces that are abnormally hard, especially those that are clearly larger in diameter than normal, tend to suggest constipation. However, the most important question in most constipated patients is whether the constipation is the primary cause of the tenesmus or if whatever caused the tenesmus ultimately resulted in constipation because the patient could not or would not defecate (Figure 23.3).

- Constipation (can be the cause of the tenesmus or secondary to whatever is causing the tenesmus – especially obstructions)
- Gastrointestinal disorders
  - Colitis
  - Anorectal neoplasia (benign or malignant)
  - Anorectal obstruction (neoplastic 'napkin ring' lesion, benign stricture)
  - Rectal prolapse
  - Ileocolic intussusception that reaches the anorectal area
- Perianal/perineal disorders
  - Perineal hernia
  - Anal furunculosis
  - Anal sac disease (inflammation, abscess, neoplasia)
  - Pseudocoprostasis
- Urogenital disorders
  - Cystitis and urethritis
  - Urethral or cystic obstruction (calculi, tumour)
  - Prostatomegaly
  - Urogenital neoplasia
- Caudal abdominal disorders
  - Abdominal cavity masses
  - Pelvic fracture

23.3 Common causes of tenesmus in the dog and cat.

Physical examination

Physical examination is the next most important diagnostic test after the history. If necessary, the clinician should not hesitate to sedate or even anaesthetize the patient in order to do a good physical examination, especially a careful evaluation of the perineal area and a thorough digital rectal examination. A good digital rectal examination is usually more valuable than imaging or an endoscopic examination of the anorectal area and lower colon.

The perineal region

The perineal region should be carefully examined for pain, perineal hernia, anal furunculosis, anal sac disease (e.g. inflammation, rupture, tumour) and perianal masses. While anal furunculosis is usually easy to find (i.e. there is an obvious draining tract around the anus), sometimes the tract only opens into the rectal lumen, and these fistulas will first be suspected by finding thickening around the anus. Anal sac disease may not be obvious until the anal sacs are expressed. Finding pus or blood in the anal sac contents strongly suggests anal sacculitis. Finding the anus covered with a tightly adherent mat of faeces and hair is diagnostic of pseudocoprostasis.

Abdominal palpation

Abdominal palpation may reveal a large, turgid bladder (indicative of urinary obstruction), a very small, obviously painful bladder (suggestive of cystitis), a distended colon filled with hard faeces (suggestive of constipation or obstipation) and/or organomegaly (e.g. prostatomegaly). Abdominal palpation is especially important in larger dogs because it can be hard to adequately examine the entire rectal lumen with a finger given the patient's size. Sometimes, the clinician can palpate what appears to be a very large, solid colon in animals with very long ileocolic intussusceptions that are filling much of the colonic lumen.

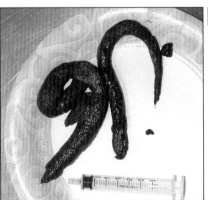

23.2 Narrow 'ribbon-like' faeces can be suggestive of an anorectal stricture.

Digital rectal examination

Digital rectal examination is performed to rule out anorectal and colonic disease, such as benign and malignant strictures, intraluminal masses (e.g. polyps or malignant tumours), perineal hernias, anorectal foreign bodies, prostatomegaly and/or caudal abdominal cavity disorders (mass, pelvic fracture). The size of the patient must be taken into consideration. It is rare that sublumbar masses can be palpated in patients larger than 10 kg. Very large dogs (e.g. >45 kg) may have a rectal lumen so large that digital examination with one finger may not detect partial strictures (it may be necessary to use two fingers in these patients). Digital rectal examination can also evaluate portions of the lower genitourinary tract. If mucosa is protruding from the anus, it is important to feel for a fornix so as to differentiate rectal prolapse (which has a fornix) from an intussusception protruding from the anus (which does not have a fornix). Such tissue must also be distinguished from rectal polyps protruding from the anus (Figure 23.4).

The penis or vagina should be examined for pain, masses or calculi.

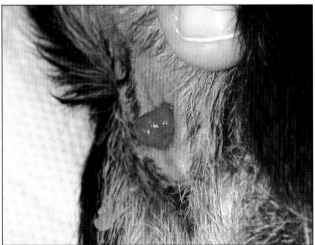

23.4 A small mass of mucosa protruding from the anus of a dog. This mass is a rectal polyp, but digital rectal examination is necessary to be sure that it is not a rectal prolapse or an intussusception.

Diagnostic tests

After a careful history and physical examination, the need for additional diagnostic tests is determined upon the localization of the cause of the tenesmus to either the genitourinary or gastrointestinal tract. Diagnostic tests that may be required to definitively diagnose genitourinary causes for tenesmus (especially cats) are outside the scope of this chapter (see the BSAVA Manual of Canine and Feline Nephrology and Urology).

Many patients (especially dogs) with tenesmus will have underlying disturbances of the anorectal area, which may in turn necessitate other tests:

* Faecal examination
* Haematology and serum biochemistry panels
* Survey and/or contrast radiography of the lower gastrointestinal tract
* Abdominal ultrasonography of the caudal abdomen, including the prostate and colon
* Proctoscopy/biopsy.

Faecal analysis

Examination of multiple faecal samples for parasites is recommended, especially in areas in which intestinal parasites are common (see Chapter 2). *Trichuris vulpis* in particular may yield false-negative results on a single faecal examination, even when there are remarkable numbers of nematodes in the colon. Evaluation of direct smears of very fresh faeces (typically mixed with warm physiological saline or warm tap water) for protozoan parasites (especially *Giardia* or *Tritrichomonas*) may be helpful, but direct examination has a very low sensitivity. Large numbers of faecal leucocytes (neutrophils) may be seen in animals with severe proctitis/colitis. Faecal cultures are very difficult to interpret because almost any pathogen (e.g. *Salmonella* spp., *Clostridium perfringens*, *Campylobacter* spp.) may be found in clinically healthy dogs or cats. Therefore, they are seldom indicated.

Diagnostic imaging

Diagnostic imaging (i.e. survey radiographs, contrast radiographs (both positive and negative contrast), and/or ultrasonography) is sometimes helpful in patients with anorectal causes for tenesmus (see Chapter 3). However, good digital rectal examination often eliminates the need for these tests except in larger animals. These imaging techniques may detect colonic foreign bodies, faecal impaction, intraluminal masses, prostatomegaly, ileocolic intussusception, and mesenteric lymphadenopathy associated with both benign and malignant (e.g. lymphoma, adenocarcinoma) infiltrative diseases, especially in animals that are not amenable to good digital rectal examination (i.e. very large or very obese patients). If genitourinary causes for tenesmus are suspected, then survey and contrast radiographs with or without abdominal ultrasonography are sometimes useful in detecting prostatomegaly, urinary masses, urinary obstruction and abdominal masses.

Proctoscopy

Proctoscopy with mucosal biopsy is sometimes helpful in evaluating animals with tenesmus due to anorectal disease. A rigid proctoscope is typically the most useful endoscope for patients with tenesmus. It is difficult to adequately examine the anorectal area with a flexible endoscope because it is impossible to adequately distend this area with air insufflation. Furthermore, when biopsy is indicated (especially for mass lesions), rigid proctoscopy allows the use of rigid biopsy forceps, which can produce far superior tissue samples compared with those obtained with the biopsy forceps used through flexible endoscopes. For anatomical lesions (e.g. a mass or a mucosal/submucosal stricture), it is critically important to obtain generous amounts of submucosa because this layer is often needed to distinguish benign from malignant lesions. In properly obtained tissue samples, the submucosa can typically be seen as a pale layer of tissue immediately below the darker superficial mucosa. Animals that are suspected of having a more diffuse proctitis or colitis (i.e. those in which a focal lesion is not found) do not need such a deep biopsy; however, proper use of rigid forceps can produce far superior mucosal tissue samples. It is usually best to take at least three or four tissue samples, even when there is an apparently 'obvious' lesion.

Clinical pathology tests

Clinical pathology tests (e.g. haematology, serum biochemistry profile and urinalysis) are sometimes helpful in animals with tenesmus due to gastrointestinal disease. They are primarily useful in patients with signs suggestive of systemic disease (e.g. anorexia, weight loss, dehydration, bilaterally symmetrical alopecia, polyuria/polydipsia) and/or severe constipation. In dogs with constipation of unknown cause, these tests may identify electrolyte abnormalities (e.g. severe hypokalaemia, hypercalcaemia) that can cause colonic weakness, or hypercholesterolaemia suggestive of hypothyroidism (which can produce severe constipation). Cytological examination of rectal scrapings is appropriate as a quick test to look for *Histoplasma* or *Prototheca* organisms and/or inflammatory cells (which are indicative of colitis). However, negative cytology results do not eliminate these disorders. Cytology of fine-needle aspiration samples from rectal and perineal masses may allow identification of neoplasms (but failure to find malignant cells does not eliminate the diagnosis of cancer).

References and further reading

Elliott J, Grauer GF and Westropp J (2017) *BSAVA Manual of Canine and Feline Nephrology and Urology, 3rd edn*. BSAVA Publications, Gloucester

Chapter 24

Ascites

Andrea Boari

Definition of the problem

A body cavity effusion is defined as the abnormal accumulation of fluid of any type within a cavity, and ascites is the accumulation of fluid in the peritoneal cavity. Effusions are traditionally classified as pure transudate, modified transudate and exudate based on the total protein concentration and total nucleated cell count (Figure 24.1). Thus, although any peritoneal fluid accumulation, including bile, blood, chyle and urine, could be classified as ascites, the term is usually best used to refer to pure transudate or modified transudate.

Recently, the more clinically useful classification has categorized effusions on the basis of their aetiology into:

- **Transudates** – subtyped into protein-rich or protein-poor (Figure 24.2)
- **Exudates** – subtyped into septic or non-septic
- **Effusion caused by a ruptured vessel or viscus** – haemorrhagic, chylous, urinary, biliary
- **Effusion caused by cell exfoliation** – mainly neoplastic.

That said, ascites mainly refers to transudates associated with either a protein-poor or protein-rich fluid accumulation.

Ascites occurs by processes that involve the forces of Starling's law, anatomical structures and lymphatic drainage. The most common mechanisms for a transudate to accumulate are passive fluid shifting caused by decreased colloid osmotic pressure, increased capillary hydrostatic pressure or ineffective lymphatic drainage. However, more than one of these mechanisms will often simultaneously contribute to the fluid accumulation, and the composition of ascitic fluid is influenced by the overlapping anatomical and vascular system abnormalities. The anatomical system is based on the gross anatomy (i.e. pre-hepatic, intra-hepatic or post-hepatic) and relates to the flow of blood to,

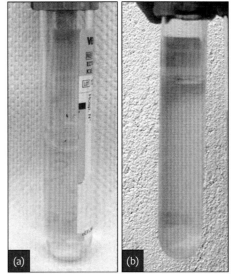

24.2 Gross appearance of effusions. (a) Protein-poor and (b) protein-rich transudate.

through and from the liver, and the vascular system related to the hepatic sinusoids (i.e. pre-sinusoidal, sinusoidal, post-sinusoidal).

In animals, the primary cause of a protein-poor transudate effusion is hypoalbuminaemia; the most common disorders that cause severe hypoalbuminaemia are shown in Figure 24.3. Hypoalbuminaemia alone would have to be severe (usually 1.5 g/dl) for ascites to develop. However, less severe hypoalbuminaemia may facilitate the formation of ascitic fluid if other causes, such as portal hypertension (PH), are also present.

The definition of PH is the sustained increase in blood pressure in the portal system and results from increased intra-hepatic resistance or portal vein obstruction, often combined with either increased or centrifugal blood flow. In PH, the composition of the ascitic fluid depends on the varying permeability of the blood vessels involved: the hepatic sinusoidal capillaries have a fenestrated endothelium and are more permeable to albumin than capillaries of the splanchnic bed. Based on these anatomical characteristics, pre-hepatic and intra-hepatic (pre-sinusoidal) PH generally produce a low-protein transudate, whereas intra-hepatic (sinusoidal and post-sinusoidal) and post-hepatic PH produce a high-protein transudate.

Type of effusion	Specific gravity	Total protein (g/l)	Total nucleated cell count (cells/μl)
Pure transudate	<1.017	<25	<1,500
Modified (protein-rich) transudate	1.017–1.025	25–75	1,000–7,000
Exudate	>1.025	>30	>7,000

24.1 Traditional classification of effusions.

Intra-hepatic PH, caused by hepatic cirrhosis, can be either pre-sinusoidal or sinusoidal. If the increased hydrostatic pressure is pre-sinusoidal, the resulting effusion is a protein-poor transudate. Sinusoidal PH may also cause a protein-poor transudate when concurrent hypoproteinaemia is severe.

Persistently increased intestinal capillary hydrostatic pressure causes transudation from intestinal lymphatics and/or capillaries, both into the peritoneal cavity and into the intestinal lumen. Intestinal lymph has a much lower protein concentration than hepatic lymph because of the relative impermeability of intestinal capillaries to proteins, and, therefore, the resulting effusion has the characteristics of a protein-poor transudate. Lymphangiectasia and mesenteric lymph node diseases are the main causes of protein-poor fluid production due to lymphatic obstruction.

Protein-rich transudates are often the least specific from a diagnostic standpoint and are generally caused by conditions that produce increases in vascular hydrostatic pressure or permeability within the capillaries, lymphatics or both. Cardiovascular disease (e.g. right-sided or biventricular failure, pericardial tamponade) and mass lesions obstructing blood flow from the hepatic vein, or caudal vena cava, into the right side of the heart are some examples of post-hepatic and post-sinusoidal hypertension leading to a protein-rich transudate in the peritoneal cavity. Ascites as a sign of right-sided heart failure in cats is relatively uncommon. With the exception of severe hypoalbuminaemia due to liver failure, a low-protein transudate present in the abdomen for any amount of time tends to become richer in protein.

Abdominal effusion is also present in some specific conditions, which cause production of fluid with variable characteristics (Figure 24.3).

Relevant history

The history is dependent on the underlying disease. Congenital diseases may be more likely in young animals, such as specific hepatopathies, congenital portosystemic shunt or hepatic fibrosis, as well as cardiac disease in some predisposed breeds. The owner may also misinterpret abdominal distension as 'weight gain'. In some cases, the animal may show neurobehavioural signs ranging from alterations of normal behaviour and lethargy to seizures and coma caused by hepatic encephalopathy. The animal can be presented with other signs of hepatic disease, such as icteric mucous membranes, anorexia, vomiting, polyuria/polydipsia, melaena, weakness and lethargy. The presence of diarrhoea may indicate a protein-losing enteropathy (PLE) or PH, but small intestinal diarrhoea may be absent even in severe cases of PLE, if the large intestine maintains sufficient capacity to absorb excess faecal water coming from the small intestine. Polyuria and polydipsia may be due to hepatic failure or other causes of abdominal enlargement (e.g. hyperadrenocorticism, pyometra), which may be mistaken for ascites on palpation. Respiratory distress, exercise intolerance and syncope may be present if there is concomitant pleural effusion or cardiovascular disease. Potential exposure to toxic substances and drugs should be investigated. Possible involvement of intestinal parasites (especially in young puppies and kittens) or heartworm may also be of importance.

Physical examination

Accumulation of abdominal fluid may be readily apparent as abdominal enlargement (Figure 24.4) with positive ballottement, weight gain and poor exercise tolerance.

Type of effusion	Gross appearance	Total protein (g/dl)	Total nucleated cell count (x 10⁶ cells/l)	Pathological mechanism	Condition or disorder
Transudate, protein-poor	Clear, colourless	<20	<1,500	Altered hydrostatic and oncotic pressures	• Hypoalbuminaemia (common) • Cirrhosis • Lymphatic obstruction • Pre-sinusoidal hepatic and pre-hepatic portal hypertension
Transudate, protein-rich	Clear to slightly cloudy, straw-coloured	≥20	<5,000	Increased hydrostatic pressure	• Congestive heart failure (common) • Sinusoidal and post-sinusoidal hepatic and post-hepatic portal hypertension • Feline infectious peritonitis[a]
Exudate, septic	Cloudy, flocculent, serosanguinous, creamy, yellow or tan-tinged	≥20	>5,000	Increased vascular permeability to plasma protein	• Bacterial effusion (common) • Fungal (*Histoplasma, Blastomyces, Coccidioides, Candida*), protozoal (*Leishmania, Toxoplasma, Neospora*) and parasitic (*Mesocestoides*) effusions
Exudate, non-septic	Cloudy, serosanguinous, yellow or red-tinged				Tissue inflammation of viscus (e.g. pancreas and liver)
Effusion from rupture of vessel or viscus	Variable	Variable	Variable	Rupture of intra-abdominal vessel or viscus	• Haemoperitoneum • Uroperitoneum • Bile peritonitis • Chylous or non-chylous lymphorrhagic effusions • *Bartonella* spp.– associated effusion
Effusion from cell exfoliation	Variable	Variable	Variable	Exfoliation due to inflammatory or neoplastic lesion	• Neoplasia (lymphoma common) • Reactive mesothelial proliferation

24.3 Classification of effusions based on aetiopathogenic mechanisms. [a] Feline infectious peritonitis-associated effusions may have variable characteristics ranging from transudate to exudate.

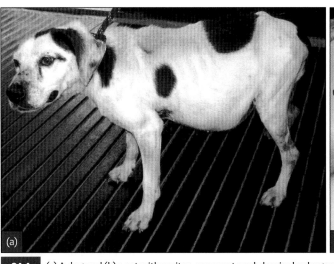
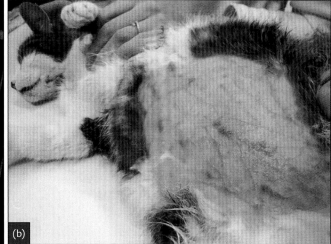

24.4 (a) A dog and (b) a cat with ascites, apparent as abdominal enlargement.

Abdominal palpation may give an impression of slippery loops of small intestine. Small amounts of abdominal fluid cannot always be detected with ballottement alone, thus, additional diagnostics may be needed.

Reduction in ventilation caused by displacement and compression of the diaphragm by severe fluid accumulation can induce tachypnoea. Other clinical signs are highly variable and dependent on the underlying disease, such as:

- Thoracic effusion, peripheral oedema and thromboembolic diseases, if the patient is severely hypoalbuminaemic
- Jaundice in severe hepatobiliary diseases
- Arrhythmia and heart murmur in right-sided heart failure
- Jugular distension or pulsation, muffled heart sounds and collapse in pericardial effusion and tamponade
- Respiratory distress, mucous membrane pallor, collapse and anaemia in haemorrhagic effusions
- Anuria and uraemic syndrome in uroperitoneum
- Fever is suggestive of an inflammatory or infectious disorder
- Lymphadenopathy may be consistent with lymphoma
- Concurrent pleural effusion can be present with post-hepatic PH (caused by right-sided cardiac disease) or pulmonary hypertension.

Additional signs may also be present, such as vomiting, acholic faeces, weakness, lethargy, melaena and others because of simultaneous conditions or complications.

Diagnosis

A correct diagnosis of the cause of ascites is essential for its successful treatment. The first important step is to assess whether abdominal distension is due to fluid accumulation (usually positive ballottement) or other causes, such as the presence of gas (e.g. gastric dilatation-volvulus, usually with a tympanic sound on abdominal percussion), organomegaly (e.g. hepatomegaly, splenomegaly, renomegaly, megacolon, neoplasia or pregnancy, usually revealed by deep palpation), fat (obesity, lipoma) or weak abdominal muscles (hyperadrenocorticism). If abdominal fluid is confirmed, it must be established whether the fluid is free in the abdomen or contained within a viscus (e.g. bladder distension, cysts, pyometra). See Figure 24.5 for specific diagnostic techniques.

Diagnostic tests

Diagnostic investigations in patients with ascites are as follows:

- Radiographic examination of the abdomen. This is rarely useful in the presence of a large volume of fluid because of a lack of contrast
- Ultrasound examination is a sensitive technique that is able to reveal even small amounts of fluid not detected clinically and can also be useful in differentiating ascites from organomegaly or fluid within a viscus. Furthermore, ultrasonography can be a useful technique for a guided diagnostic centesis
- Paracentesis with ascitic fluid analysis to establish the nature of the effusion is essential
- Diagnostic peritoneal lavage can be helpful in the presence of a small amount of fluid
- Routine laboratory tests (haematology, biochemistry and coagulation profile, serum protein electrophoresis and urinalysis), in addition to specific laboratory tests (i.e. serum or urinary bile acids, measurement of serum folate and cobalamin, urine protein:creatinine ratio, basal cortisol or adrenocorticotropic hormone stimulation test and faecal alpha$_1$-proteinase inhibitor), thoracic and abdominal imaging and histopathological investigations may be needed to further investigate for underlying conditions such as PLE, protein-losing nephropathy (PLN), infectious, hepatic, cardiovascular, immune-mediated and neoplastic diseases.

Differential diagnoses

An algorithmic approach based on the characteristics of the fluid is useful in investigations of the common causes of ascites (Figure 24.5).

Fluid appearance

- **Clear to cloudy, green-tinged (TP >20 g/l; TNCC >5,000)** → Bile peritonitis
- **Cloudy, red-tinged (TP and TNCC = blood)** → Haemoperitoneum
- **Cloudy, flocculent, creamy, serosanguineous, tan-tinged (TP >20 g/l; TNCC >5,000)** → Septic or non-septic exudate
- **Opaque, white-tinged (TP >20 g/l; TNCC variable)** → Lymphorrhagic chylous effusion
- **Slightly cloudy, yellow-tinged (TP >20 g/l)**
  - **TNCC >5,000** → Uroabdomen; Non-chylous lymphorrhagic effusion; Neoplastic effusion; Reactive mesothelial proliferation
  - **TNCC <5,000**
    - **TP >20 g/l** → Fluid/blood [crea] >2.0; Fluid/blood [potassium] >1.4; Fluid/normal blood [crea] >4.0
      - Yes → Subacute/chronic uroperitoneum
      - No → Protein-rich transudate → Altered echocardiography and electrocardiography
        - Yes → Congestive heart failure; Cardiac tamponade → Valvular heart disease; Dilated cardiomyopathy; Pericardial disease; Haemangiosarcoma; Heart base tumours; Cor triatriatum dexter; *Dirofilaria*; *Angiostrongylus*
        - No → Liver disease (altered liver laboratory tests, imaging and biopsy)
          - Yes → Non-cardiac post-sinusoidal hepatic or post-hepatic PH → Caudal vena cava obstruction (thrombosis, congenital abnormalities, dirofilariasis, neoplasia, trauma-causing kinking); Budd-Chiari-like syndrome
          - No → Neoplastic effusion; FIP → Lymphoma; Mast cell neoplasia; Mesothelioma; Carcinoma; Adenocarcinoma
- **Clear, colourless**
  - **TP <20 g/l** → Fluid/blood [crea] >2.0; Fluid/blood [potassium] >1.4; Fluid/normal blood [crea] >4.0
    - Yes → Acute uroperitoneum
    - No → Protein-poor transudate → Hypoalbuminaemia (<15 g/l)
      - Yes → ↑ Urinary protein:creatinine ratio
        - Rule out skin losses
        - Yes → Protein-losing nephropathy → Glomerulonephritis (e.g. pyometra, borreliosis, leishmaniosis, ehrlichiosis, immune-mediated polyarthritis, FIV, FeLV); amyloidosis
        - No → Altered laboratory tests for liver function (e.g. bile acids, ammonia)
          - Yes → Liver failure → Portosystemic shunt, cirrhosis
          - No → Protein-losing enteropathy → Chronic inflammatory enteropathies, lymphangiectasia, parasitism, intussusception, neoplasia
      - No → Liver disease (altered liver laboratory tests, imaging and biopsy)
        - Yes → Non-cirrhotic PH (pre-sinusoidal hepatic or pre-hepatic); Cirrhotic PH (pre-sinusoidal hepatic) → Portal vein intraluminal occlusion (thrombosis, neoplasia), extraluminal compression (abdominal masses) and anomalies (stenosis, atresia, hypoplasia)
        - No → Lymphatic obstruction → Lymphangiectasia, lymph node diseases

24.5 Algorithmic approach to ascites based on the characteristics of the fluid. [crea] = creatinine concentration; FeLV = feline leukaemia virus; FIP = feline infectious peritonitis; FIV = feline immunodeficiency virus; PH = portal hypertension; [potassium] = potassium concentration; TNCC = total nucleated cell count ($\times 10^6$ cells/l); TP = total protein.

References and further reading

Buob S, Johnston AN and Webster CRL (2011) Portal hypertension: pathophysiology, diagnosis, and treatment. *Journal of Veterinary Internal Medicine* **25**, 169–186

Dempsey DM and Ewing PJ (2011) A review of the pathophysiology, classification, and analysis of canine and feline cavitary effusions. *Journal of the American Animal Hospital Association* **47**, 1–11

Mansfield C (2013) Ascites. In: *Canine and Feline Gastroenterology*, ed. RJ Washabau and MJ Day, pp. 80–86. Saunders, St. Louis

Stockham SL and Scott MA (2008) Cavitary effusions. In: *Fundamentals of Veterinary Clinical Pathology, 2nd edn*, ed. SL Stockham and MA Scott, pp. 831–868. Blackwell Publishing Professional, Ames

Valenciano AC, Arndt TP and Rizzi TE (2014) Effusions: abdominal, thoracic, and pericardial. In: *Cowell and Tyler's Diagnostic Cytology and Hematology of the Dog and Cat, 4th edn*, ed. AC Valenciano and RL Cowell, pp. 244–265. Elsevier Mosby, St. Louis

Chapter 25

Jaundice

Andrea Boari

Definition of the problem

The terms jaundice and icterus are used interchangeably and refer to a clinical sign characterized by deposition of bilirubin pigment in tissues, including the blood, skin and mucous membranes, resulting in a yellowish discolouration of these tissues. Clinically apparent tissue icterus generally does not occur until serum bilirubin concentration exceeds between 35 and 55 mmol/l, whereas the serum or plasma is visually icteric at around 25 mmol/l (Figure 25.1).

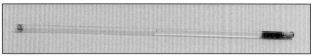

25.1 Microhaematocrit capillary tube containing a blood sample from a jaundiced dog with immune-mediated haemolytic anaemia.

Jaundice can be categorized as follows:

- Pre-hepatic jaundice
- Hepatic jaundice
- Post-hepatic jaundice.

Therefore, increased bilirubin concentrations may occur in patients with non-hepatic causes (Figure 25.2)

This classification is useful clinically, and is based on an understanding of bilirubin metabolism (see the *BSAVA Manual of Canine and Feline Clinical Pathology*). It allows clinicians to characterize hyperbilirubinaemia, leading to the correct clinical approach to the jaundiced patient (Figure 25.3).

Species	Cause
Dogs and cats	• Haemolysis (see Figure 25.4) • Acute inflammatory mediators (e.g. TNF-α) • Bacterial endotoxins • Severe inflammation • Septicaemia • Toxaemia
Cats	• Hyperthyroidism • Anorexia or dietary restriction leading to hepatic lipidosis • Feline infectious peritonitis
Dogs	• Lipaemia[a]

25.2 Causes of non-hepatic hyperbilirubinaemia in dogs and cats. [a] Cause of pseudohyperbilirubinaemia due to interference of lipid with colorimetric laboratory methods. TNF-α = tumour necrosis factor-alpha.

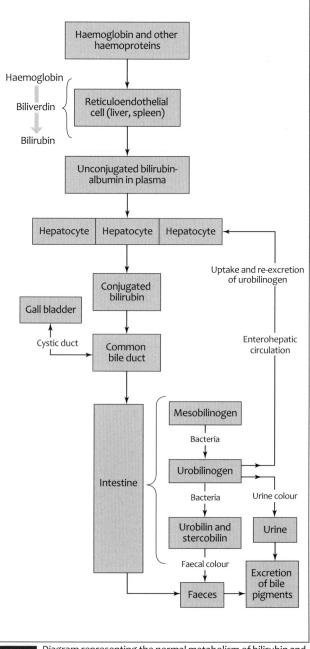

25.3 Diagram representing the normal metabolism of bilirubin and excretion of urobilinogen.
(From *BSAVA Manual of Canine and Feline Clinical Pathology*)

Pre-hepatic jaundice

Pre-hepatic jaundice results from accelerated red blood cell destruction as the primary abnormality, although secondary hepatic dysfunction may contribute. The main differential diagnoses for pre-hepatic icterus include both intravascular and extravascular haemolytic anaemias of different causes (Figure 25.4).

In severe haemolytic situations, anaemic hypoxia of hepatocytes can influence liver function and promote intra-hepatic cholestasis. In this case, icterus and hyperbilirubinaemia are due to a combination of unconjugated and conjugated bilirubin derived from both increased production and intra-hepatic cholestasis.

Pre-hepatic causes
Haemolytic anaemia
• Immune-mediated haemolytic anaemia
• Primary
• Secondary
– Dogs: some drugs[a], lymphoma, myeloproliferative diseases, ehrlichiosis, leishmaniosis, rickettsioses
– Cats: some drugs, lymphoma, FeLV, FIP, myelodysplastic syndromes, acute myelogenous leukaemia
– Associated with other immune disorders: SLE
– Associated with blood parasites: *Mycoplasma haemofelis*, *Mycoplasma haemocanis*[b], *Babesia* spp., *Cytauxzoon felis*
• Heinz body anaemia
• Dogs: onions (most common), vitamin K_3, naphthalene, propylene glycol, benzocaine, methylene blue, copper, zinc, phenylhydrazine, paracetamol (acetaminophen)
• Cats: methylene blue, paracetamol, phenacetin, phenazopyridine, propofol, propylene glycol, salmon-based diets, onions, metabolic diseases (diabetic ketoacidosis, hyperthyroidism, lymphoma)
• Other causes
• Zinc or copper toxicity
• Envenomation
• Hypophosphataemia (refeeding syndrome, insulin therapy)
• Hereditary RBC defects
• Microangiopathic RBC fragmentation
• DIC, vasculitis, haemangiosarcoma, splenic torsion, heatstroke, *Dirofilaria immitis* (postcaval syndrome)
• Blood transfusion reaction
• Neonatal isoerythrolysis (cats)
• Sepsis (cats)
Large haematoma and intramuscular haemorrhage (uncommon)

25.4 Main differential diagnoses of pre-hepatic, haemolytic icterus in dogs and cats. DIC = disseminated intravascular coagulation; FeLV = feline leukaemia virus; FIP = feline infectious peritonitis; RBC = red blood cell; SLE = systemic lupus erythematosus. [a] Levamisole, carprofen, trimethoprim/sulphonamide, cephalosporins. [b] *M. haemocanis* only causes jaundice in splenectomized dogs.

The main causes of haemolysis-induced icterus in the dog include immune-mediated haemolytic anaemia (where only 40–70% of dogs become jaundiced), adverse drug reactions and infectious disease, such as babesiosis. Some important causes of haemolysis in cats may, but do not always, cause jaundice. They are haemoplasmosis (formerly haemobartonellosis) (Figures 25.4 and 25.5), adverse drug reactions and toxins (paracetamol (acetaminophen), methylene blue, onion, copper, lead), auto-immune haemolytic anaemia (often feline leukaemia virus (FeLV)-positive), transfusion reactions and haemolytic disease of the newborn.

Hepatic jaundice

Hepatocellular injury, necrosis or dysfunction can impair hepatocyte uptake, conjugation and secretory ability, causing intra-hepatic cholestasis and jaundice, and this

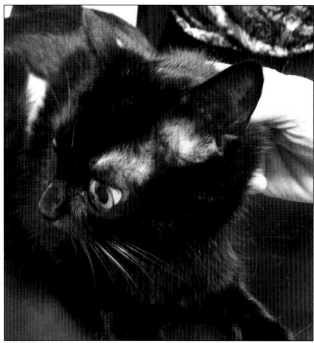

25.5 Jaundice in a young Domestic Shorthaired cat with haemolytic anaemia secondary to *Mycoplasma haemofelis* infection.

can occur with both primary and secondary causes of hepatic disease (Figure 25.6). However, it is worth emphasizing that, although intra-hepatic cholestasis occurs in most hepatobiliary diseases, in most cases there is no overt jaundice; it is observed in less than 50% of dogs and cats with hepatic disease.

As a rule, the occurrence of jaundice is more likely when the liver disorder involves the periportal hepatocytes and, while parenchymal liver disease is most

Hepatic causes
Acute liver failure
• Dogs
• Idiopathic acute hepatitis
• Toxicants: cycad palms, blue-green algae (*Microcystis aeruginosa*), *Amanita phalloides*, aflatoxins, xylitol, carprofen
• Drugs: paracetamol (acetaminophen), phenazopyridine, trimethoprim/sulphonamide, lomustine, zonisamide
• Infective: leptospirosis, CAV-1
• Cats
• Hepatic lipidosis
• Liver fluke
• Toxoplasmosis
• Drugs: stanozolol, oral benzodiazepines
Primary chronic hepatitis
• Dogs
• Drugs
– Phenobarbital, primidone, halothane
• Idiopathic chronic hepatopathy
• Breed-specific copper hepatitis: Bedlington Terrier, Dobermann, Dalmatian, West Highland White Terrier, Labrador Retriever
• Cirrhosis
• Lobular dissecting hepatitis
• Inflammatory hepatitis
• Hepatobiliary neoplasia
• Cats
• Hepatic lipidosis
• Cholangitis/cholangiohepatitis
– Triaditis syndrome
Feline infectious peritonitis
Non-specific reactive hepatitis
Hepatobiliary neoplasia

25.6 Main differential diagnoses of hepatic icterus and hyperbilirubinaemia in dogs and cats. CAV-1 = canine adenovirus 1.

common in dogs, hepatic lipidosis and inflammatory disorders involving the bile ductules and periportal hepatocytes (cholangitis/cholangiohepatitis or lymphocytic hepatitis) predominate in cats. Furthermore, in cats, triaditis (see Chapter 36), which consists of concurrent cholangitis, pancreatitis and chronic inflammatory enteropathy, can contribute to jaundice.

Post-hepatic jaundice

Post-hepatic jaundice is more common in dogs than in cats and includes those disorders that cause decreased excretion of bilirubin (see Figure 25.7). Acholic faeces are diagnostic for total obstruction to bile flow, but this sign is very rare in dogs and cats.

Finally, traumatic or pathological rupture of the gall bladder and/or bile duct near the duodenum will cause jaundice, abdominal effusion and chemical peritonitis.

Post-hepatic causes
EHBD obstruction
• Cholelithiasis/choledocholithiasis
Gall bladder disease
• Congenital atresia (dogs) (rare)
• Cholecystitis (dogs)
• Gall bladder mucocoele (dogs)
• Liver fluke (cats)
Disorders of bile ducts
• Choledochitis
• Cholelithiasis
• Choledochal cyst
• Biliary neoplasia
• Stricture (traumatic or iatrogenic)
• Liver fluke (cats)
Pancreatic disorders
• Pancreatitis
• Pancreatic carcinoma
• Pancreatic abscess
Duodenal disorders
• Duodenitis
• Duodenal neoplasia
• Foreign body
Bile duct or gall bladder rupture

25.7 Main differential diagnoses of post-hepatic icterus and hyperbilirubinaemia in dogs and cats. EHBD = extra-hepatic bile duct.

Relevant history

The history is often vague and non-specific signs (e.g. anorexia, lethargy, vomiting) are present. Genetic and breed predisposition for specific diseases (e.g. chronic hepatitis, copper hepatopathy) should be considered. Depending on the underlying disease, the owners may report changes in the colour of the urine or faeces. Marked bilirubinuria can cause orange or green discolouration of urine (pigmenturia), whereas intravascular haemolysis can cause dark red or brown urine (haemoglobinuria). In dogs, hyperbilirubinaemia can cause dark orange urine before jaundice is visible in the patient. Other complaints can include anorexia, weight loss, abdominal distension (related to hepatomegaly or ascites), vomiting, diarrhoea, polyuria/polydipsia, hepatic encephalopathy (seizures, stupor, disorientation, ptyalism), external bleeding and/or discolouration of faeces (acholic or melaena).

The possibility of exposure to potentially hepatotoxic substances and risk factors for infectious diseases (indoor versus outdoor) should be ascertained. Furthermore, drug and toxin exposure (e.g. xylitol, aflatoxin, cycad and other plants, amanita mushrooms, non-steroidal anti-inflammatory drugs, phenobarbital and many others), as well as vaccination history, should be considered.

A history of exercise intolerance, lethargy, weakness and pallor of mucous membranes can be indicative of haemolytic icterus. Moreover, investigation should be focused on previous exposure to blood transfusions, oxidant substances, zinc (contained in metallic objects (coins) or sun protectant), vector-borne parasites, snakes, insects (fleas, bees), spiders and hunting in cats (e.g. toxoplasmosis).

Insulin therapy in ketoacidotic diabetic patients, or intensive refeeding in cats, can cause hypophosphataemic haemolysis when serum phosphorus is less than 0.32 mmol/l in dogs and 0.81 mmol/l in cats.

Physical examination

Tissue icterus is first seen in the sclera of the eye and the mucosa of the soft palate (Figure 25.8), and then can be clinically evident in the skin, especially the pinnae, third eyelids and iris.

Lethargy, weakness, pale and/or yellow mucous membranes, tachypnoea, tachycardia, hyperdynamic pulses, haemic murmur and hepatosplenomegaly may suggest prehepatic icterus. Mucous membrane pallor associated with anaemia, ecchymosis and petechiation can be seen with bleeding disorders (Figure 25.9).

Abdominal palpation may reveal:

• Effusion/ascites from portal hypertension, haemorrhage, hepatic or pancreatic inflammation or feline infectious peritonitis (FIP)

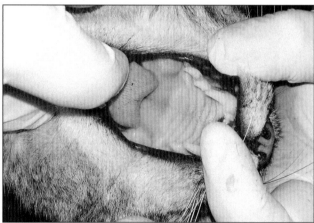

25.8 Jaundiced soft palate in a young cat during hospitalization for severe sepsis.

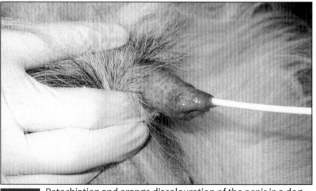

25.9 Petechiation and orange discolouration of the penis in a dog with a bleeding disorder due to hepatic insufficiency.

- Hepatomegaly can be evident in most animals with primary or secondary hepatic disease and extramedullary haematopoiesis
- Splenomegaly, due to neoplasia (such as lymphoma or mastocytosis) and extramedullary haematopoiesis
- Abdominal pain is suggestive of an obstructive intestinal or hepatic process, pancreatitis or cholangitis/cholangiohepatitis.

Fever can be seen with neutrophilic cholangitis, FIP, toxoplasmosis, pancreatitis, and immune-mediated haemolysis. Neurological signs and ptyalism (mainly in cats) may indicate hepatic encephalopathy.

In cats, a complete ophthalmological examination is mandatory to aid in identifying systemic diseases (lymphoma, FIP, systemic mycosis and toxoplasmosis).

Diagnostic tests

An initial evaluation should include haematology, serum chemistry and urinalysis. Additionally, testing for FeLV and feline immunodeficiency virus should be performed in all jaundiced cats. Serum thyroxine concentrations should be measured in all jaundiced cats older than 6 years of age, as hyperthyroidism may be a co-morbidity.

Determining the cause of jaundice requires a systematic approach (Figure 25.10) targeted at classifying the jaundice as pre-hepatic, hepatic or post-hepatic.

The first step is to consider pre-hepatic jaundice, and haematology should be obtained in order to rule out haemolytic disease. As a general rule, if a severe anaemia is not present (i.e. packed cell volume >20%) and there are no signs of red blood cell regeneration, pre-hepatic causes of jaundice can be generally ruled out.

In jaundiced animals, normal haematocrit or mild non-regenerative anaemia, associated with high serum hepatic enzyme activity (aspartate aminotransferase, alanine aminotransferase, alkaline phosphatase, gamma glutamyl transferase), are indicative of hepatobiliary disorder. However, liver enzyme activities and other liver function parameters (albumin, cholesterol, glucose, blood urea nitrogen) are not useful to differentiate between pre-hepatic and hepatic, and between hepatic and post-hepatic jaundice. Indeed, both pre-hepatic and post-hepatic icterus can cause secondary hepatocellular damage and, in order to differentiate these conditions, haematology, imaging and/or surgical evaluation are usually needed. While standard radiographs have limited utility, abdominal ultrasonography and, if available, computed tomography are invaluable for assessment of the liver, biliary system and adjacent organs, such as the duodenum and pancreas. Post-hepatic causes of jaundice can be suggested when findings of a pancreatic or gall bladder mass, cholelithiasis, dilated biliary ducts within the hepatic parenchyma or gall bladder mucocoele are present. Lastly, if any of these signs are present, exploratory laparotomy or laparoscopy may be indicated for diagnostic or therapeutic purposes.

In primary or secondary hepatobiliary disease, a definitive diagnosis is made by histopathological examination of a liver biopsy specimen. Depending on the size of the liver and the disease suspected, fine-needle aspiration (FNA), percutaneous needle biopsy (PNB) or wedge biopsy are performed. FNA and PNB are most helpful to identify diffuse hepatic neoplasia (lymphoma) and hepatic lipidosis, whereas wedge biopsy by laparoscopy or coeliotomy is preferred for all other hepatic diseases.

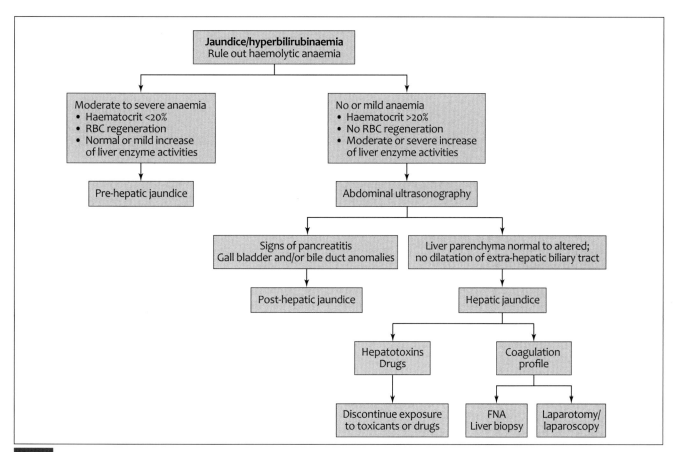

25.10 Suggested algorithm for evaluation of a dog or cat with jaundice. FNA = fine-needle aspiration; RBC = red blood cell.

Differential diagnosis

In dogs and cats, jaundice can be associated with many disorders and the two main causes are haemolytic and hepatobiliary diseases. Specific causes of jaundice are listed in Figures 25.4, 25.6 and 25.7.

Treatment

Treatment of jaundice depends on the underlying disease. For more information, see Chapters 36 and 37.

References and further reading

Cocker S and Richter K (2017) Diagnostic evaluation of the liver. In: *Textbook of Veterinary Internal Medicine, 8th edn*, ed. SJ Ettinger, EC Feldman and E Côté, pp. 59–63. Saunders, St. Louis

Sherding RG (2013) Icterus. In: *Canine and Feline Gastroenterology*, ed. RJ Washabau and MJ Day, pp. 140–147. Saunders, St. Louis

Villiers E and Ristic J (2016) *BSAVA Manual of Canine and Feline Clinical Pathology, 3rd edn*. BSAVA Publications, Gloucester

Webster CRL and Cooper JC (2014) Diagnostic approach to hepatobiliary disease. In: *Kirk's Current Veterinary Therapy XV*, ed. JD Bonagura and DC Twedt, pp. 569–575. Saunders, St. Louis

Weiss DJ and Tvedten H (2012) Erythrocyte disorders. In: *Small Animal Clinical Diagnosis by Laboratory Methods, 5th edn*, ed. MD Willard and H Tvedten, pp. 38–62. Saunders, St. Louis

Chapter 26

Systemic, neurological and uncommon presentations of gastrointestinal disease

Marcella Ridgway

The intestinal tract is the sole conduit for water and other nutrients entering the body and sustains diverse populations of micro-organisms partitioned from systemic exposure by normal mucosal barrier function and appropriate immunological responses. The liver and pancreas serve important roles in facilitating digestion of luminal contents, modulating intestinal microbial growth and intercepting harmful substances or bacteria originating from the gut. Intestinal disease may have far-reaching effects resulting from consequent malnutrition, dehydration, acid–base abnormalities or electrolyte disturbances, bacterial translocation or toxaemia, when these functions are disturbed. Hypoalbuminaemia secondary to protein-losing enteropathy (PLE) or hepatic synthetic failure may result in oedema affecting multiple tissues, as well as altered handling of drugs and endogenous substances that are highly protein-bound. Loss of immunological functions of the gut or liver, or of mucosal barrier integrity may result in systemic infection or toxaemia. In addition to these general alterations associated with loss of intestinal function, there are a number of more specific syndromes and extra-intestinal manifestations of gastrointestinal (GI) disease which may be less readily apparent as relating to underlying primary intestinal disease, presenting instead with characteristics of non-intestinal body systems.

Neurological signs

Neurological manifestations of GI disease may occur in a number of conditions.

Hyperammonaemic encephalopathies
Hepatic encephalopathy

Hepatic encephalopathy (HE) is the best known neurological manifestation of liver disease and refers to a syndrome of neurological abnormalities secondary to the liver disease, including mental dullness, disorientation, ataxia, hypersalivation (in cats), compulsive or aimless wandering, head pressing, blindness, coma and, sometimes, seizures (more common in cats than dogs). Neurological signs may be waxing and waning, and may be precipitated or worsened by a meal (especially one rich in protein), GI haemorrhage, dehydration, alkalosis, hypokalaemia, anaesthetics and sedatives. The underlying mechanisms are not known, but endogenous toxins (ammonia, mercaptans, short-chain fatty acids, gamma-aminobutyric acid and other false neurotransmitters) which are normally cleared by the liver, accumulate because of reduced hepatic metabolism due to vascular shunting (portosystemic shunt) or obstruction (portal venous thrombosis) or primary hepatocellular failure) and contribute to the development of central nervous system (CNS) signs. Recent work points to central abnormalities in glutamate metabolism at the core of HE pathogenesis. Signs correspond roughly to blood ammonia concentrations and are improved by treatments aimed at reducing blood ammonia (i.e. dietary protein restriction, lactulose, antibiotics). Patients with HE are at increased risk for cerebral oedema, which may cause acute worsening of neurological signs, bradycardia and death, if not quickly addressed.

Cobalamin (vitamin B$_{12}$) deficiency

Hypocobalaminaemia is a common consequence of severe intestinal disease (chronic inflammatory enteropathy), lymphosarcoma, other chronic enteropathies affecting the ileum), pancreatic disease (exocrine pancreatic insufficiency) or small intestinal dysbiosis (utilization by gut bacteria reducing available luminal cobalamin), leading to insufficient cobalamin absorption. It may cause hyperammonaemic encephalopathy through interference with the urea cycle, and seizures, and may also cause anaemia and organic acidaemia, which may secondarily affect the function of the nervous system.

Other causes of hyperammonaemia

As well as being caused by liver disease and hypocobalaminaemia, hyperammonaemic encephalopathies may also occur as a result of urea cycle enzyme defects, organic acidaemias (metabolic disorders of amino acid metabolism) and nutritional deficiencies. Arginine is an integral component of the urea cycle, which detoxifies ammonia, whilst carnitine is an essential co-factor in fatty acid metabolism, and deficiencies of carnitine lead to cytosolic accumulation of metabolites, which inhibit the urea cycle. Arginine and carnitine deficiencies can develop consequent to malnutrition and, thus, cause hyperammonaemic encephalopathy, which may manifest early in anorexic cats.

Pancreatic encephalopathy

Pancreatic encephalopathy (PE) is uncommon and is a less well known metabolic encephalopathy than HE. It is the most common neurological complication of severe acute pancreatitis in humans and an important cause of death in this population. Acute pancreatitis results in increased blood–brain barrier permeability (increasing exposure of brain tissue to circulating toxins) and altered brain micro-circulation (caused by pro-inflammatory cytokines) and subsequent vasogenic cerebral oedema and brain injury (diffuse encephalopathy, neuronal apoptosis, demyelination, cerebral venous thrombosis, intracerebral haemorrhage). PE manifests as disorientation/confusion, altered mentation, agitation, aphasia, seizures and other neuropsychiatric abnormalities. PE has not been described in dogs or cats but occurs reliably in rats with experimentally induced severe acute pancreatitis.

Bilirubin encephalopathy

This condition, also called kernicterus, develops in some animals (typically young) with hyperbilirubinaemia (cholestatic liver disease, extra-hepatic bile duct obstruction/acute pancreatitis). The mechanism of injury is not well understood but appears to be initiated by disruption of neuronal cellular membranes. Signs include obtundation, seizures, proprioceptive deficits, tetraparesis, opisthotonus and coma.

Circulatory disturbances

Hypercoagulability secondary to PLE with associated loss of anticoagulant proteins (e.g. antithrombin) may result in ischaemic injury secondary to thrombosis of vessels supplying nervous system tissues, precipitating neurological signs attributable to the regions served by the thrombosed vessels. Pulmonary thromboembolism that causes a significant reduction in arterial oxygen content may further cause hypoxic encephalopathy. Hyperviscosity in patients with hyperlipidaemia (pancreatic disease) or hyperglobulinaemia (Basenji enteropathy) may have similar neurological consequences (seizures, other central or peripheral neurological signs) due to vascular compromise and nervous system tissue ischaemia.

Hypoglycaemia

Prolonged low blood glucose (caused by liver synthetic failure, malnutrition or insulinoma) may cause hypoglycaemic neuropathy: brain cells are dependent on blood glucose to support cellular metabolic needs, and lack of glucose results in cellular dysfunction, neuronal necrosis and vascular constriction, leading to additional ischaemic injury. Clinical signs of hypoglycaemia are generally the signs of the resulting nervous system dysfunction: mental dullness, disorientation, weakness, seizures, tremors, blindness and coma.

Thiamine (vitamin B₁) deficiency

This can occur in dogs or cats fed diets that are thiamine-deficient, preserved with sulphur dioxide or contain uncooked thiaminase-rich fish/shellfish. Deficiency causes disruption of carbohydrate metabolism and energy production, signs of cerebral and vestibular dysfunction, and may progress to polioencephalomalacia. Clinical signs include generalized weakness, dull mentation, ataxia, stiff/spastic gait, spastic cervical ventroflexion (in cats), circling, head tremors, seizures, opisthotonus, stupor/coma and death.

Electrolyte abnormalities

These may develop in animals with GI or hepatic disease and may precipitate central or peripheral neurological signs.

Hypocalcaemia

Hypoalbuminaemia (due to liver dysfunction or PLE) is often associated with a reduced total serum calcium level, reflecting a reduction in the inactive, protein-bound calcium fraction; if the active, ionized calcium fraction is normal, which is usually the case if hypoalbuminaemia is the sole factor responsible for the low total calcium level, the hypocalcaemia is asymptomatic and inconsequential. However, ionized hypocalcaemia can occur secondary to intestinal disease, due to malabsorption of vitamin D, calcium and magnesium, or loss of vitamin D binding protein through the PLE. Ionized hypocalcaemia can also be due to acute pancreatitis through altered calcium metabolism and binding and calcium precipitation in peripancreatic tissues. Hypocalcaemia causes increased excitability of the CNS and muscle cell membranes and may result in neurological signs of face rubbing, muscle rigidity/stiff gait, tremors, tetany, ileus and seizures.

Hyponatraemia

Severe liver or intestinal disease can cause hyponatraemia and consequent cerebral oedema and diffuse encephalopathy. Rapid correction of hyponatraemia may cause osmotic demyelination syndrome with CNS signs.

Hypokalaemia

Reduced intake/absorption and increased loss of potassium in diarrhoea/vomitus can cause hypokalaemia. This may result in neuromuscular signs of generalized weakness, flaccid cervical ventroflexion (in cats), forelimb hypermetria and a wide-based hindlimb stance. Peripheral neuropathy is a common neurological manifestation of IBD in humans.

Renal/urinary signs

Azotaemia

Prerenal azotaemia develops readily in patients with GI, hepatic and pancreatic disease that have reduced fluid intake and increased loss through vomiting and/or diarrhoea; this azotaemia may be difficult to distinguish from renal azotaemia in patients with other factors (hypokalaemia, glucocorticoid therapy, liver dysfunction) influencing their ability to concentrate urine despite normal renal function.

Polyuria/polydipsia

Hypokalaemia causes a primary polyuria with compensatory polydipsia due to abnormal urine-concentrating ability. Occasionally, dogs with gastric disease will show primary polydipsia with secondary polyuria to excrete the unnecessary water load. Polyuria/polydipsia is common in dogs (less common in cats) with liver dysfunction. Potential mechanisms include alterations in neurotransmitters and CNS function, resulting in hypersecretion of adrenocorticotropic hormone and consequently cortisol in HE, abnormal aldosterone responsiveness and reduced urea synthesis leading to reduced renal medullary concentration ability.

Hepatorenal syndrome

This condition is a syndrome of acute kidney injury caused by intense renal vasoconstriction and the resulting hypoperfusion of the kidney. Renal injury occurs as a consequence of advanced (cirrhotic) liver disease and its associated circulatory changes, including increased release of endogenous vasodilators, splanchnic and systemic arterial vasodilatation, subsequent cardiac insufficiency leading to effective hypovolaemia, and renin angiotensin-aldosterone system activation in the face of increased renal circulatory sensitivity to vasoconstrictors. Clinical signs are those of renal insufficiency superimposed on existing signs of liver failure. Hepatorenal syndrome is not well identified in small animals but can be experimentally produced in dogs and may occur clinically in some dogs with cirrhosis.

Translocation of enteric bacteria and bacterial products to the systemic circulation through diseased intestinal mucosa contributes to the progression of chronic kidney disease in humans and contributes to renal injury in patients with cirrhosis. Hyperbilirubinaemia (cholestatic liver disease, extra-hepatic bile duct obstruction/acute pancreatitis) can cause injury to renal cells (cholaemic nephrosis) secondary to uptake of unconjugated bilirubin (proximal tubular damage) or by formation of intrarenal bilirubin casts (bile cast nephropathy).

Musculoskeletal abnormalities

Muscle dysfunction

Small animal patients with chronic disease of the intestine, pancreas and/or liver may show chronic generalized malnutrition with muscle wasting and weakness. Treatment with glucocorticoids generally exacerbates muscle wasting, especially in larger dogs. As a result of reduced muscle function, increased strain may be transmitted to ligaments, predisposing them to rupture. Certain nutritional deficiencies (carnitine, thiamine) and electrolyte disturbances (hypokalaemia, hypocalcaemia) secondary to intestinal disease may impair muscle function.

Arthropathies

Arthropathies are the most common extra-intestinal manifestation of inflammatory bowel disease (IBD) in humans, usually involving axial joints (sacroiliitis, ankylosing spondylitis) but sometimes causing peripheral arthritis. Concurrent manifestation of disease in other extra-intestinal sites (skin, mucous membranes, eye) is common in patients with enteropathic arthropathy. Enteropathic arthropathies are not described in small animals. Humans with IBD are at risk for developing osteoporosis and osteopenia resulting from impaired absorption of nutrients important for bone health, effects of inflammatory cytokines on bone metabolism and impact of glucocorticoid use. Similar complications have not been recognized in small animal patients.

Cutaneous abnormalities

Food-associated skin disease

Food allergy in dogs and cats may manifest as dermatological disease with non-seasonal pruritus (especially affecting the face and ears) and otitis externa; as gastrointestinal disease with inappetence, weight loss or poor body condition and diarrhoea; or with a combination of dermatological and GI signs. Food allergy often first manifests in young animals (dogs under 1 year of age, cats under 2 years of age) and the offending dietary allergen has usually been fed for months to years before signs become evident. Humans with IBD often develop dermatological manifestations (erythema nodosum, pyoderma gangrenosum) and/or oral lesions (aphthous ulcers, granular cheilitis, pyostomatitis) but such associations have not been established in small animal patients. Vitamin A deficiency, secondary to malabsorption (cholestatic liver disease, intestinal disease), is believed to contribute to the development of cutaneous and mucocutaneous lesions in humans with IBD and has the potential for dermatological manifestations in small animals as well.

Superficial necrolytic dermatitis

Superficial necrolytic dermatitis (hepatocutaneous syndrome) occurs in some animals with liver disease and is attributed to increased hepatic catabolism of amino acids, possibly driven by excess glucagon, which leads to deficient levels of circulating amino acids delivered to the cutaneous tissues and subsequent pathological changes in epidermal cells. The condition is more common in dogs than cats and characteristically manifests first with painful foot lesions (thickened/crusted/fissured footpads, erythema of interdigital skin), then crusting and ulceration of mucocutaneous junctions, ear pinnae, and skin of the ventrum and overlying pressure points. Lymph node enlargement and fever may also be present.

Paraneoplastic effects

Paraneoplastic alopecia is a rare non-pruritic symmetrical dermatological condition characterized by circumscribed but often extensive areas of alopecia with a smooth, shiny skin surface, typically involving the ventrum, and often crusted or erythematous footpad lesions. So called 'shiny skin' disease, is most commonly associated with pancreatic malignancy (adenocarcinoma) in cats, although a relationship to other malignancies (hepatocellular carcinoma, bile duct carcinoma) has been described.

Cholestatic pruritus

Hyperbilirubinaemia in humans can cause cholestatic pruritus, an often intense and unrelenting condition attributed to deposition of retained bile acids in the skin.

Respiratory signs

Regurgitation and vomiting may also result in aspiration pneumonia, but respiratory signs of tachypnoea or dyspnoea may also develop in patients with pulmonary thromboembolism secondary to hypercoagulability in PLE or with acute respiratory distress syndrome secondary to acute pancreatitis, hepatitis or sepsis resulting from bacterial translocation from a diseased intestine.

Tachypnoea may also be evident in patients with abdominal pain referable to inflammatory diseases of the GI tract, liver or pancreas, or conditions causing distension of these organs. Tachypnoea is also common in patients with significant anaemia secondary to GI bleeding or malabsorption of iron, cobalamin or other factors. In humans with IBD, extra-intestinal manifestations are common but pulmonary involvement is considered relatively rare: airway (tracheitis, chronic bronchitis, bronchiectasis, bronchiolitis obliterans with organizing pneumonia) or parenchymal (pulmonary interstitial emphysema, interstitial pneumonia, fibrosing alveolitis, granulomatous pulmonary nodules) disease may develop. More commonly, subclinical pulmonary dysfunction (impaired gas diffusion, which worsens with GI disease activity) occurs, affecting 40–60% of human IBD patients. Similar pulmonary manifestations have not been documented in small animal patients.

Cardiovascular signs

Pain, anaemia or volume depletion secondary to GI, liver or pancreatic disease may result in tachycardia, but high vagal tone induced by inflammation or distension of abdominal organs may cause bradycardia. Cardiovascular function may be altered by electrolyte disturbances such as hypocalcaemia (tachyarrhythmias, weak pulse), hypokalaemia or hyponatraemia (hypovolaemia, weak pulse, tachycardia) associated with GI disease. Carnitine deficiency resulting from anorexia or malabsorption or grain-free diets may impair cardiac muscle function.

Pulmonary thromboembolism secondary to PLE may result in increased pulmonary artery pressure and subsequent right heart dysfunction. Impaired intestinal barrier function and alterations in the gut microbiome are implicated as contributing to the pathogenesis of heart failure in humans. Cirrhotic cardiomyopathy is a condition of impaired cardiac contractility with systolic and diastolic dysfunction and conduction abnormalities in humans with advanced (cirrhotic) liver disease; this condition is not documented in small animals.

Ocular abnormalities

Humans with IBD may develop ocular manifestations including episcleritis, scleritis, uveitis, keratopathy and night blindness secondary to vitamin A malabsorption, and, less commonly, retinal or corneal disease or lid margin ulcers. Subcapsular cataracts are a common consequence of glucocorticoid therapy (used in managing IBD) in humans. Corresponding ocular abnormalities have not been described in small animals.

Haemopoietic abnormalities

Anaemia

Anaemia of chronic disease (normocytic, normochromic, non-regenerative) may result from any chronic inflammatory or neoplastic condition due to suppression of erythropoietin production by inflammatory cytokines. However, anaemia may also arise by a variety of other mechanisms in animals with GI, liver or pancreatic disease.

Blood loss through ulcerated GI mucosal lesions or intestinal parasitism (e.g. ancyclostomiasis) may result in anaemia that is regenerative but may become microcytic and hypochromic with chronicity and the development of iron deficiency. A microcytic hypochromic anaemia, characteristic of iron deficiency, may also result from malabsorption of iron in severe intestinal disease or with diffuse gastric mucosal disease (chronic gastritis, achlorhydria, helicobacteriosis, gastric neoplasia).

Malabsorption of cobalamin (secondary to GI or pancreatic disease) or folate (in GI disease), if severe, may cause a macrocytic or normocytic-normochromic anaemia. However, these haematological changes are both markedly less frequent and severe than classically seen in human patients.

Humans with IBD often have other immunological diseases of non-GI tissue, and immune-mediated haemolytic anaemia (IMHA) may be a manifestation seen in patients with Crohn's disease, a subtype of human IBD; corresponding associations have not been reported in cats and dogs.

Patients with liver disease may show anaemia due to GI blood loss (predisposition to GI mucosal ulceration), bleeding at other sites (coagulation abnormalities), abnormal iron metabolism or decreased red blood cell lifespan (abnormal phospholipid synthesis, abnormal energy metabolism).

Leucopenia and thrombocytopenia

Leucopenia and neutropenia may occur with enteric infections or systemic infectious diseases involving the gut (parvoviral enteritis, ehrlichiosis, sepsis, feline retroviral infection) and may also result from cobalamin deficiency. Thrombocytopenia may be seen in patients with liver disease, vasculitis secondary to pancreatitis or sepsis secondary to intestinal mucosal barrier dysfunction or hepatic dysfunction.

Non-GI signs related to medications

Therapeutic agents used in the treatment of GI disease may also have widespread impact and induce multisystemic signs (Figure 26.1).

In all patients under treatment, careful consideration of all therapeutic agents for any potential to precipitate observed abnormalities independent of the patient's disease process is imperative.

Drugs used to treat GI disease	Non-GI side effects
Glucocorticoids and other immunosuppressants	• PU/PD • Cutaneous changes • Muscle wasting • Secondary infections • Neoplasia
Ciclosporin	• Gingival hyperplasia • Papillomatosis • Renal or hepatic injury
Azathioprine	• Poor hair growth • Acute pancreatitis • Hepatotoxicity • Bone marrow suppression (leucopenia) • Thrombocytopenia (and associated bleeding tendencies) • Anaemia (with signs of weakness) • Tachypnoea • Exercise intolerance

26.1 Medications for the treatment of gastrointestinal (GI) disease that can create non-GI side effects. Many antimicrobial agents have the potential to cause bone marrow suppression manifesting as neutropenia with or without other haematological abnormalities. PU/PD = polyuria/polydipsia. (continues) ▶

Drugs used to treat GI disease	Non-GI side effects
Chlorambucil	• Bone marrow suppression (leucopenia) • Thrombocytopenia (and associated bleeding tendencies) • Anaemia (with signs of weakness) • Tachypnoea • Exercise intolerance

Metronidazole and ronidazole	• Severe neurological signs
	• Proprioceptive deficits
	  • Ataxia
	  • Tremors
	  • Seizures
	  • Mydriasis
	  • Lethargy
	  • Disorientation
	• Bradycardia
	• Neutropenia (or haematuria)
	• Hepatotoxicity

Metoclopramide	• Various mentation and behavioural abnormalities
	  • Hyperactivity
	  • Lethargy
	  • Disorientation
	  • Ataxia

26.1 (continued) Medications for the treatment of gastrointestinal (GI) disease that can create non-GI side effects. Many antimicrobial agents have the potential to cause bone marrow suppression manifesting as neutropenia with or without other haematological abnormalities. PU/PD = polyuria/polydipsia.

References and further reading

Contreras ET, Giger U, Malmberg JL et al. (2015) Bilirubin encephalopathy in a domestic shorthair cat with increased osmotic fragility and cholangiohepatitis. Veterinary Pathology 53, 1–4

Durand F, Graupera I, Gines P et al. (2015) Pathogenesis of hepatorenal syndrome: implications for therapy. American Journal of Kidney Diseases 67, 318–328

Lidbury JA, Ivanek R, Suchodolski JS et al. (2015) Putative precipitating factors for hepatic encephalopathy in dogs: 118 cases (1991–2014). Journal of the American Veterinary Medical Association 247, 176–183

Pahl MV and Vaziri ND (2015) The chronic kidney disease–colonic axis. Seminars in Dialysis 28, 459–463

Peluso R, Manguso F, Vitiello M et al. (2015) Management of arthropathy in inflammatory bowel diseases. Therapeutic Advances in Chronic Disease 6, 65–77

Qiu F, Lu X and Huang Y (2012) Protective effect of low-molecular-weight heparin on pancreatic encephalopathy in severe acute pancreatitic rats. Inflammation Research 61, 1203–1209

Ruaux C (2013) Cobalamin in companion animals: diagnostic marker, deficiency states and therapeutic implications. The Veterinary Journal 196, 145–152

Rylander H (2017) Neurologic manifestations of systemic disease. In: Textbook of Veterinary Internal Medicine, 8th edn, eds. SJ Ettinger, EC Feldman and E Côté, pp. 167–171. Elsevier Saunders, St. Louis

Trikudanathan G, Venkatesh P and Navaneethan U (2012) Diagnosis and therapeutic management of extra-intestinal manifestations of inflammatory bowel disease. Drugs 72, 2333–2349

Weathers A and Lewis S (2009) Rare and unusual...or are they? Less commonly diagnosed encephalopathies associated with systemic disease. Seminars in Neurology 29, 136–153

Chapter 27

Non-pharmacological therapies

Marcella Ridgway

General supportive measures for patients with gastrointestinal (GI) and hepatic disease include fluid therapy and nutritional management, and constitute a vital aspect of care to optimize patient outcomes. Manipulations of the enteric microbiome and other treatment strategies to limit ongoing cellular injury may also provide therapeutic benefit.

Fluid therapy

The GI tract is responsible for large volumes of fluid transfer, serving as the sole means of fluid uptake to meet the whole body's needs, as well as being the site of significant fluid losses in normal GI secretions. Normal fluid and electrolyte balances are also important for the maintenance of other normal GI functions, as hypoperfusion of the gut results in reduced motility and mucosal disruption. Patients with GI disease are particularly prone to volume depletion: many primary GI conditions are associated with increased secretion and decreased absorption of fluid and electrolytes by enterocytes and subsequent loss from the body. Vomiting and/or diarrhoea result in potentially extensive loss of fluid and electrolytes. Although the absorptive function of the GI tract is often maintained in the face of most disease conditions, reduced voluntary intake because of nausea or malaise, coupled with increased ongoing losses, predispose the GI patient to significant and even life-threatening volume depletion, electrolyte imbalances and acid-base abnormalities. Reduced perfusion of the gut secondary to volume depletion leads to further GI injury and worsening fluid losses.

Judicious use of antiemetics may help to minimize ongoing losses due to vomiting and alleviate nausea, which may be limiting voluntary fluid and nutrient intake. Some owners elect to restrict water intake in pets with diarrhoea, erroneously associating the increased faecal water content with increased water intake when in fact animals with diarrhoea require increased water intake to compensate for diarrhoeal losses. It is important for owners to understand this increased fluid requirement for optimal care of non-hospitalized patients. Normalization of fluid balance may result in improved secretion and motility, leading to improvement of patient status and even resolution of clinical problems (e.g. in case of constipation).

Even in completely anorexic animals, acute weight loss reflects volume depletion rather than loss of lean body mass, and these weight differences may be used to estimate fluid deficits (each change of 0.5 kg represents a volume change of approximately 500 ml). Otherwise, deficits are estimated subjectively by assessing capillary refill time (CRT), mucous membrane moisture and skin turgor/tenting, as well as more objective but less specific parameters of heart rate, pulse quality and mentation. The degree of dehydration is assessed as 5%, 7%, 10% or 12%. General guidelines for determining the degree of dehydration based on physical examination findings are outlined in Figure 27.1.

Fluid deficit is then calculated as percentage dehydration x bodyweight (kg) = ml fluid deficit. Replacement fluid volumes are added to maintenance fluid requirements to replace existing deficits over 8–24 hours, unless hypovolaemic shock dictates a more aggressive initial approach. Maintenance fluid requirements are estimated as 40 ml/kg/day for dogs >10 kg and 60 ml/kg/day for cats and dogs <10 kg. Puppies and kittens have higher (80–100 ml/kg/d) maintenance requirements than adult animals. The fluid administration volume is also adjusted to replace estimated ongoing loss to determine the total fluid dose (see the *BSAVA Manual of Canine and Feline Emergency and Critical Care* for more detailed information on fluid therapy).

Initial fluid doses are based on these general guidelines but provide only an estimate, because of uncertainty in how well the gut will function in absorbing oral fluids and inexact measurement of deficits and ongoing losses (i.e. unquantifiable volume of increased secretions and loss through vomiting or into the gut lumen in diarrhoeic patients). Monitoring the response to administration of a fluid dose is critical to ensure proper adjustment of fluid rates to guard against volume overload once initial deficits

Level of dehydration	Clinical findings
5%	Dry/tacky mucous membranes (MM)
7%	Dry MM, prolonged skin tenting
10%	Dry MM, prolonged skin tenting, sunken eyes, slow capillary refill time (CRT), tachycardia
12%	Dry MM, prolonged skin tenting, sunken eyes, slow CRT, tachycardia, decreased pulse pressure, obtundation

27.1 Estimation of dehydration. Skin tenting may be prolonged in older or underweight animals independent of hydration status and may appear normal in dehydrated young or obese animals. Oral mucous membranes may be moist in nervous, nauseated or vomiting animals despite dehydration, and may be dry in normal animals that are panting/open-mouth breathing.

BSAVA Manual of Canine and Feline Gastroenterology, third edition. Edited by Edward J. Hall, David A. Williams and Aarti Kathrani. ©BSAVA 2020

are corrected, especially if ongoing losses are over-estimated, and against under-hydration if fluid requirements are underestimated.

Parameters that are monitored to assess fluid therapy include physical examination findings, patient bodyweight (measured 2–4 times daily depending on the rate of fluid administration and patient condition), packed cell volume/total solids, and urine concentration and output. Physical examination parameters (mucous membrane moisture, CRT and skin tenting) may be misleading: mucous membranes may be moist because of hypersalivation associated with nausea rather than because of adequate perfusion; skin tent may be falsely prolonged in older or in cachectic animals independent of dehydration, and skin turgor may appear normal in obese or young animals that are dehydrated. Onset of serous nasal discharge, pulmonary crackles, gallop rhythm or dyspnoea due to pulmonary oedema may indicate over-hydration; cats are more susceptible than dogs. However, short-term weight changes better reflect fluid status: ongoing acute weight loss indicates insufficient fluid replacement. Monitoring central venous pressure via a centrally placed intravenous catheter is a potentially more objective means of assessing fluid status but is rarely performed in general practice. Serial monitoring of response to fluid administration is imperative to inform fluid dose adjustments, prevent under- or over-hydration and assure optimal patient care and safety.

Oral hydration may be employed in patients with minimal existing fluid deficits and mild ongoing losses (e.g. patients that are not vomiting), because the ability of the gut to absorb ingested fluid is retained in most disease states. If oral rehydration solutions rather than water are used, patients should be monitored for development of hypernatraemia. When fluid deficits are moderate to severe and the patient is either vomiting or there is obstructive disease or ileus, or when severity of the enteric diseases makes adequate absorption of oral fluids unlikely, parenteral (intravenous, intraosseous, subcutaneous) administration of fluids is indicated. Use of subcutaneous fluid administration (10–20 ml/kg per site) should be limited to cases of mild dehydration in tractable patients, as significantly dehydrated animals may not adequately absorb fluids from subcutaneous sites. Dextrose-containing fluids should never be given by this route due to the risk of skin sloughing. Intravenous routes are preferred in the majority of patients requiring parenteral fluids, as provision of specific fluid volumes can be assured and electrolyte and acid-base abnormalities can be specifically addressed. Intraosseous fluids are given when intravenous access is unavailable.

Animals with GI disease are predisposed to hypokalaemia due to increased potassium losses (diarrhoea, vomiting), acid-base abnormalities (acidaemia) and reduced intake (anorexia) and often require potassium supplementation of intravenous fluids; potassium supplementation should not exceed a rate of 0.5 mmol/kg/h and serum potassium concentrations should be monitored during treatment to prevent over- or under-supplementation. Oral supplementation of potassium can be effective in animals that are not vomiting.

The presence of concomitant diseases must also be taken into consideration when determining fluid volume and type; for example, abnormal cardiac or renal function may impair the individual patient's ability to tolerate what would otherwise be appropriate fluid doses. Hepatic disease may result in sodium retention and, in patients with oedema or ascites, the sodium load presented by fluid administration should be limited by selecting crystalloids with lower sodium content (i.e. 0.45% NaCl

with 2.5% dextrose). Many clinicians advocate the avoidance of lactated Ringer's solution for patients with advanced liver disease in favour of solutions containing other buffering substrates, because lactate requires hepatic metabolism to bicarbonate.

Hypoalbuminaemia, whether resulting from GI loss in patients with protein-losing enteropathy, reduced synthesis in patients with liver disease, exudative losses with pancreatitis or non-GI causes, may limit administration of crystalloid fluids as well as altering interstitial tissue volume and metabolism of protein-bound drugs and endogenous substances. Administration of colloids results in better maintenance of microcirculation relative to crystalloids in pancreatitis, and may help to mobilize ascites in patients with low plasma oncotic pressure. In patients with hypoalbuminaemia, high rates of crystalloid fluid administration may dilute already low albumin to cause problematic decreases in intravascular oncotic pressure, leading to loss of fluids from the vascular compartment, potentially causing ascites, pleural fluid accumulation or tissue oedema, further compromising the functions of the gut and other organs. Colloid administration can improve oncotic pressure and thus prevent or help reverse these effects. Plasma transfusion (6–10 ml/kg) provides oncotic support, maintaining vascular volume, and provides other benefits such as buffering activity, serine proteases and globulins of benefit to patients with pancreatitis. In patients with protein-losing diseases, transfused albumin, like endogenous albumin, is lost, making repeated transfusion or use of alternative colloids necessary. Human albumin has also been used instead of plasma to treat hypoalbuminaemic animals, but supply is very limited in some countries and administration may lead to anaphylaxis. Other colloid options include hetastarch (5–20 ml/kg/day) and dextran 70, which provide molecules larger than albumin (therefore, less likely than albumin to be lost in protein-losing diseases) to provide plasma oncotic pressure support but are no longer available in many countries: gelofusine is still available as an alternative. Anaphylaxis, acute kidney injury, coagulopathies, hepatopathies and reticulo-endothelial dysfunction are some of the potential serious side effects associated with colloid use in humans. Septic patients have been shown to be at higher risk of adverse effects. When colloids are administered, crystalloid fluid doses are typically reduced by 40–60% to prevent over-hydration.

Once ongoing losses and the underlying causative disease are controlled, supplemental fluid administration can be reduced or discontinued based on demonstration that the patient can maintain adequate fluid intake.

Nutrition

The liver, the pancreas and, particularly, the intestinal tract play vital roles in nutrient absorption and metabolism, functions that may be compromised by disease. Additionally, animals that are ill as a result of GI or hepatic disease may have altered nutritional requirements and many will be inappetent as a result of illness, further compromising the overall nutritional status. Malnutrition impairs immune function, predisposing to enteric dysbiosis and infectious disease, or worsening of existing infectious processes. Certain dietary constituents may not be tolerated or may contribute to the pathology in some disease states. Clearly, diet composition and maintaining nutritional intake are very important components of patient management.

Feeding techniques

Hyporexia and anorexia are common in patients with GI disease (see Chapter 8), and nutritional support of patients often requires specific intervention. In some patients, offering a novel, highly palatable food may suffice for a disease process not negatively impacted by these foods – often offering just a very small amount of food at a time is beneficial, or warming the food for a few seconds in a microwave may improve acceptability. In debilitated patients, it is important to facilitate access (e.g. hand-feeding) lest weakness or other physical problems discourage the patient from accessing food and water. Uneaten food should be immediately removed from the patient area – food that is less than fresh or that remains uneaten in the vicinity of the inappetent patient counters efforts to improve intake. Force-feeding is generally discouraged, as it can promote development of food aversions and carries the risk of injury or aspiration pneumonia in the animal struggling to avoid being fed. Food games or feeding toys may sometimes improve interest in food by an inappetent pet.

Appetite stimulants such as diazepam, mirtazapine, cyproheptadine and capromorelin (see Chapter 28), are variably effective in inappetent patients with GI disease, but trial administration is warranted in relatively stable patients. In some inappetent pets, treatment with an antiemetic may result in improved appetite by controlling nausea manifesting as anorexia (even if vomiting is not present). Similarly, cobalamin supplementation may increase appetite if anorexia is caused by hypocobalaminaemia.

In patients that are unresponsive to initial efforts to improve food intake, more aggressive measures are indicated. An enteric route of nutrition should be prioritized as enterocytes derive their nutrition directly from gut luminal contents, and normal gut microbial populations are also sustained by enteric nutrients. Appetite stimulants can be tried, but placement of any feeding tube is highly beneficial as a reliable route for enteral feeding, fluids and easy administration of oral medications. Options include naso-oesophageal/nasogastric, oesophagostomy, gastrostomy or jejunostomy feeding tubes, based on the site of introduction of the tube and the patient's requirements (see the *BSAVA Guide to Procedures in Small Animal Practice*). However, except naso-oesophageal/nasogastric tubes, placement does require general anaesthesia. Parenteral nutrition may be considered in non-septic patients, particularly as an initial approach in those with severe enteric disease where the absorptive capacity of the gut is severely compromised or in patients with intractable vomiting or diarrhoea.

Naso-oesophageal/nasogastric tubes are usually of too small a diameter to allow prolonged feeding. An oesophagostomy feeding tube is preferred unless contraindicated by general anaesthesia, oesophageal disease, frequent vomiting or the presence of disease proximal to the small intestine, which would restrict oesophageal feedings from reaching the gut. Oesophagostomy feeding tube placement is a relatively simple procedure, requiring short-duration anaesthesia, and allows utilization of tubes of sufficient calibre to permit use of most commercial diets after processing in a food blender with added water to achieve a consistency suitable for tube feeding. Any water added to the diet or used to flush the tube after feeding should be taken into account as contributing toward the patient's fluid needs.

Canned critical care diets are nutrient-dense and often of a consistency appropriate for tube feeding as packaged or after mixing with a small volume of water. However, such diets are typically rich in fat and protein, which may make them inappropriate for some patients. Feeding plans should be individualized and based on calculation of basal or resting energy requirements (RER) estimated by the equation RER = 70 x bodyweight(kg)$^{0.75}$ = kcal/day required. Feeding should begin with 25% of the calculated RER daily and increased by 25% increments q24h if feedings are well tolerated. Dogs and cats should not be fed more than 100% RER whilst hospitalized to prevent complications associated with over-feeding.

Postural (elevated) feeding is a mainstay of management of animals with megaoesophagus or oesophageal dysmotility and may be helpful in those with gastro-oesophageal reflux. For this to be beneficial, food should be provided at a level of at least 45 degrees higher than the lower oesophageal sphincter, and, ideally, in an upright position to maximize the benefit of gravitational pull in aiding proper directional movement of food through the oesophagus into the stomach. The upright position should be maintained for a period of 20–30 minutes following the meal. Dogs can often be trained to feed from and maintain an elevated position or can be placed in a Bailey chair, a specialized feeding enclosure designed to maintain the animal in an upright position. Instructions for the construction of a Bailey chair can be found at many online sites identified by searching 'Bailey chair construction plans'. Placement in an owner-worn papoose-style baby carrier may be effective for cats and small dogs, as long as the owner remembers to remain upright for the recommended period.

Withholding of food is no longer recommended in ill patients, including those with pancreatitis and GI disease, unless the patient is unable to swallow safely (e.g. stuporous) or actively vomits when food is presented or swallowed. Evidence confirms that enteral feeding is vital for maintenance and restoration of GI health and withholding food delays resolution of GI disease and predisposes to bacterial translocation. That being said, withholding food for 24 hours in an otherwise healthy adult dog with acute non-specific diarrhoea is probably not harmful and may allow resolution of signs by 'resting the gut' (i.e. reducing secretion and peristalsis, removing exposure to ingested bacteria and dietary antigens, and reducing vomiting triggered by GI distension or gastric mucosal irritation). Osmotic diarrhoea generally improves when food is withheld, returning when feeding resumes. Complete restriction of food is not recommended in cats, mainly due to the concern for hepatic lipidosis.

Enteral diets

Diets used in managing GI, pancreatic and hepatic diseases are modified in protein, fat, carbohydrate and fibre content and type, and are generally of particularly high digestibility. Some specialized diets provide nutrients in partially hydrolysed (proteins in hydrolysed diets) or elemental (simple sugars and amino acids in elemental diets) forms to reduce antigenicity and increase ease of digestion and absorption for animals with food allergy/intolerance or malabsorption due to severe small intestinal disease. In animals with intestinal disease, any diet change (irrespective of specific diet composition) may effect an improvement in clinical signs due to resulting shifts in intestinal microbial populations, so just changing the diet has potential benefits, although 'trial and error' may be needed to find which specific diet best controls signs. Generally, changes to a diet with specific compositional characteristics are recommended based on the underlying disease condition.

Diets for acute GI disease

For dogs with acute non-specific GI disease, 'bland' diets are typically recommended. The bland diet is fed in small amounts at more frequent intervals until clinical signs are controlled, then the patient may be transitioned back to the usual diet and feeding frequency. The primary characteristics of a diet considered to be 'bland' are high digestibility (low in non-fermentable fibre) and, usually, reduced fat content. Fat is the most complex nutrient to digest, involving many steps and relying on normal functioning of the liver, pancreas, small intestine and lymphatics. Fats that are not properly digested and absorbed become hydroxylated by luminal bacteria: hydroxylated fatty acids are injurious to the colonic mucosa and can trigger secretory diarrhoea. Dietary fat may also promote inflammation: n-6 fatty acids are metabolized to proinflammatory compounds. Fat (and fibre) delay gastric emptying, which may exacerbate vomiting. The author prefers a formulation of low fat and high fermentable fibre for dogs with acute non-specific diarrhoea.

Low-fat/GI diets

Low-fat diets are considered to be those containing less than 10% fat on a dry matter basis or with less than 20% of calories from fat. Commercially available weight-loss-promoting or reduced-fat diets for dogs include Purina Pro Plan Veterinary Diets OM, Royal Canin Veterinary Diet Gastrointestinal Low Fat and Hill's Prescription Diet i/d Low Fat. The reader should refer to the specific manufacturer's product guide for up to date information on the percentage fat on a dry matter and calorie basis. Dietary fat restriction may be beneficial for multiple reasons in patients with chronic as well as acute GI disease, and is generally recommended for dogs with chronic diarrhoea and animals with pancreatitis or hepatobiliary (especially cholestatic) disease. Ultra-low-fat diets, with restricted amounts of long-chain fatty acids, which normally require uptake through the lymphatics, are recommended for animals with intestinal lymphangiectasia. However, because fat is the most energy-dense nutrient, reduction of fat levels in the diet may make it difficult to meet a patient's energy needs. In fat-reduced diets, the principal energy source is usually complex carbohydrates. At this time, it does not appear that fat restriction is beneficial in managing GI or pancreatic disease in cats.

Protein in diets for GI patients should be highly digestible, a function of protein source and processing and factors related to other dietary components. In addition to manipulation of protein types to address food allergy or intolerance, total protein content may be varied to address specific disease conditions. Diets high in protein and low in carbohydrate appear to be beneficial in managing chronic diarrhoea in cats. Protein restriction is often promoted for patients with hepatic disease to prevent or manage hepatic encephalopathy but may not always be appropriate, as some hepatic diets may not meet the energy and protein requirements for maintenance and cell regeneration in liver disease.

Exclusion diets

Exclusion (elimination) diets are intended to identify a specific dietary component (generally protein) that is responsible for an adverse food reaction leading to clinical signs, so that exclusion of that component from the patient's diet becomes the principal treatment. The most important characteristic of an exclusion diet is that it is formulated from ingredients that the patient has not received before, and hence are theoretically not responsible for an existing dietary sensitivity (i.e. limited antigen/novel protein diets), or ingredients unlikely to trigger an adverse dietary response (i.e. hydrolysed diets). These diets should contain highly digestible protein.

There are a number of commercially available therapeutic diets for dogs which may be used, including Hill's Prescription Diet z/d dry and tinned food, Hill's Prescription Diet d/d dry and tinned food (multiple formulations), Purina Pro Plan Veterinary Diets HA dry food, Royal Canin Veterinary Diet Hypoallergenic dry and tinned food, Royal Canin Veterinary Diet Anallergenic (Ultamino) dry food; options for cats include Hill's Prescription Diet z/d dry and tinned food, Hill's Prescription Diet d/d dry and tinned food, Purina Pro Plan Veterinary Diets HA dry food, Royal Canin Veterinary Diet Hypoallergenic dry food and Royal Canin Veterinary Diet Anallergenic (Ultamino) dry food. Homemade novel ingredient diets may be employed, but consultation with a specialist (board-certified) veterinary nutritionist to assess nutritional balance should be sought. When exclusion diets are initiated, it is critical that the patient receives no other foods, including treats or flavoured chewable medications (including heartworm and flea/tick preventative medications) or supplements. Animals with dietary sensitivities generally respond within the first 2–4 weeks of receiving the exclusion diet, but the exclusion diet alone should be fed for at least 10 weeks to provide adequate time for all animals to show a response and to ensure that remission of signs is sustained and due to the diet change rather than the natural fluctuation in the severity of signs common in GI disease. If the animal responds to the diet, then other ingredients can be added back to the diet one at a time to identify which one(s) is (are) responsible for recurrence of clinical signs and, therefore, which specific ingredient(s) must be excluded from that patient's diet: signs generally recur within 3–7 days of reintroduction of the offending ingredient. Commonly, owners are pleased with the positive response and opt to stay with the effective exclusion diet rather than proceeding with specific identification of the problematic ingredient, which requires a relapse of their pet's signs. If the animal does not respond to the diet, either dietary sensitivity is not the cause of clinical signs or the exclusion diet itself contains the causative ingredient and a trial with another diet may be indicated. Here, initial use of a hydrolysed diet may offer significant advantage over limited-antigen diets, as these are formulated to provide proteins hydrolysed to be too small to trigger a type 1 hypersensitivity response. Even so, different hydrolysed diets utilize different protein sources and, if one hydrolysed diet is not effective, changing to another hydrolysed diet formulated with a different protein base may be effective.

Fibre

Dietary fibre plays a significant role in GI health and disease, although it is not directly digested by dogs and cats, which lack the necessary enzymes, but by enteric microbes. Dietary fibre is classified as fermentable or non-fermentable, depending on the degree to which it is metabolized by intestinal bacteria. Fermentable fibre is metabolized by luminal bacteria to release short-chain fatty acids (SCFAs), which in turn provide a range of beneficial effects. SCFAs are the primary energy source for colonocytes, promote colonocyte turnover and function, facilitate fluid and electrolyte exchange, support normal motility of the distal small intestine and colon, support beneficial intestinal bacterial populations, leading to exclusion of pathogens, and influence nutrient absorption rate in the small intestine. Non-fermentable fibre is not well metabolized by luminal bacteria and remains intact as it traverses the gut, providing bulk and enhancing motility. All fibre binds water to some degree and, in so doing, can effect improvement in faecal consistency in small or large intestinal diarrhoea; use of a fibre-rich diet is favoured by the author for management of acute to subacute non-specific diarrhoea in dogs.

Vitamins

Malabsorption or loss of vitamins may occur in GI, pancreatic and hepatobiliary disease. Deficiencies should be recognized and appropriate supplementation given.

Water-soluble vitamins:

Folic acid: Folate deficiency is a marker for proximal small intestinal disease, although serum concentrations are affected by dietary folate content and intestinal bacterial synthesis with 100–400 μg of either synthetic folic acid or the naturally-occuring biologically active moiety 5-methyltetrahydrofolate ('folate'). Deficiencies are addressed by oral supplementation.

Cobalamin: Dogs and cats with chronic GI or pancreatic disease quite frequently have malabsorption of vitamin B12 and develop cobalamin deficiency. As well as being a diagnostic marker, this deficiency contributes to systemic consequences of disease and interferes with resolution of GI disease.

Cobalamin deficiency has traditionally been addressed via parenteral (subcutaneous) administration of cyanocobalamin (250 μg–1 mg s.c. weekly) until gut absorption of vitamin B_{12} is restored. However, recent studies have clearly shown that even if the normal absorptive pathway in the ileum (receptor-mediated endocytosis) is impaired, a small amount of cobalamin can still be absorbed by other pathways. Daily oral cobalamin (0.25–2.0 mg orally once daily) has been shown to be effective not only at restoring serum cobalamin concentrations, but also at normalizing one of the metabolic abnormalities (methylmalonic acidaemia) associated with hypocobalaminaemia. A veterinary commercial product (Cobalaplex; Cobalaquin in USA) combining cobalamin, folate and prebiotic is now available.

Fat-soluble vitamins:

Vitamin A: Low serum vitamin A has been used historically as a marker of malabsorption, but has not been associated with clinical signs.

Vitamin D: Ionized hypocalcaemia is sometimes recognized in protein-losing enteropathy. It is thought to occur as a result of calcium and vitamin D malabsorption and probably loss of serum vitamin D binding protein. It occasionally causes neuromuscular clinical signs that need to be addressed by calcium and vitamin D supplementation.

Vitamin E (tocopherol): Vitamin E deficiency has been documented in dogs with pancreatic insufficiency and in cases of intestinal malabsorption, and can be supplemented at a dose of 100–400 IU orally q24h for 30 days, then as needed for dogs, and 30 IU orally q24h for 30 days, then as needed for cats.

Vitamin K: Malabsorption of vitamin K is occasionally seen in biliary disease and pancreatic insufficiency, especially in cats, and can cause prolonged coagulation times and, rarely, even overt bleeding. Deficiencies can be corrected by parenteral vitamin K, administered subcutaneously as 0.5–1.0 mg/kg q12h for a maximum of four doses to avoid inducing haemolysis.

Manipulation of gut microbiota

The GI microbiota serves important roles in normal function and health of the GI tract, and GI disease conditions are associated with shifts in GI microbial populations, so-called dysbiosis. The integral interrelationship of microbes and GI health support the concept that manipulation of GI microbiota offers potential targets for managing GI disease, which has been borne out in many studies of GI and other diseases in humans. Veterinary studies are fewer but still indicate that manipulating intestinal microbiota can have beneficial effects on disease outcome. Options for manipulating the GI microbiota include the use of prebiotics and non-fermentable dietary fibre, probiotics, faecal microbiota transplantation (FMT) and administration of antimicrobials.

Antimicrobials

Antimicrobials have traditionally been used to manipulate GI microbial populations with the intent to reduce overall bacterial numbers (treatment of hepatic encephalopathy, 'small intestinal bacterial overgrowth' (SIBO), shift an abnormal microbial balance (dysbiosis), control specific bacterial and protozoal pathogens or for beneficial effects beyond their direct antimicrobial activity (e.g. modulation of inflammation by doxycycline and metronidazole), although this may at least in part relate to their impact on microbial populations. Use of prebiotics and probiotics and, potentially, FMT has allowed a reduction in the use of antimicrobial drugs to control endogenous GI bacterial populations (see also Chapter 29).

Prebiotics

Prebiotics are fermentable fibres, which serve as a substrate for fermentation by beneficial bacteria in the gut and, when ingested by the animal, selectively promote replication and/or activity of beneficial GI bacteria. Examples of prebiotic fibre sources include beet pulp, chicory (inulin), aleurone, soya hulls, psyllium and various other grain, vegetable and fruit fibre sources. Prebiotics are generally administered by incorporating them into the diet and commercial diets, including maintenance as well as intestinal diets, often include prebiotics in their formulations.

Probiotics

Probiotics are live microorganisms that, when administered in adequate amounts, provide a health benefit to the animal. The mechanisms by which these organisms exert their beneficial effect are, for the most part, poorly defined, but appear to include fermentation of fibre to SCFAs, anti-inflammatory effects, promotion of normal intestinal motility, prevention of bacterial translocation and inhibition of pathogenic organisms. Studies in dogs and cats demonstrate improvement in faecal quality and reduction in duration of non-specific diarrhoea in working dogs and in dogs and cats in animal shelters. In the European Union, human probiotics are regulated by Health Claim Regulations and animal probiotics by additional Safety Regulations. In the USA they are classified as supplements and are not regulated by the Food and Drug Administration.

Products vary considerably, and studies of probiotic products used in small animals in North America have shown that few products actually contain the types and numbers of organisms claimed on the label and some contain no live bacteria at all. Of products tested, only two were accurately labelled (i.e. contained the indicated organism species and met or exceeded the numbers claimed on their labels): FortiFlora™ (Purina) and the synbiotic (a synbiotic is a combination of probiotic and prebiotic) Proviable® (Nutramax). Use of probiotics offers a high degree of safety, with the only potential contraindications being marked or prolonged immunosuppression and animals with severe disruption of the GI mucosal barrier and bacterial translocation. Probiotics show little residual effect after administration is discontinued and must be given continuously for sustained benefit.

Faecal microbiota transplantation

FMT is proven to be effective in humans with colitis associated with post-antibiotic *Clostridium difficile* overgrowth, a clinical entity not recognized in dogs or cats. It may have some efficacy in other human intestinal disorders, including ulcerative colitis, irritable bowel syndrome and Crohn's disease, as well as in some non-GI conditions, including autism, obesity, insulin resistance and metabolic syndrome. FMT has been utilized for some time in veterinary medicine but principally as a means of immune inoculation in production animal management (pigs). Therapeutic use in small animal patients is only recently being addressed in controlled investigations, and evidence of efficacy is purely anecdotal so far. A suspension of faeces from a healthy donor is inoculated via nasogastric tube, gastroduodenoscopy, colonoscopy or enema with the goal of establishing a healthy bacterial microbiota in the recipient. Optimized protocols have yet to be established.

Other strategies to reduce GI injury

As described above, maintaining hydration and dietary manipulation are important strategies for limiting progression of injury in GI disease. Dietary protein modification reduces antigenicity and subsequent inflammation. n-3 polyunsaturated fatty acids (PUFAs), which are present in high concentrations in fish oils, are metabolized to non-inflammatory eicosanoids, whereas n-6 PUFAs generate pro-inflammatory metabolites: diets enriched with n-3 fatty acids may reduce inflammation in the gut. Manipulation of the GI microbiota with probiotics or FMT shows anti-inflammatory effects. Some antimicrobials (metronidazole, doxycycline) used to control enteric bacterial populations show anti-inflammatory properties, although the extent to which this is due to their impact on gut microbial species *versus* their direct anti-inflammatory effect is unclear.

Administration of supplemental antioxidants is indicated in conditions such as paracetamol (acetaminophen)-induced hepatotoxicity, where oxidative stress is the predominant pathophysiological mechanism. Use of antioxidants is often advocated in treating other hepatic diseases because oxidative stress contributes to the pathogenesis of many inflammatory diseases, although studies of efficacy are lacking. Administration of antioxidants, such as silymarin, *S*-adenosylmethionine (SAMe), vitamin C or vitamin E, is relatively safe and may confer as yet undocumented benefit in hepatic or other inflammatory diseases by acting as free-radical scavengers (vitamin C, vitamin E) or increasing endogenous antioxidants through increases in the activity of superoxide dismutase (silymarin) and concentrations of glutathione. Commercial diets contain antioxidants (vitamin C, vitamin E, beta-carotene) that are absorbed and provide antioxidant support. Use of these compounds as separate antioxidant supplements should be employed with caution as excesses may cause deleterious effects (e.g. excess vitamin C may increase the risk of calcium oxalate urolithiasis in susceptible individuals and may increase tissue damage in patients with high hepatic copper and iron levels). Zinc, used therapeutically in some hepatic diseases to limit copper absorption from the gut, also has antioxidant properties, but over-supplementation may cause zinc toxicity (haemolytic anaemia, acute GI signs, potential liver or kidney injury). Ursodeoxycholic acid, also used therapeutically in hepatic disease, has antioxidant properties as well as immunomodulatory effects, helping to limit inflammation.

Summary

Adjunctive therapies complement more specific treatments in the management of GI, pancreatic and hepatic diseases and serve as effective tools in managing acute non-specific GI-related illnesses. Maintaining hydration and nutrition are universally important in achieving good patient outcomes, and other therapies contribute enhanced benefit in a multimodal approach to treatment. These therapies may be implemented prior to determination of a specific diagnosis and are generally safe and beneficial across a range of disease entities, sometimes constituting all the treatment that is necessary to allow complete resolution of disease.

References and further reading

Bexfield N and Lee K (2014) *BSAVA Guide to Procedures in Small Animal Practice, 2nd edn.* BSAVA Publications, Gloucester

King LG and Boag A (2018) *BSAVA Manual of Canine and Feline Emergency and Critical Care, 3rd edn.* BSAVA Publications, Gloucester

Toresson L, Steiner JM, Olmedal G *et al.* (2017) Oral cobalamin supplementation in cats with hypocobalaminaemia: a retrospective study. *Journal of Feline Medicine and Surgery* **19**, 1302–1306

Toresson L, Steiner JM, Razdan P *et al.* (2018) Comparison of efficacy of oral and parenteral cobalamin supplementation in normalizing low cobalamin concentrations in dogs: a randomized controlled study. *The Veterinary Journal* **232**, 27–32

Toresson L, Steiner JM, Spodsberg E *et al.* (2019) Effects of oral versus parenteral cobalamin supplementation on methylmalonic acid and homocysteine concentrations in dogs with chronic enteropathies and low cobalamin concentrations. *The Veterinary Journal* **243**, 8–14

Chapter 28

Non-specific drug therapy

Edward J. Hall

This chapter describes drugs used non-specifically to manage signs associated with gastrointestinal (GI) and liver diseases, their proposed modes of action, interactions and potential side effects in dogs and cats. Information and recommendations on specific treatments of specific conditions are given in the relevant chapters, and the very important roles of fluid therapy and dietary modification and the potential benefits of pre- and probiotics are covered in Chapter 27. The uses of antibacterial and antiparasitic drugs are described in Chapters 29 and 30, respectively. Names of drugs with a UK marketing authorization and non-licensed drugs are included here; dosages are available from the *BSAVA Small Animal Formulary*.

Whilst these symptomatic therapies are available, most GI disturbances are acute and self-limiting, and so the need for some of them is debatable. Furthermore, their mechanism of action is often uncertain and their efficacy frequently unproven. Ideally, such remedies are only used *after* a diagnosis has been made and specific treatment has been initiated. If a definitive diagnosis has not been made, then they should be used only for a short period (maximum of 48 hours) without re-assessment, so that definitive treatment is not dangerously delayed. For example, using antiemetics can mask the signs of an intestinal obstruction, delaying surgery and endangering the patient.

Antiemetics

These drugs inhibit the vomiting reflex, controlling emesis by peripheral and/or central actions. They are indicated for the prevention of vomiting in predictable circumstances (e.g. motion sickness, after chemotherapy) and for the control of vomiting, especially when protracted and profuse, causing water and electrolyte disturbances and patient distress. They are contraindicated when there is GI obstruction, or after ingestion of caustics and some toxins, or when hypotension exists.

Centrally acting antiemetics

These drugs act on the central nervous system (CNS) to inhibit the vomiting reflex. Depending on which neurotransmitter they block and at which site they act, centrally acting antiemetics have either a narrow or a broad spectrum of activity.

Maropitant

This is a veterinary licensed antiemetic and anti-nausea drug for dogs and cats. It is also licensed, at higher doses, for the control of motion sickness in dogs but not cats. A related molecule, aprepitant, is used in humans, but one of the veterinary licensed products should be used in cats and dogs. Maropitant (Cerenia™, Prevomax™) is a very effective, broad-spectrum antiemetic, as it blocks NK$_1$ (substance P) receptors, the final common pathway in the vomiting centre when vomiting is triggered. Cerenia™ has been shown to be effective at inhibiting vomiting due to various chemotherapy agents, chronic kidney disease, the canine emetic apomorphine, opioids given postoperatively and in acute gastroenteritis. In cases of refractory vomiting, higher doses can be tried, or maropitant can be given in combination with other antiemetics, such as metoclopramide, that act on an alternative neurotransmitter pathway.

Experimental studies of acute pancreatitis in mice indicate that maropitant may have some anti-inflammatory effect as well as being an antiemetic. Furthermore, through its action on NK$_1$ receptors blocking substance P involved in neurogenic pain sensation, there is a suggestion that maropitant may also be an analgesic. Studies so far have only examined surgical pain, and at best maropitant appears to be a weak analgesic, which is unlikely to be adequate on its own. However, these potential additional mechanisms mean that its value in managing acute pancreatitis may have been underestimated.

Maropitant can be given orally, but treatment is usually initiated by subcutaneous or slow intravenous injection that is then followed by oral dosing once vomiting is controlled. A pain reaction is quite frequently seen after subcutaneous injection of Cerenia™: the maropitant molecule separates from cyclodextrin, its vehicle, as it warms and is completely dissociated above 20°C (Narishetty *et al.*, 2009), and it is the free drug which can cause this pain. Therefore, Cerenia™ should be stored at 4°C in the refrigerator and administered cold when injected subcutaneously; minimal pain reaction is seen if it is given slowly intravenously. A new formulation (Prevomax™) uses a different preservative (benzyl alcohol) to Cerenia™, and it is claimed that its injection does not produce a pain response.

Maropitant is only 50% bioavailable from the GI tract so the oral dose is twice the injectable dose (2 mg/kg orally or 1 mg/kg s.c. or i.v.). It is highly protein-bound, and so it persists in plasma, and once-daily dosing is effective: it reaches a plateau after approximately 7 days of daily dosing. It is metabolized by the liver, although by different pathways in dogs and cats, and the dose should be reduced in liver disease in both species as a precaution. The safety of maropitant in puppies less than 8 weeks of age and kittens less than 16 weeks has not been established. There were concerns of leucopenia when it was tested for efficacy against vomiting in naturally occurring gastroenteritis in puppies, although this may have been a coincidence because parvoviral infection may have been the cause of the gastroenteritis and the leucopenia.

At higher doses (8 mg/kg orally q24h), maropitant can inhibit motion sickness, but as this involves the presumed conscious perception of nausea, it must also be acting at sites other than the vomiting centre.

Metoclopramide

Metoclopramide (Emeprid™, Vomend™) is recognized as a relatively safe antiemetic in dogs, although animal studies are limited, and most information is extrapolated from humans. Like all antiemetics, it is contraindicated if there is a GI obstruction. Historically it was the first-choice antiemetic in dogs until the original veterinary licensed product was withdrawn and maropitant was marketed. However, it is now available again as a veterinary licensed antiemetic as both oral and injectable formulations; the latter is light-sensitive, and when used as a constant rate infusion, obscuring the infusion bag contents is recommended.

At low doses metoclopramide is a D_2 dopamine receptor antagonist and at higher doses it antagonizes 5-HT_3 receptors and, thus, is effective against emetic substances that stimulate the chemoreceptor trigger zone (CRTZ) in dogs. It is particularly effective as a constant rate infusion in puppies with parvoviral enteritis. It is much less effective in cats as D_2 receptors are not the predominant receptor in their CRTZ. It is also prokinetic in the upper GI tract (see later).

Dose-dependent side effects, linked to dopaminergic CNS activity (e.g. excitement, muscle tremors), were often seen historically because of an error in the published recommended dosage. They were most notable in cats, and were another reason not to recommend metoclopramide for this species. Metoclopramide undergoes urinary excretion, so dose reduction is indicated in renal insufficiency, and it is potentiated by glucocorticoids, phenothiazines and fluoxetine.

Ondansetron

By blocking 5-HT_3 receptors, ondansetron is a very potent antiemetic and was developed for the control of emesis in humans receiving chemotherapy. It is more likely to prevent vomiting (i.e. when given before chemotherapy) than stop ongoing vomiting, and it is effective in postoperative nausea.

It appears to be effective in dogs but is expensive in some countries and not licensed in animals, and is generally reserved for cisplatin toxicity and refractory vomiting. Side effects are mild but include sedation and head shaking. Related molecules (e.g. azestron, dolasetron, granisetron, palanosetron, tropisetron) are sometimes used in veterinary medicine.

Anticholinergics

Atropine-like drugs act as antiemetics by blocking muscarinic receptors in higher centres and the vomiting centre, and so they must be able to cross the blood–brain barrier.

Scopolamine (hyoscine hydrobromide) and propantheline tend to be more effective in humans, antagonizing M_1 receptors, thereby blocking muscarinic effects of acetylcholine. They consequently have peripheral side effects, such as dry mouth, constipation, mydriasis and tachycardia. There are no veterinary licensed preparations. Butylscopolamine (see below) cannot cross the blood–brain barrier and is, therefore, not directly antiemetic.

Antihistamines

Histamine H_2-receptor antagonists are used to block gastric acid production (see later), and are not directly antiemetic. H_1-receptor antagonists block transmission from the vestibular apparatus via the CRTZ and have some efficacy in motion sickness and vestibular disease. They are more effective in humans than dogs, and are ineffective in cats. They are also ineffective against other causes of vomiting in both dogs and cats.

There are no veterinary licensed H_1-receptor antagonists, but human drugs can be used, e.g. diphenhydramine, meclizine or promethazine. Meclizine and promethazine have a longer duration of action but can cause drowsiness and a dry mouth. Other H_1-receptor antagonists, such as chlorphenamine, clemastine and hydroxyzine have less sedative effect but are largely used to help control pruritus in allergic skin disease, as they are not very potent antiemetics.

Phenothiazines

Prochlorperazine, acepromazine and chlorpromazine are broad-spectrum antiemetics blocking vomiting in the CRTZ and possibly the vomiting centre, by blocking D_2 dopamine receptors. However, they are considered 'dirty' or broad-spectrum drugs, as they can also antagonize α_1 adrenergic, 5-HT_3, H_1 and M_1 receptors. Consequently, they can cause vasodilation and may be hypotensive, and so should only be used once any dehydration is resolved. They can all cause drowsiness, but this effect is least with prochlorperazine. However, a tranquillizing effect can be helpful if the vomiting patient is distressed.

Prochlorpromazine and chlorpromazine are available for humans, but there are no veterinary licensed products. Phenothiazines can have significant interactions with organophosphates and CNS depressants (barbiturates, narcotics); antidiarrhoeals and antacids may impair absorption and they are incompatible in the syringe with penicillin, chloramphenicol or hydrocortisone. Prochlorperazine is only available in some countries in a combination product with an anticholinergic, isopropamide (see below).

Sedatives

Barbiturates and benzodiazepines have antiemetic properties. Phenobarbital and a variety of benzodiazepines have been used to control psychogenic and behavioural vomiting, and so-called limbal epilepsy. Phenobarbital is also useful for controlling sialoadenosis/sialoadenitis/salivary infarction, although the mechanism of action is unclear (see Chapter 31).

Others

A number of other drugs are potential antiemetics, but are rarely used in veterinary medicine. Butyrophenones are potent antidopaminergic antiemetics; corticosteroids can also be antiemetic and this effect may be useful during chemotherapy; cannabinoids are antiemetic but not used in animals.

Peripherally acting antiemetics

Occasionally, drugs used for their locally protective effect on the GI tract will also stop vomiting, examples are protectants and acid blockers, which are discussed later. Prokinetics, such as metoclopramide, can physically reduce the triggers for emesis by increasing lower oesophageal sphincter tone and emptying the stomach.

Anticholinergics

Butylscopolamine: Butylscopolamine (hyoscine butylbromide) is licensed in combination with metamizole (a non-steroidal anti-inflammatory drug (NSAID): it causes smooth muscle relaxation in the GI tract, but does not cross the blood–brain barrier, so it will only indirectly reduce vomiting due to reduction of abdominal pain. It is often used in practice, but often inappropriately, as it can cause gastric atony and intestinal ileus, which may potentiate vomiting and absorption of toxins. However, it is useful in patients with mild, colicky abdominal pain.

Others: Glycopyrronium bromide (glycopyrrolate), propantheline, methscopolamine, isopropamide and aminopentamide are anticholinergics which do not cross the blood–brain barrier and are antiemetic because they inhibit efferent vagal stimuli, relieve smooth muscle spasm and dry GI secretions. They can also cause dry mouth, constipation, tachycardia and urine retention. None are recommended for cats.

Prokinetics

Prokinetics are drugs that stimulate motility in part or all of the GI tract, and are indicated when there is ileus not related to electrolyte imbalances. They are contraindicated in intestinal obstruction.

Cholinergics

The use of cholinergics is limited by their tendency to cause systemic effects. Pilocarpine, arecoline and carbachol are purgatives and cause marked abdominal cramping and pain.

Bethanechol

This drug acts exclusively on M_2 muscarinic receptors and increases contractions throughout the GI tract, but mostly at the lower oesophageal sphincter and in the rectum. As it increases lower oesophageal sphincter tone, it is contraindicated in idiopathic megaoesophagus. It has been used to treat megacolon and dysautonomia; it is poorly prokinetic in the small intestine, but can also cause abdominal cramps, diarrhoea, salivation and bradycardia.

Anticholinesterases

Neostigmine and pyridostigmine are used to treat focal myasthenia gravis affecting the oesophagus, potentiating the action of acetylcholine at the neuromuscular junction and allowing peristalsis.

Metoclopramide

In addition to its central antiemetic effect (see earlier), metoclopramide acts peripherally as an antidopaminergic and a cholinergic agent. This activity is abolished by antimuscarinics such as atropine. Although its activity is confined to the upper GI tract, it can be useful in preventing gastro-oesophageal reflux and promoting gastric emptying. It is not effective in treating gastric dilatation, intestinal ileus or constipation.

Cisapride

This is the most effective GI prokinetic ever marketed. Cisapride stimulates GI 5-HT_4 receptors, resulting in:

- Contraction of oesophageal smooth muscle
- Increased lower oesophageal sphincter tone
- Decreased pyloric tone
- Propulsive peristaltic waves in the stomach, duodenum, jejunum and colon.

As the canine oesophagus is largely striated muscle, cisapride is not effective in idiopathic megaoesophagus, but it is indicated for gastro-oesophageal reflux and GI smooth muscle motility disorders, including dysautonomia and feline idiopathic megacolon.

However, cisapride was withdrawn because of its effect on myocardial calcium channels, with QT prolongation and the risk of fatal cardiac arrhythmias (torsades de pointes) in humans; this is not a concern in canine patients because of differences in myocardial physiology. The risk was enhanced when co-administered with drugs inhibiting cytochrome P450. Some stocks are still available and they can be obtained in the UK on a Special Import Certificate. Newer, related 5-HT_4 prokinetics, prucalopride and mosapride, have been developed. They have prokinetic activity but not the cardiac side effect. Mosapride is available in Japan but, like metoclopramide, its activity is limited to the stomach and duodenum; prucalopride is available in Europe.

Domperidone

This is a dopamine antagonist with similar prokinetic activity to metoclopramide in humans. However, it cannot cross the blood–brain barrier so does not have central antiemetic activity or cause CNS side effects. Its activity in dogs has not been fully studied.

H_2-antagonists

Ranitidine and nizatidine are gastric acid blockers (see later) but are also weak prokinetics. Consequently, they may be an appropriate choice in gastritis, where their ability to stimulate gastric emptying will complement their acid-blocking activity. They are also effective in the lower GI tract *in vitro* and so have been recommended for feline idiopathic megacolon when cisapride is not available, although their efficacy *in vivo* seems poor.

Erythromycin

Vomiting as a side effect of antibacterial doses of erythromycin (i.e. 10 mg/kg) is well known. It occurs through hyperstimulation of motilin receptors in the GI tract. At much lower doses (i.e. 1–2 mg/kg), it stimulates motility resembling normal migrating motor complexes, and this can be used as a helpful prokinetic effect. However, the peristalsis it causes most resembles the interdigestive motility pattern and not normal digestive motility, and the public health concern of using chronic low doses of antibacterials means it is rarely used for this purpose.

Azithromycin is equivalent to erythromycin in accelerating the gastric emptying of adult humans with gastroparesis (Potter and Snider, 2013). Furthermore, its longer duration of action, better side effect profile and lack of P450 interaction may make it more suitable, but further evaluation in dogs and cats is needed.

Mucosal (cyto)protectants

Protectants aid the mucosal barrier function when oesophageal or gastric ulceration exists, and may act as cytoprotective agents or chemical diffusion barriers or both. Cytoprotective agents enhance the viability of GI epithelial cells, particularly through the delivery or generation of beneficial prostaglandins.

Prostaglandins

Cytoprotective prostaglandins are crucial to the health of the gastric mucosal barrier by:

- Increasing gastric mucosal blood flow
- Increasing gastric mucus secretion
- Stabilizing histamine-containing enterochromaffin-like cells
- Decreasing gastric acid secretion.

It is the inhibition of the constitutive gastric cyclooxygenase enzyme (COX-1) by NSAIDs that leads to a deficiency of cytoprotective prostaglandin E (PGE) and gastric ulceration. Misoprostol, a synthetic PGE1, can protect against such damage, whilst the NSAIDs still exert their beneficial anti-inflammatory effect against the inducible COX-2 enzyme. Misoprostol has been shown in dogs to protect the gastric mucosa from aspirin and meloxicam-induced ulceration, but it is not very effective at healing pre-existing ulcers. It is indicated in dogs that must take NSAIDs for chronic inflammatory disease but suffer gastro-erosive side effects. Misoprostol does not have a UK veterinary licence. It is given orally; diarrhoea and abdominal cramping are side effects that are usually self-limiting, and actually lessened if NSAIDs are being co-administered. Being a prostaglandin, misoprostol will cause abortions and, therefore, must not be used in pregnancy.

Antacids

Compounds such as aluminium hydroxide, calcium carbonate, sodium bicarbonate, and magnesium oxide and hydroxide are relatively safe and effective orally administered protectants. As well as neutralizing gastric acid, they decrease pepsin activity, bind bile acids, stimulate bicarbonate secretion and, possibly, increase endogenous prostaglandin production.

Most available preparations usually contain combinations of aluminium and magnesium hydroxide to maximize the buffering capacity and minimize side effects. Calcium and sodium carbonate have the shortest duration of action, magnesium hydroxide is more prolonged and aluminium hydroxide has the most persistent effect. Aluminium hydroxide is also helpful in the vomiting uraemic patient, as it reduces hyperphosphataemia. Antacids are sometimes combined with local anaesthetic (oxethazine), another protectant (sodium alginate) or an antifoaming agent (activated dimethicone) to enhance their utility in gastro-oesophageal disease. Over-the-counter preparations are readily available.

All antacids can interfere with the absorption of drugs such as digoxin, tetracyclines and fluoroquinolones. They may also alkalinize the urine, increasing the excretion of weak acids such as NSAIDs and phenobarbital. Calcium and sodium carbonate may produce large volumes of gas (CO_2). Calcium-containing antacids tend to promote constipation and predispose to metabolic alkalosis, soft tissue calcification and urolithiasis. Magnesium salts tend to promote diarrhoea through increased intestinal motility, whilst aluminium salts reduce GI motility. They are frequently combined so that these effects counteract each other. Long-term use of aluminium compounds may cause hypophosphataemia and, perhaps, neurotoxicity.

Antacids are not popular choices in veterinary medicine, because oral administration is problematic in a vomiting patient and a high volume must be administered four to six times daily. If not given frequently, reflex increases in gastrin stimulate rebound secretion of acid, when the next dose is due, and gastric pH becomes even lower.

Bismuth salts

Compounds such as bismuth subcarbonate, bismuth subnitrate, tripotassium dicitratobismuthate and bismuth subsalicylate have a cytoprotective effect in the stomach (i.e. they stimulate bicarbonate and prostaglandin production) and are antibacterial against *Helicobacter* spp. They make the colour of faeces darker, which can potentially be mistaken for melaena. They are also used as antidiarrhoeals (see below). Long-term use should be avoided, as absorbed bismuth is neurotoxic.

Sucralfate

Sucralfate is an orally administered complex of sucrose octasulphate and aluminium hydroxide, usually available as tablets and suspension. In some countries, the suspension is not available and the large 1 g tablets can be crushed and suspended in water. Sucralfate has no EU veterinary licence and was unavailable in the UK for several years due to a manufacturing problem of Antepsin®, although it can be imported.

At a simplistic level, sucralfate aids healing of gastro-oesophageal ulcerations by binding to the tissue, forming a barrier against gastric acid penetration. In an acidic gastric environment, the sucrose is freed from the aluminium hydroxide and cross-polymerizes the proteinaceous exudates over ulcerated tissue. Whilst this mechanism is important, it is known that sucralfate also:

- Inactivates pepsin
- Binds refluxed bile acids
- Is cytoprotective through stimulation of endogenous prostaglandin synthesis
- Increases mucosal blood flow
- Binds and concentrates epidermal growth factor, stimulating GI epithelial cell proliferation
- Binds antibiotics, such as tetracyclines, at the ulcer site.

Its safety is well accepted: less than 5% is absorbed and excreted unchanged in urine, and constipation is the only reported side effect. The controversy concerning sucralfate relates to its drug interactions. There is no doubt that the aluminium component blocks the absorption of fluoroquinolones, tetracyclines, theophylline, aminophylline, digoxin, azithromycin and perhaps cimetidine. It is, therefore, recommended that these drugs are administered 2 hours before sucralfate. However, there is a hypothetical argument that not only does co-administration with acid blockers prevent their absorption, but also that their acid blockade may prevent sucralfate precipitation. These arguments appear to have little basis in fact: interaction with ranitidine has been shown to be insignificant (Mullersman *et al.*, 1986), but studies in dogs and cats are lacking. Thus, it is still recommended that these drugs be given 30–60 minutes apart, although which should be given first is rarely made clear! Antibiotics must be given 2 hours before sucralfate, but it seems sensible to give sucralfate both before and after feeding (i.e. on an empty stomach) to coat ulcerated areas, with acid blockers given 30 minutes before food to prevent food-related stimulation of acid secretion. By using an acid blocker, which is recommended to be given once or twice daily (e.g. famotidine, omeprazole), problems of co-administration can more easily be avoided.

Acid blockers (anti-ulcer drugs)

Acid blockade is an important part of healing oesophageal and gastric ulceration. Although effective drugs have been available for over 40 years, recently more potent drugs, potentially needing just once-daily administration, have become available. An increase in intragastric pH to ≥4 is recommended as necessary to heal gastric ulcers in humans, but the cut-off is not established in dogs and cats, which also have a much lower basal acid secretion than humans. Even an increase from pH 1 to pH 3 is a hundred fold decrease in acid concentration.

Reduced acid secretion may enhance the activity of exogenous pancreatic enzyme in exocrine pancreatic insufficiency, but raising the gastric pH can reduce the absorption of metoclopramide, digoxin, itraconazole and ketoconazole, which should, therefore, be given two hours prior. Chronic use may predispose to bacterial overgrowth.

H$_2$-antagonists

The four available H$_2$-antagonists, cimetidine, ranitidine, nizatidine and famotidine, differ in their potency and pharmacokinetics (see below), but no studies have demonstrated enhanced clinical benefit in gastric ulceration, providing equipotent doses are used. However, the only UK veterinary licensed H$_2$-receptor antagonist is cimetidine, and under the prescribing cascade this must be dispensed if oral cimetidine is prescribed; there is no intravenous formulation of Zitac and a human preparation of cimetidine can be given if intravenous administration is required. Nevertheless, a clinical decision can be made to prescribe any of the other H$_2$-antagonists. They are all reversible competitive antagonists and can block histamine-induced gastric acid and pepsin secretion. However, recent studies suggest that they are poor at increasing intragastric pH, they may have a short duration of action, and that tolerance may develop with continued use as they only produce competitive inhibition, which is overcome by increased gastrin and histamine secretion.

Cimetidine

As well as blocking histamine-induced gastric acid secretion, cimetidine may also have immunomodulatory effects by blocking H$_2$-receptors on T-cells. It can be given orally and parenterally, with an oral bioavailability of 70%. However, its plasma half-life is short and its acid blockade

may last less than 6 hours. Thus, it needs to be given at least three times daily. It undergoes hepatic metabolism and is excreted in urine both changed and unchanged. The dose should be reduced by 50% in liver disease or renal insufficiency.

Through its effects on hepatic cytochrome P450 activity, cimetidine has significant drug interactions: it decreases the breakdown of chloramphenicol, metronidazole, lidocaine, procainamide, theophylline, warfarin, propranolol, diazepam and others, and can therefore cause unexpected toxicities. It also decreases sex hormone degradation, and gynaecomastia is a recognized complication in men. Cimetidine reduces hepatic blood flow significantly, which is another good reason not to choose it to treat gastric ulceration in chronic hepatic disease. Ranitidine, nizatidine and famotidine do not have the hepatic side effects, and can be given less frequently, although studies of their efficacy in clinical cases are lacking for dogs and cats.

Ranitidine

Ranitidine has lower oral bioavailability (50%) than cimetidine but is reported to be 5 to 10 times more potent. It has a longer duration of action, needing to be given only two or three times daily. It does not have the hepatic side effects of cimetidine, and has the added bonus of mild prokinetic activity (see earlier). The intravenous preparation should be administered slowly as it may cause cardiac arrhythmias if given rapidly.

Nizatidine

At least 10 times more potent than cimetidine, nizatidine may require only once-daily dosing. Oral nizatidine is almost completely absorbed and then excreted in urine, and is a theoretically better choice in liver disease. It also has a mild prokinetic effect (see earlier).

Famotidine

Famotidine is 20 to 50 times more potent than cimetidine, and, although it is poorly absorbed orally (37% bioavailable), its duration of action may allow only once-daily administration. It is completely excreted in urine. The intravenous preparation provides rapid-onset acid blockade in critical patients, although the dose should be halved if there is renal impairment. It is often preferred in cats because of better palatability, but the efficacy of once-daily administration is debated, and many experts recommend twice-daily administration.

Proton pump inhibitors

Proton pump inhibitors (PPIs) are substituted benzimidazoles that irreversibly bind the proton pump, the final step in acid secretion (i.e. H$^+$K$^+$-ATPase), and so are very potent inhibitors of gastric acid secretion. Their advantages over most H$_2$-antagonists of greater potency and less frequent administration, with only marginally greater cost, means they are being used more frequently, although none are licensed for dogs or cats. They are the drug of choice for severe reflux oesophagitis, severe gastritis and gastric ulcers, and rare conditions such as gastrinomas.

Omeprazole

This was the first PPI to be marketed, and is 30 times more potent than cimetidine. Omeprazole is a weak base and is unstable in an acid environment, so it is formulated as encapsulated enteric-coated granules or a multiple unit pellet system, which dissolve in the more alkaline intestinal pH. The granules must not be crushed. As acid secretion is progressively blocked and gastric pH rises, oral bioavailability increases and so plasma concentrations increase over the first 5 days. Molecules selectively partition into the acidic environment of the gastric parietal cell and, after protonation, irreversibly bind the proton pump. The gradual accumulation in the parietal cell results in a lag phase of up to 5 days before maximal effect, but activity starts within hours and continues after the drug is discontinued. However, recent studies indicate that twice-daily administration may be required for optimal acid suppression, at least initially until maximal acid suppression is achieved. A concern of rebound hyperacidity on withdrawal of omeprazole appears overstated when the gradual decline in accumulated drug is considered.

Omeprazole is probably the only PPI needed in small animal practice, being available in convenient 10 and 20 mg capsules, and as an intravenous preparation. The human drug can be used even though there is a licensed equine omeprazole product, as its formulation is too concentrated to allow accurate dosing in dogs and cats. Diluting the paste in oil has been suggested, but it is preferable to use a quality-controlled product. Omeprazole is inactive at physiological pH and only inhibits ATPase in gastric parietal cells. It does inhibit the P450 elimination of some drugs, such as warfarin and diazepam, but has fewer side effects than cimetidine. There is a risk of interaction with tacrolimus, mycophenolate mofetil, clopidogrel, digoxin and itraconazole. However, because of its potency, it can cause reflex hypergastrinaemia, which has been linked to the induction of carcinoid tumours in rodents. A similar consequence has not been seen in humans, dogs or cats, but gastric acid secretory capacity is increased after treatment. Paradoxically, some patients appear nauseous when given omeprazole and become inappetent.

Second-generation PPIs

Lansoprazole, pantoprazole and rabeprazole appear to have little additional benefit over omeprazole. Pantoprazole was the first PPI to be available for intravenous use, but the data sheet reports it causes pulmonary oedema in dogs at high (7 mg/kg) doses.

Esomeprazole

Omeprazole is a racemic mixture of two isomers, of which only one is active. The active S-isomer, esomeprazole, is available as a pure preparation.

Antidiarrhoeals

Intestinal protectants and adsorbents

Antidiarrhoeal products can contain one or more of a number of compounds including kaolin, aluminium hydroxide, aluminium phosphate, calcium carbonate, pectin, activated charcoal, magnesium trisilicate and hydrated magnesium-aluminium trisilicate (activated attapulgite); even microfine barium sulphate suspensions, used for radiological examination, appear to have an antidiarrhoeal effect. Such products have been used for years to manage acute diarrhoea but their efficacy is unproven, as most cases are naturally self-limiting.

The concept that antidiarrhoeals merely act by coating the mucosa, protecting it from irritation, has been challenged, as most possess both protectant and adsorbent properties.

Their positive actions probably include:

- Binding water and making diarrhoea less fluid
- Direct anti-secretory effect
- Binding toxins and pathogenic bacteria.

They are all likely to interfere with the absorption of other orally administered drugs.

Kaolin and pectin

Kaolin is aluminium silicate, whilst pectins are natural polygalacturonic acids extracted from fruit pith, and their combination suspended in 20 parts of water is a demulcent and adsorbent. Their efficacy for treating diarrhoea in small animals is unproven, but their safety and use have withstood the test of time. They are sometimes combined with antibacterials and/or anticholinergics and/or morphine, but such polypharmacy may be inappropriate, and therefore a kaolin with morphine preparation is not available in the UK. Montmorillonite is a trilaminar smectite clay with superior adsorbent properties to regular kaolin, and is marketed in combination with simple sugars and electrolytes (Diarsanyl™).

Activated charcoal

Activated charcoal is an adsorbent that is primarily used for treating intoxications. It possesses more pores and increased binding capacity compared with charcoal. Its efficacy in treating diarrhoea and odoriferous flatulence is unproven.

Bismuth

As well as their use in treating gastric disease (see above), insoluble bismuth salts (bismuth subcarbonate, bismuth subnitrate and bismuth subsalicylate) may be beneficial in acute diarrhoea. The subsalicylate-containing preparation can be useful in acute inflammation, but such compounds should be used cautiously in cats, as nearly all the salicylate is systemically available.

Colestyramine (cholestyramine)

This is a basic anion exchange resin that binds bile acids that may be stimulating intestinal secretion, and thus can reduce diarrhoea associated with increased intraluminal concentrations of primary bile acids in patients with dysbiosis or ileal resection. It should be administered with food or water. Nausea and constipation are possible side effects.

Motility modifiers

Modification of intestinal motility can be a useful symptomatic treatment for acute diarrhoea. Motility is often inextricably linked with GI secretion, and many of these motility modifiers are also antisecretory. Thus, as well as delaying transit time, relieving abdominal pain and tenesmus, and reducing the frequency of defecation, they may also decrease the volume of diarrhoea. However, they are rarely essential, as most acute diarrhoea is self-limiting, and slowing intestinal transit may actually be deleterious if toxin-producing bacteria are retained rather than being purged.

Anticholinergics

Antimuscarinics are not recommended in the management of diarrhoea in small animals, although they are frequently included in combination products. As most diarrhoea is associated with intestinal hypomotility they are likely to worsen ileus, especially if concurrent hypokalaemia is present. And as they inhibit only gastric and not intestinal secretion and preferentially decrease segmental intestinal contractions, any propulsive peristalsis is unimpeded and diarrhoea will occur. They may also have undesirable systemic effects (see antiemetics).

Agents used include atropine, homatropine, butyl-scopolamine (hyoscine), aminopentamide, dicyclomine, glycopyrrolate, propantheline and clidinium. They may be justified in the short term for the relief of tenesmus and pain in acute colitis. Butylscopolamine is commonly combined with metamizole (dipyrone), and a combination of clidinium bromide and a benzodiazepine (chlordiazepoxide) has been recommended for treating irritable bowel syndrome, although it is not available in the UK. Anticholinergics are not recommended in cats.

Opioids

The ability of opiates to cause constipation is well known, and opioids are effective antidiarrhoeals. They increase segmental intestinal contractions, delay transit and have an antisecretory effect. They are indicated for temporary, non-specific relief of acute diarrhoea, and may be of benefit in faecal incontinence. Paregoric (tincture of opium) is used occasionally, but kaolin with morphine is no longer available in the UK.

Diphenoxylate: As well as its motility-modifying effect, this opioid also increases fluid and water absorption and inhibits the activity of secretagogues such as *Escherichia coli* enterotoxin. Diphenoxylate is a pethidine (meperidine) derivative marketed in combination with atropine to discourage substance abuse, but at therapeutic doses the atropine has no clinical effect. It is currently unavailable in the UK.

Loperamide: Loperamide is available, and has a similar mechanism of action to diphenoxylate. It is relatively safe, as it does not normally cross the normal blood–brain barrier. It can cross into the brain in dogs with the *MDR-1* (ABCB1 transporter) mutation and cause sedation. Its use in at-risk breeds, such as collies, is best avoided.

Antispasmodics

Painful intestinal spasm in acute GI disease can be relieved by antimuscarinic agents. Butylscopolamine is used symptomatically (see above). Repeated intestinal spasm (irritable bowel syndrome) is better treated with dietary modification and perhaps anxiolytics. Mebeverine (an antispasmodic derived from peppermint oil) and its natural oil source are used in humans to treat irritable bowel syndrome, but their efficacy in dogs is untested.

Laxatives and cathartics

Both laxatives and cathartics (Figure 28.1) promote defecation by increasing the frequency, fluidity and volume of the faeces, and are used to treat constipation and aid the elimination of toxins. Laxatives (aperients) promote

Simple bulk laxatives
- Bran (wheat husk)
- Prunes
- Psyllium seeds, psyllium/ispaghula (*Plantago*, plantain)
- Sterculia (Mallow)
- Methylcellulose
- Carboxymethylcellulose sodium

Emollient laxatives
- Paraffin paste
- Liquid paraffin (mineral oil)
- Docusate sodium (dioctyl sodium sulphosuccinate, DSS)
- Poloxamer (in combination with dantron: codanthromer)

Osmotic laxatives
- Mannitol
- Lactulose
- Magnesium salts
  - Magnesium citrate
  - Magnesium hydroxide
  - Magnesium oxide (milk of magnesia)
  - Magnesium sulphate (Epsom salts)
- Sodium salts
  - Sodium sulphate (Glauber's salt)
  - Sodium picosulphate
  - Sodium phosphate, sodium acid phosphate
  - Sodium chloride
  - Sodium citrate
  - Sodium potassium tartrate (Rochelle's salt)
  - Sodium lauryl sulphate
- Polyethylene glycol

Irritant cathartics
- Aloe
- Senna
- Cascara
- Arachis oil
- Glycerol
- Bisacodyl
- Olive oil
- Linseed oil
- Castor oil
- Dantron (in combination with poloxamer: codanthromer)

Enemas
- Warm water
- Warm soapy water
- Saline (isotonic and hypertonic)
- Sorbitol
- Glycerol
- Sodium lauryl sulphate
- Olive oil
- Lactulose
- Polyethylene glycol
- Bisacodyl
- Phosphate (NOT in cats)

28.1 Laxatives, cathartics and enemas available for treating dogs and cats.

elimination of faeces by increasing the hydration and, consequently, the softness of the faecal mass. Increase in faecal bulk may also stimulate intestinal peristalsis. In contrast, cathartics (purgatives) alter intestinal electrolyte transport, thereby increasing faecal water, and/or stimulate, local myenteric reflexes, and tend to produce a more violent and more fluid bowel evacuation. Excessive or constant use of cathartics can be deleterious, with continual diarrhoea, dehydration and electrolyte disturbances, with the potential to develop megacolon.

Bulk laxatives

These simple substances (e.g. bran, ispaghula, sterculia and methylcellulose) are hydrophilic in nature and are not digested. They absorb water and swell: the resultant increase in bulk stimulates reflex peristalsis and defecation. Some fibres are fermentable and the resultant volatile fatty acids exert an osmotic laxative effect as well. However, if excess fibre is given, diarrhoea, flatulence and bloating may occur.

Emollient laxatives

These are lubricants that pass unchanged and act as faecal softeners. They are mild but not reliably effective.

Paraffin

Paraffin is available as a paste or as liquid paraffin (mineral oil). The paste is used as a mild treatment for hairballs and constipation in cats. If it is smeared on the cat's nose or feet, it will be licked off and ingested. Liquid paraffin is tasteless, and if given orally by syringe there is a significant danger of inhalation and lipoid pneumonia. Its use is no longer recommended.

Docusate sodium

Previously called dioctyl sodium sulphosuccinate, docusate is an anionic surfactant and detergent that acts as a faecal softener. It is sometimes combined with dantron (co-danthramer), an irritant cathartic.

Poloxamers

These are non-ionic co-polymers of a central hydrophobic polypropylene oxide chain flanked by two hydrophilic polyethylene oxide chains that can have surfactant properties, softening faeces and easing its passage. They are often combined with cathartics such as dantron.

Osmotic laxatives and cathartics

These work by drawing water into the faeces, making it softer and encouraging expulsive movement. Sugar alcohols, such as mannitol and sorbitol, found both naturally in food and added as sugar-free sweeteners, have this effect, but are rarely used intentionally as laxatives.

Lactulose

Lactulose is an indigestible synthetic disaccharide that is fermented in the large intestine to acetate and lactate, with consequent osmotic laxative effect. In hepatoencephalopathy, it helps by eliminating fermenting material and acidifying the colon to prevent ammonia absorption. It is a relatively gentle, physiological laxative, but a patient's response is variable and the dose must be titrated to the individual to produce two to three soft bowel movements per day without diarrhoea.

Saline purgatives

Magnesium and sodium salts that are not (or incompletely) absorbed are osmotic laxatives, and even large volumes of saline are an effective purgative. Solutions containing magnesium ions (e.g. magnesium citrate) may also stimulate peristalsis directly as a cathartic. Although they are small in volume to administer, they frequently cause vomiting, abdominal discomfort and dehydration, and sometimes cause hypermagnesaemia. It is imperative that the patient has water to drink after their administration, and they should never be given to a dehydrated patient or to cats.

Colonic cleansers

Oral lavage solutions are the preferred preparation for colonoscopy, and can also be used as laxatives. They are iso-osmotic solutions of polyethylene glycol and electrolytes that produce osmotic diarrhoea to wash out gut contents. A number of products are available. The patient is given two to four doses of 25–30 ml/kg, each at least 2 hours apart, and ideally the last dose is given 12 hours before colonoscopy. As large volumes must be given, a stomach tube is used for administration to dogs. In cats the solution can be administered via a naso-oesophageal tube, as a slow infusion of 20 ml/kg/h for 4 hours. Particular care should be taken in patients with dysphagia or delayed gastric emptying.

Irritant cathartics

Contact or irritant cathartics stimulate the local myenteric plexus and intestinal secretion to provoke fluid accumulation and expulsion. Natural irritant compounds include aloe, senna and cascara. Glycerol and bisacodyl have the mildest action, whilst a combination of sodium picosulphate and magnesium oxide is powerful.

Vegetable oils

These are hydrolysed by pancreatic lipase to irritant fatty acids: castor oil to highly irritant ricinoleates, linseed oil to less irritant linoleates, and olive oil to mild oliveates.

Dantron (danthron)

This is a synthetic anthroquinone derivative that is a stimulant. It is often combined with a faecal softener (e.g. poloxamer, docusate).

Enemas
Warm water

Repeated warm water enemas are cheap and do not cause histological artefacts if used in preparation for colonscopic biopsy, but the method is unpleasant and the quality of colonic cleansing is poor. In medium-sized dogs, at least 1 litre of warm water should be used for each enema; the volume is doubled for patients weighing more than 30 kg. The enema tube is well lubricated and gently inserted to the level of the last rib. Warm water is instilled either by gravity from an enema bucket, or gently by a Higginson pump. During instillation the tube is moved back and forth to loosen the faeces. Liquid may escape from the anus during the procedure when the colon is full: more fluid should not be forced in, especially if the patient vomits. Enemas are repeated until the liquid runs clear and contains no particulate matter. In normal-sized cats, about 20 ml/kg of warm water is given as an enema through a soft, flexible urinary catheter attached to a large syringe. Instillation should be gradual or vomiting will occur. Oral lavage (see above) is more suitable, especially if there is anorectal pain, and can be followed by a single enema before colonoscopy.

Irritant laxative enemas

Enemas containing substances such as soap, bisacodyl and phosphate should never be used before colonoscopy as they may cause artefactual inflammatory changes in mucosal biopsies. They are used to stimulate colonic evacuation for other purposes such as radiographs. Phosphate enemas can cause fatal hyperphosphataemia in cats and small dogs.

Immunosuppressive/ anti-inflammatory agents

Non-steroidal anti-inflammatory drugs

Some beneficial effects of NSAIDs may be noted in GI inflammation, and the efficacy of bismuth subsalicylate and sulfasalazine is recognized in acute inflammatory intestinal disease. However, the deleterious effects of NSAIDs on the GI tract and kidneys, particularly in dehydrated patients, predominate and, in general, NSAIDs should **not** be used in GI disease.

5-aminosalicyclic acid and its derivatives

Sulfasalazine: This is a pro-drug: a diazo bond binding sulfapyridine to 5-aminosalicyclic acid (5-ASA) is cleaved by colonic bacteria to release free 5-ASA, which acts locally in high concentrations in the colon as an anti-inflammatory. It is used to treat colitis. Hepatoxicity can occur, but the major side effect is keratoconjunctivitis sicca (KCS), and regular Schirmer tear tests should be performed. KCS is believed to be a complication of the sulfa moiety, although it has been seen with olsalazine, which contains no sulphonamide (see below).

Olsalazine: This is two 5-ASA molecules joined by a diazo bond and which again are released by colonic bacteria. It was developed in an attempt to reduce the frequency of KCS, which was considered to be attributable to the sulfapyridine in sulfasalazine. It has been used successfully in dogs, although occasional KCS has still been reported. The dose is one-half the dose of sulfasalazine, as it contains twice the amount of active ingredient.

Balsalazide: A newer pro-drug, balsalazide (4-amino-benzoyl-β-alanine-mesalamine), is activated to 5-ASA by the same mechanism as sulfsalazine, but its safety and efficacy have not been evaluated in small animals.

Mesalazine: Native 5-ASA is termed mesalazine, and slow-release enteric formulations are available for humans. Premature release in the small intestine is likely to cause absorption and nephrotoxicity, but at human intestinal pH the majority of the 5-ASA is released in the colon. The safety of oral formulations in dogs and cats is unclear. Mesalazine enemas and suppositories, available for humans, would be safe but impracticable.

Corticosteroids

Prednisolone

Prednisolone and methylprednisolone are the first choice immunosuppressive agents in dogs and cats. Dexamethasone has similar immunosuppressive effects in equipotent doses. However, it has deleterious effects on brush border enzyme activity in some laboratory species, compared with prednisolone, which increases brush border enzyme and transport protein expression. It is, therefore, not the first choice unless a depot preparation is needed because the patient cannot be dosed daily. An initial dose of 2–4 mg/kg/day of prednisolone is used and then tapered; whether the higher dose confers greater efficacy is unproven. Its mechanism of action is via blockade of a nuclear transcription pathway, NF-κB (nuclear factor kappa-light-chain-enhancer of activated B cells), which is involved in the transcription of pro-inflammatory cytokines such as tumour necrosis factor alpha. The aim of therapy is always to find the minimum effective dose, which hopefully is either zero or at least low-dose administration every other day. The cushingoid side effects of prednisolone are well known, and so if the minimum effective dose still causes significant side effects, adjunctive agents should be introduced for their steroid-sparing effect.

Budesonide

An enteric-coated version of this novel steroid is available. Budesonide is largely metabolized by first pass through the liver and thus the systemic side effects are minimized. However, steroid hepatopathy has been noted in dogs, and there is certainly some depression of the adrenal axis. There are anecdotal reports of budesonide's efficacy in canine and feline chronic enteropathy, but some studies used the non-enteric-coated formulation from asthma inhalers, and in others the required dose was very variable. It is no more effective than prednisolone and is usually reserved for those patients in which steroid side effects are problematic.

Others

Azathioprine

In humans, this immunosuppressive agent is not effective unless the patient is already on steroids, takes 2–4 weeks to be fully effective, and its premature withdrawal may result in relapse. Thus, its major use is not as a first-line agent, but as a steroid-sparing drug.

Bone marrow toxicity (neutropenia, anaemia) is uncommon in dogs, but it will occur within weeks in some individuals. They probably lack thiopurine methyl transferase (TPMT), the enzyme necessary to degrade 6-mercaptopurine, azathioprine's active metabolite. TPMT activity is naturally low in cats, explaining why the recommended dose in cats is so much lower than in dogs. As the smallest formulation available in the UK is 25 mg, and splitting of this coated cytotoxic agent is prohibited, azathioprine is not a good choice for cats. In some countries reformulation is available, but there are still health concerns about the excretion of this cytotoxic drug in the home.

Chlorambucil

In cats, chlorambucil is a much safer immunosuppressive drug than azathioprine if prednisolone alone is not effective. One study has also demonstrated efficacy in canine chronic enteropathy with protein-losing enteropathy (Dandrieux *et al.*, 2013).

Ciclosporin

Ciclosporin A (CsA) is a potent immunosuppressive drug for human transplantation and selective (auto)immune diseases. In veterinary gastroenterology, CsA has been used as a sole agent to treat anal furunculosis. Its activity can be potentiated by co-administration with ketoconazole, which inhibits its hepatic metabolism.

In early studies CsA's efficacy in chronic inflammatory enteropathies was variable, but it is a suitable choice if prednisolone causes excessive side effects or is not effective. It may also be effective in lymphangiectasia. CsA can be nephrotoxic, and monitoring of trough serum concentrations is usually recommended. However, as it undergoes enterohepatic recycling, serum concentrations cannot be used to predict the effective concentration in the GI tract.

Mycophenolate mofetil

This is an immunomodulator used to prevent transplant rejection, being an antimetabolite inhibiting purine synthesis in lymphocytes. It has been reported to have successfully treated myasthenia gravis (MG), including focal MG of the oesophagus. However, its use is not widespread, and spontaneous improvement may give a false impression of efficacy.

Tacrolimus

Tacrolimus is a macrolide antibiotic produced by *Streptomyces* that inhibits T-cell activation and is used to stop transplant rejection. In dogs, it is more toxic than ciclosporin, but has been used topically to treat anal furunculosis.

Appetite stimulants

Glucocorticoids used to treat chronic inflammatory enteropathies may increase the patient's appetite as well as having an immunosuppressive effect on the intestinal immune system. This is an added benefit in those patient's with hyporexia that is not seen with other immunosuppressive agents. Treatment with acid blockers, anti-emetics, prokinetics and analgesics may improve appetite by reducing nausea and pain. Supplementation of cobalamin can improve appetite in patients that are hypocobalaminaemic, although it is not an appetite stimulant *per se*.

As enteral nutrition is considered the optimal route by which to provide nutrition even when the GI tract is diseased, some drugs are administered specifically just to increase voluntary food intake. However, feeding tubes should be considered if the amount eaten remains inadequate as the efficacy of various appetite stimulants is variable and also depends on the disease and its severity.

Diazepam

Low doses of diazepam can trigger cats (and some dogs) to start eating. However, they often become drowsy and fail to consume the desired caloric quantity. The small amount they do eat may be enough to observe what type of dysphagia they may be suffering, and even allow fluoroscopic evaluation of one or two swallows. However, diazepam can also cause idiosyncratic hepatic failure in cats and so cannot be recommended.

Cyproheptadine

Cyproheptadine (Periactin™) is a first-generation antihistamine with additional anticholinergic, antiserotonergic, and local anaesthetic properties that has a side-effect of increasing appetite in cats. There is only weak evidence for its efficacy in children and none in cats, and its use has fallen out of favour.

Mirtazapine

Mirtazapine (Zispin) is a tricyclic antidepressant used in humans acting on central alpha-2 receptors and also inhibiting several types of serotonin and histamine (H_1) receptors, one of the side effects of mirtazapine is increased appetite and weight gain. It has also been found to stimulate appetite in cats and dogs when used at low doses and has been shown to be effective in cats with stable chronic kidney disease. It can be used in GI diseases causing anorexia, but side effects may be marked, especially if the dose is increased (Ferguson *et al.*, 2016). Sedation is common and can be profound, and behaviour may be altered, with increased vocalisation and interaction with others.

Capromorelin

Capromorelin (Entyce®) is an agonist for receptors in the hypothalamus normally stimulated by the hormone ghrelin to increase appetite. It is the most physiological of the appetite stimulants with minimal side effects (Rhodes *et al.*, 2018). It is currently is only licensed in the USA for treating dogs, although can be used off-label in cats.

References and further reading

Dandrieux JRS, Noble P-J, Scase T, Cripps PJ and German AJ (2013) Comparison of chlorambucil-prednisolone combination with azathioprine-prednisolone combination for treatment of chronic enteropathy with concurrent protein-losing enteropathy in dogs: 27 cases (2007–2010). *Journal of the American Veterinary Medical Association* **242**, 1705–1714

Ferguson LE, McLean MK, Bates JA and Quimby JM (2016) Mirtazapine toxicity in cats: retrospective study of 84 cases (2006–2011). *Journal of Feline Medicine and Surgery* **18**, 868–874

Mullersman G, Gotz VP, Russell WL and Derendorth (1986) Lack of clinically significant in vitro and in vivo interactions between ranitidine and sucralfate. *Journal of Pharmaceutical Sciences* **75**, 995–998

Narishetty ST, Galvan B, Coscarelli E *et al.* (2009) Effect of refrigeration of the antiemetic Cerenia (maropitant) on pain on injection. *Veterinary Therapeutics* **10**, 93–102

Potter TG and Snider KR (2013) Azithromycin for the treatment of gastroparesis. *Annals of Pharmacotherapy* **47**, 411–415

Ramsey IR (2017) *BSAVA Small Animal Formulary, 9th edn.* BSAVA Publications, Gloucester

Rhodes L, Zollers B, Wofford J and Heinen E. (2018) Capromorelin: a ghrelin receptor agonist and novel therapy for stimulation of appetite in dogs. *Veterinary Medicine and Science* **4**, 3–16

Chapter 29

Antibacterials

Ian A. Battersby

Antibacterials are prescribed due to their effects on bacteria, either killing them or preventing them from growing, reproducing or spreading. Most importantly, this assists the patient's immune system in controlling an active infection. In chronic gastrointestinal disease, antibacterials may also be prescribed for their effects on the microbiome.

Increasing resistance to antibacterials is well documented and recognized across the health professions (human and veterinary), and with the lack of new classes of antibiotics being readily available this is understandably a concern for all patients. So, regularly reviewing the principles of antibiotic usage is prudent and, whenever possible, their use should be avoided.

Antibiotic resistance

Impact of antibiotic prescribing on the development of resistance

Mutations which cause antibiotic resistance genes do not require the presence of antibiotics for their generation. The introduction of an antibacterial will result in preferential selection of the bacterial strain that bears an advantageous genotype, and the longer the exposure to the antibacterial the more rigorous the selection process. Therefore, the presumption that long courses of antibiotics prevent resistance is incorrect; prolonged courses eliminate the sensitive bacteria and exert a positive selection pressure, favouring resistant strains. Furthermore, since plasmids may encode resistance to several antibiotic classes, the use of one antibiotic may result in selection for strains with resistance to multiple antibiotic classes.

Observations have also shown that in the presence of sub-therapeutic levels of antibacterial agents, bacteria can become hypermutable. This transient state adds a further twist to the selection pressure exerted by antibiotics, and may explain why multiple mutations have emerged more rapidly than predicted (Livermore, 2003).

Ways in which prescribing can help reduce the prevalence of antibiotic resistance

- Reviewing one's own prescribing: 'Are antibiotics really indicated or am I prescribing them just in case?'.
- Choosing the right drug for the target bacteria based on its spectrum of activity (preferably a narrow spectrum) and its pharmacokinetics.

- Treating for long enough, but not too long. In human medicine, a large number of studies are being undertaken to determine the shortest duration of course required. In veterinary medicine, these studies are currently lacking.
- Reserving specific classes of antibiotics as second- or even third-line choices.
- Developing a practice policy for empirical antibiotic use – these schemes are beneficial in optimizing patient outcome and reducing unnecessary prescribing. Practice policy schemes have been developed by a variety of organizations (e.g. the BSAVA/Small Animal Medicine Society (SAMSoc) PROTECT ME scheme is available to download free of charge).

Gastrointestinal conditions in which antibiotics are not indicated

Figure 29.1 details the gastrointestinal conditions for which antibiotics are not indicated.

Antibiotic requirements	Gastrointestinal condition
Not indicated	• Acute vomiting • Acute diarrhoea (including acute haemorrhagic cases) in patients that are systemically well • Pancreatitis • Most gastric *Helicobacter* infections • Most *Campylobacter* infections • Most *Salmonella* infections • Most *Clostridium perfringens* or *Clostridium difficile* infections • Chronic diarrhoea (except as part of a treatment trial; see below)
May be indicated on an individual case basis	• *Helicobacter* infections • *Campylobacter, Salmonella, C. perfringens* or *C. difficile* infections in a small number of situations • Hepatic encephalopathy (if dietary modification and lactulose are insufficient to control signs)
Indicated	• Bacterial cholangitis • Acute diarrhoea with signs of systemic involvement (i.e. sepsis, immunosuppression). Note: systemic signs due to hypovolaemia/dehydration are not indications for antibiotics • Chronic diarrhoea, as part of a treatment trial when other differential diagnoses have been excluded, i.e. following a diet trial and in some cases after an immunosuppression trial • Granulomatous (histiocytic ulcerative) colitis, only after confirmation by biopsy and culture

29.1 Overview of the gastrointestinal conditions in which antibiotics are and are not indicated.

Acute vomiting

Each vomiting patient will have its individual presentation, some requiring more interventions than others. In the majority of systemically well patients the cause is non-bacterial and, in those cases, the vomiting is frequently self-limiting. As a consequence, and similar to the situation in humans, antibiotics are not indicated.

Pancreatitis

Acute/chronic pancreatitis in the dog and cat is typically a sterile inflammatory process. Pancreatic abscessation is rarely reported in the literature; as such, antibiotics are not indicated in patients that are systemically stable. In systemically unwell patients with prolonged anorexia due to necrotizing pancreatitis, bacterial translocation may occur. Antibiotics may be prescribed in severely debilitated patients if the combination of clinical and haematological signs suggests systemic involvement (systemic inflammatory response syndrome), but alongside other measures to manage hypovolaemia and blood pressure. However, in the author's experience this situation is very rare.

Systemically well with acute diarrhoea (including haemorrhagic diarrhoea)

Acute diarrhoea is a frequent presentation and may be a complication of treatment for other diseases. It is not uncommon for veterinary surgeons (veterinarians) to prescribe antimicrobials for patients with acute diarrhoea, but this may not always be necessary or appropriate. A study published in 2010 (German et al., 2010) demonstrated that 71% of patients were prescribed antimicrobials at the first consultation and that this prescribing practice did not always follow current guidelines.

In a more recent surveillance study in 2018 by SAVSNET indicated that this has since fallen to 37% (Singleton et al., 2019). Yet there are comparisons between the prescribing decisions for the treatment of diarrhoea in small animals and in humans. In both instances the causes of acute diarrhoea are many and include a number of non-bacterial aetiologies, meaning that antibiotics will have a limited effect. Most infectious causes of diarrhoea (viral, bacterial or protozoal) are self-limiting and therefore do not require therapy with antimicrobials. Antibiotics are indicated for only a small number of specific infections and are therefore not prescribed routinely in humans; as such, recommendations are similar for dogs and cats (see Enteropathogens below).

The presence of blood in the faeces (indicating breakdown of the mucosal barrier) can be a prompt indication to prescribe antimicrobials. A combination of penicillins and metronidazole (and even fluoroquinolones) to provide four quadrant cover have been used historically. Yet, recent study of dogs with haemorrhagic diarrhoea treated in first-opinion practice (Ortiz et al., 2018) demonstrated no difference in outcome when the dogs were treated with co-amoxiclav alone or in combination with metronidazole. A prospective, blinded, randomized study of 60 dogs with idiopathic haemorrhagic gastroenteritis without clinical or laboratory evidence of sepsis demonstrated no difference between dogs treated with co-amoxiclav and those that were not (Unterer et al., 2011). This study suggests that antibiotics may not always be necessary in dogs with haemorrhagic diarrhoea if signs of sepsis are absent.

Gastrointestinal conditions in which antibiotics may be indicated

This section outlines conditions in which antibiotics may be indicated based on the individual presentation (see Figure 29.1). In the author's experience the need to prescribe antibacterials in these conditions is very infrequent. For further information on these topics see Chapter 27.

Enteropathogens

The bacterial agents listed in Figure 29.2 are potential pathogens in dogs and cats but can also be isolated from healthy animals. Therefore, interpretation of faecal culture, immunoassay and polymerase chain reaction detection of the organisms or their enterotoxins is problematic. This raises the difficult question of when antimicrobials should be prescribed following a positive culture result, particularly taking into consideration the fact that such infections are often self-limiting with supportive care (as outlined in human medicine). The reader is directed to Chapters 34 and 35 and the American College of Veterinary Internal Medicine (ACVIM) consensus statement on enteropathogens (Marks et al., 2011) to assist with decision-making.

The author may perform faecal cultures when:

- The diarrhoea involves more than one in-contact animal
- There is an association with sepsis
- The pet is immunosuppressed
- The pet is consuming a raw food diet
- The pet is in close contact with immunocompromised human beings.

Organism	Antibacterial therapy (Reserved for septic, bacteraemic or immunocompromised patients)
Campylobacter	• Erythromycin • Fluoroquinolone
Clostridium difficile	• Metronidazole
Clostridium perfringens	• Metronidazole • Ampicillin • Erythromycin
Escherichia coli	• Co-amoxiclav • Trimethoprim/sulphonamide • Fluoroquinolone
Salmonella	• Ampicillin • Fluoroquinolone

29.2 Enteropathogens that can be isolated from the faeces of dogs and cats with gastrointestinal disease. However, it should be noted that these pathogens can also be isolated from the faeces of healthy animals.

Helicobacter

The pathogenicity of Helicobacter species in humans, ferrets and mice is accepted but seems unlikely in dogs and cats since, despite investigation, similar evidence has not been forthcoming. So, when finding the organisms in biopsy samples, it is often unclear whether they should be treated. This is further confounded by studies demonstrating that dogs treated for Helicobacter appear to be recolonized despite no recurrence of clinical signs. Even when seeming to be effective, the treatment may be helping with co-existing disease. The reader is directed to Chapter 33 for a detailed discussion and a summary of treatment protocols.

Hepatic encephalopathy

Hepatic encephalopathy can occur with congenital hepatic vascular abnormalities (e.g. portosystemic shunts) or due to advanced acquired liver disease (see Chapter 37). Treatment strategies focus on the reduction of blood toxin levels, in particular ammonia. Current evidence suggests that glutamine metabolism by the enterocytes is a significant contributor to blood ammonia concentrations (Rama Rao, 2014), in addition to food breakdown and production by enteric bacteria (see Chapter 37). In the author's experience, the majority of patients can be managed with small frequent meals to reduce spikes of glutamine metabolism and reduced protein load (with or without a commercial therapeutic hepatic diet) and lactulose. Antimicrobials (metronidazole or amoxicillin) can be used to reduce ammonia-producing bacteria in the colon. However, in a number of cases antimicrobials are not required.

Conditions in which antibiotics are indicated

The conditions for which antibiotics are indicated are detailed in Figure 29.1.

Acute diarrhoea with systemic signs indicating actual (or risk of) bacteraemia or sepsis

The time to consider antimicrobial usage in acute diarrhoea is when the patient is systemically unwell (note: not due to dehydration and/or hypovolaemia) or immunosuppressed (e.g. parvovirus infection, chemotherapy-induced diarrhoea). Frequently listed markers that could suggest systemic involvement of a bacterial infection include fever, neutropenia or neutrophilia. However, it should be noted that these changes are not specific for a bacterial infection – for example viraemia could also cause a fever and does not justify the prescription of antibacterials.

Bacterial translocation is also a consideration when electing to prescribe antimicrobials in cases of acute diarrhoea. Interestingly, studies have demonstrated that approximately 50% of healthy dogs undergoing hysterectomy had positive cultures from mesenteric lymph node samples. This figure could be even higher given the limitations of current culture methodologies. Bacterial translocation to the mesenteric lymph node is therefore likely to represent part of the intestine's normal immunosurveillance. However, rather than the bacteria entering the lymphatic or systemic circulation, it may instead be the bacterial toxins or cytokines that cause the systemic inflammatory response. As the mesenteric lymph nodes drain into the thoracic duct, these products can bypass the Kupffer cells and, as a consequence, result in a more virulent systemic inflammatory response. Bacterial translocation (and subsequent septicaemia) can manifest as a variety of clinical signs, including melaena, ileus, arrhythmias, hypotension, hypothermia, tachycardia and bradycardia. These signs understandably warrant aggressive management and, in these patients, antimicrobial treatment is essential.

Chronic enteropathy – following other treatment failure

Dietary manipulation (hydrolysed or novel protein source diets) can alleviate signs in 60–80% of chronic enteropathy patients. Antibiotic-responsive diarrhoea (a form of SI dysbiosis) has been described in young large-breed dogs (especially German Shepherd Dogs) and these cases warrant empirical antibacterial treatment (metronidazole, oxytetracycline or tylosin). The role of the antibacterial in these cases is not clear; however, a change in the bacterial population of the gastrointestinal tract (the microbiome) would seem logical. Nowadays, this may be most easily accomplished by dietary change.

An antibacterial therapeutic trial may also be considered in other breeds with chronic enteropathy, although most clinicians now advocate prior dietary trials with one or more of the numerous and diverse therapeutic diets available, and also perhaps a trial with glucocorticoid treatment or other immunosuppressants.

Alternatives to antibiotic trials include probiotics and faecal microbiota transplantation (FMT) (see Chapter 27). There are a variety of probiotic products available for which initial clinical trials have been performed, with varied impacts of clinical outcome. At the time of writing, there are no published studies reporting the outcomes in canine and feline patients with chronic enteropathy treated with FMT. However, there are anecdotal reports and case series presented in abstract form showing a positive response. The author has seen a variable response to FMT in chronic enteropathies in dogs and cats, and, in general, anecdotal reports support transient clinical improvements at best in most cases (see Chapter 27). This likely reflects a lack of understanding of which microbiome is optimal for which recipient and which cases of chronic enteropathy may benefit from FMT. In humans, the National Institute for Health and Care Excellence (NICE) guidelines now include the use of FMT in the treatment of *Clostridium difficile* colitis (NICE, 2009), but a similar enteropathy has not been reported in dogs or cats.

Granulomatous (histiocytic ulcerative) colitis

Granulomatous (histiocytic ulcerative) colitis is a condition typically associated with young Boxers; however, there have been cases reported in other breeds, such as the French Bulldog. Clinical signs do not respond to immunosuppression; however, studies have identified an association between adherent and invasive *Escherichia coli* and the resolution of clinical signs with 6 weeks of antibiotic treatment (Mansfield, *et al.* 2009). This is a relatively rare condition in the UK, and treatment with antibiotics should only commence following biopsy confirmation and culture and sensitivity testing in order to tailor the antibiotic treatment. Initial cases were treated successfully with enrofloxacin; however, there are increasing anecdotal reports of disease caused by fluoroquinolone-resistant *E. coli*.

Cholangitis/cholangiohepatitis

Common hepatobiliary bacterial isolates from dogs with cholecystitis include *E. coli*, *Enterococcus* spp. and *Clostridium* spp. Resistance to cefalexin and co-amoxiclav has been reported (Tamborini, *et al.* 2016). *E. coli* is the most common organism cultured from the bile of cats.

Obtaining a sample for culture by cholecystocentesis is optimal but should be attempted by an experienced ultrasonographer. Bile peritonitis is a serious life-threatening sequela of this technique; empirical therapy should reflect anticipated pathogens and their potential resistance profile. Treatment options include co-amoxiclav, ampicillin or cefalexin in dogs; metronidazole can also be added to the regimen for dogs if needed.

List of antibacterials for treatment of gastrointestinal disease

For up-to-date dosage recommendations, please refer to the *BSAVA Small Animal Formulary*.

Tetracyclines
- Tetracycline
- Oxytetracycline
- Doxycycline
- Minocycline

The tetracyclines are a group of drugs with a broad spectrum of activity against both Gram-positive and Gram-negative bacteria in addition to *Chlamydia*, *Rickettsia*, *Mycoplasma* and some forms of protozoa. They may also have an anti-inflammatory effect. Oral absorption can be unpredictable but is a sufficient route for treatment in animals. Co-administration with calcium and other divert cations can chelate the drug (less of an issue with doxycycline).

Side effects
Diarrhoea, risk of oesophagitis/stricture in cats, if not followed with food or water.

Macrolides
- Tylosin
- Erythromycin

Tylosin
The activity of this drug is better for Gram-positive than Gram-negative bacteria. Gram-positive bacteria accumulate this class of drug almost 100 times more effectively than Gram-negative bacteria. As a consequence, activity can be poor against Gram-negative bacterial groups such as the Enterobacteriaceae. When prescribing in cases of tylosin-responsive diarrhoea, the target microbes are not known, but an increase in faeces of potentially probiotic Enterococci are found.

Side effects: Anorexia and diarrhoea are rarely reported.

Erythromycin
This drug has more activity against Gram-positive than Gram-negative bacteria. Oral absorption in dogs and cats is poor and inconsistent. Stimulation of gastric motility occurs due to the activation of motilin receptors via release of endogenous motilin or cholinergic stimulation of the upper gastrointestinal tract. As a consequence, this drug may be used in cases of gastric atony.

Side effects: Diarrhoea is common.

Nitroimidazoles
- Metronidazole

This is the most commonly prescribed drug of the group for antibacterial effects. Metronidazole has very little activity against aerobes; it is very effective against anaerobic organisms, but not facultative anaerobes. Following uptake into the bacteria, metronidazole is metabolized into cytotoxic compounds.

Side effects
Neurological signs caused by the inhibition of the neurotransmitter gamma-aminobutyric acid. This side effect is most commonly seen in dogs but has been reported in cats and is dose-dependent (>50 mg/kg per day for >7 days – although there are anecdotal reports at lower dosages). Recovery is possible following withdrawal of the drug but can take 7–10 days.

Aminopenicillins
- Amoxicillin
- Ampicillin

Amoxicillin and ampicillin are synthetic derivatives of penicillin, which have better oral absorption and better Gram-negative activity than penicillin.

Side effects
Diarrhoea is possible due to disruption of gastrointestinal flora.

Fluoroquinolones
- Enrofloxacin
- Marbofloxacin
- Pradofloxacin
- Orbifloxacin

This drug group is used in gastrointestinal disease primarily for its activity against Gram-negative bacteria (especially the Enterobacteriaceae). With the exception of pradofloxacin, these drugs have weak activity against anaerobes and, as a consequence, are less likely to disrupt the anaerobic bacterial population. Concurrent oral administration of magnesium-, aluminium- and calcium-containing products (e.g. antacids, sucralfate or nutritional supplements) can inactivate fluoroquinolones.

Side effects
Use in growing dogs is associated with the development of an arthropathy and dosages of enrofloxacin exceeding 5 mg/kg in cats can cause blindness. Neurological side effects (including seizures) are described in dogs, but are rare.

Sulphonamides
- Trimethoprim/sulphonamide

Trimethoprim/sulphonamide is a broad-spectrum combination product.

Side effects
Keratoconjunctivitis sicca has been reported in dogs. Acute hepatitis, immune-mediated polyarthritis and immune-mediated thrombocytopenia have all been reported in the dog. In cats, anorexia, ptyalism and bone marrow dyscrasia have been reported. Sulphonamide crystal formation can occur in the urine. Dobermanns appear to be susceptible to the development of immune-mediated side effects.

References and further reading
BSAVA/SAMsoc PROTECT ME (2018) Available from www.bsavalibrary.com/protectme

German AJ, Halladay LJ and Noble P-JM (2010) First-choice therapy for dogs presenting with diarrhoea in clinical practice. *Veterinary Record* **167**, 810–814

Livermore DM (2003) Bacterial resistance: origins, epidemiology and impact. *Clinical Infectious Diseases* **36**, 11–23

Mansfield C, James FE, Craven M *et al.* (2009) Remission of histiocytic ulcerative colitis in Boxer dogs correlates with eradication of invasive intramucosal *Escherichia coli. Journal of Veterinary Internal Medicine* **23**, 964–969

Marks SL, Rankin SC, Byrne BA and Weese JS (2011) Enteropathogenic bacteria in dogs and cats: diagnosis, epidemiology, treatment, and control. *Journal of Veterinary Internal Medicine* **25**, 1095–1208

NICE Guidelines (2009) Diarrhoea and vomiting caused by gastroenteritis. Diagnosis, assessment and management in children under 5 years old. National Collaborating Centre for Clinical Guideline CG84. Women's and Children's Health, London

Ortiz V, Klein L, Channell S *et al.* (2018) Evaluating the effect of metronidazole plus amoxicillin-clavulanate *versus* amoxicillin-clavulanate alone in canine haemorrhagic diarrhoea: a randomised controlled trial in primary care practice *Journal of Small Animal Practice* **59**, 398–403

Rama Rao KV and Norenberg MD (2014) Glutamine in the pathogenesis of hepatic encephalopathy: the Trojan Horse hypothesis revisited. *Neurochemical Research* **39**, 593–598

Ramsey I (2017) *BSAVA Small Animal Formulary, 9th edn, Part A: Canine and Feline.* BSAVA Publications, Gloucester

Singleton DA, Arsevska E, Smyth S *et al.* (2019) Small animal disease surveillance: gastrointestinal disease, antibacterial prescription and tritrichomonas foetus. *Veterinary Record* **184**, 211–216

Tamborini A, Jahns H, McAllister H *et al.* (2016) Bacterial cholangitis, cholecystitis, or both in dogs. *Journal of Veterinary Internal Medicine* **30**, 1046–1055

Unterer S, Strohmeyer K, Kruse BD, Sauter-Louis C and Hartmann K (2011) Treatment of aseptic dogs with hemorrhagic gastroenteritis with amoxicillin/clavulanic acid: a prospective blinded study. *Journal of Veterinary Internal Medicine* **25**, 973–979

Chapter 30

Parasiticides and gastrointestinal parasites of dogs and cats

Maggie Fisher and Peter Holdsworth

The focus of this chapter is parasiticides targeting eukaryotic parasites. Therefore, helminths and protozoans are considered in this chapter, while bacteria and fungi are excluded. Parasitic protozoans are unicellular organisms that can only divide within the host. Parasitic helminths (roundworms and tapeworms) are elongated, soft-bodied multicellular invertebrates (Figures 30.1 and 30.2). The term 'parasiticides' refers to compounds/products that kill parasites. 'Nematicides', 'cestocides', 'coccidiocides' and 'anthelmintics' kill nematodes, cestodes, coccidial protozoans and helminths, respectively.

Therapeutic parasiticides target established parasite populations in a host and deliver an immediate (relatively) 'cidal' effect. Preventive parasiticides offer a prophylactic or a residual effect beyond their initial killing (therapeutic) impact on parasites after administration. They provide some degree (length) of protection (measured as time) against reinfection by affected parasites. Where the presence of adult parasites is deemed undesirable, treatments may be timed to prevent the development of adult parasites or patent infections; for example, monthly treatment with an anthelmintic effective against larval stages of the worm *Toxocara canis* will largely prevent patent infection in dogs.

'Broad-spectrum' and 'narrow-spectrum' (Figure 30.3) refer to the number or range of parasite species a parasiticide can kill or control. Parasiticides that kill only one or a

Nematode group	Cat	Dog
Ascarids	*Toxocara cati*	*Toxocara canis*
	Toxascaris leonina	*Toxascaris leonina*
Hookworms	*Ancylostoma tubaeforme*	*Ancylostoma caninum**
	Uncinaria stenocephala	*Uncinaria stenocephala*
Whipworms	–	*Trichuris vulpis*

30.1 Major intestinal nematodes of dogs and cats. *Currently not in the UK.

Species	Final host	Approximate prepatent period (weeks)	Intermediate host	Intermediate stage – metacestode[a]
Taenia pisiformis	Dog and fox	6–8	Rabbit	Cysticercus pisiformis
				Abdomen or liver
Taenia hydatigena	Dog and fox	7–10	Cattle, sheep	Cysticercus tenuicollis
				Abdomen or liver
Taenia multiceps	Dog	4–6	Sheep, cattle	Coenurus cerebralis
				Brain and spinal cord
Taenia ovis	Dog and fox	6–8	Sheep and goat	Cysticercus ovis
				Muscle
Taenia serialis	Dog	–	Rabbit	Coenurus serialis
				Connective tissue
Taenia taeniaeformis	Cat	7	Mouse	Strobilocercus
				Liver
Echinococcus granulosus	Dog	7	Sheep and other mammals	Hydatid cyst
				Liver
Echinococcus multilocularis[b]	Fox, dog and cat[c]	4	Normally small rodents	Alveolar cyst
				Liver
Dipylidium caninum	Dog and cat	3	Fleas and biting lice on dogs	Cysticercoid
				Abdomen

30.2 Species of tapeworms found in dogs and cats. [a] The genus and species-type names for these stages are gradually being phased out as it is recognized that they represent simply the immature stage of the tapeworm in the final host, and they are no longer put into italic to denote they are not regarded as species names. [b] Not present in the UK and forms the basis for the mandatory tapeworm treatment prior to entry into the UK. [c] The fox is the best of the hosts with the cat the least, with markedly fewer worms establishing and reaching maturity in cats.

Product	Spectrum of activity				
	Protozoa	*Cestoda*	*Nematoda*	*Insecta*[a]	*Acarina*[a]
Piperazine			Dog, cat		
Pyrantel			Dog		
Benzimidazoles	Dog[b]	Dog, cat	Dog, cat		
Nitroscanate		Dog	Dog		
Praziquantel		Dog, cat			
Pyrantel and praziquantel		Cat	Cat		
Pyrantel, febantel and praziquantel		Dog	Dog		
Pyrantel and febantel			Dog		
Selamectin			Dog, cat	Dog, cat	Dog, cat
Lufenuron and milbemycin			Dog	Dog	
Milbemycin and praziquantel		Dog, cat	Dog, cat		
Moxidectin and imidacloprid			Dog, cat	Dog, cat	Dog, cat
Oxantel, pyrantel and praziquantel		Dog	Dog		
Emodepside and praziquantel		Cat	Cat		
Fipronil, S-methoprene, eprinomectin, praziquantel		Cat	Cat	Cat	Cat
Spinosad and milbemycin oxime			Dog	Dog	

30.3 The spectrum of activity of antiparasitic compounds against key canine and feline parasites. [a]Some genera only – see individual data sheets for more information. [b]*Giardia* only. Note: The table is based on the data sheet claims for the products.

few parasite species generally are termed narrow spectrum parasiticides, while those that have multiple parasite genus/species effectiveness are termed broad spectrum, which may be achieved by a single active ingredient or a combination of active ingredients. There are no universally accepted scientific definitions of narrow- or broad-spectrum status of parasiticides. Some antiparasitics have a spectrum of activity that includes some ectoparasite species or protozoans in addition to having gastrointestinal anthelmintic activity, and some are active against helminths present in other organs (Figure 30.3).

Overview of parasiticides

The active ingredients used in anthelmintic parasiticides are shown in Figure 30.4 together with a brief description of their mode of action. Formulation chemistry is an integral part of each parasiticide and plays a major role in determining the route of administration, distribution and duration of efficacy. Parasiticides with gastrointestinal activity may be administered orally, parenterally (e.g. praziquantel) or topically. Over the past decade the number of generic parasiticides has increased. Both the parasiticide originator and any generic would be required to achieve a minimum of 90% efficacy for most gastrointestinal parasite species,

with the exception of *Echinococcus* species, where 100% efficacy is required.

There are far fewer treatments available for the treatment of protozoal infections (Figure 30.5), with the majority of these being used off-label where treatment is necessary. Unlike the situation with anthelmintic parasiticides, which may be used in a preventive manner, antiprotozoals are normally used where there is a diagnosis of a particular infection. Where clinical signs are severe, for example, with isosporosis, which is typically a disease of young puppies or kittens, then additional supportive therapy may be necessary.

In the UK, anthelmintic parasiticides traverse the legal categories of veterinary pharmaceuticals, from prescription to over-the-counter (OTC) products. A number of parasiticides fall within the remit of the Suitably Qualified Person. With the increase in OTC anthelmintics in some countries being used without veterinary oversight, there are concerns that this is contributing to anthelmintic resistance (AR) development. The availability of OTC anthelmintics is believed to lead not only to an increased frequency of treatments, but also to a decreased interaction of pet owners with veterinary surgeons (veterinarians) and fewer opportunities to implement effective worm control programmes based on veterinary insight into parasite biology.

Active ingredient	Chemical group	Mode of action	Administration route
Febantel, fenbendazole	Benzimidazoles	Prevent tubulin construction	Oral
Oxantel, pyrantel	Tetrahydropyrimidines	Neuromuscular paralysis	Oral
Milbemycin oxime, moxidectin, selamectin	Macrocyclic lactones	Inhibit glutamate-gated chloride channels	Oral or spot-on
Nitroscanate	Isothiocyanate	–	Oral
Piperazine	–	Affects neuromuscular transmission	Oral
Praziquantel	Isoquinoline	Damage to parasite tegument and other effects	Oral, spot-on, injection[a]

30.4 Anthelmintic agents. [a]Not currently available in the UK, although available in some other European countries.

Disease	Host	Treatment
Giardiosis	Dog Cat	Fenbendazole 50 mg/day for 3 days (licensed for use in the dog only)
Isosporosis	Dog Cat	Toltrazuril or diclazuril (off-label use) Sulphonamides (off-label use)
Neosporosis	Dog	Clindamycin or trimethoprim/ sulphonamide (off-label use)
Toxoplasmosis	Cat	Clindamycin (off-label use)
Tritrichomonosis	Cat	Ronidazole (off-label use)

30.5 Gastrointestinal protozoans, hosts and available treatments.

Puppies, kittens and pregnant or lactating queens and bitches are all groups where parasiticidal treatment requires special consideration. Some parasiticides are not licensed for use in particularly young animals or pregnant or lactating dams. Data sheets for individual products should be consulted for this information. Control of *T. canis*, *Toxocara cati* and *Ancylostoma caninum*, where transplacental (*T. canis*) or transmammary (all species) infection can occur from the dam to the offspring, requires particular consideration, as many standard anthelmintics will not have any effect on this transfer from the dam to the offspring, which can result in young animals carrying intestinal infections with these parasites. The treatment regimen currently authorized for prevention of perinatal transmission to puppies is fenbendazole at a dose-rate of 25 mg/kg from day 42 of pregnancy to 2 days postpartum. With or without this treatment of bitches, it is recommended that puppies are treated beginning at 2 weeks of age, and for kittens, beginning at 3 weeks of age.

A wide variety of factors contribute to parasiticide resistance, including parasite management and parasiticide-specific factors. AR is the heritable ability of helminths to withstand the normal effects of a parasiticide when administered at the approved dosage. To date there are few proven cases of AR in cats and dogs, with the only confirmed resistance to pyrantel in canine hookworms in Australia (Kopp *et al.*, 2007). Detection of 'true' AR in parasites of cats and dogs remains problematic, as the detection/diagnostic techniques in use are not definitive in the results offered. It is believed by some that long-acting parasiticides are more prone for AR development compared with short-acting parasiticides. It is likely that the highest selection pressure that could lead to the development of AR would occur in kennel and cattery situations.

Anthelmintic treatment is generally regarded as a routine treatment and so adverse events following treatment would be expected to be rare. Exceptionally, collies and related breeds, due to the *MDR-1* mutation, lack a P-glycoprotein-based transportation system, which renders them susceptible to toxicosis with ivermectin and other macrocyclic lactones (Geyer and Janko, 2012). Tolerance of macrocyclic lactones by affected dogs varies according to the route of administration, dose-rate, the particular macrocyclic lactone and whether the dog is a homozygous or heterozygous for the mutation. For example, low-dose ivermectin has been developed as a heartworm preventive and is well tolerated, but is not legally available in the UK. Particular care should be taken with collies to ensure that macrocyclic lactones are not used off-label and that label instructions are followed for these dogs.

Alternatives to parasiticides, including vaccinology and bespoke therapy (e.g. gene therapy), are a long way off in this area, therefore, reliance on parasiticides will continue. Few vaccines are marketed that target parasites. Eukaryotic parasites are vastly more complex than viruses or bacteria, hence developing effective vaccines is problematic. Vaccines may have a role in the future.

Treatment

Parasiticides are one part of effective gastrointestinal parasite control. Other management factors, such as only feeding cooked food, picking up and disposal of faeces, providing a clean environment and preventing hunting and access to carcases where possible, are also important. Preventive regimens should involve a frequency of repeat parasiticide treatment and choice of treatment that is customized to the needs of the client and pet. Catteries and kennels may benefit from the development of programmes that consider the infections present and the possibility of resistance developing to particular parasiticide active ingredient groups.

Any infection requiring therapy should be suitably treated, together with supportive treatment and nursing where necessary. This is particularly the case for protozoal infection, where there are relatively few products available for treatment of infections (Figure 30.5).

References and further reading

Geyer J and Janko C (2012) Treatment of *MDR1* mutant dogs with macrocyclic lactones. *Current Pharmaceutical Biotechnology* **13**, 969–986

Kopp SR, Kotze AC, McCarthy JS and Coleman GT (2007) High-level pyrantel resistance in the hookworm *Ancylostoma caninum*. *Veterinary Parasitology* **143**, 299–304

Chapter 31

Oral cavity, oropharynx and salivary glands

Edward J. Hall

The integrated activities of the oral cavity, oropharynx and salivary glands enable the prehension, mastication and swallowing of food at the start of its passage through the digestive tract. Dental and periodontal diseases are the most common problems in the mouth; specific dental conditions are detailed in the *BSAVA Manual of Canine and Feline Dentistry and Oral Surgery* and are not discussed further here. However, other structural or functional abnormalities of the oral cavity, oropharynx or salivary glands can cause similar signs of dysphagia, drooling, halitosis, anorexia and oral pain.

Structure and function

The mouth, tongue and throat perform physiological functions such as taste, thermoregulation (panting) and immune surveillance (through the tonsils), but with respect to gastroenterology, eating and swallowing are the key functions. The oropharyngeal phase of swallowing can be subdivided into three stages:

- The first, or oral, stage begins with the prehension and chewing of food by the teeth and tongue, and the formation, mixed with saliva, of a food bolus at the base of the tongue
- In the second (pharyngeal) stage, rostral to caudal pharyngeal contractions propel the bolus from the base of the tongue to the upper oesophageal sphincter opening
- The cricopharyngeus muscle relaxes during the third (cricopharyngeal) stage, and the bolus passes into the upper oesophageal body. The cricopharyngeus subsequently contracts, pharyngeal muscles relax and the oropharyngeal phase is repeated over and over again.

The innervation of the mouth, tongue and pharynx is complex, with ordinary sensory function provided by the maxillary and mandibular branches of the trigeminal nerve and by the glossopharyngeal nerves caudally; taste sensation by branches of the facial (chorda tympani) and glossopharyngeal nerves; and motor function of the muscles closing the jaw by the mandibular branch of the trigeminal nerve, the pharyngeal muscles by the glossopharyngeal and vagus nerves, and the tongue by the hypoglossal nerve. The palatine, pharyngeal, hyoid and laryngeal muscles, with the epiglottis, are also critical in closing the nasopharynx and glottis during swallowing. The cricopharyngeus muscle is innervated by the vagus and acts as the upper oesophageal sphincter.

Oral cavity

The lips and buccal mucosa form the rostral and lateral outer boundaries of the mouth, and help retain ingested food and water. The oral cavity is bounded dorsally by the hard palate and ventrally by the tongue and floor of the mouth. The oropharynx is bounded by the soft palate and pharyngeal mucosa, with the glottis opening past the epiglottis into the larynx.

It is the teeth and tongue within the oral cavity that are pivotal in the prehension, chewing and maceration of food and the delivery of food boluses to the oropharynx for swallowing. The teeth of dogs and cats have been developed to prehend prey (canines), tear and slice meat (incisors and carnassials, respectively) and grind bones (molars). Flattened premolars and molars for grinding plant material are not as developed as in herbivores. The tongue helps form boluses against the palate and moves them to the oropharynx.

Oropharynx

The oropharynx receives food boluses and liquids and delivers them to the upper oesophageal sphincter. Dysfunction or incoordination of pharyngeal peristalsis with the relaxation of the cricopharyngeus muscle leads to structural or functional dysphagia, respectively (see Chapter 12). Simultaneously, with the swallowing of a bolus from the oropharynx, there is normally a reflex closure of the nasopharynx, the epiglottis over the glottis and the laryngeal folds to prevent nasal reflux and inhalation (Figure 31.1).

Salivary glands

The paired salivary glands (sublingual, mandibular, parotid and orbital/zygomatic) and small accessory glands within the oral mucosa provide fluid to enable maceration of food to increase the surface area available for the action of digestive enzymes, and to lubricate its passage down the oesophagus (Figure 31.2). Salivation is stimulated by the anticipation, smell and taste of food, and is mediated by parasympathetic and sympathetic branches within the trigeminal or facial nerves. Canine saliva does contain a

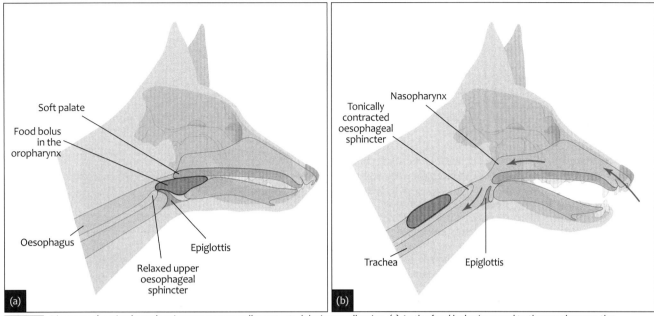

31.1 Diagrams showing how the airways are normally protected during swallowing. (a) As the food bolus is moved to the oropharynx, the nasopharynx and trachea are protected by closure of the soft palate and glottis. (b) After the bolus has entered the oesophagus, the upper oesophageal sphincter closes and the airways open.

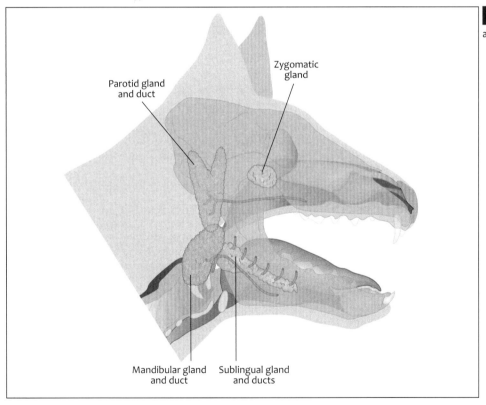

31.2 Diagram showing the position of the paired salivary glands and their ducts.

small amount of the enzyme amylase (Iacopetti *et al.*, 2017; Pasha *et al.*, 2018); this has not been studied in cats. However, as neither dogs nor cats chew food for long, the role of this enzyme in digestion is negligible. Many of the other components of saliva, antibody (immunoglobulin A), carbonic anhydrase, lysozyme, lactoperoxidase, mucins and minerals, are important for lubrication, maintaining oral and dental health and for taste. Saliva also contains a number of hormones including epidermal growth factor, which stimulates epithelial renewal in the gastrointestinal (GI) tract, and salivary cortisol, which can be measured as a marker of stress in dogs.

Understanding the anatomy of the duct system is important when surgical excision of specific glands is needed to eliminate sialocoeles (see later).

Pathophysiology

Anorexia, drooling, halitosis and dysphagia (see Chapters 8 and 10–12) are the most common signs caused by problems in the mouth and throat. These signs can be caused by both morphological conditions and functional disorders. Morphological conditions are typically visible or, at least identifiable on biopsy; functional disorders may show no physical abnormalities on direct observation.

Dental and periodontal diseases are the most common problems, causing either pain or tissue inflammation/infection/necrosis with putrefaction of any necrotic tissue and retained food. Painful dental lesions (e.g. severe gingivitis, tooth fractures, retained dental roots, caries and pulp exposure, apical abscesses and feline odontoclastic resorptive lesions) can lead to hyporexia. Most often, the patient will try to eat and then drop the food if chewing is painful, and so complete anorexia is rarely a sign of dental disease. Indeed, other inflammatory, neoplastic and physical lesions in the oral cavity and oropharynx, as well as functional disturbances, can cause similar signs. Even if the patient wants to eat, dysfunction or physical interference can lead to failure of swallowing and weight loss (see Chapters 8 and 9). Functional disorders of eating and swallowing are caused by neuromuscular disorders, with aspiration pneumonia a common and serious consequence of oropharyngeal and oesophageal dysfunction (see Chapter 32).

Failure to produce saliva leads to a dry mouth (xerostomia), which predisposes to oral infections, and disruption of the salivary ducts leads to leakage within tissues, causing a sialocoele. More commonly, increased production of saliva (ptyalism) can cause drooling, whereas deformities of the lips and mouth (congenital, breed-related and acquired, e.g. due to an oral mass) cause pseudoptyalism, the failure to swallow normal amounts of saliva (see Chapter 10).

Diagnostic approach

Algorithms for the diagnostic approach to the problems of dysphagia, halitosis, and hypersalivation with drooling that are associated with oropharyngeal disease are detailed in Chapters 10–12. An overview of potential investigations for conditions of the mouth, oropharynx and salivary glands follows.

The diagnostic approach to morphological disorders of the mouth and pharynx is straightforward, but the diagnosis of functional disorders causing oropharyngeal dysphagia is generally made on the basis of clinical signs and by exclusion of other oropharyngeal and oesophageal pathology; videofluoroscopy and manometry, the diagnostic tools of choice for functional disorders, are rarely available in general practice. However, once an oropharyngeal dysphagia is suspected, it can be further classified into an oral, pharyngeal or cricopharyngeal stage disorder.

- Oral stage dysphagias with prehension deficits or dropping of food from the mouth are mainly due to loss of tongue function (Figure 31.3).
- Pharyngeal stage dysphagias, with transport deficits, are mainly due to loss of cranial and caudal pharyngeal constrictor function.
- Cricopharyngeal stage dysphagias are associated with cricopharyngeal opening deficits (achalasia), or incoordination (asynchrony) between pharyngeal contraction and cricopharyngeal sphincter relaxation.

History

Dysphagia and hypersalivation are the most important clinical signs indicative of oropharyngeal disorders, and can lead to drooling, halitosis and anorexia. Halitosis

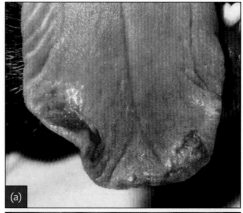
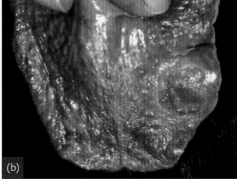

31.3 (a) Dorsal and (b) ventral aspects of the tongue of a Golden Retriever with a deficit in trigeminal sensation. The dog could prehend food but would then drop it from its mouth during mastication. The ulcerated lesions on both aspects of the tongue are where the dog bit it because of lack of sensation.

may result if food is retained in the mouth or if a lesion is infected/necrotic (see Chapter 11). Pet owners may also describe related signs such as:

- Gagging/choking, difficulties in drinking water or forming a solid bolus
- Excessive mandibular or head motion
- Persistent forceful ineffective swallowing efforts
- Dropping of food from the mouth
- Nasal discharge due to misdirection of food into the nasopharynx
- Excessive salivation
- Foaming from the mouth
- Coughing
- Failure to thrive
- Reluctance to eat (see Chapter 12).

Regurgitation, a common sign of oesophageal disease (see Chapter 13), is less frequently reported with oropharyngeal dysphagias.

Physical examination

Findings on physical examination are dependent upon the pathogenesis and severity of the dysphagia. Weight loss is a non-specific finding related to decreased successful food intake. Many morphological abnormalities (e.g. neoplasia, inflammation, foreign body) are usually obvious on examination of the oropharynx, although sedation or even general anaesthesia may be needed for a complete examination.

Animals with functional oropharyngeal dysphagias, on the other hand, may have no or few morphological abnormalities, although dry mucous membranes, a failure to clear food from the mouth or a nasal discharge may give clues. Focal or generalized muscle atrophy and a diminished or absent gag reflex may be the only abnormal findings in animals with neuromuscular disease, and a neurological examination should be performed before sedation/anaesthesia to examine the mouth.

Laboratory tests

The diagnosis of a morphological abnormality is usually straightforward through direct observation, and specific laboratory tests are often unnecessary, except for tissue biopsy or culture. For example, suspected neoplastic lesions should always undergo incisional or excisional biopsy, and pharyngeal swabbing for calicivirus and feline herpesvirus is indicated in cats with evidence of oropharyngeal inflammation/ulceration with or without respiratory and conjunctival disease. Swabbing inflamed tissue for bacterial culture is often not helpful as the oropharynx contains a large population of commensal bacteria, making interpretation of results difficult, but any abscesses should be cultured.

A routine minimum database may be helpful: it will document anaemia and/or thrombocytopenia if there has been extensive oral/oropharyngeal bleeding, and may identify infectious/inflammatory diseases. Serum biochemistry is important to rule out some systemic causes of oropharyngeal conditions, such as uraemic ulcers. For neuromuscular problems, specific tests may help in reaching a diagnosis: temporal myositis can be confirmed by measurement of 2M antibody titres, and focal myasthenia gravis (MG) affecting the pharynx (with or without oesophageal involvement) can be tested for by measuring the acetylcholine receptor antibody titre (see Chapter 32; Useful websites). Other diagnostic tests that may be warranted after an oropharyngeal dysphagia has been diagnosed include antinuclear antibody titre measurement, thyroid function testing, serum creatine phosphokinase activity, muscle biopsy and brainstem magnetic resonance imaging (MRI).

Diagnostic imaging

Survey radiography, ultrasonography, computed tomography (CT) and/or MRI (see Chapter 3) may be performed to assess the severity of local conformational, neoplastic or traumatic lesions, and to look for distant metastasis. Aspiration pneumonia is not a typical finding in oral stage dysphagias but is in pharyngeal stage dysphagias as well as oesophageal regurgitation.

Videofluoroscopy is the diagnostic test of choice for functional problems of swallowing since it is impossible to classify these disorders on the basis of physical examination or plain radiography. However, it may only be available in referral practices. The videofluoroscopic findings of oral stage dysphagias are typified by:

- Weak tongue-thrust action
- Retention of contrast medium in the oropharynx
- Loss of contrast medium from the mouth.

Videofluoroscopic findings consistent with a pharyngeal stage dysphagia include:

- Slow induction and slow progression of peristaltic-like contractions from the rostral to the caudal pharynx
- Asynchrony: incomplete pharyngeal contraction with adequate cricopharyngeal relaxation, or incomplete cricopharyngeal relaxation with adequate pharyngeal contraction
- Laryngotracheal aspiration.

Electromyography

This may be useful in distinguishing oropharyngeal dysphagia from cricopharyngeal achalasia (see later). Fibrillation and positive sharp waves observed in the oropharyngeal musculature suggest that the disorder involves the structures of the oral cavity and pharynx instead of the cricopharyngeus.

Histopathology

Unless the diagnosis is apparent on direct observation (e.g. luminal foreign body), any visible lesions should be sampled by incisional or excisional biopsy; the method depends on the size and nature of the lesion and the ability to remove all or part of any mass without the risk of uncontrollable bleeding or iatrogenic bone fracture. Touch impressions will be contaminated with oral bacteria but, along with fine-needle aspirates of masses, they may give a quicker answer than biopsy. Obtaining fine-needle aspirates of the submandibular lymph nodes to look for metastasis is an important part of staging of oral masses.

Specific conditions of the oropharynx

Abnormalities in any of the oropharyngeal stages of swallowing can produce dysphagia and other signs of local disease, and can be either functional or morphological in origin. Most functional disorders consist of failure, spasticity or incoordination of muscular contractions and are due to neuromuscular disease. Morphological disorders that interfere with the oropharyngeal phase of swallowing include foreign bodies and neoplastic, traumatic and inflammatory processes of the oral cavity and pharynx.

Morphological conditions

As mentioned previously, dental and periodontal diseases are the most common causes of morphological problems in the mouth, but are not discussed further here (see the *BSAVA Manual of Canine and Feline Dentistry and Oral Surgery*). Other morphological conditions can often be diagnosed by direct observation and the methods described above, and can be classified based on their aetiology.

Congenital and developmental disorders

Conformational abnormalities: Abnormal conformation of the mouth and lips often leads to pseudoptyalism and drooling, and is typically seen in certain breeds, that is those with brachygnathism or excessive lip folds.

Cleft palate:
- A primary cleft palate, or 'harelip', is a congenital split in the upper lip and gums.
- A secondary cleft palate is a congenital opening between the mouth and the nose in the hard and/or soft palate, which may occur concurrently with a primary cleft palate (Figure 31.4).

Purebreed animals have a higher incidence of cleft palate, with a predisposition seen in Boston Terriers, Pekingese, Bulldogs, Miniature Schnauzers, Beagles,

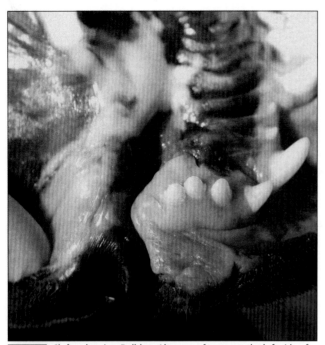

31.4 Cleft palate in a Bulldog. Absence of rugae on the left side of the hard palate is a consequence of a previous failed repair.
(Reproduced from the *BSAVA Manual of Canine and Feline Head, Neck and Thoracic Surgery, 2nd edn*)

Cocker Spaniels, Dachshunds and Siamese cats. Although congenital and probably inherited, nutritional deficiencies, viruses and exposure to toxins during pregnancy may also increase the risk. Secondary (palatine) cleft palates may cause sneezing and nasal discharge, as food and saliva will pass into the nose, and neonates may fail to thrive if they cannot suckle effectively. The diagnosis is straightforward with a thorough oral examination: as well as a palatine cleft and/or a primary cleft palate, protruding incisors and deformed nostrils may be apparent. Treatment is surgical (see the *BSAVA Manual of Canine and Feline Head, Neck and Thoracic Surgery*), but cleft palate closure is difficult in very young patients, and oesophagostomy tube feeding may be required until they have grown enough to undergo surgery.

Ankyloglossia: Colloquially known as 'tongue-tie', ankyloglossia is a rare congenital oral anomaly in dogs. A complete attachment of the lingual frenulum to the floor of the oral cavity leads to limited mobility of the tongue, causing problems during suckling, eating and swallowing. The condition is treated surgically.

Macroglossia: Puppies born with an extremely long and/or thick tongue are commonly seen in brachycephalic breeds (and those patients that cannot retract the tongue due to a neurological deficit) and may show difficulties of prehension, as well as desiccation and ulceration of the tongue surface. Resection of the rostral portion of an over-long tongue may be of benefit. Enlargement of the tongue is also sometimes seen in acromegaly where, more commonly, hypertrophy of pharyngeal soft tissues can cause dysphagia and/or increased respiratory noise.

Temporomandibular joint disorders: The bilateral temporomandibular joints (TMJ) are condylar synovial joints between the mandibular condyles and the mandibular fossae of the zygomatic processes of the temporal bones that enable opening and closing of the mouth with, in dogs and cats, limited lateral chewing motion. Congenital

dysplasia of the TMJ can cause difficulties eating, and is seen mostly in Basset Hounds and Irish Setters. However, TMJ dysplasia is very common in other breeds, such as Cavalier King Charles Spaniels, yet is not always associated with dysfunction. It is uncommon in cats.

Two forms of TMJ dysplasia are recognized (Gemmill, 2008). The more common involves cranial displacement of a dysplastic articular process, resulting in lateral deviation of the mandible and locking of the coronoid process of the mandible lateral to the zygomatic arch with the mouth locked open. Diagnosis is achieved by examination under anaesthesia and radiography, and treatment is by excision of the ventral aspect of the zygomatic arch. The second type occurs without impingement between the coronoid process and the zygomatic arch. It may arise after yawning, repetitive chewing of rawhide chews or bones, or playing and can result in considerable distress to the patient as the jaw is locked open. Treatment is by excision arthroplasty. Neuropraxia is a major differential diagnosis but is not usually painful and the jaw can be closed manually; it usually resolves within 48 hours.

Craniomandibular osteopathy: Craniomandibular osteopathy (CMO) is a disease mainly affecting West Highland White Terriers and is also known as 'Westie jaw' or 'lion jaw'. It also occurs occasionally in Scottish, Cairn, Parson Russell and Boston Terriers, and in Lancashire Heelers and Australian Shepherd Dogs. It results in excessive growth of skull bones, particularly the mandible, which may prevent the jaw from opening and closing normally and even cause total immobility if the TMJ fuses. Cycles of abnormal bone growth occur during the first year of life and often cause pain, hyporexia and pyrexia. Diagnosis is made by observation of characteristic radiographic changes (Figure 31.5), which sometimes are mistaken for bony neoplasia or osteomyelitis. CMO is an autosomal recessive disorder with a c.1332C→T mutation in the *SLC37A2* gene, which encodes for the glucose-6-phosphate transporter that is produced mainly in osteoclasts, and for which there is now a genetic test (Hytönen *et al.*, 2016). By the time of skeletal maturity (approximately 12 months), the abnormal bone growth usually slows, and may regress or even recede completely, although some jaw function impairment typically persists. There is no known treatment to prevent or stop this condition, and therapy is aimed solely at reducing any pain and swelling; in cases of complete jaw fusion, palliative surgery or euthanasia may be required. Affected dogs and their relatives should not be bred from.

Calcinosis circumscripta: An abnormal discrete area of soft tissue calcification, calcinosis circumscripta usually occurs in the subcutaneous tissues overlying bony prominences such as the elbow joint. However, lesions can arise in the tongue, although they rarely cause significant clinical signs (Figure 31.6). Lesions are circumscribed granulomatous masses containing chalky, putty-like matrix embedded in fibrous tissue. German Shepherd Dogs and other large-breed dogs appear predisposed. Treatment involves resection of affected tissue and apposition of the incised edges with synthetic absorbable suture material.

TMJ osteoarthritis and ankylosis: Congenital dysplasia, luxation or fracture of the TMJ can initiate the development of osteoarthritis (Gemmill, 2008). It may be asymptomatic but is likely to be painful and, in severe cases, may cause complete ankylosis, preventing normal eating. Severe cases can be treated by excision arthroplasty.

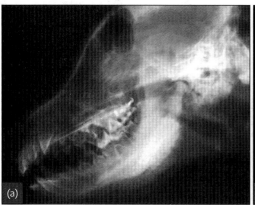
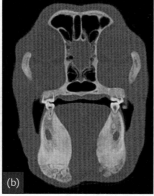
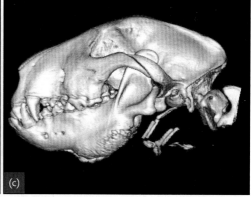

31.5   Craniomandibular osteopathy in West Highland White Terriers. (a) Lateral skull radiograph showing excessive new bone, particularly around the mandible and temporomandibular joint. (b) Transverse computed tomographic (CT) image showing new bone around the mandible. (c) Reconstruction of the CT image in (b) again showing the mandibular new bone.
(Courtesy of Chris Warren-Smith, Langford Vets)

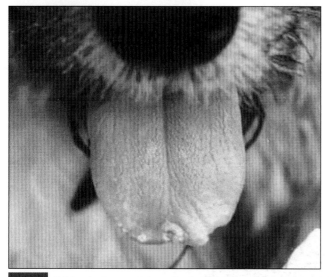

31.6   Calcinosis circumscripta on the tip of the tongue in a dog.

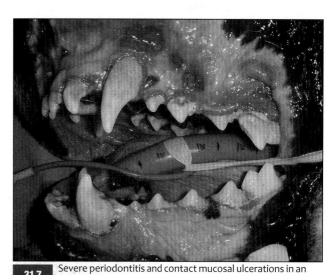

31.7   Severe periodontitis and contact mucosal ulcerations in an 11-year-old Basset Hound.
(© Dr Margherita Gracis and reproduced from the BSAVA Manual of Canine and Feline Dentistry and Oral Surgery, 4th edn)

Infectious/inflammatory diseases

Inflammation of the mouth (stomatitis), gums (gingivitis), pharynx (pharyngitis), tonsils (tonsillitis) and even lips (cheilitis) can cause signs of oropharyngeal dysfunction, and again dental and periodontal diseases are the most common underlying reasons. Chronic ulcerative para-dental stomatitis, also known as contact mucositis (Figure 31.7), is often overlooked as the cause of buccal mucosal lesions until it is recognized that the close proximity of dental plaque to the buccal mucosa in the closed mouth is causing the lesions. Nevertheless, specific inflammatory conditions of the mouth are also seen.

Viral infections: Canine distemper can cause enamel hypoplasia of the teeth, and parvovirus inclusions can be found in tongue tissue, but neither infection specifically causes signs of oropharyngeal disease alone.

Feline respiratory viruses: Feline calicivirus and feline herpesvirus can cause ulcerative lesions in the mouth, which may lead to anorexia as a result of pain associated with feeding and swallowing, as well as loss of appetite due to the temporary loss of the sense of smell if cat flu develops. Further information on the diagnosis and management of these infections can be found in the *BSAVA Manual of Feline Practice: A Foundation Manual.*

Oral papilloma virus: This virus causes an infection that may induce formation of single or multiple papillomas in the mouth of dogs (Lange and Favrot, 2011). These cauliflower-like, exophytic or wart-like growths are benign and may simply be unsightly incidental findings, although they can interfere with eating (Figure 31.8).

Papillomas initially appear on the oral mucosa as pale, smooth elevations that develop a rough surface early in

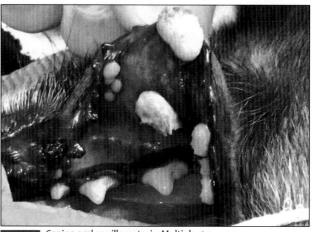

31.8   Canine oral papillomatosis. Multiple grey, verrucous masses are seen on the oral mucosa.

the disease process. Older lesions of 3–4 weeks' duration usually have deep and closely packed fronds, and lesions observed during regression appear shrivelled and dark grey. They typically resolve spontaneously, but complete regression may take several weeks and usually leaves no scar. However, they may be persistent, and may even transform into an oral squamous cell carcinoma. Azithromycin seems to have an accelerating effect on the regression of papillomas (Yağci *et al.*, 2008).

Bacterial infections:
Gingivostomatitis: Primary bacterial stomatitis is rare. Most commonly, gingivostomatitis is associated with bacterial plaque and periodontal disease, but any ulcerated or neoplastic lesion in the oropharynx may be secondarily infected with bacteria, some of which may normally be commensals. Treatment of secondary bacterial stomatitis is by dental scaling, dilute chlorhexidine mouth rinses and, sometimes, antibiotics if the underlying cause persists.

Pharyngitis and tonsillitis: Primary bacterial pharyngitis and tonsillitis are rare. Secondary enlargement of tonsils is seen in animals that are persistently vomiting or regurgitating, or that have perianal disease and lick the affected area.

Eosinophilic and pyogranulomatous stomatitis:
Eosinophilic stomatitis with oral ulceration has been reported in Cavalier King Charles Spaniels in association with other eosinophilic diseases, such as eosinophilic bronchopneumopathy and eosinophilic enteritis, and in other breeds such as the Siberian Husky. A sterile pyogranulomatous stomatitis is recognized in English Springer and Cocker Spaniels and may be associated with sterile pyogranulomatous lymphadenitis occurring in these breeds (Ribas Latre *et al.*, 2019). The finding of pyogranulomatous inflammation in the mouth often dictates that infectious agents are looked for by staining and culturing biopsy samples, or by applying fluorescence *in situ* hybridization. However, in the UK, the lesions are usually sterile. Both eosinophilic and sterile pyogranulomatous stomatitis are either self-limiting or respond to an exclusion diet or steroid therapy.

Eosinophilic granuloma complex:
Lesions in the eosinophilic granuloma complex in cats can sometimes be found in the mouth. Most typically developing on the lips (so-called 'rodent ulcers'), they can also occur on the palate (Figure 31.9). The differential diagnoses include neoplasia,

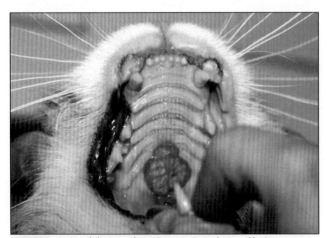

31.9 Eosinophilic granuloma in a cat. Two ulcerated lesions are seen on the upper lip adjacent to the canine teeth, and one on the hard palate.

and incisional biopsy is necessary to confirm the diagnosis. The cause is not certain, but flea and food allergic diseases have been incriminated. Strict flea control and an exclusion diet trial are indicated, but treatment with either immunosuppressants or immunostimulants may be required.

Necrotizing ulcerative gingivitis: 'Trench mouth' (so called because it was first recognized in humans during World War I), but better termed necrotizing ulcerative gingivitis, is a rare disease in humans with even rarer reports in dogs. It has an acute, painful, destructive presentation often with severe halitosis. It is the result of an opportunistic bacterial infection and is predominantly associated with spirochaetes (Figure 31.10).

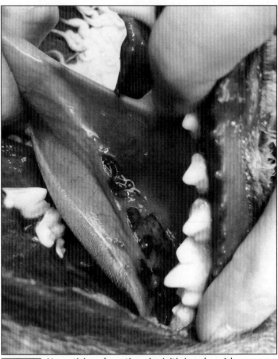

31.10 Necrotizing ulcerative gingivitis in a dog. A large necrotic lesion is seen at the base of the tongue.

Candidiasis: Secondary oral infection with *Candida albicans* can occur after prolonged antibiotic use and/or immunosuppression, and typically causes multiple white spots on the tongue and oral mucosa. Treatment with topical nystatin suspension 2–3 times daily is usually effective if the underlying predisposition is addressed. Nystatin is not absorbed from the GI tract.

Immune-mediated diseases

Mucocutaneous diseases: Autoimmune skin diseases, such as pemphigus vulgaris (PV), are very rare, but can affect the mucocutaneous junctions of the oral cavity and at other sites (i.e. perineum, prepuce, vulva). In PV, autoantibodies to the desmosomal glycoprotein desmoglein-3 cause vesicles to develop due to loss of keratinocyte cell–cell adhesion in the deeper epidermis. The vesicles often rupture and ulcerate before they are observed. Lesions may be painful and cause signs of anorexia and drooling. Diagnosis is by histopathology and immunofluorescence, and treatment is with immunosuppressants.

Feline plasma cell gingivitis: Bilateral, proliferative, ulcerated tissue occurring in the caudal mouth (fauces and gingiva) is seen quite commonly in cats (Figure 31.11)

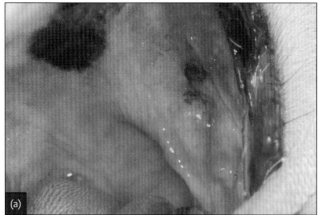

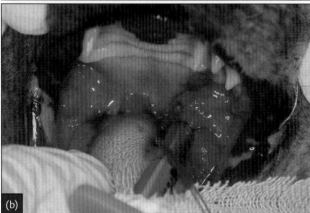

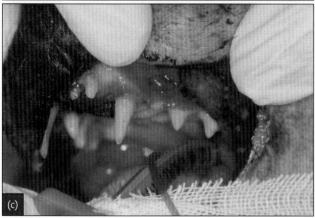

31.11 Plasma cell gingivitis in a cat. (a) Mild faucitis. (b) Severe proliferative inflammation in the fauces of the mouth. (c) Smaller lesion on the maxillary gingiva of the same cat as in (b).
(Courtesy of L Boland, University of Sydney)

and may cause pain on eating and consequent hyporexia. Differential diagnoses for these visible lesions include eosinophilic granuloma and squamous cell carcinoma, but the bilateral nature of this condition makes plasma cell gingivitis more likely. It can be confirmed on biopsy, as the plasma cell infiltration is characteristic. It seems most likely this is an immune-mediated response to bacterial plaque. Optimal treatment is unclear but immunosuppression, immunomodulation, dental cleaning and even total dental extraction (edentulation) have all been tried.

Direct injury

Trauma: Facial trauma and jaw fractures can prevent normal eating, and patients may require feeding via an oesophagostomy tube until healing has occurred. In cats, separation of the mandibular symphysis is a common

sequel to road traffic accidents and falls from high-rise buildings, and often requires simple stabilization with a cerclage wire. Large lacerations and lip avulsion require surgical correction. Stick injuries to the oropharynx and/or proximal oesophagus most commonly occur when dogs impale themselves on the end of a stick that has been thrown for them to chase. The visible damage may be limited (Figure 31.12), but CT can show the extent of any tract and the presence of foreign material, and it is considered best practice to explore any site of penetration.

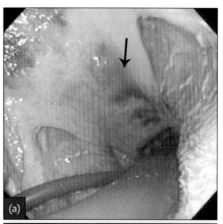

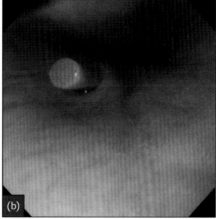

31.12 Stick injury in dogs. (a) Abrasions are seen on the soft palate (arrowed) where the dog ran on to the end of a stick.
(b) Self-impalement of the proximal oesophagus with a kebab stick in a Labrador Retriever.

Chewing lesions: Chewing lesions may result from chronic self-induced trauma to the sublingual mucosa or the labial and buccal mucosa. Usually, no treatment is required, but surgical resection is indicated for excessive hyperplastic tissue that continues to be traumatized.

Oral foreign bodies: Foreign bodies (mainly sticks) and lumps of food can get wedged between teeth but may not be noticed until halitosis due to putrefaction and secondary infection occurs. Short sticks can also become wedged between the left and right upper dental arcades against the hard palate if dogs gnaw them. The patient is usually quite distressed by this, but the diagnosis and treatment is simple, as the stick is visible on opening the mouth and can usually be flicked out of the mouth even without sedation. Rings of marrow bones can become trapped over the mandible in dogs (Figure 31.13). They can be removed either by tensing the submandibular skin caudally or by osteotomy of the marrow bone.

Linear foreign bodies arise when a piece of string/ thread gets caught either around the base of the tongue or

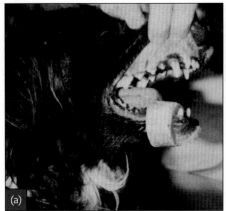

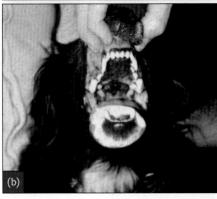

31.13 Ring of marrow bone stuck on the mandible of a Border Collie. (a) Lateral and (b) frontal views.

at the pylorus. Signs are largely related to intestinal obstruction or perforation if the diagnosis is delayed. However, linear foreign bodies starting in the mouth can cause gagging and distress in the patient, and should be identifiable by looking under the tongue during the physical examination (Figure 31.14).

Local irritants: A large number of substances can cause oral irritation if the patient attempts to ingest them. The diagnosis is typically based on the history, and most cases are self-limiting and require no treatment except, perhaps, oral lavage.

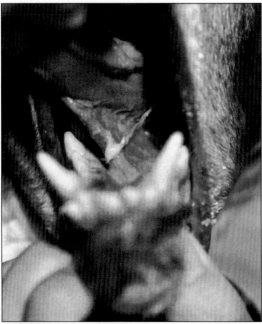

31.14 Linear foreign body: a loop of string under the tongue of a dog.

Phytochemicals: Many plant leaves and stems contain compounds, such as insoluble calcium oxalate, that can cause oral irritation, for example, *Philodendron, Dieffenbachia, Calladium, Poinsettia, Euphorbia,* and seeds of the Kentucky coffee tree (*Gymnocladus dioicus*) found in North America.

Processionary moth caterpillars: Caterpillars of the pine and the oak processionary moths are found in mainland Europe and form distinctive clusters on trees. The oak processionary moth is a recent invader into the UK and is currently found largely within the area encircled by the M25. The caterpillars are covered in urticating hairs that embed in the lips, tongue and oral mucosa when licked by an animal. These hairs cause intense irritation and inflammation and can even cause the tongue epithelium to slough. The hairs require painstaking removal under general anaesthesia as they are very fine and difficult to identify.

Toads: Toads (*Bufo* spp.) secrete toxic substances on their skin, which cause hypersalivation in any dog that tries to pick them up in their mouth. This most often occurs at night when toads are active and dogs may not be observed to interact with them, but signs are self-limiting.

Bitter medications: Bitter drugs, such as metronidazole, trimethoprim/sulphonamide, tylosin and tramadol, can cause hypersalivation and are usually administered in coated tablets or capsules to avoid direct contact with the oral mucosa.

Burns:
Thermal burns: Burns caused by the ingestion of hot substances are typically seen in dogs that steal freshly cooked food that is still too hot for safe ingestion: barbecued meat and baked potatoes are the most common. Because the food is often gulped with minimal contact in the mouth, thermal injury is actually more common in the oesophagus, and causes severe oesophagitis and stricture formation (see Chapter 32).

Chemical/caustic contact injuries: Cats are at risk of caustic burns to the tongue and oropharynx if their coat comes into contact with chemicals that they then attempt to remove by grooming. Tars and other petroleum compounds are most commonly seen as the cause.

Electrical burns: Animals surviving electrocution may seizure and develop non-cardiogenic pulmonary oedema in the dorsal lung fields. However, if they survive longer, over the subsequent few days transverse, linear, oral burns may develop as necrosis occurs where electrical contact was made.

Neoplastic conditions

Benign and malignant tumours of the oropharynx are equally common in dogs, but the majority of oral tumours in cats are malignant. In dogs, periodontal ligament tumours, malignant melanoma, fibrosarcoma and squamous cell carcinoma (SCC) are most commonly diagnosed. In cats, the predominant tumours are SCC and fibrosarcoma. Other malignant neoplasms of the oropharynx include malignant peripheral nerve sheath tumours, osteosarcomas, multilobular tumours of bone, mast cell tumours, lymphosarcoma and undifferentiated tumours.

Depending on the size, position and presence of ulceration and secondary infection, any of these tumours is capable of causing drooling through lip and mouth deformity, halitosis, oral bleeding, dysphagia and anorexia. Diagnosis is by incisional or excisional biopsy, with staging involving examination of fine-needle aspirates of the mandibular lymph nodes and imaging of the lungs (preferably by CT). The biological nature and management of these varied tumours is detailed in the *BSAVA Manual of Canine and Feline Oncology* and the *BSAVA Manual of Canine and Feline Head, Neck and Thoracic Surgery.*

Oral bleeding

Owners often recognize bleeding from the mouth when they see drooling of blood stained saliva, or blood in a water bowl after drinking. Local sources of bleeding are mostly ulcerated inflammatory or neoplastic or traumatic lesions, or the bleeding may be sign of a coagulopathy.

Generalized bleeding disorders: Oral bleeding can be a sign of a coagulopathy. Petechiation in the mucous membranes is suggestive of thrombocytopenia, whilst vitamin K antagonist rodenticides can cause bleeding from the gum margins. In both conditions, bleeding at other sites is evidence that the bleeding is not due to local disease, and the diagnosis can be confirmed by checking the platelet count and the prothrombin and activated partial thromboplastin times.

Menrath's ulcer: This is an unusual lesion seen in cats (Figure 31.15). A small but deep ulcer in the hard palate can erode through the palatine artery and cause life-threatening haemorrhage (Menrath and Miller, 1995). The aetiology is uncertain, but abrasion by the cat's rough tongue probably perpetuates bleeding. Lesions are sometimes difficult to visualize if the mouth is examined when the ulcer is not bleeding. Treatment involves ligation of the ipsilateral palatine artery.

Neuromuscular disorders

Neurological disorders typically result in dysfunction but with no physical manifestation or visible lesions. However, conditions directly affecting the muscles of mastication may produce physical findings.

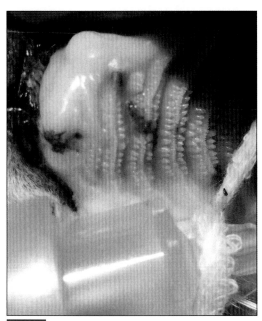

31.15 Menrath's ulcer in the hard palate of a cat.

Masticatory muscle myositis: Masticatory muscle myositis (MMM) is a relatively common inflammatory myopathy (i.e. myositis) in dogs and affects their ability to open their mouth. Originally called temporal muscle myositis, and sometimes eosinophilic myositis, it is now known that this presumed autoimmune condition can affect all the muscles of mastication, that is the temporalis, masseter, lateral and medial pterygoids (Figure 31.16); the frontalis muscle is not involved in mastication and is not affected.

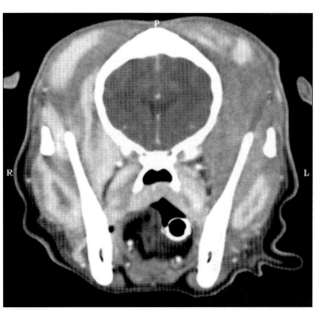

31.16 Computed tomographic image of the skull of a dog with masticatory muscle myositis. Note that abnormal attenuation is seen in all masticatory muscles.

Diagnosis:

Clinical signs: Initially, acute swelling of the temporalis and masseter muscles causes pain and dogs are reluctant to open their mouths. This stage lasts 2–3 weeks, during which time patients are lethargic, reluctant to eat, and show signs of pain on yawning or when prehending and chewing food. As the disease continues, it may appear quiescent, but ultimately progressive fibrosis restricts jaw movement physically and the dog is unable to eat.

Physical examination: In the acute phase of MMM, the temporal muscles may be markedly swollen. Affected dogs can show fever, regional lymphadenopathy and exophthalmos, as well as swelling of the temporal and masseter muscles, which are painful on palpation: the dog resists opening of the mouth because of pain but it can be opened under general anaesthesia. In the chronic phase, marked muscle atrophy over the temporal region becomes apparent (Figure 31.17), and a classic sign of chronic MMM is the inability to open the jaw even under anaesthesia because of the fibrosis that has developed.

Differential diagnoses: Differentials for marked temporal muscle atrophy include hyperadrenocorticism or iatrogenic glucocorticoid administration, hypothyroidism and disorders of the TMJ affecting joint mobility. Polymyositis can also cause temporal muscle atrophy with subclinical involvement of limb muscles only being apparent on electromyography. The inflammatory polymyopathy seen in Hungarian Vizslas typically affects the jaw muscles preferentially. In MMM, muscle atrophy is almost always bilateral, although rare cases of unilateral disease are reported. However, unilateral temporal muscle atrophy is much more

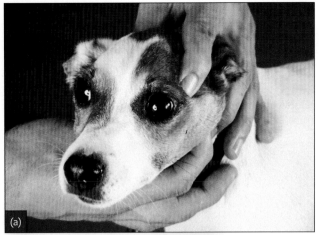

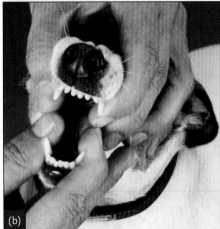

31.17 Masticatory muscle myositis. (a) A Jack Russell Terrier with severe temporal muscle atrophy. (b) Maximum opening of the mouth in the same dog.

suggestive of a trigeminal nerve root sheath tumour or an extra-axial mass affecting the cerebellopontine angle (Milodowski *et al.*, 2019).

Imaging: Radiography is unhelpful, but CT aids in ruling out most differentials of MMM, may allow guided fine-needle aspiration (FNA) of surgically inaccessible pterygoid muscles, and shows changes in size, tissue attenuation and heterogeneous contrast enhancement in affected muscles, as well as the presence of regional lymphadenopathy (see Figure 31.16).

Minimum database: Haematology and routine serum biochemistry may show no significant changes or just non-specific changes consistent with inflammation. However, serum creatine kinase (CK) and/or aspartate aminotransferase (AST) activities should be determined. If increased initially, CK and/or AST are worth tracking to monitor treatment.

2M antibody: Type 2M muscle fibre myosin is only present in muscles supplied by the mandibular branch of the trigeminal nerve (i.e. the masticatory muscles). Thus, the 2M antibody assay, an enzyme-linked immunosorbent assay incubating serum from a dog suspected as having MMM with masticatory muscle antigens, is quite specific; it is negative in cases of polymyositis affecting both masticatory and limb muscles. A serum type 2M fibre antibody titre of <1:100 is considered negative, 1:100 is borderline and >1:100 is positive. False-negatives may occur if the dog has been on immunosuppressive doses of corticosteroids for longer than 7–10 days or if the MMM is end-stage with marked fibrosis. Thus, the test is not 100% sensitive, and contemporaneous muscle biopsy is recommended (see Useful websites).

Muscle biopsy: Biopsy of affected temporal and/or masseter muscle can confirm myositis and provide prognostic information from the degree of fibrosis. Care must be taken when anaesthetizing patients for biopsy because an inability to open the jaw may make intubation very tricky. Another potential problem is that the frontalis muscle may be biopsied by mistake.

Treatment: As MMM is believed to be an autoimmune condition, treatment with immunosuppressants is indicated. Prednisolone at 2 mg/kg/day is the first choice, but other cytotoxic agents (e.g. azathioprine) can be added if steroid side effects are intolerable, as prolonged therapy may be needed. The dosage of prednisolone is tapered until the minimum dose that maintains remission is noted, and this dose is then given for at least 6 months. The owner can judge whether relapse is occurring by periodic measurement of how far the mouth can be opened.

Prognosis: Early diagnosis and treatment generally give a good prognosis, but if treatment does not start until there is marked atrophy and fibrosis, the clinical outcome can be poor.

Functional disorders

Neuromuscular disease is an important underlying pathogenic mechanism of oropharyngeal dysphagia, but the precise aetiologies are rarely identified. Some cases have been associated either with diseases originating outside the oropharynx (e.g. brainstem diseases) or with systemic diseases (e.g. rabies, pseudorabies (Aujeszky's disease), peripheral neuropathy, generalized MG, polymyositis, muscular dystrophy and possibly hypothyroidism). A unique form of oropharyngeal dysphagia bearing some resemblance to muscular dystrophy was described in the Bouvier des Flandres breed of dog in 1994 (Peeters and Ubbink, 1994).

Treatment

Functional disorders causing oropharyngeal dysphagia are all treated medically. Cricopharyngeal myotomy appears to be of no benefit in oral and pharyngeal stage dysphagia except for true cricopharyngeal achalasia; indeed, oropharyngeal dysphagia may be worsened by cricopharyngeal myotomy. The medical therapy for functional oropharyngeal dysphagia is mostly supportive and consists of nutritional support (i.e. tube feeding) on a temporary or permanent basis. Elevated feedings and different food consistencies may be trialled, but these efforts are often of little clinical benefit. Thyroid hormone replacement therapy should be given in animals with documented hypothyroidism.

Prognosis

In general, the prognosis for functional oropharyngeal dysphagias is guarded to poor. Only those associated with MG, polymyositis and hypothyroidism may show some clinical improvement with therapy. Bouvier des Flandres dogs may have a better prognosis, particularly if the disorder is confined to the oesophagus instead of the oropharynx.

Cricopharyngeal achalasia

Aetiopathogenesis: Cricopharyngeal achalasia is a neuromuscular disorder of young dogs. It is characterized by persistent hypertension of the cranial oesophageal sphincter and consequent inadequate relaxation of the sphincter during swallowing. However, the aetiology, pathogenesis and breed predisposition of this disorder are unknown: dysfunction of the inhibitory neurons mediating sphincter relaxation has been postulated, but true stenosis is also possible. Thus, it is not always clear whether this is a morphological or a functional disorder. What is clear is that the cricopharyngeus muscle cannot relax at any time during swallowing, which distinguishes it from the functional disorder where there is asynchrony between pharyngeal contraction and cricopharyngeus relaxation. Thus, this condition should be distinguished from the purely functional problem of asynchrony, because only true achalasia appears to benefit from myotomy of the cricopharyngeus muscle, and indeed this procedure may be detrimental in cases of asynchrony.

Diagnosis:
Clinical signs: Affected animals show progressive dysphagia and regurgitation soon after weaning. They typically make repeated, unproductive swallowing attempts that culminate in regurgitation of undigested food. Coughing and pulmonary crackles may develop as a consequence of food being aspirated into the airways. Physical examination is otherwise usually unremarkable.

Imaging: Survey and static barium-contrast radiography are not useful in diagnosing this disorder because of their inability to evaluate the rapid and complex series of events that occur during swallowing. Definitive diagnosis of cricopharyngeal achalasia requires the use of videofluoroscopy and, ideally, manometry. The videofluoroscopic finding of multiple, unproductive attempts at swallowing barium liquid or paste is consistent with a diagnosis of cricopharyngeal achalasia. This should be supported by the manometric demonstration of elevated basal pressures and inadequate relaxation. If manometry is unavailable and the diagnosis is still questionable, electromyography of the oropharyngeal musculature should be performed to exclude the possibility of a more proximal oropharyngeal dysphagia.

Treatment: It is difficult to generalize based on the small number of cases that have been reported, but the disorder is probably best treated with cricopharyngeal myotomy. Most animals experience immediate relief following surgery. Effective medical management has not been described for this disorder, although injection of botulinum toxin may be used both to test whether the diagnosis is likely and myotomy indicated, and to provide temporary relief.

Prognosis: The prognosis is guarded to poor without surgery. Untreated animals will suffer from malnutrition and recurrent bouts of aspiration pneumonia. Significant and longstanding improvement has been reported with cricopharyngeal myotomy.

Cricopharyngeal asynchrony

Aetiopathogenesis: For unknown reasons cricopharyngeal relaxation does not occur when pharyngeal contractions deliver a bolus to be swallowed. This condition should be distinguished from cricopharyngeal achalasia, where the sphincter never relaxes because of either increased muscle tone or true stenosis.

Diagnosis:
Clinical signs: Affected animals show progressive dysphagia and regurgitation soon after weaning. They typically make repeated, unproductive swallowing attempts that culminate in regurgitation of undigested food. Coughing and pulmonary crackles may develop as a consequence of food being aspirated into the airways. Physical examination is usually unremarkable except for signs of inhalation and malnutrition.

Imaging: Survey and static barium-contrast radiography are not useful in diagnosing the disorder. Definitive diagnosis of cricopharyngeal asynchrony requires the use of videofluoroscopy and oesophageal manometry. The videofluoroscopic finding of multiple, unproductive attempts at swallowing barium liquid or paste is consistent with a diagnosis if the cricopharyngeus muscle is observed to be able to open at other times.

Manometry: Videofluoroscopic findings ideally should be supported by the manometric demonstration of asynchronous relaxation with swallowing. If manometry is unavailable and the diagnosis is still questionable, electromyography of the oropharyngeal musculature should be performed to exclude the possibility of a more proximal oropharyngeal dysphagia.

Treatment: It is difficult to generalize based on the small number of cases that have been reported, but the disorder is probably best not treated with cricopharyngeal myotomy, yet effective medical management has not been described for this disorder.

Prognosis: The prognosis is guarded to poor, as surgical myotomy is not helpful and may even predispose to inhalation.

Myasthenia gravis

This autoimmune disease, with autoantibodies targeting nicotinic acetylcholine receptors, can affect all striated muscle. The oropharynx and oesophagus may be affected when there is generalized MG acting on the skeletal muscle, but focal disease affecting just the pharynx or just the oesophagus or both can occur. Myasthenia affecting the oesophagus is the most common presentation and is described in detail in Chapter 32.

Diagnosis: Diagnosis of focal MG can only be made by measuring acetylcholine receptor antibody titres. The edrophonium response test, which can be used to diagnose generalized MG, is insensitive, probably because, even with videofluoroscopy, it is impossible to determine whether pharyngeal function is temporarily restored. Manometry might be helpful in detecting subtle changes in muscle strength but is rarely available.

Treatment: In early cases of MG, acetylcholinesterase inhibitors (e.g. pyridostigmine) may yield substantial clinical improvement. Glucocorticoid therapy (prednisolone) may also improve clinical signs in many myasthenia and polymyositis patients, but it must be used cautiously if there is a risk of inhalation pneumonia. However, some cases of canine MG resolve spontaneously without immunosuppressant therapy.

Feline orofacial pain syndrome

Considered to be a neuropathic pain disorder of cats, feline orofacial pain syndrome (FOPS) can lead to euthanasia on welfare grounds (Rusbridge *et al.*, 2010). Recurrent episodes of typically unilateral discomfort seem to be triggered in many cases by mouth movements. There may be a familial predisposition in Burmese cats. Sensitization of trigeminal nerve endings as a consequence of oral disease or tooth eruption appears to be an important factor, sometimes exacerbated by situations causing anxiety. Affected cats show behavioural signs of oral discomfort with exaggerated licking and chewing movements, and pawing at the mouth. More severe cases of FOPS may self-mutilate the tongue, lips and buccal mucosa, and consequently may be anorexic or dysphagic. Traditional analgesics aren't effective but management with phenobarbital may help.

Salivary glands

Diseases of the salivary glands are uncommon but may interfere with oropharyngeal function. A review of 245 cases (160 dogs, 85 cats) in which salivary gland tissue had been evaluated histologically reported that 89% of salivary gland submissions were allotted to one of five major categories: malignant neoplasms (30%), sialadenitis (26%), normal salivary gland (16%), sialocoele (9%) and salivary gland infarction (8%) (Spangler and Culbertson, 1991). The prevalence of sialocoeles may have been underestimated, as salivary gland tissue may not be submitted routinely after surgery. The remaining 11% of submissions included various degenerative or fibrotic lesions, ductal ectasia, sialolithiasis, oedema, benign neoplasia and secondary salivary involvement with lymphoma or fibrosarcoma in the head and neck.

Sialocoeles may be unsightly but rarely cause oropharyngeal dysfunction. However, there are a number of conditions that cause salivary gland enlargement, some of which are painful and cause anorexia and drooling, and some stimulate reflex vomiting via the glossopharyngeal nerve input to the vomiting centre (see Chapter 14). Some causes also involve other glandular tissue, such as the lacrimal glands, and may result in both 'dry eye' (xerophthalmia) and 'dry mouth' (xerostomia).

Sialocoeles

Siaolocoeles are caused by accumulation of saliva in tissue due to salivary duct rupture, sometimes following obstruction by calculi, although sialolithiasis is rare in dogs and cats. They can also develop secondary to salivary gland neoplasia (Figure 31.18). Initially, they may be painful and the surrounding tissue swollen due to local inflammation, but they typically become large, usually non-painful, swellings. Depending on the location of the duct rupture, sialocoeles may be associated with dysphagia, gagging, dyspnoea or no clinical signs. Rupture of the sublingual gland duct leads to a ranula, an accumulation of saliva in the tissues under the tongue, and is seen more commonly in cats. The most common problem in dogs is rupture of the duct of the mandibular gland. Sialocoeles arising from the parotid gland are very rare, and problems are more likely to be caused by leakage directly from the gland due to a traumatic injury. Sialocoeles of the zygomatic gland containing mucoid secretions (mucocoeles) tend to cause exophthalmos rather than oropharyngeal signs.

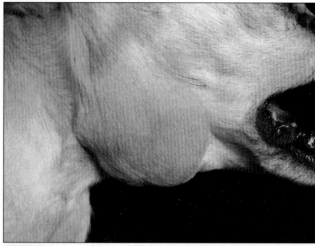

31.18 Tumour of the mandibular salivary gland with an associated mucocoele.
(Reproduced from the *BSAVA Manual of Canine and Feline Oncology*, 3rd edn)

Diagnosis of a sialocoele is based on the gross appearance (stringy, mucoid saliva) and cytological evaluation of aspirated fluid. These 'pockets' of saliva are lined not with epithelium but with connective tissue and often contain foamy macrophages. The lesion is usually unilateral, and the initial position of the sialocoele may identify its side of origin. However, over time, the saliva will tend to accumulate in the ventral midline, making identification of its origin more difficult. In such cases, sialography under anaesthesia may be helpful, but cannulation of the salivary ducts is not easy. Complete surgical removal of the affected salivary ducts and associated gland should result in complete resolution. The removal of the mandibular salivary gland also involves excising the normal ipsilateral sublingual gland; this lateral approach technique is described in the *BSAVA Manual of Canine and Feline Head, Neck and Thoracic Surgery*.

Enlarged salivary glands

Differential diagnoses for non-neoplastic causes of enlarged salivary glands include sialadenosis, sialadenitis and salivary gland infarction. It is not clear whether these three conditions are unrelated or whether they represent a spectrum of severity of the same condition. Secondary salivary gland infection and malignant neoplasia occur rarely.

Sialadenosis

Sialadenosis is a chronic, non-painful, afebrile enlargement of the salivary glands, primarily reported in dogs (Alcoverro *et al.* 2014), but a cat with suspected sialadenosis responding to phenobarbital therapy has been reported. One canine case was reported to be transitory following general anaesthesia, and one case with concurrent cricopharyngeal achalasia has been reported. Clinical signs include frequent retching, gulping, ptyalism and poor appetite; signs are often worse when the dog is excited. Cytological and histological examination of the salivary glands does not reveal any significant changes.

It has been suggested that this condition is a manifestation of neurogenic over-stimulation, or so-called limbic or visceral epilepsy. The prognosis is good, as most patients respond well to treatment with phenobarbital. In resistant cases, monitoring phenobarbital levels to assure a therapeutic range and using potassium bromide may be necessary for complete control.

Sialadenitis

Primary sialadenitis is characterized on FNA cytology or histopathological examination by an inflammatory response with no evidence of infection. Common presenting signs include gagging, coughing, inappetence, lethargy and fever. Enlarged painful salivary glands distinguish this condition from sialadenosis. Refractory vomiting is common, and control may require combinations of maropitant, metoclopramide and ondansetron. Affected dogs usually respond to glucocorticoid therapy, although phenobarbital is often added anyway and may be of benefit.

Salivary gland infarction

This is a potentially fatal disease seen most commonly in terriers. In the original case report, the main changes were ischaemic necrosis, capsular fibrosis and regenerative hyperplasia of surviving ductal epithelium. Necrosis of arterial tunica media and thrombosis were found, but only in the infarcted parts of the salivary glands. The lesions appeared to be confined to the salivary glands and no cause for the infarction was found. More recent studies have also found necrosis, and the term 'necrotizing metaplasia' has been applied. The aetiology is unknown, but one study identified a variety of concurrent oesophageal diseases in the vast majority of cases (Schroeder and Berry, 1998). Optimal treatment is also unknown and the prognosis is guarded.

Salivary gland infection

Bacterial infection: Infection of salivary glands with bacteria and abscessation can be secondary to a tooth root abscess, direct trauma or migration of a foreign body (e.g. grass awn) up a salivary duct from the mouth.

Mumps: This is a paramyxovirus related to canine distemper. Although a primary pathogen in humans, where it causes parotid gland enlargement, mumps can also infect dogs, presumably as a reverse zoonosis. Infected dogs may be asymptomatic or just have swollen salivary glands. Spontaneous resolution can take a few weeks; there is no known treatment. It is so rare that it seems likely that either the canine distemper vaccine offers cross-protection or dogs are generally resistant to infection.

Salivary gland neoplasia

Fortunately, neoplasia of the salivary glands is rare, as the majority are malignant and there is no effective treatment. Mucoepidermoid tumours, SCC, malignant mixed tumours, adenoid cystic carcinoma, acinic cell carcinoma, adenocarcinoma, undifferentiated carcinoma and sarcoma have been reported: adenocarcinoma is the most common. Surgical resection is usually not possible, as the tumour most often arises in the parotid salivary glands and surrounds adjacent vessels and cranial nerves, and combination chemotherapy is palliative at best.

Xerostomia

Failure of saliva secretion leads to a dry mouth (xerostomia) with secondary accumulation of food and consequent stomatitis. The dryness may be appreciated by rubbing a gloved finger along the gums. Failure to secrete saliva may be part of a more generalized dysautonomia or be caused by irradiation of the head for cancer treatment. However, a primary autoimmune attack on the salivary glands has also been postulated. This condition may resemble Sjögren's syndrome in humans, as it may occur with concurrent xerophthalmia (dry eye) causing keratoconjunctivitis sicca. This comparison was made in one affected cat (Canapp et al., 2001). Symptomatic treatment of xerostomia with dilute chlorhexidine washes is indicated, but as so few cases are reported, it is not known whether immunosuppression would be effective.

References and further reading

Alcoverro E, Tabar MD, Lloret A et al. (2014) Phenobarbital-responsive sialadenosis in dogs: case series. Topics in Companion Animal Medicine **29**, 109–112

Brockman DJ, Holt DE and ter Haar G (2018) BSAVA Manual of Canine and Feline Head, Neck and Thoracic Surgery, 2nd edn. BSAVA Publications, Gloucester

Canapp SO, Cohn LA, Maggs CJ et al. (2001) Xerostomia, xerophthalmia, and plasmacytic infiltrates of the salivary glands (Sjögren's-like syndrome) in a cat. Journal of the American Veterinary Medical Association **218**, 59–65

Cannon MS, Matthew S, Paglia D et al. (2011) Clinical and diagnostic imaging findings in dogs with zygomatic sialadenitis: 11 cases (1990–2009). Journal of the American Veterinary Medical Association **239**, 1211–1218

Dobson J and Lascelles D (2011) BSAVA Manual of Canine and Feline Oncology, 3rd edn. BSAVA Publications, Gloucester

Gemmill T (2008) Conditions of the temporomandibular joint in dogs and cats. In Practice **30**, 36–43

Harvey A and Tasker S (2013) BSAVA Manual of Feline Practice: A Foundation Manual. BSAVA Publications, Gloucester

Hytönen MK, Arumilli M, Lappalainen AK et al. (2016) Molecular characterization of three canine models of human rare bone diseases: Caffey, van den Ende-Gupta, and Raine syndromes. PLOS Genetics **12**, e1006037

Iacopetti I, Perazzi A, Badon T et al. (2017) Salivary pH, calcium, phosphorus and selected enzymes in healthy dogs: a pilot study. BMC Veterinary Research **13**, 330–336

Lange CE and Favrot C (2011) Canine papillomaviruses. Veterinary Clinics of North America: Small Animal Practice **41**, 1183–1195

Menrath VH and Miller R (1995) The repair and prevention of bleeding palatine erosive lesions in the cat. Australian Veterinary Practitioner **25**, 202–205

Milodowski EJ, Amengual-Batle P, Beltran E et al. (2019) Clinical findings and outcome of dogs with unilateral masticatory muscle atrophy. Journal of Veterinary Internal Medicine **33**, 735–742

Pasha S, Inui T, Chapple I et al. (2018) The saliva proteome of dogs; variations within and between breeds and species. Proteomics **18**, 1700293

Peeters ME and Ubbink GJ (1994) Dysphagia-associated muscular-dystrophy – a familial trait in the Bouvier des Flandres. Veterinary Record **134**, 444–446

Reiter AM and Gracis M (2018) BSAVA Manual of Canine and Feline Dentistry and Oral Surgery, 4th edn. BSAVA Publications, Gloucester

Ribas Latre A, McPartland A, Cain D et al. (2019) Canine sterile steroid-responsive lymphadenitis in 49 dogs. Journal of Small Animal Practice **60**, 280–290

Rusbridge C, Heath S, Gunn-Moore DA et al. (2010) Feline orofacial pain syndrome (FOPS): a retrospective study of 113 cases. Journal of Feline Medicine and Surgery **12**, 498–508

Schroeder H and Berry WL (1998) Salivary gland necrosis in dogs: a retrospective study of 19 cases. Journal of Small Animal Practice **39**, 121–125

Spangler WL and Culbertson MR (1991) Salivary gland disease in dogs and cats: 245 cases (1985–1988). Journal of the American Veterinary Medical Association **198**, 465–469

Yağci BB, Ural K, Ocal N et al. (2008) Azithromycin therapy of papillomatosis in dogs: a prospective, randomized, double-blinded, placebo-controlled clinical trial. Veterinary Dermatology **19**, 194–198

Useful websites

Comparative Neuromuscular Laboratory, UC San Diego, USA:
http://vetneuromuscular.ucsd.edu/

Dogwellnet:
https://dogwellnet.com/ctp/

Chapter 32

Oesophagus

Peter Kook

The oesophagus is a hollow muscular tube responsible for transporting liquid and ingesta from the oropharynx to the stomach. The majority of oesophageal disorders result in variable degrees of neuromuscular dysfunction and can be grouped into degenerative/idiopathic, inflammatory and immune-mediated diseases. Less common entities, such as endocrine disease, toxicities, congenital neurological dysfunctions and acquired brainstem disease, also manifest themselves clinically as motility disorders. The second group of oesophageal disorders comprises structural disorders causing obstruction, such as foreign bodies, vascular malformations, strictures and, rarely, neoplasia.

Structure and function

The oesophagus consists of the upper oesophageal sphincter (UOS), the tubular oesophageal body and the lower oesophageal sphincter (LOS). The entire length of the canine oesophagus is composed of striated muscle; the smooth muscle in the lamina muscularis mucosae does not contribute to peristalsis. Longitudinal mucosal folds are seen in the canine oesophagus (Figure 32.1a), whereas the distal one-third of the feline oesophagus is composed of both longitudinal and transverse smooth muscle, resulting in the characteristic herringbone pattern in cats (Figure 32.1b). The LOS, in turn, consists of smooth muscle. The lining of the oesophagus is a robust, stratified squamous epithelium, which terminates abruptly at the point of entry into the stomach, becoming a simple columnar lining.

Unlike most other parts of the gastrointestinal (GI) tract, coordinated motor function depends on an extrinsic nervous system: branches of the vagus nerve innervate the oesophagus. The neural coordination comprises somatic motor nerves from the nucleus ambiguus in the brainstem to the oesophageal striated muscle, autonomic nerves to the oesophageal smooth muscle and general visceral afferent nerves from the oesophageal sensory receptors. The act of swallowing consists of a series of sequential, well coordinated events that transport food and liquids from the oral cavity to the stomach and can be divided into the oropharyngeal, oesophageal and gastro-oesophageal phases (see Chapter 31). The oesophageal phase of swallowing begins with relaxation of the UOS, thus allowing the food bolus into the proximal oesophagus. The first peristaltic wave initiated in the pharynx carries the bolus further aborally. If the primary peristaltic wave is insufficient to

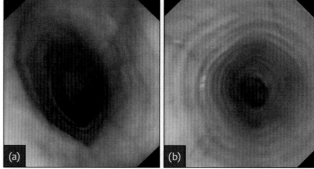

32.1 (a) Normal oesophagus of a healthy dog showing the typical longitudinal folds. (b) Normal oesophagus of a healthy cat. There are longitudinal and transverse folds from the level of the heart base distally. This combination of folds gives the characteristic herringbone pattern as seen on a barium swallow study.

propel the bolus into the stomach, a second wave is generated cranial to the bolus by oesophageal distension-sensitive receptors that complete the bolus transport. The LOS finally relaxes in advance of tubular oesophageal pressures and contracts again after the bolus has passed, thereby preventing reflux of gastric contents. The LOS resting pressure is maintained by two excitatory neural influences (vagal cholinergic, as well as non-vagal mechanisms mediated by alpha-adrenergic and cholinergic receptors). Baseline pressures vary in awake dogs between 14 and 45 mm Hg (median ≈ 30 mmHg) (Kempf et al., 2013; Kempf et al., 2014b), which is considerably higher than in humans.

Pathophysiology

Inflammation, dysmotility and obstruction are the major pathophysiological processes in the oesophagus of dogs and cats. These processes are often interwoven, and it can be difficult to readily recognize the primary mechanism. Any interference with the sensory reinforcement of the swallowing reflex can result in disordered oesophageal motor activity, illustrating why oesophageal inflammation in itself may also cause oesophageal hypomotility. This pathophysiological mechanism also applies to primary obstructive lesions such as lodged foreign bodies, and to congenital vascular ring anomalies that lead to adjacent oesophageal inflammation and hypomotility.

History

A careful history can help in differentiating clinical signs of oesophageal disease from oral, pharyngeal or GI disease, and can guide the clinician when selecting diagnostic tests for the individual patient. Before initiating testing, it should be ascertained that the patient is indeed regurgitating and not vomiting. Regurgitation is characterized by a passive retrograde and typically soundless expulsion of oesophageal contents (undigested food and liquids). The frequency and timing of regurgitation after feeding can vary considerably and can usually be differentiated from vomiting by the lack of forceful abdominal contractions. Also, the regurgitated material should not have a bilious (yellowish-green) appearance.

At times, it can be difficult to differentiate regurgitation from vomiting clearly, and some animals, particularly with oesophagitis, show both signs. Even though regurgitation is widely considered the clinical hallmark of oesophageal disease, dogs with oesophageal diseases may present with histories and clinical signs that may not be readily identified as being caused by oesophageal disease; these can include halitosis, licking surfaces, drooling, empty swallowing or gulping, lip-smacking, odynophagia (painful swallowing), belching, retching, or simply inappetence or anorexia. Depending on the cause and magnitude of additional oesophageal inflammation, vomiting may also be seen. Clinical signs of individual oesophageal disorders have not been evaluated in-depth so far, most likely because clinical signs can be overshadowed by the underlying primary disease. Respiratory clinical signs such as coughing and wheezing may be the major presenting sign in some animals that have developed aspiration pneumonia. Additional clinical signs detected in dogs with oesophageal disease might be weakness and gait abnormalities, pointing to polymyopathies, exercise intolerance with neuromuscular disease, GI signs with Addison's disease or, rarely, neurological signs with lead intoxication.

Physical examination

Results of the clinical examination are often normal in cats and dogs with oesophageal disease. Prolonged repeated regurgitation or anorexia may cause weight loss. Some animals with underlying neuromuscular disease may present with pronounced muscle weakness or wasting. Fever and pulmonary crackles identified during auscultation point to aspiration pneumonia. Crusty nares, dilated pupils, a distended urinary bladder and reduced anal tone can be found with dysautonomia. Concurrent skin lesions (alopecia, scaling) can be seen with underlying dermatomyositis. Occasionally, palpation of the cervical oesophagus may reveal a diverticulum (palpable food-filled pouch) or foreign body.

Laboratory tests

Even though primary oesophageal diseases are rarely associated with laboratory abnormalities, it is worthwhile to perform a routine haematology and serum biochemistry panel in order to exclude systemic or metabolic disease as a cause for secondary oesophageal clinical signs. In particular, serum creatine kinase activity should always be included in the database, as it can be a useful clue for an underlying primary myopathy. While an inflammatory leucogram may point to aspiration pneumonia, increased numbers of erythroid precursors (normoblasts) are indicative of lead toxicity. Hyponatraemia and hyperkalaemia may be seen in regurgitating dogs with hypoadrenocorticism and secondary oesophageal hypomotility, while in rare cases, hyperlipidaemia can be suggestive of underlying hypothyroidism.

Diagnostic imaging

Survey radiography of the thorax and the cervical part of the oesophagus should be performed in every patient suspected of having oesophageal disease. Radiography allows a definitive diagnosis for conditions such as radiopaque foreign bodies or persistent right aortic arch. A persistent right aortic arch is typically seen in young dogs that regurgitate after eating solid food and is usually associated with focal leftward deviation of the trachea near the cranial border of the heart in dorsoventral or ventrodorsal radiographs (Buchanan, 2004). Evidence in support of a diagnosis may also be found in cases of diverticula, other vascular anomalies or hiatal hernias with gastric prolapse. It should be noted that oesophageal dilatation can also be caused by excitement (panting), coughing, aerophagia/dyspnoea, general anaesthesia or persistent vomiting, although in these situations dilatation is normally mild. The degree of radiographic oesophageal dilatation is not helpful in differentiating idiopathic megaoesophagus from oesophageal dilatation secondary to an underlying primary disease. Thoracic radiographs will also identify potential complications of oesophageal disease, such as aspiration pneumonia, pneumomediastinum or pleural effusion.

Disorders not readily diagnosed by survey radiographs (i.e. radiolucent foreign bodies, diverticula, stricture, intramural masses) may be diagnosed with contrast radiographs. However, this technique is neither sensitive nor specific for diagnosing oesophagitis or gastro-oesophageal reflux. Videofluoroscopy and/or manometry are helpful in cases of suspected motility disorders, and oesophagoscopy is the diagnostic procedure of choice to examine the inner mucosal lining of the oesophagus, as well as to diagnose strictures, diverticula, foreign bodies and masses. Oesophagoscopy is also therapeutic in cases where foreign bodies can be removed or strictures can be dilated. In selected cases, endoscopic ultrasonography can help in assessing the extent of intramural oesophageal masses.

Inflammatory disorders of the oesophagus

Oesophagitis

Aetiology

Oesophagitis denotes a localized or diffuse inflammation of the oesophageal mucosa. It can occur after ingestion of hot food objects causing a thermal burn, but it is thought to result usually from a caustic or chemical injury. The most common scenario for increased oesophageal acid exposure in small animals is peri-anaesthetic reflux, with clinical signs usually beginning a couple of days post anaesthesia. Other causes are medication-induced oesophagitis, lodged foreign bodies, frequent vomiting, malpositioned oesophageal feeding tubes and distal oesophageal neoplasia. Cats appear particularly susceptible to pill-induced oesophagitis when receiving peroral medication, especially doxycycline hyclate or doxycycline hydrochloride formulations, as they are acidic in solution (Schulz *et al.*, 2013). Clindamycin has also been incriminated in cats. Thus, routine administration of a 5 ml water bolus to facilitate oesophageal clearance is recommended in this species (Westfall *et al.*, 2001). Spontaneous reflux oesophagitis due to LOS incompetence is frequently suspected based on a variety of clinical signs (see below); however, it is still controversial whether it truly is a disease in cats and dogs (Kook *et al.*, 2014). Reflux oesophagitis is seen secondary to hiatal hernias.

Diagnosis

Historical signs seen in cats and dogs with oesophagitis can comprise lip-smacking, odynophagia, increased empty swallowing motions, extension of the head and neck while swallowing, retching, vomiting, regurgitation, sudden unexplained discomfort, belching, drooling, excessive grass eating or surface licking, refusal to eat despite interest and halitosis. By extrapolation from humans, it is surmised that oesophagitis may also cause inflammatory airway disease and intermittent cough. Physical examination is mostly unremarkable, although salivation, laryngitis and tonsillitis may be detected.

Diagnostic imaging

Radiography is of limited use for the detection of oesophagitis; sometimes oesophageal air and fluid accumulation are noted. However, underlying foreign bodies, hiatal hernias, oesophageal dilatation, vascular ring anomalies or masses may be detected, and a pathological lung pattern may reflect aspiration injury to the lungs. Mediastinal or pleural air or liquid accumulation may indicate oesophageal perforation. Endoscopic examination is the most sensitive method to diagnose oesophagitis, but mild cases may appear normal on endoscopy, and mucosal biopsy will be necessary to confirm the suspicion. Biopsies are best performed with standard forceps manufactured for single use with working diameters >2 mm and ellipsoid cups with a spike or lancet. Due to the composition of the oesophageal mucosa with its tough stratified squamous epithelium, it can be difficult to obtain adequate oesophageal biopsy samples, but structural abnormalities can be found in biopsy samples comprising only the squamous epithelium and the lamina propria mucosae (Münster *et al.*, 2013, Münster *et al.*, 2017). Endoscopic signs include increased vascularity (Figures 32.2 and 32.3), as enlarged capillaries develop in response to acid near the mucosal surface. Mucosal striations with visible submucosal vascularity may be seen in the distal third of the oesophagus.

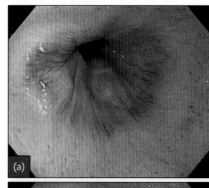
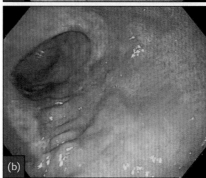

32.3 (a) Distal oesophagitis in a 12-year-old Labrador Retriever presented for halitosis and lip-smacking. (b) Gastric body and antrum with irregularly puckered and reddened mucosa. Histopathology of gastric biopsy samples revealed severe lymphocytic gastritis, but the diagnosis was ultimately confirmed as lymphoma.

Another common sign is increased granularity; the mucosal surface appears rough and puckered (Figure 32.4). Findings compatible with severe oesophagitis are areas of exudative pseudomembranes and ulcerated mucosa. Circular reddening just above the LOS should not be confused with the squamocolumnar junction (i.e. the demarcation line between the squamous oesophageal lining and the reddened columnar gastric lining), which should appear sharply delineated in cats and dogs (Figures 32.2 and 32.5). This is seen especially with oesophageal overinsufflation causing the LOS to be open.

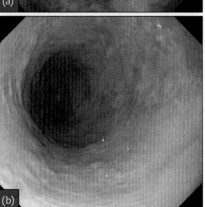
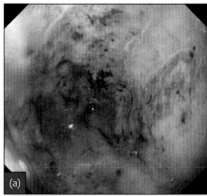

32.4 (a) Severe oesophagitis in a 7-year-old Husky. No cause was identified but there was suspicion of reflux oesophagitis. (b) The same case following treatment for 5 weeks with omeprazole at a dose of 1 mg/kg orally q12h. (Courtesy of M. Münster)

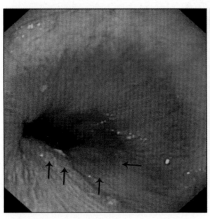

32.2 Distal oesophagitis in a 9-year-old Bernese Mountain Dog presented for a decreased appetite and lip-smacking. The gastro-oesophageal junction (Z-line), which marks the border between the oesophagus and the stomach, is denoted by the arrows.

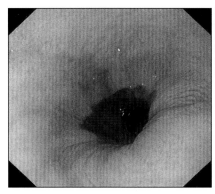

32.5 Sharp demarcation line (Z-line) between the oesophageal and reddened gastric mucosa in a dog.

In order to diagnose reflux oesophagitis definitively, wireless intraoesophageal pH-monitoring devices are available that can relatively easily be attached to the distal oesophageal mucosa (Figure 32.6) during oesophagoscopy, and oesophageal pH can be measured for up to 96 hours (Kook *et al.*, 2014). The main indication in dogs would be endoscopic evidence of oesophagitis without apparent causes (prior anaesthesia, foreign body, hiatal hernia). Because of the associated cost of this diagnostic approach, a therapeutic trial with proton pump inhibitors (e.g. omeprazole 1–1.5 mg/kg q12h over 3–4 weeks) seems a reasonable alternative.

Treatment

Treatment should ideally be directed at the underlying causes of the oesophagitis, and it is important to eliminate predisposing factors (e.g. oral medication). As anaesthesia is the most common time for oesophagitis to be initiated, it is desirable to prevent acid reflux in patients undergoing anaesthesia, especially in those that already have a history of anaesthesia-related oesophagitis. Pretreatment with high doses of metoclopramide yielded conflicting results, and the administration of ranitidine prior to surgery also did not reduce the incidence of gastro-oesophageal reflux (Wilson *et al.*, 2006; Favarato *et al.*, 2011). While preanaesthetic administration of cisapride and esomeprazole together decreased the number of reflux episodes in anaesthetized dogs in one study, administration of omeprazole alone was felt to be less effective, as it decreased only the acidity of refluxes but not the overall quantity of reflux episodes (Panti *et al.*, 2009; Zacuto *et al.*, 2012). A recent study in cats suggested pre-anaesthetic administration of two doses of omeprazole at higher than usual dosage orally (1.45–2.20 mg/kg) in order to significantly increase the gastric and oesophageal pH within 24 hours (Garcia *et al.* 2017).

The principle of increasing LOS pressure together with gastric acid suppression in order to prevent further injury and allow oesophageal healing is currently recommended

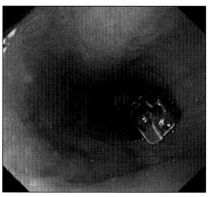

32.6 Capsule in the distal oesophagus for continuous recording of oesophageal pH in a dog with suspicion of reflux disease.

in the treatment of suspected reflux oesophagitis, because it has been shown that oesophageal inflammation in itself may cause oesophageal hypomotility. In cats, experimentally induced oesophagitis decreases oesophageal peristalsis, reduces LOS pressure and diminishes oesophageal clearance. These changes are reversible with the healing of the oesophagus (Zhang *et al.*, 2005). Contrary to common belief, orally administered metoclopramide did not result in significant changes in LOS pressure in dogs. Only cisapride administration significantly increased LOS pressure in a recent placebo-controlled study (Kempf *et al.*, 2014b). Because cisapride has been withdrawn from some national markets (see Chapter 28), available treatments for patients with suspected oesophagitis are generally limited to a combination of gastric acid suppression and sucralfate.

In dogs and cats, proton pump inhibitors (e.g. omeprazole) provide superior gastric acid suppression compared with H_2-receptor antagonists (e.g. ranitidine, famotidine) and should, therefore, be considered more effective for the treatment of acid-related disorders (Bersenas *et al.*, 2005; Tolbert *et al.*, 2011; Parkinson *et al.*, 2015; Šutalo *et al.*, 2015). While twice-daily dosing with omeprazole (1 mg/kg) is advised in order to maximize gastric acid suppression in more severe oesophagitis cases in dogs (Tolbert *et al.*, 2011), in cats omeprazole should routinely be administered twice daily (1 mg/kg), as once-daily dosing did not differ from placebo in a recent study (Šutalo *et al.*, 2015). Recent evidence showed that fractionated enteric-coated omeprazole tablets remain efficacious despite disruption of the enteric coating, allowing for more convenient, titratable dosing in small patients (Parkinson *et al.*, 2015).

Sucralfate, an aluminium salt of sulfated sucrose, is a mucosal protectant that binds to inflamed/ulcerated tissue to create a protective barrier. It is supposed to block diffusion of gastric acid and pepsin across the oesophageal mucosa and inhibit the erosive action of pepsin and possibly bile. Although the rationale for its effectiveness is based on its protective adherence to denuded mucosal surface in an acidic environment, whilst the canine oesophageal milieu is weakly alkaline, clinically it appears to soothe the patient's discomfort when dosed multiple times daily. In humans, intensive high-dose sucralfate therapy has been shown to be beneficial in enhancing mucosal healing and preventing stricture formation in advanced-grade corrosive oesophagitis (Gümürdülü *et al.*, 2010). In the UK, when sucralfate was unavailable, a homemade concoction of aluminium and magnesium hydroxide suspension (Maalox) at 0.5 ml/kg, mixed with 0.2 ml/kg of 2% lidocaine, known colloquially as 'Pink Lady', has anecdotally been helpful in oesophagitis.

Prognosis

Mild oesophagitis generally has a favourable prognosis, while cases of ulcerative (foreign body and pill-induced) oesophagitis may progress to stricture formation that will require dilation. It is difficult to foresee which cases will result in stricture, but generally the extent of mucosal damage is a good predictor (i.e. >180-degree lesions have a higher risk of forming a stricture).

Oesophageal fistula

Aetiology

Communication between the GI and respiratory systems can occur as a fistula. Both broncho-oesophageal and tracheo-oesophageal fistulae have been reported in the dog and cat, but they are rare. Most are acquired from penetrating foreign bodies rather than being congenital. Reported cases of broncho-oesophageal fistulae largely involved small breeds, and Miniature Poodles and terriers appear over-represented (Della Ripa *et al.*, 2010). Congenital oesophageal fistula may be seen more commonly in Cairn Terriers. In acquired cases, a traction diverticulum can develop at the site of the fistula because of the associated inflammatory reactions between the oesophagus and the airway. Histological criteria for identifying congenital broncho-oesophageal fistula in human infants are the presence of squamous or columnar epithelial lining that can be ciliated or non-ciliated, and lack of inflammation in tissue surrounding the fistula. In the dog, reported cases of congenital fistula have had epithelial lining as described above, but have also had inflammatory reaction surrounding them.

Clinical signs

Affected dogs present because of coughing that typically worsens after eating and drinking. Some dogs show regurgitation and anorexia. Concurrent pyrexia and dyspnoea may be seen in cases of concurrent pneumonia or pleuritis. Whilst clinical signs would be presumed to occur shortly after weaning in congenital cases, protracted courses of disease with a history of recurrent pneumonia lasting for months have also been described (Basher *et al.*, 1991; Nawrocki *et al.*, 2003).

Diagnostic imaging

Radiographically, focal densities are typically seen in the right caudal lung lobes, the oesophagus can be locally dilated and oesophageal foreign bodies can be trapped at the fistula site. Pleural fluid can also be present. Diagnosis has usually been accomplished by contrast radiography. The selection of contrast material should be decided based on the anticipated site of the fistula according to survey radiographs. A non-ionic aqueous iodine agent should be selected if mediastinal involvement is suspected due to iodine's low tissue reactivity. Barium suspension is preferred if communication with the bronchi is suspected because of its lower reactivity in airways. Contrast material will accumulate in the adjacent diverticulum and reflux into the bronchi. Small fistulae may be missed if contrast material does not readily enter the bronchus, and videofluoroscopy may be necessary. Bronchoscopic examination can help reveal the presence of an abnormal bronchial opening (Nawrocki *et al.*, 2003).

Treatment and prognosis

Surgical repair of the fistula and lung lobectomy are the most successful treatments for broncho-oesophageal fistula. Without secondary complications (e.g. pleuropneumonia, pulmonary abscessation), the prognosis has been described as good.

Oesophageal motility disorders

Megaoesophagus

Aetiology

The term megaoesophagus (MO) describes a syndrome of segmental or diffuse oesophageal dilatation. Congenital and acquired forms of the disorder have been described:

acquired MO is subclassified into idiopathic and secondary forms. Congenital and idiopathic acquired forms are suspected to result from a combination of neurological dysfunction within the afferent vagal arm of the swallowing reflex and insufficient vagal responsiveness to intraluminal oesophageal distension.

Secondary acquired MO can be caused by any disease interfering with oesophageal peristalsis. This can be due to disruption of central (e.g. brainstem disease) efferent or afferent neuronal pathways (e.g. lead or thallium toxicity, snake envenomation), or by diseases affecting the oesophageal musculature. While idiopathic acquired MO is the most common cause of regurgitation in dogs, it is a rare finding in cats, and an underlying disease can more often be identified in this species (Byron *et al.*, 2010; DeSandre-Robinson *et al.*, 2011; Schneider *et al.*, 2015).

Diagnosis

History and clinical signs: When regurgitation occurs in a puppy, congenital MO, vascular malformation (e.g. persistent right aortic arch) or a syndrome of delayed oesophageal maturation should be considered. In older animals with acquired MO, the timing and frequency of regurgitation are usually more variable. Weight loss and halitosis are also commonly reported by owners. Cough or fever and lethargy are suggestive of aspiration pneumonia.

Congenital megaoesophagus: The congenital form has been reported in Newfoundlands, Samoyeds, Springer Spaniels, Parson Russell Terriers and Miniature Schnauzers. Congenital MO is extremely rare in cats and has been suspected in a Siamese kitten. Congenital MO reported in Smooth Fox Terriers may be due to congenital myasthenia gravis (MG). An important differential diagnosis would be congenital hiatal hernia with secondary reflux oesophagitis – especially in predisposed breeds (Shar Pei, brachycephalic breeds). Even if the cause of the oesophageal hypomotility is as yet unclear in congenital MO, it has been speculated that this hypomotility is due to a delayed maturation of oesophageal function (Bexfield *et al.*, 2006). Some puppies presenting with regurgitation and radiographic evidence of a dilated oesophagus improve clinically over time when consistently fed in a vertical position (Figure 32.7).

At the author's clinic this phenomenon is seen in Berger Blanc Suisse, Irish Setters, Labrador Retrievers and German Shepherd Dogs. Interestingly, the author and colleagues have documented continuous improvement in oesophageal function via high-resolution manometry, accompanied by improvement in clinical signs but no radiographic normalization. Currently, the only way to find out whether a puppy with evidence of oesophageal hypomotility will improve clinically or not, is to strictly feed and keep the dog after each meal for 20–30 minutes in a fixed vertical position and monitor over time. Results of a study on associations of clinical features with outcome in dogs with generalized MO were encouraging insofar as age at the onset of clinical signs (regurgitation) was significantly associated with survival time. Young dogs (<13 months) were more likely to survive (McBrearty *et al.*, 2011). Ongoing oesophageal maturation and resulting improvement in clinical signs was thought to reduce risk of death in young dogs.

Concurrent generalized weakness that cannot be explained by pneumonia may be indicative of congenital MG. These dogs have a deficiency or functional abnormality of acetylcholine receptors at the motor endplate and the prognosis is usually poor. A recent study evaluated the

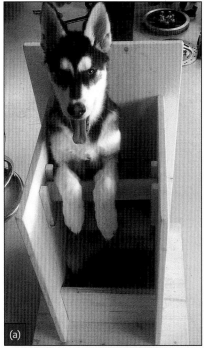

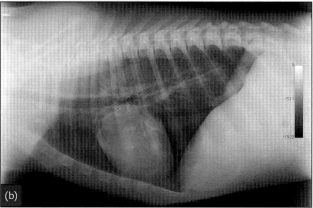

32.7 (a) A 3-month-old Husky/Berger Blanc Suisse crossbreed dog, presented with regurgitation and failure to thrive, in a Bailey chair. (b) Radiography revealed generalized megaoesophagus. Gradual normalization of bolus transport and oesophageal function was noted over time on high-resolution manometry, and the dog stopped regurgitating, but the oesophagus continued to appear dilated on radiography. At 17 months, the dog could be fed normally, manometric evaluation was near normal, however on radiographs the oesophagus was still dilated.

therapeutic efficacy of sildenafil (1 mg/kg q12h) in dogs with congenital MO, on the premise that a decreased LOS tone would facilitate the entry of the ingesta into the stomach. Sildenafil ameliorated clinical and radiographic signs in these patients by reducing the LOS tone. This could represent a novel therapeutic tool for the treatment of this disease (Quintavalla *et al.*, 2017).

Acquired megaoesophagus: Most cases of adult-onset MO have no known aetiology and are referred to as acquired idiopathic MO. The syndrome occurs spontaneously in middle-aged to old (7–15 years old) dogs. Any breed can be affected, although large and giant breed dogs, especially Golden Retrievers and German Shepherd Dogs, have an increased prevalence. Acquired idiopathic MO is a frustrating disease because treatment is limited to supportive and symptomatic care. Thus, attempts should be made to rule out possible underlying neuromuscular, immune-mediated, endocrine, paraneoplastic and toxic diseases. MG is the

most important differential diagnosis, and some cases of MG present only with regurgitation without generalized muscle weakness.

The second largest group comprises generalized neuromuscular diseases (myositis, dystrophic polymyopathies and degenerative neuropathies). This disease category is particularly important in dogs because the canine oesophagus is predominantly composed of striated muscle. Approximately 14% of dogs with generalized inflammatory myopathies present with MO (Evans *et al.*, 2004). In most acquired secondary cases, regurgitation is only one of many clinical signs (Figure 32.8). For example, patients with organophosphate poisoning may regurgitate and have radiographic evidence of oesophageal dilatation, but will also show signs of a cholinergic crisis (such as salivation, lacrimation, defecation and urination). Dogs with generalized tetanus and oesophageal dysfunction will have a stiff gait and risus sardonicus, whereas dogs with dermatomyositis and MO will regurgitate but also show multifocal alopecia and ulcerative skin disease (Bresciani *et al.*, 2014). In recent years, outbreaks of acquired MO in association with a peripheral neuropathy have been reported in both Latvia and Australia. There is a suspicion that these disease clusters relate to pet food contamination with an unknown toxin.

Acquired secondary MO has also been associated with a variety of miscellaneous conditions. Even though these diagnoses are only sporadically associated with MO, they should be investigated so as not to miss a potentially treatable cause. Hypoadrenocorticism and hypothyroidism can be associated with reversible MO. The oesophageal hypomotility rarely seen in hypoadrenocorticism patients is most likely due to oesophageal muscular glycogen depletion secondary to cortisol deficiency. In fact, the majority of reported cases were due to glucocorticoid-deficient hypoadrenocorticism, and the underlying disease might be missed if no further testing (e.g. baseline cortisol concentration, adrenocorticotropic hormone stimulation test) is pursued due to the presence of normal electrolytes. The association between MO and hypothyroidism is still controversial. However, complete resolution of clinical and radiographic signs has been reported in single cases (Fracassi and Tamborini, 2011). Because aspiration pneumonia may cause euthyroid sick syndrome, while a normal serum thyroxine concentration rules out hypothyroidism, a low value potentially reflecting hypothyroidism should be backed up by evaluation of serum canine thyroid-stimulating hormone (cTSH) with thyroxine, free thyroxine (T4), or a TSH stimulation test.

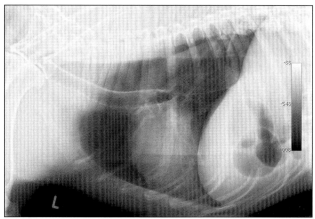

32.8 Lateral radiograph of a 12-year-old female neutered Boxer presented with regurgitation. Extensive investigation revealed a degenerative (demyelinating) neuropathy.

Oesophageal neoplasia, especially when located more distally within the caudal oesophagus, may mimic MO (Kook *et al.*, 2009; Arnell *et al.*, 2013). Although carcinoma and sarcoma carry a poor prognosis, it should be noted that oesophageal leiomyoma (Figure 32.9) can be completely excised and dogs can fully recover (Arnell *et al.*, 2013). Achalasia, the best defined oesophageal motility disorder in humans, characterized by the absence of distal oesophageal peristalsis and inadequate LOS relaxation, was often suspected to be responsible for cases of (presumably idiopathic) MO in the older literature. However, true achalasia has been documented convincingly recently in only one dog presenting with MO so far, and should be considered a rare cause of MO (Kempf *et al.*, 2014a). Successful response to botulinum toxin injection into the LOS and mechanical dilation has recently been described in regurgitating dogs that had fluoroscopic evidence of delayed, or even failed, opening of the LOS (Grobman *et al.*, 2019). Rarely, intermittent regurgitation and transient radiographic oesophageal dilatation in older dogs can be subtle first hints for underlying brainstem disease (e.g. neoplasia) (Figure 32.10). The space-occupying lesions interfere with the vagal neuromuscular reflex arc necessary for the swallowing process.

Laboratory tests: A complete blood count, serum biochemistry panel that includes creatine kinase activity and urinalysis should be performed in all regurgitating patients, especially in cases where MO is suspected. In addition, an acetylcholine receptor antibody test should

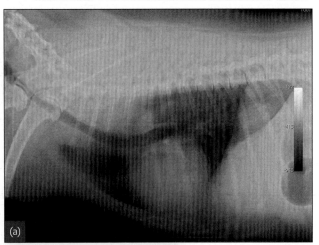

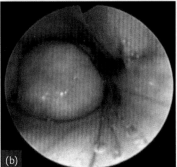

32.9 A 12-year-old male neutered Labrador Retriever was presented with acute vomiting and retching. (a) A lateral radiograph revealed an ill-defined soft tissue space-occupying lesion in the cranial mediastinum dorsal to the trachea. Note the displacement of the trachea ventrally and the accumulation of gas cranial to the lesion. There is mild narrowing of the intrathoracic trachea. The cardiac silhouette is of normal size and the pulmonary vessels are at the lower limit of normal size. (b) Endoscopic view of the mass. Histopathology confirmed a leiomyoma.

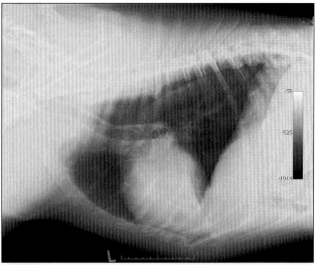

32.10 Lateral thoracic radiograph of a dog showing moderate megaoesophagus and aerophagia and an associated severe interstitial pattern in the right middle lung lobe and a mild interstitial pattern in the right cranial lung lobe. A large intracranial extra-axial space-occupying lesion was identified in the pons and myelencephalon on magnetic resonance imaging. The diagnosis of meningothelial meningioma and multifocal to diffuse non-purulent meningitis was confirmed at post-mortem examination.

be performed in all cases of acquired MO, as it is the most commonly identified underlying disease. A baseline cortisol concentration is helpful to rule out Addison's disease, which is less likely; measurement of thyroxine/canine thyroid-stimulating hormone is indicated in dogs with suspicion of hypothyroidism.

Diagnostic imaging: Survey radiography is diagnostic for most cases of MO, and causes such as vascular ring anomalies, foreign bodies, neoplasia or hiatal hernia can be detected. The concurrent finding of a distended GI tract or urinary bladder should raise suspicion for dysautonomia. A barium contrast oesophagogram is rarely indicated, but may help highlight the presence of either an intraluminal mass or obstructive lesion. Its benefit should be weighed against the risk for aspirating contrast agent. Fluoroscopy evaluates pharyngeal and oesophageal peristalsis but is not essential for the diagnosis of MO, although it can be helpful in rare cases of oesophageal achalasia when manometry is not available (Kempf *et al.*, 2014a). The decision as to whether to perform oesophagoscopy is difficult, but in rare cases treatable oesophagitis or obstructive disease, such as leiomyoma, may be found. Oesophagoscopy cannot differentiate the type of underlying vascular ring anomaly, whereas computed tomography angiography is ideal for this purpose.

Treatment

Treatment for acquired idiopathic MO is largely supportive with the objective of meeting the caloric needs of the patient and minimizing regurgitation. While periodic thoracic radiographs can help to evaluate possible aspiration pneumonia and oesophageal foreign bodies, which idiopathic MO patients may be predisposed to as most have a ravenous appetite and are not fastidious eaters, following the progression of oesophageal dilatation has no prognostic value.

Managing feedings and assuring adequate caloric intake can be difficult for owners (especially with large dogs). Specially made feeding chairs (Bailey Chair, see

Figure 32.7) minimize the client's frustration: only when the patient is in a vertical position can gravity effectively help move food into the stomach. Currently, the best diet consistency and ideal duration of time needed for upright feeding in dogs with MO is unknown. It is recommended to keep the patient in a vertical position for at least 20–30 minutes after feeding. In some patients, food in a meatball consistency may facilitate quicker oesophageal transit, and individual experimentation is generally encouraged. Anecdotal case reports suggest that dogs with dedicated owners can live long and active lives with appropriate management. In weak and debilitated patients (i.e. at risk of aspiration), feeding through a gastrostomy tube may be indicated (see *BSAVA Manual of Endoscopy and Endosurgery*). Low-profile gastrostomy tubes (Figure 32.11) can be effective long term (e.g. years) in some patients (Yoshimoto *et al.*, 2006). However, gastrostomy tubes

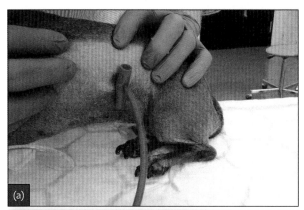

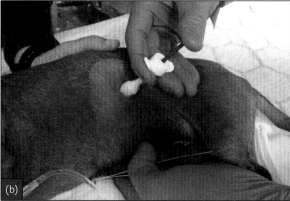

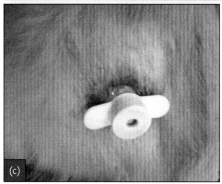

| 32.11 | Low-profile gastrostomy tube. (a) A normal percutaneous endoscopic gastrostomy (PEG) tube is in place initially and has created a stoma. (b) The PEG tube has been removed and is being replaced by a low-profile gastrostomy tube inserted through the stoma. (c) A low-profile gastrostomy tube is in place for long-term feeding in a Golden Retriever with idiopathic megaoesophagus which could not be managed otherwise. The patient lived for 3.5 years with no incidents of aspiration pneumonia. The tube had to be replaced approximately every 9 months due to valve leakage.

cannot be regarded as a universal remedy because, unpredictably, some dogs will continue to regurgitate even with tube feeding. These are the dogs that develop massive accumulation of mucoid fluid from inflamed oesophageal mucus glands to a degree that regular suctioning of the mucus is required. Promotility drugs (metoclopramide, cisapride) that act on smooth muscle have no benefit in the management of canine MO, but may be beneficial in cats with MO, because the distal third of the feline oesophagus is composed of smooth muscle. Cisapride would in fact be contraindicated in canine MO patients, as it increases LOS pressure (Kempf *et al.*, 2013), an undesirable effect as it may interfere with oesophageal emptying.

Treatment of acquired secondary MO is based on a definitive diagnosis. For example, dogs with MG are treated with pyridostigmine or with immunosuppressive drugs (e.g. azathioprine, ciclosporin, mycophenolate) if the condition is not satisfactorily controlled with anticholinesterase therapy alone. Corticosteroids have the potential to worsen muscular weakness, and clinical deterioration may occur by commencing with immunosuppressive doses, and lower doses are generally recommended. Spontaneous remission may occur (Shelton, 2014), and there is no evidence for efficacy of mycophenolate (Dewey *et al.*, 2010).

Prognosis

The prognosis depends on the underlying aetiology, the presence of complications such as pneumonia and malnutrition and, most notably, on the owner's dedication and commitment. Congenital MO carries a guarded prognosis; however, supportive treatment should always be tried, as it is impossible to predict future oesophageal motility at the time of diagnosis. Improvement of oesophageal motility with maturity up to 1 year has been demonstrated (Bexfield *et al.*, 2006). This is also reflected in a higher overall survival time in dogs with onset of clinical signs at a young age (McBrearty *et al.*, 2011). Acquired idiopathic MO is a devastating disease, carrying a guarded to poor prognosis. In recent studies from Scotland and Germany, the outcome in dogs with generalized MO was a median survival time of 90 days from the time of diagnosis and almost 27% died before discharge (McBrearty *et al.*, 2011; Schönfelder *et al.*, 2011). The prognosis for MO secondary to MG can be good with early diagnosis and appropriate treatment (Shelton, 2014), and if dogs survive the initial month following onset of clinical signs, chances are good for spontaneous remission. Clinical improvement of oesophageal function is also commonly seen with polymyositis cases, underlining the value of taking muscle biopsy samples early in the course of the disease.

Hiatal hernia
Aetiology

Hiatal hernia is defined as the protrusion of abdominal contents through the oesophageal hiatus of the diaphragm into the thorax. Two types of hiatal hernia have been described in dogs and cats:

- Type I (sliding axial hernia), in which the abdominal segment of the oesophagus and parts of the stomach are displaced cranially into the caudal mediastinum. Type I hiatal hernias can be intermittent, complicating definitive diagnosis. It is most commonly found in puppies and young dogs and cats (congenital form), with Chinese Shar Peis, English and French Bulldogs, as well as Boston Terriers and Pugs being the most commonly affected breeds (Sivacolundhu *et al.*, 2002). The congenital form is the result of incomplete closure of the diaphragm during embryonic development and the acquired form of type I hiatal hernia results from traumatic events or in association with severe upper respiratory obstruction, including brachycephalic obstructive airway syndrome and laryngeal paralysis

- Type II (paraoesophageal hiatal hernia), in which the gastro-oesophageal junction remains in place, but the fundus slides through the hiatus into the thorax. Type II is less frequently found than type I.

Diagnosis

Clinical signs: Dogs and cats with hiatal hernia present with regurgitation, hypersalivation, vomiting, odynophagia and, sometimes, in cases of congenital hiatal hernia, with slow growth. These signs can be mistaken for MO, but it is very likely that the associated oesophageal hypomotility (and radiographically visible mild MO) results from reflux oesophagitis secondary to a reduced LOS tone. Respiratory signs indicate brachycephalic obstructive airway syndrome (BOAS) or aspiration (tracheitis and/or pneumonia). In dogs and cats with acquired hiatal hernia, clinical signs are similar but usually more discrete and intermittent. Inspiratory stridor can be found with laryngeal paralysis.

Diagnostic imaging: Diagnosis is based on plain thoracic radiographs and barium oesophagogram, with fluoroscopy facilitating detection of intermittent herniation in most cases. Definitive diagnosis is based on the presence of a caudodorsal, often oval, intrathoracic gas- or fluid-filled, soft tissue opacity. Although hiatal hernia can present with concurrent MO, the radiographic dilatation is usually mild and the oesophagus can also be normal. In rare cases of a marked dilatation, a misdiagnosis of congenital MO can be made if hiatal herniation is not readily apparent. Endoscopy allows evaluation for concurrent oesophagitis and sliding hernias may be visualized, particularly if the endotracheal tube is occluded for three breaths, provoking herniation and/or reflux (Broux *et al.*, 2016).

Treatment

The two main treatment options are medical therapy and surgery. Medical therapy is recommended initially and includes prokinetics (metoclopramide or, preferably, cisapride if available), gastric acid suppressants (e.g., omeprazole) and a cytoprotective agent (i.e. sucralfate). Feeding small amounts of a low-fat diet in a vertical position may also help. The goal of medical management is to resolve reflux oesophagitis and associated MO. Surgical management involves several stabilization procedures, including left fundic gastropexy, oesophagopexy, fundoplication and oesophageal hiatus plication (phrenoplasty). Early surgical intervention is recommended in Shar Peis with congenital hiatal hernia (Guiot *et al.*, 2008). In cases of acquired intermittent axial hernia, the primary intent is to treat the underlying cause (e.g. surgical treatment of BOAS or laryngeal paralysis), together with treatment for reflux oesophagitis.

Dysautonomia
Aetiology

Dysautonomia is a sporadic idiopathic disease that results in a progressive clinical disease of the autonomic nervous system. Dysfunction or failure of the sympathetic and parasympathetic nervous systems is due to chromatolytic degeneration of the autonomic nervous ganglia. First reported in cats in the 1980s in the UK, it has now been reported worldwide in dogs and cats. To date, most reported feline cases have occurred in the UK and Scandinavia. Residence in rural areas has been identified as a risk factor, possibly suggesting an association with rainfall. However, the exact cause is unknown, and auto-immunity, environmental toxins and microorganisms or biotoxins are suspected.

Diagnosis

Clinical signs: Commonly reported clinical findings, due to widespread degeneration of neurons, include depression, anorexia, dysphagia, regurgitation or vomiting, constipation, dilated unresponsive pupils, prolapsed nictitating membranes, dry mucous membranes, reduced lacrimation, bradycardia (fixed heart rate), MO, absent or reduced anal tone, and distended urinary bladder. The frequency and severity of MO varies between reports from common to rare (Kidder *et al.*, 2008; Novellas *et al.*, 2010). A clinical diagnosis is made in most cases based on anamnestic and clinical findings. Autonomic nervous system function tests that can be performed in practice comprise: Schirmer tear testing, local administration of diluted pilocarpine ophthalmic solution, atropine response test and histamine response test. A definitive diagnosis is based upon demonstration of characteristic histological lesions in the autonomic ganglia.

Treatment

No definitive therapy is currently available. Supportive care comprises elevated feeding, artificial tears, expressing the urinary bladder, antacids, antibiotics and prokinetics (ideally cisapride). Gastrostomy tube feeding may bridge the gap until neurological recovery occurs in some animals.

Prognosis

Dysautonomia typically carries a grave prognosis, and recovery rates are lower in dogs than cats. In a study of 40 cats, complete resolution occurred in about 25% of affected cats and partial recovery was noted in some cats. Mildly affected dogs (with dysuria as the only major clinical sign) without GI signs may have a better prognosis.

Oesophageal diverticula
Aetiology

Oesophageal diverticula are pouch-like sacculations of the oesophageal wall. Depending on their size, they can interfere with the orderly movement of ingesta through the oesophagus. Generally, diverticula are rare in small animals. Both congenital and acquired forms have been reported. Congenital diverticula are caused by developmental abnormalities involving broncho-pulmonary-foregut malformations. Acquired oesophageal diverticula can be divided into traction or pulsion diverticula.

- Traction diverticula are very rare and are caused by cervical soft tissue or mediastinal disease secondarily affecting the oesophagus. Perioesophageal inflammation leads to fibrosis and contraction, thereby pulling the oesophageal wall out, forming a pouch.

- Pulsion diverticula are caused by disorders within the oesophagus that increase intraluminal pressure, such as obstruction by strictures or foreign bodies (e.g. trichobezoars) (Durocher *et al.*, 2009), or food impaction associated with hypomotility or oesophagitis. A more common example for pulsion diverticula would be the development of pouch-like lesions cranial to the heart base in cases of vascular ring anomalies.

Diagnosis

Clinical signs: Clinical signs noted in oesophageal diverticula cases do not differ from clinical signs associated with other oesophageal disorders and include regurgitation, halitosis, odynophagia and retching. Smaller diverticula may be incidental findings not associated with clinical signs. Cervical diverticula can be palpated when filled with food feeling like a goitre (Figure 32.12).

Diagnostic imaging: Diverticula can be identified radiographically, endoscopically or fluoroscopically (Figure 32.13). Thoracic radiographs show the air-, fluid- or food-filled oesophageal sacculation or pouching, and contrast radiography demonstrates pooling of barium in the diverticulum. Confusion with a mediastinal mass is possible when the diverticulum is of soft tissue opacity (i.e. fluid-filled). Diverticula are usually seen in the cranial mediastinal and epiphrenic regions of the oesophagus. Oesophagoscopy reveals a sac-like outpouching of the oesophageal lumen, often with erosive oesophagitis of the mucosa lining the diverticulum. Food, fluid or hair may have to be removed from the diverticulum before it can be adequately visualized. If a diverticulum is small, the only obvious finding may be a focal pooling of fluid. Because of the thin diverticular

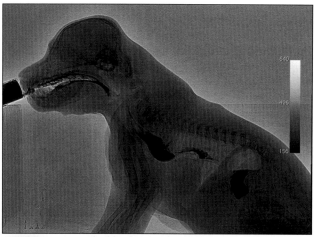

32.13 A 2.5-month-old male Labrador Retriever was presented with regurgitation. Fluoroscopy revealed precardial formation of oesophageal diverticula and raised suspicion of a persistent right aortic arch (which was confirmed at surgery). The patient did well following surgery.

wall, caution must be used to avoid perforation during oesophagoscopy. Whenever an acquired diverticulum is identified, the patient should be carefully evaluated for an underlying cause. A redundant flexure or deviation of the oesophagus at the thoracic inlet seen on radiographs or fluoroscopy is a common incidental finding in clinically normal brachycephalic and Shar Pei dogs and should not be mistaken for a diverticulum. These false diverticula lack pooling of food and fluid and decrease or even disappear with extension of the neck.

Treatment

Surgical excision and reconstruction of the oesophageal wall are the preferred treatment methods for diverticula in humans. Small diverticula can be managed conservatively with measures that minimize the likelihood of food impaction, such as feeding a liquid or semi-liquid diet. In cats, trichobezoar prevention is recommended.

Prognosis

Even with conservative management, continuous food impaction may cause small diverticula to enlarge, ultimately necessitating surgery. As diverticula may be a sequela of idiopathic oesophageal hypomotility disorders, owners should be advised that dysmotility may persist after surgery. Also, stricture formation after corrective surgery must be considered.

Oesophageal obstructions

Oesophageal stricture

Oesophageal stricture is an abnormal narrowing of the oesophageal lumen. Congenital strictures in the form of a fibrous narrowing orad to the gastro-oesophageal junction have been described in kittens (Schneider *et al.*, 2015), and in the form of a stricturing membranous web in puppies (Fox *et al.*, 2007). Congenital strictures can be misdiagnosed as congenital MO if oesophagoscopy is not performed in these cases. Aetiologies of acquired benign strictures are chemical or thermal injury from swallowed substances, mechanical pressure from lodged foreign bodies, oesophageal surgery and, less commonly, intra- or

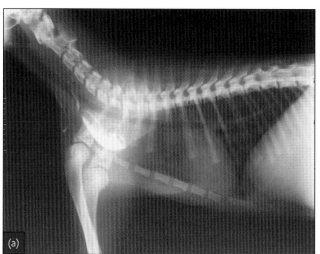

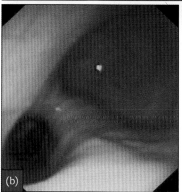

32.12 A food-filled diverticulum could be palpated on extension of the neck in a 6-month-old Maine Coon kitten. (a) A lateral thoracic radiograph reveals focal oesophageal dilatation with accumulation of contrast material in the area of the thoracic inlet. (b) Endoscopic view of the diverticulum (top right) and normal oesophagus (lower left).

extraluminal mass lesions (abscesses, *Spirocerca lupi* granuloma). Anaesthesia-related gastro-oesophageal reflux may cause oesophagitis and subsequent stricture formation in animals with LOS weakness. Cats may be more susceptible to doxycycline hyclate or hydrochloride-associated oesophagitis and stricture. Doxycycline monohydrate does not cause this problem. Usually, oesophageal neoplasia does not lead to classical stricture formation *per se*, but luminal mass compression can ultimately cause oesophageal stenosis with the same clinical effect.

Diagnosis

Clinical signs: The severity of clinical signs (regurgitation, dysphagia) is related to the severity, location (cervical *versus* thoracic) and extent of the stricture. Most animals have a ravenous appetite and may attempt to re-ingest the regurgitated material, and liquid food is often better tolerated. With progressive oesophageal narrowing, aspiration pneumonia may develop.

Diagnostic imaging: Thoracic radiographs are usually normal in animals with benign fibrosing strictures. There may be oesophageal dilatation and or fluid/food accumulation cranial to the stricture, and cases with distal strictures may, thus, be misdiagnosed as MO if contrast radiography or oesophagoscopy are not performed. Endoscopy should be performed in order to assess the site and the severity of the stricture (Figure 32.14) and also to examine for intraluminal neoplasia. Care should be taken not to overlook partial stricture formation (Figure 32.15), as some animals may present with regurgitation due to pooling of food in pouch-like sacculations cranial to such a partial stricture.

Treatment

In mild or partial strictures, semi-liquid feeding may be sufficient to control clinical signs. In cases of severe strictures, feeding by means of a temporary gastrostomy tube may be necessary to provide adequate nutrition. Oesophageal strictures are best managed with mechanical dilation. This can be achieved through ballooning and bougienage. Balloon dilation is performed with a catheter involving an inflatable balloon. The balloon is positioned in the stricture and then expanded with fluid. Often, multiple dilations are needed at 4–7-day intervals, until the stricture orifice is increased sufficiently. Bougienage involves the use of rigid instruments of different diameters pushed longitudinally through the narrow point. Because it allows more force to be applied to the stricture, bougienage seems most appropriate for tough, fibrous strictures, or strictures so small that balloons cannot be inserted through them (Bissett *et al.*, 2009). Some clinicians administer corticosteroids to inhibit fibroblastic proliferation and contraction associated with healing in order to avoid stricture re-formation. Generally, oral corticosteroids are not considered effective, and endoscopically guided submucosal triamcinolone injections at the stricture site prior to ballooning are likely to be effective for preventing stricture reformation (Mayer-Roenne *et al.*, 2009), but controlled studies are lacking. Thoracic radiographs should be performed after difficult procedures, or if there is evidence of respiratory compromise, to check for pneumomediastinum secondary to oesophageal tearing. Feeding with a liquid diet can be initiated 24 hours after a dilation procedure. All animals with oesophagitis or distal strictures post dilation should be treated with proton pump inhibitors, cisapride (if available) and sucralfate. Surgical resection of oesophageal strictures should be considered the last resort. These invasive procedures are complicated by difficult surgical exposure, tension on the anastomosis and poor healing properties of the thoracic oesophagus. Oesophageal stenting has recently been described for the treatment of refractory benign oesophageal strictures in dogs, but was found to be associated with a high complication rate and poor long-term success for the majority of dogs (Lam *et al.*, 2013).

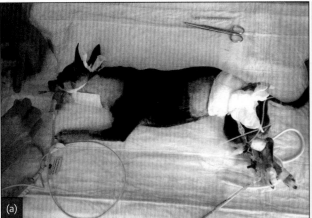
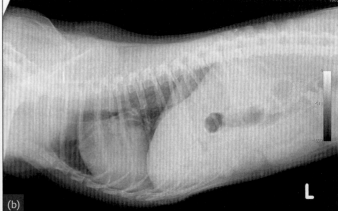
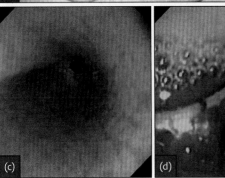
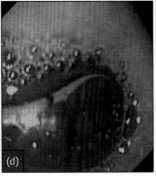

32.14 (a) A 12-year-old Chihuahua presented with regurgitation due to the presence of a bony foreign body. (b) Lateral radiograph showing the foreign body at the level of the second intercostal space. Following surgery, a percutaneous endoscopic gastrostomy tube was placed in the hope that the oesophagus would heal without stricture formation. (c) The dog, presented 2 weeks later with recurring regurgitation and a stricture over the heart base was diagnosed on endoscopy. Note the presence of inflamed oesophageal mucosa proximal to the stricture. (d) A balloon dilation procedure was performed using a 15 mm diameter balloon. A second ballooning procedure was performed 2 weeks later and the outcome for the patient was good.

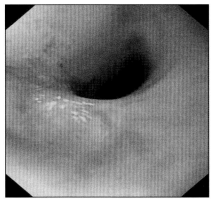

32.15 A 10-year-old female neutered Cavalier King Charles Spaniel presented with a partial stricture in the mid-thoracic oesophagus following removal of a foreign body. Food collected proximal to the partial stricture and ultimately caused regurgitation. The dog improved after two balloon dilation procedures.

Prognosis

Pet owners should be advised that strictures can recur despite multiple dilation procedures. The major complication is oesophageal perforation, which usually occurs at the time of dilation. Rarely, perforation occurs several days afterwards.

Oesophageal neoplasia
Aetiology

Primary oesophageal tumours are rare in cats and dogs. The most common tumour types include squamous cell carcinoma (Figure 32.16), leiomyosarcoma, leiomyoma, fibrosarcoma and osteosarcoma. Adenomatous polyps have also been reported in the distal oesophagus (Gibson *et al.*, 2010). In dogs, sarcomas can also develop secondary to *Spirocerca lupi* infection in indigenous areas. Oesophageal lymphoma in cats is very rare. Other paraoesophageal tumours involving the heart base, thymus or thyroid glands may invade the oesophagus. Oesophageal metastasis can occur but it is rare.

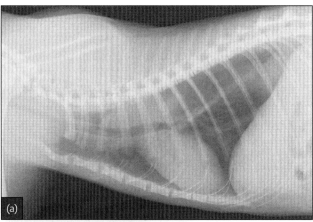

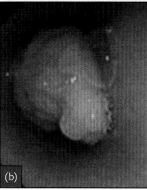

32.16 A 10-year-old male neutered Domestic Shorthaired cat presented with chronic vomiting, lethargy, hypersalivation and lip-smacking. (a) A lateral radiograph revealed a soft tissue mass in the dorsal heart base, extending cranially to the third thoracic vertebra, demarcated by oesophageal gas accumulation. Note also the mild tracheal deviation and fluid in the caudal oesophagus. (b) Endoscopic view of the mass. Squamous cell carcinoma was confirmed on histology at post-mortem examination.

Diagnosis

Clinical signs: Primary clinical signs comprise regurgitation, dysphagia, halitosis, odynophagia, vomiting and weight loss. Some dogs present with an acute onset of clinical signs but large lumen-occluding tumours have already developed (see Figure 32.9). Physical examination is mostly normal or can merely reveal weight loss. Cervical oesophageal neoplasia can sometimes be palpated.

Diagnostic imaging: Depending on the tumour size, oesophageal masses may be readily apparent on plain radiographs. Identification of an oesophageal mass may be hindered by fluid accumulating proximal to it. Similarly, air is often retained within the oesophageal lumen cranial to the tumour, and both segmental and complete dilatation of the oesophagus are possible sequelae (Kook *et al.*, 2009; Arnell *et al.*, 2013), illustrating why these cases can be mistaken for idiopathic MO if endoscopy (Figure 32.16) (Kook *et al.*, 2009) is not performed. Oesophagoscopy has the additional advantage of differentiating masses from strictures or foreign bodies, can assess the extent of concurrent oesophagitis, especially with masses just orad to the gastro-oesophageal sphincter, and offers the possibility of mucosal biopsy. However, with non-ulcerated intramural masses (especially leiomyoma) results of biopsies are often too superficial to be diagnostic.

Treatment

Benign oesophageal masses (e.g. leiomyoma) generally have a favourable prognosis following surgical resection (Arnell *et al.*, 2013). Osteo- and fibrosarcoma associated with *Spirocerca lupi* infection have recently been shown to be amenable to transendoscopic laser or electrocauterization. Transendoscopic mass ablation was feasible, and was associated with low complication rates, high perioperative survival and a survival time comparable to that of dogs undergoing tumour excision via open thoracic surgery (Shipov *et al.*, 2015). Radiation therapy, chemotherapy or multimodality therapy are possible palliative treatments, however no data have been published.

Oesophageal foreign bodies
Aetiology

Lodged oesophageal foreign bodies are a frequent clinical problem in dogs and cats that can have serious consequences in terms of morbidity and mortality, as well as cost. They should always be considered an emergency and immediate removal should be pursued. The severity of oesophageal mucosal damage is dependent upon size and composition of the foreign body and on the duration of the obstruction. Although angular and sharply pointed foreign bodies are intuitively considered detrimental, wedged foreign bodies with diffuse mucosal contact with the oesophagus further increase the tightness of the impaction. The pressures that the foreign body exerts on the oesophageal wall may ultimately cause pressure necrosis and perforation, requiring immediate surgical management. Terrier breeds, and specifically West Highland White Terriers, are at increased risk for oesophageal foreign bodies (Figure 32.17). This has been a consistent finding in multiple studies throughout the past 50 years (Gianella *et al.*, 2009; Juvet *et al.*, 2010; Jankowski *et al.*, 2013; Deroy *et al.*, 2015). It is likely that some form of as yet undefined occult oesophageal dysmotility puts dogs of terrier breeds at risk for oesophageal foreign bodies (Bexfield *et al.*, 2006).

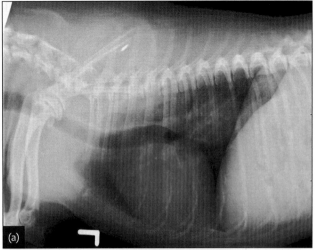

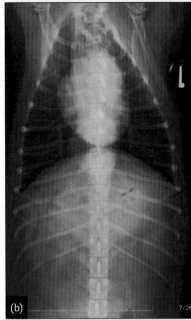

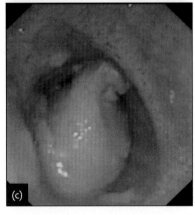

32.17 (a) Lateral and (b) ventrodorsal views of a 7-year-old West Highland White Terrier presented with acute foreign body ingestion. (c) Endoscopy revealed a boiled potato that the dog had ingested before it was mashed.

Diagnosis

Clinical signs: The diagnosis is straightforward in cases where foreign body ingestion has been witnessed. The more difficult presentations are dogs or cats where foreign body ingestion went unnoticed and the only clinical signs are anorexia and apathy. The onset and severity of regurgitation depends on the extent of oesophageal obstruction. Animals with complete obstruction present with acute regurgitation, whereas animals with partial obstruction (particularly pieces of lamb vertebrae) may be presented with signs of several days' duration. Generally, typical clinical signs include regurgitation, odynophagia, tachypnoea, drooling and anorexia.

Diagnostic imaging: Because most foreign bodies become lodged in the thoracic oesophagus (distal oesophagus> heart base> thoracic inlet), definitive diagnosis requires radiography. Rarely, radiolucent foreign bodies require contrast radiography, although ultimately oesophagoscopy is needed to confirm and, ideally, remove the foreign body. In a recent study, radiographic findings were not helpful in predicting the success of endoscopic removal (Juvet *et al.*, 2010).

Treatment

An oesophageal foreign body should be removed as soon as possible. Prolonged retention increases the likelihood of mucosal damage, ulceration and perforation. Rigid or flexible endoscopic retrieval are the modalities of choice for retrieving oesophageal foreign bodies. Those with smooth contours, lacking pointed irregular surfaces, can be difficult to retrieve even with state-of-the-art grasping forceps. These and foreign bodies with sharp endings that cannot be safely removed, can be pushed into the stomach; they can then be removed by gastrotomy if deemed harmful, although most chew treats or bones will be safely digested. Post retrieval, a 24-hour fast is generally sufficient. Longer periods may be required with extensive ulcerative lesions and assisted gastrostomy tube feeding may be necessary. However, in the author's experience this is very rarely indicated. Intensive sucralfate therapy (1 g sucralfate as suspension q4–6h) seems to provide the best relief for affected patients. Patients with ulcerative lesions, particularly in the distal oesophagus, should also be treated with omeprazole (1–1.5 mg/kg q12h) in order to prevent ongoing mucosal damage. Analgesic medication (opioids, non-steroidal anti-inflammatory drugs) may be necessary with ulcerative lesions. Surgery becomes necessary if endoscopy fails, or in cases of oesophageal perforation. Gastrotomy is preferred to oesophagotomy for very distal oesophageal foreign bodies, as thoracotomy is a major surgical procedure, and oesophageal surgery can be associated with life-threatening complications. However, results of a recent study suggest that prompt surgical removal of oesophageal foreign bodies after failed endoscopic removal was associated with a low overall complication rate that was similar between the two methods (Deroy *et al.*, 2015). The authors concluded that rapidly selected oesophagotomy was an effective and valuable method with a good outcome.

Prognosis

The prognosis for promptly removed oesophageal foreign bodies is generally good. In unrecognized cases retained for a prolonged period of time, surgical intervention is more likely to be required. Complication rates are also higher in small (<10 kg bodyweight) dogs and dogs that ingested bone foreign bodies (Gianella *et al.*, 2009). Aspiration pneumonia, oesophageal perforation, haemorrhage and formation of a stricture or diverticulum at the foreign body site are further complications. The risk reported of oesophageal stricture formation varies in the literature, with up to 25% of animals developing regurgitation up to 14 days post foreign body removal. Most can be managed with dietary modification, and dilation manoeuvres are needed in only a small percentage. Even though intuitively stricture formation would be assumed to be more likely in cases of 180-degree, or greater, transmucosal ulceration, in the author's experience this is difficult to predict. Severe oesophageal lesions may heal satisfyingly, while subjectively mild mucosal damage may result in severe strictures.

Vascular ring anomalies

Aetiology

Vascular ring anomalies are congenital malformations of the major arteries exiting the heart that entrap the oesophagus and trachea and lead to oesophageal constriction; they are a common cause of regurgitation in young dogs. Persistent right aortic arch (PRAA), aberrant right or left subclavian arteries, double aortic arch, left aortic arch and right ligamentum arteriosum have all been described in cats and dogs. Purebreed dogs considered at risk for the most common vascular malformation, PRAA, include German Shepherd Dogs and Irish Setters. A genetic predisposition has been shown in German Shepherd Dogs and has been investigated in Greyhounds (Gunby et al., 2004).

Diagnosis

Clinical signs: Clinical signs (i.e. regurgitation, failure to thrive) are typically seen shortly following weaning in most animals, although late-onset regurgitation in adult dogs is also rarely encountered. Most affected dogs and cats are smaller compared with littermates, but they usually show great appetite, unless there is evidence of aspiration pneumonia. Physical examination findings may comprise malnourished puppies that are normal otherwise.

Diagnostic imaging: Diagnosis is typically based on compatible history and thoracic radiography. Barium oesophagograms have traditionally been performed to differentiate generalized MO from vascular ring anomalies in which the stricture site is over the base of the heart and oesophageal enlargement occurs only cranial to the heart (see Figure 32.13). However, barium oesophagograms sometimes are not diagnostic of vascular ring anomalies because of inadequate filling or minimal dysfunction and enlargement. Focal leftward curvature of the trachea near the cranial border of the heart in dorsoventral or ventrodorsal radiographs is often a reliable sign of PRAA in young dogs that regurgitate after eating solid food, and contrast oesophagograms may not be necessary any more to confirm the diagnosis (Buchanan, 2004). Endoscopy or computed tomography angiography can be performed to differentiate between benign strictures and vascular malformation, but are rarely indicated as the typical history and radiography are usually diagnostic, and so they tend to be reserved for animals presented as adults. CT angiography is the diagnostic test of choice to assess for additional vascular malformation, such as aberrant left subclavian artery or persistent left cranial vena cava (for more information, see the *BSAVA Manual of Canine and Feline Thoracic Imaging*)

Treatment

Aortic arch and possible concurrent vascular malformations, such as persistent right ductus arteriosus and aberrant right subclavian artery, are best approached by right intercostal thoracotomy. Correction of a PRAA is best managed by thoracotomy through the left fourth intercostal space. Surgical ligation and division of the ligamentum

arteriosum is the treatment of choice in cases of PRAA. Sometimes, it may be necessary to reduce areas of perioesophageal fibrosis and, in addition, to dilate the strictured site with a balloon catheter (for more information, see the *BSAVA Manual of Canine and Feline Head, Neck and Thoracic Surgery*).

Prognosis

Some animals may have persistent oesophageal hypomotility and clinical signs after corrective surgery. This is most likely when surgery was delayed, but the majority can still be managed with elevated feeding of a blended or liquid diet. Results of a recent study on the outcome of 52 dogs undergoing surgery for PRAA suggested that surgical treatment is highly rewarding but does not necessarily lead to complete resolution of clinical signs (Krebs et al., 2014). Long-term outcome for the dogs was excellent in 30%, good in 57% and poor in 13%. Owners need to be informed that continued medical management may be needed throughout the life of the dog. However, in that study, the owner's satisfaction was high despite the presence of some degree of clinical signs or the requirement for continued dietary modification, such as continued need for elevated feeding or tinned food.

References and further reading

Arnell K, Hill S, Hart J and Richter K (2013) Persistent regurgitation in four dogs with caudal esophageal neoplasia. *Journal of the American Animal Hospital Association* **49**, 58–63

Basher AW, Hogan PM, Hanna PE et al. (1991) Surgical treatment of a congenital bronchoesophageal fistula in a dog. *Journal of the American Veterinary Medical Association* **199**, 479–482

Berghaus RD, O'Brien DP, Thorne JG and Buening GM (2002) Incidence of canine dysautonomia in Missouri, USA, between January 1996 and December 2000. *Preventive Veterinary Medicine* **54**, 291–300

Bersenas AM, Mathews KA, Allen DG and Conlon PD (2005) Effects of ranitidine, famotidine, pantoprazole, and omeprazole on intragastric pH in dogs. *American Journal of Veterinary Research* **66**, 425–431

Bexfield NH, Watson PJ and Herrtage ME (2006) Esophageal dysmotility in young dogs. *Journal of Veterinary Internal Medicine* **20**, 1314–1318

Bissett SA, Davis J, Subler K and Degernes LA (2009) Risk factors and outcome of bougienage for treatment of benign oesophageal strictures in dogs and cats: 28 cases (1995–2004). *Journal of the American Veterinary Medical Association* **235**, 844–850

Bresciani F, Zagnoli L, Fracassi F et al. (2014) Dermatomyositis-like disease in a Rottweiler. *Veterinary Dermatology* **25**, 229–232

Brockman D, Holt D and ter Haar G (2018) *BSAVA Manual of Canine and Feline Head, Neck and Thoracic Surgery, 2nd edn*. BSAVA Publications, Gloucester

Broux O, Clercx C, Etienne AL et al. (2018) Effects of manipulations to detect sliding hiatal hernias in dogs with brachycephalic airway obstructive syndrome. *Veterinary Surgery* **47**, 243–251

Buchanan JW (2004) Tracheal signs and associated vascular anomalies in dogs with persistent right aortic arch. *Journal of Veterinary Internal Medicine* **18**, 510–514

Byron JK, Shadwick SR and Bennett AR (2010) Megaesophagus in a 6-month-old cat secondary to a nasopharyngeal polyp. *Journal of Feline Medical Surgery* **12**, 322–324

Della Ripa MA, Gaschen F, Gaschen L and Cho DY (2010) Canine bronchoesophageal fistulas: case report and literature review. *Compendium: Continuing Education for Veterinarians* **32**, E1–E10

Deroy C, Corcuff JB, Billen F and Hamaide A (2015) Removal of oesophageal foreign bodies: comparison between oesophagoscopy and oesophagotomy in 39 dogs. *Journal of Small Animal Practice* **56**, 613–617

DeSandre-Robinson DM, Madden SN and Walker JT (2011). Nasopharyngeal stenosis with concurrent hiatal hernia and megaesophagus in an 8-year-old cat. *Journal of Feline Medicine and Surgery* **13**, 454–459

Dewey C (2010) Mycophenolate mofetil treatment in dogs with serologically diagnosed acquired myasthenia gravis: 27 cases (1999–2008). *Journal of the American Veterinary Medical Association* **236**, 664–668

Durocher L, Johnson SE and Green E (2009) Esophageal diverticulum associated with a trichobezoar in a cat. *Journal of the American Animal Hospital Association* **45**, 142–146

Evans J, Levesque D and Shelton GD (2004) Canine inflammatory myopathies: a clinicopathologic review of 200 cases. *Journal of Veterinary Internal Medicine* **18**, 679–691

Favarato ES, de Souza MV, Costa PR *et al.* (2011) Ambulatory esophageal pHmetry in healthy dogs with and without the influence of general anesthesia. *Veterinary Research Communications* **35**, 271–282

Fox E, Lee K, Lamb CR *et al.* (2007) Congenital oesophageal stricture in a Japanese shiba inu. *Journal of Small Animal Practice* **48**, 709–712

Fracassi F and Tamborini A (2011) Reversible megaoesophagus associated with primary hypothyroidism in a dog. *Vet Record* **168**, 329b

Garcia RS, Belafsky PC, Della Maggiore A *et al.* (2017) Prevalence of gastroesophageal reflux in cats during anesthesia and effect of omeprazole on gastric pH. *Journal of Veterinary Internal Medicine* **31**, 734–742

Gianella P, Pfammatter NS and Burgener IA (2009) Oesophageal and gastric endoscopic foreign body removal: complications and follow-up of 102 dogs. *Journal of Small Animal Practice* **50**, 649–654

Gibson CJ, Parry NM, Jakowski RM and Cooper J (2010) Adenomatous polyp with intestinal metaplasia of the esophagus (Barrett esophagus) in a dog. *Veterinary Pathology* **47**, 116–119

Guiot LP, Lansdowne JL, Rouppert P and Stanley BJ (2008) Hiatal hernia in the dog: a clinical report of four Chinese shar peis. *Journal of the American Animal Hospital Association* **44**, 335–341

Gümürdülü Y, Karakoç E, Kara B *et al.* (2010) The efficiency of sucralfate in corrosive esophagitis: a randomized, prospective study. *Turkish Journal of Gastroenterology* **21**, 7–11

Gunby JM, Hardie RJ and Bjorling DE (2004) Investigation of the potential heritability of persistent right aortic arch in Greyhounds. *Journal of the American Veterinary Medical Association* **224**, 1120–1122

Jankowski M, Spuzak J, Kubiak K, Glińska-Suchocka K and Nicpoń J (2013) Oesophageal foreign bodies in dogs. *Polish Journal of Veterinary Sciences* **16**, 571–572

Juvet F, Pinilla M, Shiel RE and Mooney CT (2010) Oesophageal foreign bodies in dogs: factors affecting success of endoscopic retrieval. *Irish Veterinary Journal* **63**, 163–168

Kempf J, Beckmann K and Kook PH (2014a) Achalasia-like disease with esophageal pressurization in a myasthenic dog. *Journal of Veterinary Internal Medicine* **28**, 661–665

Kempf J, Heinrich H, Reusch CE and Kook PH (2013) Evaluation of oesophageal high-resolution manometry in awake and sedated dogs. *American Journal of Veterinary Research* **74**, 895–900

Kempf J, Lewis F, Reusch CE and Kook PH (2014b) High-resolution manometric evaluation of the effects of cisapride and metoclopramide hydrochloride administered orally on lower esophageal sphincter pressure in awake dogs. *American Journal of Veterinary Research* **75**, 361–366

Kidder AC, Johannes C, O'Brien DP, Harkin KR and Schermerhorn T (2008) Feline dysautonomia in the Midwestern United States: a retrospective study of nine cases. *Journal of Feline Medicine and Surgery* **10**, 130–136

Kook PH, Kempf J, Ruetten M and Reusch CE (2014) Wireless ambulatory esophageal pH monitoring in dogs with clinical signs interpreted as gastroesophageal reflux. *Journal of Veterinary Internal Medicine* **28**, 1716–1723

Kook PH, Wiederkehr D, Makara M and Reusch CE (2009) Megaesophagus secondary to an esophageal leiomyoma and concurrent esophagitis. *Schweizer Archiv für Tierheilkunde* **151**, 497–501

Krebs IA, Lindsley S, Shaver S and MacPhail C (2014) Short- and long-term outcome of dogs following surgical correction of a persistent right aortic arch. *Journal of the American Animal Hospital Association* **50**, 181–186

Lam N, Weisse C, Berent A *et al.* (2013) Esophageal stenting for treatment of refractory benign esophageal strictures in dogs. *Journal of Veterinary Internal Medicine* **27**, 1064–1070

Lhermette P and Sobel D (2008) *BSAVA Manual of Canine and Feline Endoscopy and Endosurgery.* BSAVA Publications, Gloucester

Mayer-Roenne B, Fraune C, Ryan KA and Gaschen FP (2009) Successul treatment of benign oesophgeal strictures with balloon dilation and submucosal triamcinolone injection in five dogs and one cat. *Journal of Veterinary Internal Medicine* **23**, 760

McBrearty AR, Ramsey IK, Courcier EA, Mellor DJ and Bell R (2011) Clinical factors associated with death before discharge and overall survival time in dogs with generalized megaesophagus. *Journal of the American Veterinary Medical Association* **238**, 1622–1628

Münster M, Hoerauf A and Vieth M (2017) Gastro-oesophageal reflux disease in 20 dogs (2012–2014). *Journal of Small Animal Practice* **58**, 276–283

Münster M, Vieth M and Hörauf A (2013) Evaluation of the quality of endoscopically obtained esophageal biopsies in the dog. *Tierärztliche Praxis. Ausgabe K, Kleintiere Heimtiere* **41**, 375–382

Nawrocki MA, Mackin AJ, McLaughlin R and Cantwell HD (2003) Fluoroscopic and endoscopic localization of an esophagobronchial fistula in a dog. *The Journal of the American Animal Hospital Association* **36**, 257–261

Novellas R, Simpson KE, Gunn-Moore DA and Hammond GJ (2010) Imaging findings in 11 cats with feline dysautonomia. *Journal of Feline Medicine and Surgery* **12**, 584–591

Panti A, Bennett RC, Corletto F *et al.* (2009) The effect of omeprazole on oesophageal pH in dogs during anaesthesia. *Journal of Small Animal Practice* **50**, 540–544

Parkinson S, Tolbert K, Messenger K *et al.* (2015) Evaluation of the effect of orally administered acid suppressants on intragastric pH in cats. *Journal of Veterinary Internal Medicine* **29**, 104–112

Quintavalla F, Menozzi A, Pozzoli C *et al.* (2017) Sildenafil improves clinical signs and radiographic features in dogs with congenital idiopathic megaoesophagus: a randomised controlled trial. *Veterinary Record* **180**, 404

Schneider J, Ames M, DiCicco M *et al.* (2015) Recovery of normal esophageal function in a kitten with diffuse megaesophagus and an occult lower esophageal stricture. *Journal of Feline Medicine and Surgery* **17**, 557–561

Schönfelder J, Schönfelder A and Neiger R (2011) Survival duration for different forms of canine megaesophagus. *Schweiz Arch Tierheilkd* **153**, 236–238

Schulz BS, Zauscher S, Ammer H, Sauter-Louis C and Hartmann K (2013) Side effects suspected to be related to doxycycline use in cats. *Veterinary Record* **172**, 184

Schwarz T and Johnson V (2008) *BSAVA Manual of Canine and Feline Thoracic Imaging.* BSAVA Publications, Gloucester

Shelton GD (2014) Treatment of autoimmune myasthenia gravis. In: *Kirk's Current Veterinary Therapy, XV,* eds JD Bonagura, DC Twedt, pp. 1109–1112. Saunders Elsevier, St Louis

Shipov A, Kelmer G, Lavy E, *et al.* (2015) Long-term outcome of transendoscopic oesophageal mass ablation in dogs with *Spirocerca lupi*-associated oesophageal sarcoma. *Veterinary Record* **177**, 365

Sivacolundhu RK, Read RA and Marchevsky AM (2002) Hiatal hernia controversies – a review of pathophysiology and treatment options. *Australian Veterinary Journal* **80**, 48–53

Šutalo S, Ruetten M, Hartnack S, Reusch CE and Kook PH (2015) The effect of orally administered ranitidine and once-daily or twice-daily orally administered omeprazole on intragastric pH in cats. *Journal of Veterinary Internal Medicine* **29**, 840–846

Tolbert K, Bissett S, King A *et al.* (2011) Efficacy of oral famotidine and 2 omeprazole formulations for the control of intragastric pH in dogs. *Journal of Veterinary Internal Medicine* **25**, 47–54

Vangrinsven E, Broux O, Claeys S, Clercx C and Billen F (2016) Endoscopic investigation of gastro-oesophageal junction dynamics in dogs with brachycephalic syndrome. *Journal of Veterinary Internal Medicine* **30**, 379

Westfall DS, Twedt DC, Steyn PF, Oberhauser EB and VanCleave JW (2001) Evaluation of esophageal transit of tablets and capsules in 30 cats. *Journal of Veterinary Internal Medicine* **15**, 467–470

Wilson DV, Evans AT and Mauer WA (2006) Influence of metoclopramide on gastroesophageal reflux in anesthetized dogs. *American Journal of Veterinary Research* **67**, 26–31

Yoshimoto SK, Marks SL, Struble AL and Riel DL (2006) Owner experiences and complications with home use of a replacement low profile gastrostomy device for long-term enteral feeding in dogs. *Canadian Veterinary Journal* **47**, 144–150

Zacuto AC, Marks SL, Osborn J, *et al.* (2012) The influence of esomeprazole and cisapride on gastroesophageal reflux during anesthesia in dogs. *Journal of Veterinary Internal Medicine* **26**, 518–525

Zhang X, Geboes K, Depoortere I *et al.* (2005) Effect of repeated cycles of acute esophagitis and healing on esophageal peristalsis, tone, and length. *American Journal of Physiology: Gastrointestinal and Liver Physiology* **288**, G1339–1346

Chapter 33

Stomach

Thomas Spillmann and Marcus V. Candido

Structure and function of the stomach

Macro- and micro-anatomy

The single-chambered stomach of dogs and cats serves as a reservoir for food, initiates digestion and regulates the passage of ingesta into the duodenum. The stomach has five distinct areas: the cardia, fundus, corpus, antrum and pylorus (Figure 33.1).

The gastric wall is covered by peritoneal serosa. Its longitudinal, circular and oblique smooth muscle layers allow dilatation for food storage while maintaining a constant intraluminal pressure. The circular muscle layer forms the lower oesophageal and pyloric sphincters, physically controlling the flow of ingesta in and out of the stomach.

The luminal side of the gastric wall is lined by mucosa comprising columnar epithelium, glandular lamina propria and muscularis mucosae. It is connected to the muscular wall by the submucosa, which consists of connective tissue, blood vessels, nerves and immune cell populations. It allows the mucosa to fold when the stomach is empty and to stretch flat with distension.

The gastric mucosa contains tubular branched cardiac, gastric and pyloric glands (Figure 33.1). Cardiac glands are considered undifferentiated gastric glands. The acid-producing gastric glands of the fundus and corpus terminate in gastric pits and contain cell types with different secretory functions:

- Neck cells secrete mucus and gastric lipase
- Parietal cells for hydrochloric acid
- Chief cells for pepsinogen A (and B in dogs)
- Enterochromaffin-like (ECL) cells for histamine
- D-cells for somatostatin.

Pyloric glands lack chief and parietal cells and produce mainly mucus, but also contain G-cells that secrete gastrin.

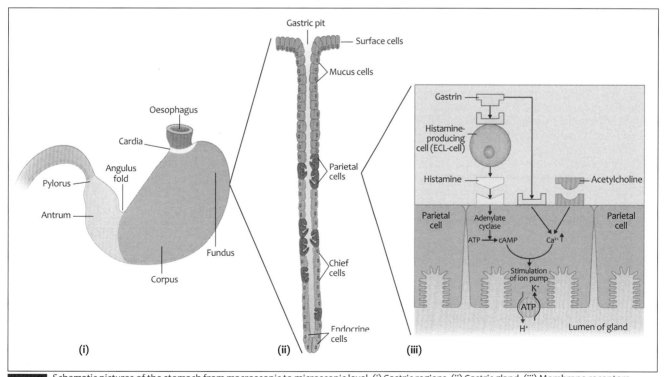

33.1 Schematic pictures of the stomach from macroscopic to microscopic level. (i) Gastric regions. (ii) Gastric gland. (iii) Membrane receptors stimulating acid secretion. ATP = adenosine triphosphate; Ca²⁺ = calcium ion; cAMP = cyclic adenosine monophosphate; ECL = enterochromaffin-like; H⁺ = hydrogen ion.

Gastric function

Gastric motility

The motility of the stomach is coordinated by the auto-nomic enteric nervous system (ENS). The ENS facilitates sensation and regulation of luminal conditions through a wide network of mechano- and chemoreceptors, inter-neurons, motor neurons and primary afferent neurons. It communicates with the central nervous system via para-sympathetic (vagus) and sympathetic pathways.

During digestion, muscle contractions break down food and transport food particles into the small intestine. The gastric emptying of liquids is faster than that of solids. Food-associated factors that reduce the gastric emptying rate are its viscosity, caloric density, particle size, and carbohydrate, amino acid and fat content. In the interdigestive (fasted) state, the migrating motor complex initiates regular waves of gastrointestinal (GI) contrac-tions for 'intestinal housekeeping'. During this process, large, indigestible solids are also expelled from the stomach; this is when gastric foreign bodies most likely pass into the small intestine.

Digestion

The digestive functions of the stomach include grinding the food and initiating lipid and protein digestion, as well as vitamin and mineral absorption. Lipid digestion is initi-ated by gastric lipase. For protein digestion, pepsinogen is converted by hydrochloric acid into pepsin that breaks down proteins into polypeptides and releases dietary cobalamin. In dogs, some cobalamin binds to an intrinsic factor produced by parietal cells, but the main source of this factor in dogs, and exclusively in cats, is the exo-crine pancreas.

Gastric secretions

Acid production: Gastrin, acetylcholine and histamine are the main stimulants of gastric acid production, binding to specific receptors at the basolateral surface of parietal cells (see Figure 33.1). Gastrin is released in response to luminal peptides, digested proteins, acetylcholine and increased gastric luminal pH. Acetylcholine derives from cholinergic fibres stimulated by the anticipation, sight, smell and taste of food, and by gastric distension. Histamine is released by the ECL cells, after gastrin and acetylcholine bind to membrane receptors. Somatostatin, secretin and prostaglandin E2 are physiological inhibitors of gastric acid secretion.

Proton pumps (H^+/K^+ ATPase) on the canalicular mem-brane (luminal side) of parietal cells exchange intracellular hydrogen for intraluminal potassium, decreasing gastric luminal pH to around pH 1 (see Figure 33.1). Parietal cells also regulate the transport of chloride and potassium into the gastric lumen.

Self-protection: The self-protection mechanisms of the gastric mucosa against the harsh acidic luminal environ-ment are very elaborate. The gastric mucosal barrier main-tains mucosal cytoprotection by several factors mainly regulated by mucosal prostaglandins (Figure 33.2).

Other peptides that influence gastric function

Ghrelin mainly regulates appetite and energy balance (orexigenic effect). Motilin co-regulates the migrating motor complex. Both stimulate gastric emptying and are

Component of gastric mucosal barrier	Physiological properties
Hydrophobic mucus layer	• Secreted by neck cells and surface mucosal cells • Forms a water-insoluble glycoprotein gel adhering to mucosal surfaces • Functions as a lubricant to prevent mechanical damage • Traps bicarbonate from mucous neck cells to keep gastric mucosal pH at 4–6 (luminal pH is 1–2)
Mucosal bicarbonate secretion	• Accumulates in mucus layer • Protects gastric epithelium from back-diffusion of free hydrogen (H^+) ions from the gastric lumen

Salivary epidermal growth factor	• Helps prevent and heal mucosal damage probably by
	  • Increasing secretion of mucin (glycoprotein)
	  • Scavenging oxygen metabolites
	  • Increasing mucosal blood flow

Mucosal cell hydrophobicity	• Phospholipids in surface cell membranes repel water-soluble contents • Prevents acid and pepsin back-diffusion
High rate of mucosal blood flow	• Supplied by a dense submucosal capillary network • Regulated by prostaglandins • Supplies oxygen and nutrients to surface cells for metabolism and renewal • Provides bicarbonate for mucosal surface to prevent back-diffusion of H^+

Restitution and rapid epithelial cell turn over	• Continuous and quick repair of gastric epithelium
	  • Seals small erosions and re-establishes intact epithelium in <1 hour
	  • Aided by local growth factors such as epidermal growth factor

Prostaglandins	• Prostaglandins E and I from gastric mucosal cells
	  • Increase mucus and bicarbonate secretion
	  • Enhance mucosal blood flow
	  • Stimulate epithelial cell growth
	  • Inhibit acid secretion

33.2 Components of the gastric mucosal barrier and their physiological properties. H^+ = hydrogen ion.
(Data modified from Henderson and Webster, 2006a)

structurally related, as are their receptors (Ogawa *et al.*, 2012). Trefoil factors are involved in rapid restitution of epi-thelial integrity after mucosal damage, and interact with the immune system.

Gastric microbiota

The stomach harbours a variety of microbes, either transient (swallowed from the oral cavity after a meal or coprophagia) or permanent. Acid secretion and gastric emptying regulate bacterial transition or colonization of the superficial mucosa, gastric glands and parietal cells. The microbiota comprises proteobacteria (e.g. *Helico-bacter* spp.) and, in a minority of cases, Firmicutes. Bacterial ability to buffer gastric acid by producing urease, which converts urea to ammonia, facilitates their survival. An interaction of *Helicobacter* species with other microbial components seems to determine the actual pathogenesis of gastric inflammation and tumour devel-opment in humans.

Pathophysiology of gastric diseases

The pathophysiology of gastric diseases is generally divided into inflammatory (non-ulcerative and ulcerative), obstructive, neoplastic or functional.

Gastritis

Gastritis is an umbrella term for an inflammatory syndrome rather than a defined disease. In pathology, the term is also used for different types of acute or chronic changes, either with prominent histological evidence of true gastritis (i.e. inflammatory, vascular and structural changes) or without (i.e. mucosal necrosis and ulceration caused by mechanical, chemical, uraemic or ischaemic insults).

Acute gastritis

Acute gastritis is induced either by primary gastric disorders (dietary indiscretion, food intolerance or allergy and infections) or by systemic diseases (systemic infections, intoxications, uraemia, hepatobiliary diseases, hypoadrenocorticism and diabetic ketoacidosis). Conversely, systemic clinical signs can result from local gastric injury caused by drugs (e.g. non-steroidal anti-inflammatory drugs (NSAIDs), high-dose glucocorticoids), ingestion of toxins (chemical, biological) or perforating foreign bodies (Figure 33.3). The response of the gastric mucosa to acute mechanical or chemical injuries is rapid (minutes to hours). Flattened surface cells and foveolar cells migrate to the damaged area. Mucosal blood flow increases to dilute injurious substances and back-diffusing gastric acid. Mucus, exfoliated cells and fibrin coat the defect, supporting mucosal restitution.

Chronic gastritis

Chronic gastritis is characterized by persistent mucosal inflammation, which may be associated with ulceration. Histologically, true chronic gastritis has been sub-classified by the predominant cellular infiltrate (lymphoplasmacytic, eosinophilic, granulomatous and lymphoid follicular) and its severity (mild, moderate, severe). It remains debatable whether mild infiltration truly reflects gastric pathology or is merely a response to the gastric microbiome, due to the complexity and variability of the microscopic anatomy of the healthy stomach, and the often patchy distribution of lesions. Persistent inflammation can lead to structural changes such as fibrosis, decrease or loss of normal cell mass (mucosal atrophy, ulceration), excessive development (hyperplasia, hypertrophy) or abnormal re-arrangement (metaplasia, dysplasia). The aetiology of chronic gastritis remains mostly idiopathic.

Potential causes of chronic gastritis: Foreign material such as grass can be associated with gastritis, but the existence of any cause-and-effect relationship remains speculative. Gastric infections are far less common than chemical (drug-induced) or mechanical insults.

- **Bacteria** implicated in the development of follicular gastritis include *Helicobacter* spp. However, an association with chronic ulcerative gastritis (or gastric carcinoma) has not been established in small animals, in contrast to *Helicobacter pylori* infection in humans. However, even *H. pylori* does not seem to act as a single, predictable pathogen, since there is evidence that the composition of non-*H. pylori* gastric microbiota may influence whether disease develops.
- **Parasites** differ across geographical regions and cause subclinical or clinical gastritis of variable severity (Figure 33.4).

Generic classification	Agent	Comments
Inert material • Foreign body • Trichobezoar • Particulate material	Plastic, wood, hair, leather, rope, stone, sand	Intermittent obstruction Mucosal ischaemia (local compression) Mechanical mucosal damage Removal of mucus layer, mucosal abrasion
Drugs • Antibiotics • Digitalis • NSAIDs • Corticosteroids	Cephalosporins Doxycycline Digoxin Acting on COX-1	Irritation Chemical burns GI signs, death due to cardiac arrest Suppression of protective prostaglandin Ulcerogenic at high dose, and exacerbate NSAID-induced damage by inhibiting repair
Toxins • Heavy metals • Toads • Plants • Household chemicals	Lead, zinc *Bufo* spp. *Bombina* spp. Araceae Euphorbiaceae Detergents Bleach Fertilizers Herbicides	Chemical irritation Chemical irritation, neurotropic alkaloids Bombesin is a gastrin analogue Oxalic acid causes chemical burns Proinflammatory diterpenes Removal of mucus layer Removal of mucus, chemical burn Irritation Interference with cell metabolism
Topical antiseptics	Peroxide, iodine	Irritation, removal of mucus, chemical burn
Contaminated food • Fungal toxins • Bacterial products	Vomitoxin (Aflatoxin, others) Various	Stimulation of vomiting centre Toxicosis causing gastric signs and/or chronic liver damage

33.3 Common causes of acute gastritis. COX-1 = cyclooxygenase-1; GI = gastrointestinal; NSAIDs = non-steroidal anti-inflammatory drugs.

Gastric parasite and host	Distribution	Faecal examination	Endoscopy with biopsy	Treatment
Ollulanus tricuspis Cat > dog	Europe, North and South America, Australasia, Middle East	Non-diagnostic due to lack of eggs or larvae in faeces	Occasional finding of 0.7–1 mm long worms if vomitus examined Mild to severe gastritis; hyperplastic mucosa with heavy infections	Levamisole, ivermectin, oxfendazole[a] (dose rate for oxfendazole: 10 mg/kg q12h for 5 days)
Gnathostoma spinigerum Cat, dog	Thailand, Japan, South-east Asia, India, China, Mexico	Greenish oval eggs with a thin cap at one pole; often absent from faeces	Spiroid nematodes in gastric biopsy samples Thick-walled fibrous cysts of up to 3–4 cm diameter, containing a worm (1–3 cm long) and fluid	Not fully investigated; surgical removal of cysts
Physaloptera praeputialis Cat > dog	China, Africa, North and South America	Elongated eggs, thickened at either pole, often not present in faeces	Adult worms of 1–60 mm length causing focal gastric ulceration and haemorrhage	Benzimidazoles over 5 days Pyrantel, praziquantel, febantel effective in increased or repeated doses
Physaloptera rara Cat > dog	North America	Thick-shelled, ellipsoid eggs 42–53 x 29–35 μm	Adult worms 2.5–6 cm	Same as *Physaloptera praeputialis*
Capillaria putorii (*Aonchotheca putorii*) Cat, dog	Europe, New Zealand, Russia	Oval, elongated eggs 60 x 30 μm; broad flat poles with two protruding semi-transparent polar plugs; contain granular unsegmented contents	Thin, filamentous worms 5–15 mm long Chronic hyperplastic ulcerated pyloric gastritis with eggs in pyloric mucus and glands	Levamisole 7.5 mg/kg at 2-week intervals Ivermectin 300 μg/kg Surgery
Cylicospirura felineus (*Cylicospirura subaequalis*) Cat	North America, Asia, Africa, Australia	No reports	Gastric nodules with intact mucosal surface containing multiple nematodes extending through an individual central pore. Histology: reactive fibroplasia, mimicking feline gastrointestinal eosinophilic sclerosing fibroplasia	No reports

33.4 Gastric parasites and their host, geographical distribution, detection methods and treatment. [a]Oxfendazole is not available in the UK.

- **Oomycete infection** with *Pythium insidiosum* leads to granulomatous and eosinophilic inflammation with transmural thickening (see Chapter 34).
- **Uraemic gastropathy** is characterized by mucosal congestion, haemorrhage and mineralization (McLeland *et al.*, 2014), but rarely ulceration. Severity correlates with the course of chronic kidney disease.

Ulcerative gastritis: Ulcerative gastritis varies from acute superficial ulcers (often termed erosions) to subacute or chronic deep ulcers, with a depressed base and a ring-wall-like contour of granulation tissue of variable thickness. The common pathophysiology of peptic ulcers is an imbalance between the efficacy of the protective gastric mucosal barrier and the necrotizing effects of gastric acid and pepsin. The differentiation between benign and malignant peptic ulcers has prognostic importance.

Causes of compromised mucosal protection: These include NSAIDs, high-dose glucocorticoids, mechanical erosion (foreign bodies; Figure 33.5), reflux of duodenal contents, and reduced mucosal perfusion or ischaemia in connection with stress, shock, trauma to the spinal cord, neurosurgery or burns.

- **NSAIDs** selectively or non-selectively inhibit cyclooxygenase-1 (COX-1), decreasing the production of gastric prostaglandin E2. This inhibits bicarbonate production, causes gastric hypermotility, alters microvascular blood flow and reduces the mucosal response to injury.
- **Glucocorticoids** delay healing of pre-existing ulcers and can also be ulcerogenic with prolonged high-dose treatment. However, increased endogenous glucocorticoids can have gastroprotective effects. The combination of NSAIDs with glucocorticoids can be hazardous in susceptible animals.

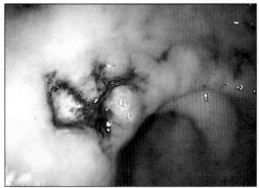

33.5 Endoscopic image of acute mechanical ulceration due to a gastric foreign body in a dog.

- **Reflux of duodenal content** exposes the gastric mucosa to bile salts and lysolecithin, leading to morphological changes, increased permeability and acid back-diffusion.
- **Acid hypersecretion** can be induced by gastrin-producing tumours (gastrinoma), histamine-releasing mast cell tumours and the neurotransmitter acetylcholine.
- **Exercise-induced gastric ulceration in athletic dogs** is possibly caused by a combination of stress-induced hyperacidity and reduced mucosal perfusion, or by exercise-induced hyperthermia and loss of gastric barrier function. A state of increased serum gastrin and decreased cortisol might also be involved.

Complications of gastric ulceration:

- **Gastric bleeding**, which can range from minor (occult) to massive, with haematemesis and melaena. Severe, acute bleeding can cause hypovolaemic shock. Chronic gastric bleeding eventually leads to microcytic, hypochromic anaemia due to iron deficiency.

- **Gastric perforation**, which occurs as a consequence of deep ulcerations or sharp foreign objects. Gastric perforation can lead to septic peritonitis with severe clinical signs, or to less severe local peritonitis and abscess formation, when gastric serosa and omentum succeed in covering the defect and limit the extent of the inflammation.

Atrophic gastritis: Structural changes in gastric wall components can occur in addition to inflammation. Atrophic gastritis (Figure 33.6) is characterized by the reduction of parietal cells, with marked infiltration of inflammatory cells. In dogs and cats, atrophic gastritis has been only sporadically reported without association with natural *Helicobacter* spp. infections. However, cats with experimental long-term *H. pylori* infections developed chronic diffuse lymphofollicular atrophic gastritis, and long-term *Helicobacter felis* infections caused atrophic gastritis in mouse models. In dogs, atrophic gastritis was described in Norwegian Lundehunds with gastric neuroendocrine carcinoma. There can be substantial variation in mucosal thickness along the various sections of the stomach, which may influence the accuracy of histological interpretation regarding atrophy.

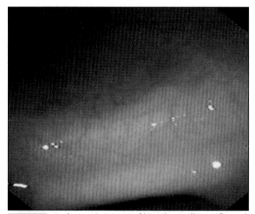

33.6 Endoscopic image of histologically confirmed atrophic gastritis in the lesser curvature.

Metaplasia and hyperplasia

Mucosal changes, such as metaplasia and dysplasia, have been rarely reported in dogs and cats. However, there is some evidence that they might be underdiagnosed. Recent advances in endoscopic imaging (e.g. narrow-band imaging chromo-endoscopy) may improve diagnosis (see the *BSAVA Manual of Canine and Feline Endoscopy and Endosurgery*).

- **Mucous metaplasia** is characterized by a replacement of parietal cells by mucous (neck) cells and increased lymphoplasmacytic cell infiltration, and has been described in Norwegian Lundehunds. This can also be found around the margins of chronic ulcers. The Tervuren (Belgian Shepherd Dog) and Shetland Sheepdog reportedly have an increased risk for being diagnosed with mucous metaplasia.
- **Gastric intestinal metaplasia** is defined as the replacement of the gastric glandular epithelium by intestine-like epithelium, and is rare in dogs and cats (Figure 33.7).
- **Gastric epithelial dysplasia** is considered a premalignant lesion of gastric carcinoma in humans. In dogs and cats, it seems to be rare but Tervurens appear to be at increased risk (Figure 33.8).

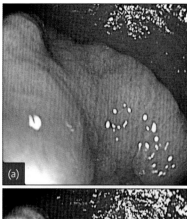

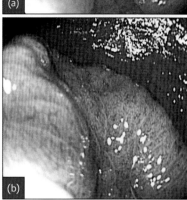

33.7 Endoscopic images of histologically confirmed intestinal metaplasia in the greater curvature of the gastric body. (a) White-light endoscopy. (b) Narrow-band imaging.

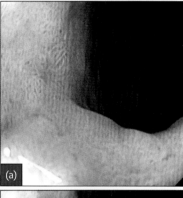

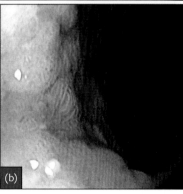

33.8 Endoscopic images of histologically confirmed gastric epithelial dysplasia in a female Tervuren (Belgian Shepherd Dog). (a) White-light endoscopy. (b) Chromoendoscopy with indigo carmine 0.2%.

- **Gastric mucosal hypertrophy** has been reported sporadically in dogs (and even less frequently in cats) with and without gastrinoma. Focal lesions are most prevalent (e.g. papillary proliferations of the antral mucosa; Figure 33.9).
- **Diffuse, hypertrophic gastritis** (Ménétrier's disease-like gastritis; Figure 33.10) and **hypertrophic antritis** are less common. Hypertrophic gastritis is characterized by marked rugal fold hypertrophy resembling cerebral gyri and involving the corpus and fundus. Feline hypertrophic gastritis was reported in association with *Ollulanus tricuspis* infection.

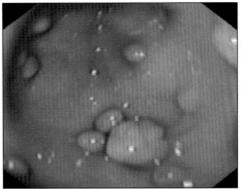

33.9 Endoscopic image of multiple papillary proliferations in the antrum of a dog.

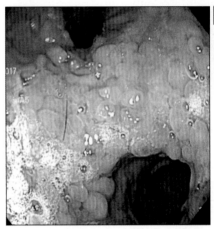

33.10 Endoscopic image of confirmed Ménétrier's-like disease (giant hypertrophic gastritis) in a dog.

Gastric neoplasia

Gastric neoplasms are most commonly epithelial, haemopoietic or mesenchymal, but neuroendocrine, secondary and unclassified tumours, and tumour-like lesions also occur.

Epithelial tumours

Epithelial tumours are either benign (adenoma) or malignant (adenocarcinoma). An adenocarcinoma, the most common primary GI neoplasm in dogs, arises from the mucosa (Figure 33.11). Local invasion is common and infiltrates are often found beneath a normal mucosal layer. The pathogenesis of canine gastric carcinoma is currently unknown but is suspected to be complex, with a genetic predisposition in certain breeds. The Tervuren, Collie and some other breeds have an increased risk for adenocarcinoma, and Norwegian Lundehunds have an increased risk for gastric neuroendocrine carcinoma.

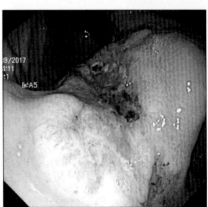

33.11 Endoscopic image of an ulcerated, invasive mucinous adenocarcinoma in the lesser curvature.

Haemopoietic tumours

Haemopoietic neoplasms include lymphoma (Figure 33.12) and extramedullary plasmacytoma. The growth pattern of lymphoma is variable, and its gross appearance can be diffuse or localized. Localized lymphoma can be solitary or multifocal, and intraluminal or intramural. Solitary gastric lymphomas tend to be B-cell type, and it has been hypothesized that *Helicobacter heilmannii* or *H. felis* may play a causative role in cats. GI small cell lymphoma is more common in cats than in dogs and can also affect the stomach. It has a better treatment response and survival rate than large-cell lymphoma (see Chapter 34). Diffuse lymphocytic proliferation appearing as a tumour can also be associated with infections and immunological disorders. This poses a challenge when differentiating infection or inflammation from neoplasia.

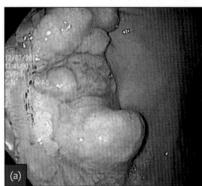

33.12 (a) Endoscopic image of a large (B-) cell lymphoma in a dog. (b) Extramedullary plasmacytoma.

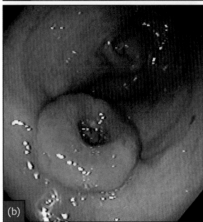

Mesenchymal tumours

Both benign and malignant smooth muscle neoplasms (leiomyoma, leiomyosarcoma) and GI stromal tumours (GISTs) can occur in the stomach. In dogs, leiomyoma and leiomyosarcoma often develop at the lower oesophageal sphincter, causing clinical and radiological signs of megaoesophagus (see Chapter 32).

Gastric outflow obstruction

Gastric outflow obstruction is more commonly reported in dogs than in cats. It should be suspected when the animal vomits food more than 8–10 hours after a meal, and when there is severe gastric distension with food and/or fluid several hours after eating or drinking.

- **Congenital outflow obstruction** can result from pyloric hypertrophy of the smooth muscles or tonic stenosis of the sphincter.

- **Acquired outflow obstructions** can be total or partial and occur with foreign bodies, gastric ulceration, polyps or tumours in the antrum, acquired pyloric stenosis, hypertrophic gastritis or pylorogastropathy, and duodenogastric intussusception.

Gastric foreign bodies

Swallowing foreign bodies occurs in dogs and cats accidentally during playing, eating and grooming (hairballs in cats), or because of pica (abnormal craving and eating of substances that are not normally eaten) in connection with primary gastroenteropathies, states of nutritional deficiency and neurological or behavioural disorders. When not causing obstruction in the oesophagus, foreign bodies collecting in the stomach can remain subclinical or cause acute or chronic signs of gastritis and gastric ulceration. Delayed gastric emptying or outflow obstruction occurs when foreign bodies block the pyloric antrum or duodenum.

Gastric motility disorders

Delayed gastric emptying and defective propulsion must be differentiated from mechanical outflow obstructions of intraluminal and intramural origin. Defective propulsion can occur secondary to pancreatitis, peritonitis, metabolic disturbances (hypokalaemia, hypocalcaemia), endocrine disorders (hypoadrenocorticism) and nervous inhibition (trauma, pain and stress). Other causes include gastric inflammation and ulceration, recent abdominal surgery, prolonged general anaesthesia, diabetes mellitus, and drugs (anticholinergics, opioids). GI wall disorders causing pseudo-obstructive effects (see Chapter 34) are either local (leiomyositis, visceral smooth muscle alpha-actin deficiency) or systemic (dysautonomia). Other motility disorders include accelerated gastric emptying, retrograde transit and delayed emptying without morphological changes; such disorders are poorly defined and regarded as idiopathic in aetiology.

Gastrointestinal pseudo-obstruction

GI pseudo-obstruction without evidence of mechanical causes can involve the stomach. This is usually a visceral myopathy and is described in association with leiomyositis and visceral smooth muscle alpha-actin deficiency. Case reports of young dogs (4 months to 4 years) with visceral myopathy have described degeneration and loss of leiomyocytes, lymphocytic leiomyositis and fibroplasia with or without neuronal atrophy. The loss of immunoreactivity for muscle alpha-actin but an intact autonomic nervous system was reported in one Bengal cat (6 years) with persistent megaoesophagus and ileus. Ganglioneuritis in the myenteric plexus causing a visceral neuropathy is very rarely described in dogs.

Dysautonomia

This condition is characterized by the degeneration of various autonomic nervous ganglia. The cause of dysautonomia is unknown, but local clustering (e.g. in the UK, Scandinavia, Midwest USA) suggests an environmental cause, with botulinum type C neurotoxin being suspected. Gastric dilatation and hypomotility is one of many multisystemic signs related to sympathetic and parasympathetic nervous system dysfunction, which affects the eyes, tear and salivary glands, and urinary and GI tracts.

Gastric dilatation-volvulus

Gastric dilatation-volvulus (GDV) is a common and very serious disorder in dogs, but it is very rare in cats. Large- and giant-breed deep-chested dogs are mainly affected (Figure 33.13). Predisposing factors include increased age, having a first-degree relative with a history of GDV, laxity of the hepatogastric ligament, feeding small food particles, fast eating, using a raised food bowl, recent kennelling, reverse sneezing and gastric motility disorders. The role of splenectomy in the development of GDV remains controversial.

Gastric bloating is attributable to aerophagia, intragastric gas production and the inability to remove accumulated gas, fluids and food from the stomach. This results in gastric dilatation, which can eventually convert to volvulus by clockwise gastric rotation up to 360 degrees around its long axis. The pylorus and duodenum move cranially to the right around the oesophagus, which is finally completely occluded.

Depending on the degree of torsion, the spleen may be displaced, undergoing congestion, infarction and even rupture. Circulatory collapse occurs as hypovolaemic shock (fluid sequestration in the stomach), obstructive shock (decreased venous return via portal vein and caudal vena cava), distributive shock (altered perfusion of abdominal organs and over-expression of micro-vascular dilating agents) and cardiogenic shock (reduced cardiac output) develop. Compromised respiratory volume results from intra-abdominal pressure affecting the diaphragm.

Ischaemia occurs in the gastric wall, pancreas and heart. The gastric wall becomes ischaemic due to increased intragastric pressure, resulting in the obliteration of vessels and tearing of short gastric arteries, leading to necrosis and, ultimately, rupture. Pancreatic ischaemia leads to the release of a myocardial depressant factor, which, along with cardiac ischaemia, causes cardiac arrhythmia. Further metabolic consequences, such as marked acid-base and electrolyte disturbances, are also seen.

Severe cases of GDV are life-threatening without rapid intervention. The most serious complications are associated with ischaemia–reperfusion injury and consequent systemic inflammatory response syndrome with multiple organ dysfunction syndrome. Other complications include hypotension, acute kidney injury, disseminated intravascular coagulation (DIC), gastric ulceration and cardiac arrhythmias. In rare cases, gastric volvulus is not associated with dilatation, and can be chronic, leading to weight loss, chronic vomiting, lethargy and abdominal pain. For further information on the management of GDV, see the *BSAVA Manual of Canine and Feline Abdominal Surgery*.

Gastric disease	Predisposed dog breeds
Gastric dilatation-volvulus	Deep-chested dogs, Great Dane, St. Bernard, Irish and Gordon Setters, Wolfhound, Borzoi, Weimaraner, Bloodhound, Dachshund
Hypertrophic gastropathy	Basenji, Drentse Patrijshond, Shih Tzu
Atrophic gastritis	Norwegian Lundehund
Mucous metaplasia	Norwegian Lundehund, Tervuren, Shetland Sheepdog
Gastric neuroendocrine carcinoma	Norwegian Lundehund
Gastric adenocarcinoma	Tervuren, Collie, Staffordshire Bull Terrier, Beagle

33.13 Canine gastric diseases and predisposed dog breeds.

Diagnostic investigation of gastric disorders

The signalment, disease history and physical examination findings can be used to create a list of clinical problems which, combined with a minimum database (MDB) of laboratory test results, help rule out non-gastric causes of vomiting, may allow a preliminary tentative diagnosis to be made and support initial treatment decisions. They may also indicate which specific laboratory tests and imaging procedures are required to establish the final diagnosis and initiate a more directed treatment.

Signalment

Age associations show that younger dogs have a higher probability of having gastric foreign bodies, congenital pyloric stenosis or pythiosis. Older dogs tend to have neoplasms more often. Breed associations have been reported for a variety of gastric disorders (see Figure 33.13).

History

The history should focus on the duration of clinical signs (acute/chronic) and their severity (local/systemic; mild to severe), as well as on housing/environmental conditions as possible aetiological factors. Clinical signs of gastric diseases vary in type, duration, combination and severity (Figure 33.14). Severe cases can lead to depression or shock. Other accompanying signs, such as polyuria, polydipsia, weight loss, diarrhoea, coughing, sneezing and exercise intolerance, point towards the involvement of other organs or systemic diseases.

General clinical signs
Inappetence
Anorexia
Nausea
Retching
Burping (eructation)
Hypersalivation
Vomiting
• Without blood
• With blood (haematemesis)
Melaena
• Dark, black, tarry faeces (marked bleeding in the upper gastrointestinal tract)
Anaemia
• With melaena
• Without melaena (occult bleeding in the upper gastrointestinal tract)
Abdominal distension
Abdominal pain
Weight loss

Signs and causes of systemic illness
Signs of clinical illness
• Mucosal pallor
• Dehydration
• Hypovolaemia
• Fever or hypothermia
• Tachycardia
• Abdominal pain
Causes of systemic illness
• Gastric dilatation-volvulus
• Gastric outflow obstruction
• Gastric ulceration
• Gastric perforation

33.14 General clinical signs and signs of systemic illness seen with canine and feline gastric diseases.

Vomiting needs to be differentiated from regurgitation (a sign of an oesophageal disorder; see Chapter 32). The combination of non-productive vomiting, retching, abdominal distension and intragastric gas accumulation is the hallmark of GDV. Haematemesis is rare in GDV, but may reflect mucosal ischaemia and sloughing (see Chapter 19). Vomiting more than 8–10 hours after feeding indicates gastric outflow disorders. Environmental factors include feeding habits, such as a raw meat diet, access to foreign bodies, medications and toxins, or the risk of infection (vaccination status, living outdoor/indoor, single/multiple animal household, inter-animal contact, exhibitions, breeding, sport/free-time events).

Physical examination

Findings on physical examination depend on the severity and any systemic effects of gastric disease. They are often unremarkable or non-specific. Abdominal/gastric distension and tympany are signs of GDV or delayed gastric emptying. A low body condition score suggests chronic disease. Signs and causes of systemic illness are summarized in Figure 33.14.

Minimum database

Animals can mask signs of illness and it is advisable to perform a MDB laboratory test panel to differentiate disorders with similar clinical signs, to assess systemic involvement, and to obtain basic data for comparisons during follow-up visits. The MDB should include haematology with a complete blood count (to assess anaemia, dehydration and inflammation), clinical chemistry (to assess the kidneys, liver and pancreas) and electrolyte status/imbalances. Urinalysis with sediment examination provides evidence of diabetic ketoacidosis or renal disease including chronic kidney disease and pyelonephritis.

Specific laboratory tests

Figure 33.15 summarizes indications for specific laboratory tests and their possible findings and interpretations in connection with clinical signs of gastric disease. These tests are used not only to identify but also to rule out certain conditions for individually tailored treatment decisions.

Diagnostic imaging

For further information on diagnostic imaging, the reader is referred to Chapter 3.

Radiography

Plain abdominal radiographs are indicated to identify gastric displacement (hiatal hernia, diaphragmatic rupture, GDV) (Figure 33.16), foreign bodies and GI perforation (peritonitis, pneumoperitoneum). They are of lower diagnostic value than ultrasonography for detecting gastric wall changes.

Contrast studies: These studies use barium sulphate to detect obstructed or delayed gastric emptying when access to ultrasonography and endoscopy is limited. Pneumogastrography uses air as a negative contrast medium, allowing assessment of gastric positioning (displacement) and wall thickness (neoplasia, hypertrophy), as well as the detection of foreign bodies or gastric perforation. Double-contrast techniques (barium contrast medium plus air/effervescent granules) can help detect ulcers. Iodinated contrast media are indicated to search for GI perforation (Figure 33.17).

Indication	Laboratory test	Possible findings	Interpretation in connection with signs of gastric disease
Excessive vomiting	• Acid–base status determination	Metabolic acidosis Metabolic alkalosis	Majority of cases when pylorus is patent Obstruction in gastric outflow tract or proximal duodenum Acid hypersecretion (gastrinoma) and emesis

Haematemesis, melaena	• Coagulation tests
	  • Activated clotting time
	  • Prothrombin time
	  • Partial thromboplastin time
	  • Platelet count
		Increased clotting times
		
		Thrombocytopenia
			Coagulopathies
			
			Primary haemostasis affected

Anaemia	• Red blood cell morphology
	  • Blood smear
	  • Automated cell analyser
	• Thrombocyte count
	• Serum urea/BUN
	
	• Faecal examination
	  • Macroscopic
	
	  • Occult blood test (o-toluidine test less influenced by processed dietary meat than guaiac test)
		Microcytosis and hypochromasia
		
		Thrombocytosis
		Thrombocytopenia
		Increased in absence of creatinine increase
		
		Melaena
		
		Occult blood
			Chronic gastrointestinal bleeding (iron deficiency)
			Gastrointestinal bleeding
			Primary cause of gastric bleeding
			Gastrointestinal bleeding
			
			Upper gastrointestinal tract bleeding of ≥350 mg/kg bodyweight haemoglobin (≥3 ml/kg blood when blood haemoglobin =
			150 g/l/9.3 mmol/l)
			Upper gastrointestinal tract bleeding of ≥10 mg/kg haemoglobin

Vomiting and diarrhoea	• Faecal examination for pathogens • Serum examination for pathogens (cats) • Cortisol, basal • (ACTH stimulation test for differentiation)	Viral, parasitic or bacterial FeLV, FIV Decreased ≤55 nmol/l Unaffected	Gastrointestinal infection Systemic infection Hypoadrenocorticism Pseudohypoadrenocorticism
Weight loss, behavioural changes	• Total T4	Increased	Hyperthyroidism • Cat: primary > alimentary • Dog: alimentary > primary
Abdominal pain (dog) Lethargy, inappetence (cat)	• Serum pancreatic lipase (PL) concentration • Serum DGGR lipase activity	Increased	Consistent with pancreatitis Consistent with pancreatitis but less specific than serum PL
Gastric dilatation-volvulus	Serum lactate	Increased	Negative prognostic factor

33.15 Indications for and the interpretation of specific laboratory tests for the diagnostic investigation of gastric diseases in dogs and cats. ACTH = adrenocorticotropic hormone; BUN = blood urea nitrogen; DGGR = 1, 2-o-dilauryl rac-glycero glutaric acid -(6'-methylresorufin) ester; FeLV: feline leukaemia virus; FIV: feline immunodeficiency virus; T4 = thyroxine.

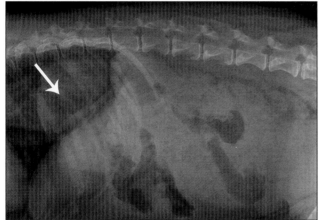

33.16 Right lateral radiographic view showing a hiatal hernia with prolapse of the stomach (arrowed) into the thoracic cavity of a dog.

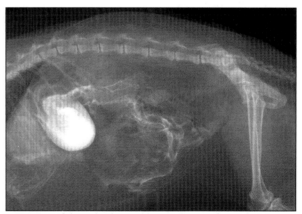

33.17 Left lateral radiographic view showing free iodine contrast medium in the abdominal cavity of a cat with gastrointestinal perforation.

Fluoroscopy

Fluoroscopy has been used to investigate gastric emptying in healthy conscious dogs, but lacks application in clinical cases.

Computed tomography

Contrast-enhanced cross-sectional imaging can help locate and define local invasiveness of gastric wall lesions, and differentiate surgical from non-surgical acute abdominal conditions (e.g. 93% sensitivity for perforated ulcers).

Ultrasonography

Standard transabdominal ultrasonography has proven useful for assessing gastric wall thickness, layering and masses (polyps, tumours), as well as for the evaluation of other abdominal organs. However, caution should be exercised not to interpret variations in wall thickness due to normal gastric contractions as abnormal findings reflecting true lesions. In addition, its diagnostic value for wall lesions is limited because imaging of the whole gastric wall is not possible due to the presence of gas and food. The sensitivity of ultrasonography for detecting ulceration is limited, but is markedly increased when there is perforation. There is a marked overlap in the ultrasonographic appearance of GI inflammation and neoplasia, with, for example, lymphoma sometimes showing only non-specific findings.

Ultrasound-based assessment of gastric emptying: This has been successfully performed in experimental studies in healthy and diabetic dogs, but has not yet entered clinical practice.

Endoscopy

Diagnostic endoscopy

Endoscopy allows direct visualization and sampling of the gastric lumen and mucosal surface. It is far superior to ultrasonography for detecting peptic and neoplastic ulcers, gastric lymphoma and benign polyps. The ability to take multiple mucosal biopsy samples allows for a certain degree of differentiation between inflammatory and neoplastic changes. Limitations include the need for general anaesthesia (and its associated risks) and missing or limited assessment of deeper wall changes, anatomical relationships and gastric function.

The extent and severity of macroscopic changes are not always consistent with the respective histopathological findings from endoscopic biopsies. Possible reasons for such discrepancies are the patchy distribution of gastric lesions and the possibility to miss flat, inconspicuous changes when using non-directed or too superficial biopsy techniques in standard endoscopic approaches with white light. Contrast enhancing techniques, such as chromoendoscopy or endoscopic narrow-band imaging, have improved endoscopic diagnostic yield in human medicine and also show promise in small animal gastroenterology. First attempts to use confocal endomicroscopy have also produced encouraging results.

Measuring the pyloric diameter of cats with endoscopic olive probes allows the diagnosis of pyloric narrowing or stenosis as possible results of chronic idiopathic inflammation. The introduction of staging protocols for the extension and severity of gastric pathologies promises further improvement.

For further information on endoscopy, see Chapter 4 and the *BSAVA Manual of Canine and Feline Endoscopy and Endosurgery.*

Therapeutic endoscopy

Therapeutic endoscopy has mainly been applied for the retrieval of gastric foreign bodies. Electrosurgical procedures such as endoscopic mucosal resection or submucosal dissection are useful for minimally invasive removal of benign polyps or pre-neoplastic changes such as metaplasia or dysplasia.

Diagnostic laparotomy

Surgical full-thickness biopsy (Figure 33.18) is indicated to diagnose pyloric muscular hypertrophy, leiomyositis and stromal tumours (leiomyoma, leiomyosarcoma, GISTs). For more information, see the *BSAVA Manual of Canine and Feline Abdominal Surgery.*

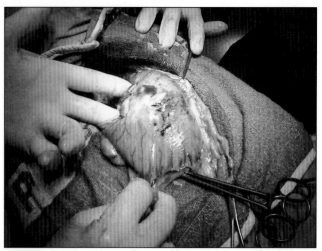

33.18 Gastric carcinoma diagnosed by laparotomy and full-thickness biopsy.

Gastric function and permeability tests

Gastric function testing aims at measuring the rate of gastric emptying and intragastric pH to diagnose gastric dysmotility and investigate the effects of diseases, diets and medications on gastric acid secretion. Gastric emptying rate determination has been performed so far by radioactive or stable isotopic methods (scintigraphy, isotope tracer studies), fluoroscopy and dynamic ultrasonography. Intragastric pH can be measured by gastric intubation (orogastric, percutaneous) or radiotelemetric techniques. Accessibility to all these methods is limited to specialist centres.

Sucrose permeability testing may be commercially available in the future: intact sucrose is not absorbed across in the normal stomach wall, but can be when there is gastric disease.

Specific diseases of the stomach

Acute gastritis

Diagnosis

Results of the MDB should rule out involvement of other intra-abdominal organs. Specific laboratory examinations to test for pancreatitis and less common disorders, and to determine severity are tailored to the individual case (see Figure 33.15).

Radiography (plain and positive or negative contrast) helps to locate foreign bodies and to assess gastric filling and positioning. Iodinated contrast medium or air should be used instead of barium sulphate when perforation is suspected or endoscopy is planned. Ultrasonography can help identify foreign material and evaluate wall thickness and layering, to reveal gastric ulcers or changes indicative of acutely deteriorating chronic processes, including neoplasia.

Treatment

Dietary management: In adult patients, withholding food and water for 12–24 hours may suffice in mild cases. Spontaneous re-alimentation should begin 6–12 hours after cessation of vomiting by offering a liquid diet to assess whether vomiting has fully resolved. Diets with positive effects in acute gastritis are rice-based, fat-restricted and contain highly digestible protein sources. They are commercially available or homemade (e.g. white rice and boiled skinless, boneless chicken breast or low-fat cottage cheese).

Medical treatment: The aim is to stabilize and support the patient, control vomiting and, in selected cases, provide gastroprotection. Volume depletion and electrolyte imbalances are corrected by intravenous fluid therapy when oral rehydration is inappropriate or insufficient due to persistent vomiting. Metoclopramide is effective for centrally induced vomiting in dogs and for stimulating progressive gastric motility in dogs and cats; ondansetron is more effective for peripherally induced vomiting; maropitant acts on both pathways. In cats, the combination of ondansetron and maropitant seems to have faster effects to decrease nausea and improve clinical wellbeing. Gastric protectants, such as histamine (H_2)-receptor antagonists, and proton pump inhibitors (PPIs) are useful in non-erosive and erosive gastritis, but mucosal protective agents such as sucralfate are indicated only when ulceration is suspected or identified (see Chapter 28).

Endoscopic removal of foreign bodies: This can be very effective to manage acute mechanical injuries if the foreign body is not too large; otherwise surgical removal is indicated. In pets with pica and gastric mucosal changes, biopsy samples should be obtained to assess for chronic gastric disease.

Prognosis

Disease outcome is highly variable and depends on the individual presentation and progression. Milder cases can recover spontaneously with dietary and medical support. Signs of more severe disease include the presence of persistent vomiting that is unresponsive to antiemetic treatment, profuse haematemesis, severe dehydration and systemic illness or early relapse. Severely affected animals may not recover spontaneously, and diagnostic steps need to be taken to determine any underlying non-gastric diseases or severe gastropathies with systemic effects that may require more aggressive intervention (e.g. obstructing foreign body, gastric perforation, chronic inflammation and neoplasia).

Chronic gastritis

The diagnosis of chronic gastritis starts with the exclusion of diseases of other organs and systemic disorders such as uraemic gastropathy. A diagnosis of chronic idiopathic gastritis is established only by the exclusion of infectious and neoplastic gastric diseases.

Infectious chronic gastritis

Bacterial infections include the controversial *Helicobacter*-associated gastritis and feline gastric actinomycosis. The likelihood of parasitic and fungal gastritis and the need to assess for them in the diagnostic investigation varies geographically and depends on the pet's lifestyle (i.e. indoor, outdoor, free-roaming, travel history, stray animal).

Helicobacter-*associated gastritis (Figure 33.19):*

Diagnosis: Both indirect and direct (biopsy-based) methods can be applied to search for *Helicobacter* spp. Indirect tests, such as the urea breath test and serology for anti-*Helicobacter* immunoglobulin G antibodies, are of lower diagnostic value than biopsy-based diagnosis by polymerase chain reaction (PCR), impression smear cytology or histopathology using haematoxylin and eosin or Warthin–Starry silver staining methods. Rapid urease tests using biopsy samples are positive not only for *Helicobacter* but also for other urease-producing, often transient, bacteria. For routine practice, the histological confirmation of *Helicobacter* spp. in connection with marked chronic and follicular gastritis seems to provide some evidence of possible *Helicobacter*-associated gastritis.

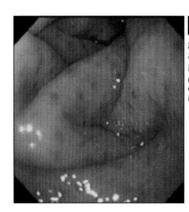

33.19 Lymphoid follicles may be seen in the gastric mucosa as darker spots and have been associated with *Helicobacter* infection.
(Reproduced from the *BSAVA Manual of Canine and Feline Endoscopy and Endosurgery*)

Treatment: Controversy lingers around the value of attempts to eradicate *Helicobacter* spp., due to the lack of a significant association between *Helicobacter* infection and pro-inflammatory cytokine expression, severity of gastritis or pathogenicity of different *Helicobacter* species. Long-term eradication has not been successful in studies of pets and recrudescence appears to be the rule even when clinical signs abate. Some consensus exists that *Helicobacter* infections should be treated only when there is massive colonization in gastric pits or intracellularly in connection with marked (follicular) inflammation. For dogs, several treatment regimens have been reported using, for 7–14 days, combinations of amoxicillin, metronidazole and bismuth subcitrate with or without famotidine; tetracycline and omeprazole; clarithromycin, amoxicillin and lansoprazole. In asymptomatic, *Helicobacter*-positive cats, quadruple therapy with amoxicillin, metronidazole, clarithromycin and omeprazole for 14 days has not been effective in eradicating naturally acquired infections.

Prognosis: Treatment of *Helicobacter* infection sometimes leads to clinical improvement in both dogs and cats; however, the bacteria remain or recur. Since most *Helicobacter* spp. probably belong to the normal gastric microbiota and spontaneous *H. pylori* infections do not occur in dogs and cats, indiscriminate use of antimicrobials should be avoided. Triple or quadruple therapies may be applicable when dietary change and gastroprotective therapy (e.g. PPIs) fails, or before treating idiopathic gastritis with immunosuppressive drugs.

Feline gastric actinomycosis:

Diagnosis: Abdominal ultrasonography can reveal focal hypoechoic transmural thickening with loss of normal wall layering and hyperechoic speckles. Gastroscopy reveals a gastric mass with an ulcerated depression. Endoscopic biopsy samples do not seem to be diagnostic, but a full-thickness specimen can identify transmural pyogranulomatous inflammation. Culture from gastric wall aspirates, biochemical testing and PCR of the *16s ribosomal RNA* gene allowed detection of *Actinomyces hordevulneris* in one case (Pietra *et al.*, 2016).

Treatment and prognosis: Surgical resection and cefovecin (8 mg/kg s.c. every 14 days for 4 months) led to a full recovery in one case. Clinical signs and abdominal ultrasonography helped to provide evidence of treatment success.

Parasitic gastritis:

Diagnosis: The epidemiological situation or a history of travel to certain geographical regions need to be considered before searching for gastric parasites. Figure 33.4 summarizes gastric parasites, their geographical distribution, different detection methods and treatments.

Treatment and prognosis: Parasitic gastritis is treated in accordance with the individual diagnosis (see Figure 33.4). Prognosis depends on the availability and efficacy of antiparasitic drugs and the severity of parasite-induced changes.

Fungal gastritis:
Transmural infection of the GI tract with the fungus-like oomycete *P. insidiosum* (pythiosis) is seen in certain geographical locations (e.g. southern USA, Brazil) and can occasionally be found concurrently with infection by the ascomycete *Blastomyces dermatitidis*. There is one case report of *Cryptococcus neoformans* causing a tumour-like gastric ulcer.

Diagnosis: Abdominal palpation, radiography and ultrasonography reveal an abdominal mass and segmental thickening of the wall, especially in the antrum. The enzyme-linked immunosorbent assay (ELISA) for anti *P. insidiosum* serum antibodies has high sensitivity and specificity, allowing early diagnosis and monitoring of the response to treatment. Endoscopy reveals hypertrophy in the antrum, but endoscopic biopsy samples may miss the fungus as the inflammatory processes tend to be localized in the submucosal and muscular layers. Resected gastric wall or full-thickness biopsy samples have a higher diagnostic value than endoscopic specimens. Fungal gastritis may be suspected on the basis of histology, but identification of the associated organisms can be difficult and generally relies on submission of tissue samples to specialized laboratories for immunohistochemical and PCR testing. Differentiation from similar fungi can be achieved by PCR or *ribosomal RNA* gene sequencing of infected tissue.

Treatment: Aggressive surgical resection is the treatment of choice, with a minimum margin of 5 cm and biopsy of local lymph nodes when enlarged. In addition, medical treatment with a combination of itraconazole (10 mg/kg orally q24h) and terbinafine (5–10 mg/kg orally q24h) is recommended for 3 months when the 5 cm margin is not achievable. Conservative medical treatment is impaired by the lack of effective drugs. There has been at least one case report of clinical remission in a dog with pythiosis treated with terbinafine plus itraconazole for 12 months and immunotherapy with a vaccine based on inactivated antigens from cultured *P. insidiosum* (Pereira *et al.*, 2013) and other cases of dogs with colonic pythiosis, treated successfully using itraconazole and terbinafine plus anti-inflammatory steroids (Reagan *et al.*, 2019).

Prognosis: Local postsurgical recurrence commonly results from inadequate margins. ELISA serology should be performed both before and 2–3 months after surgery: a decrease in the serum antibody titre by ≥50% is a sign of complete resection without recurrence, indicating that antifungal medication can stop.

Idiopathic chronic gastritis

In cases of chronic gastritis, the actual cause often remains unknown. Idiopathic lymphoplasmacytic gastritis is the most commonly reported type of chronic gastritis (Figure 33.20). Other types include eosinophilic, atrophic and hypertrophic gastritis, non-neoplastic polyps and feline acquired pyloric stenosis.

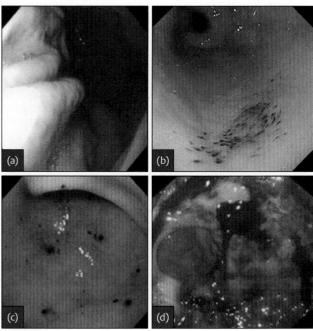

33.20 Endoscopic appearance of lymphoplasmacytic gastritis. (a) Subtle irregularities in the mucosa of the rugal folds, consistent with chronic gastritis. (b) 'Paintbrush' haemorrhages in the antrum. (c) Multiple superficial gastric ulcers (erosions) associated with chronic gastritis showing small amounts of changed (brown) blood. (d) Severe, diffuse ulceration with significant bleeding in chronic gastritis (fresh blood is dripping down).
(c, Reproduced from the *BSAVA Manual of Canine and Feline Endoscopy and Endosurgery*)
(a, b, d, Courtesy of Edward J. Hall)

Lymphoplasmacytic gastritis:

Diagnosis: Histology reveals an inflammatory infiltrate comprising predominantly lymphocytes and plasma cells. Such infiltrates are also reported as the inflammatory component of other pathological changes relevant to the differential diagnosis (e.g. gastric mucosal atrophy, metaplasia, dysplasia, hypertrophy and neoplasia). The clinical significance of mild lymphoplasmacytic infiltration in the absence of other changes remains debatable. Moderate to severe infiltration is often associated with concurrent chronic enteropathies attributable to a disturbed immune tolerance to alimentary or bacterial antigens, and evaluation of enteric function (serum cobalamin and folate) should be considered. Severe lymphoplasmacytic infiltrations might be difficult to differentiate from intestinal lymphoma when assessing endoscopic biopsy samples only.

Treatment and prognosis: Lymphoplasmacytic gastritis is considered to have an immunological aetiology. It is primarily managed with dietary changes and acid blockers, and secondarily with immunosuppressive drugs. Changing to a diet with a low food antigen load (limited-ingredient novel protein or hydrolysed diets) generally leads to an improvement within 2–5 days in cats and 10–14 days in dogs if the inflammation is diet-related. Antiemetics and gastroprotective drugs, such as H_2-receptor antagonists, are used for initial and short-term (days to weeks) supportive treatment. PPIs are generally indicated for the treatment of ulcerative gastritis or for long-term use (weeks to months) in patients with chronic lymphoplasmacytic gastritis.

If the animal is unresponsive to dietary changes and acid blockers, immunosuppressive treatment is usually started with prednisolone. In cases with hypoalbuminaemia, or when the response to glucocorticoids is poor, chlorambucil, ciclosporin, mycophenolate mofetil or azathioprine can be added. Combination protocols allow a reduction in the prednisolone dosage, especially when severe steroid sensitivity causes polydipsia, polyuria and lethargy. Azathioprine has become the least favoured of these drugs due to its slow onset of action and its side effects, which can be lethal in cats. Good evidence for the efficacy of any of these drugs in gastritis is lacking.

An effective treatment protocol and clinical outcome cannot be predicted by the clinical signs, laboratory markers or histology at the time of initial diagnosis. A stepwise treatment approach should be devised to achieve the best possible results whilst minimizing side effects. The majority of animals respond to dietary change and/or acid blockers. In unresponsive animals, glucocorticoid and immunosuppressive drugs can produce long-lasting improvement. The treatment is started with a higher loading dose until clinical improvement occurs. This is followed by tapering down to the lowest effective dose for long-term maintenance therapy (several months). Using low-dose prednisolone alone every second day or in exchange with chlorambucil on alternating days aims to keep the balance between positive and negative side effects. Occasionally, cats and dogs can become non-responsive to immunosuppression and may develop gastric lymphoma.

Eosinophilic gastritis and feline gastrointestinal eosinophilic sclerosing fibroplasia: Eosinophilic gastritis/gastroenteritis, canine eosinophilic GI masses and feline GI eosinophilic sclerosing fibroplasia are characterized histologically by a predominantly eosinophilic infiltration. They can manifest as local changes in the stomach or other parts of the GI tract, being either diffuse, mass-forming or ulcerative without predilection sites and mimicking neoplasia.

Diagnosis: A MDB may or may not reveal eosinophilia. Ultrasonography can help verify normal wall structure or may indicate gastric and/or intestinal changes, such as thickening, loss of layering and mass formation. Endoscopy can show either grossly normal-appearing mucosa or diffuse or local mass-forming, ulcerative lesions, which can cause an obstruction when affecting the antrum and pylorus. Histology reports state different degrees of tissue infiltration with eosinophilic granulocytes. Full-thickness biopsy samples or resected tissue allow for histological distinction between idiopathic inflammation and infectious/neoplastic diseases. Cytology of specimens from other organs (liver, spleen, bronchoalveolar lavage) allows exclusion of hypereosinophilic syndrome when negative for tissue eosinophilia.

Treatment: Diffuse mucosal eosinophilic gastritis is treated similarly to lymphoplasmacytic gastritis (hydrolysed or limited-ingredient novel protein diets; glucocorticoids).

Canine mass-forming eosinophilic gastritis has been treated with a combination of glucocorticoids and ivermectin, even without evidence of parasitism, and surgically. Feline GI eosinophilic sclerosing fibroplasia has been treated with surgery or antibiotics, either alone or with prednisolone.

Prognosis: Idiopathic eosinophilic gastritis and gastroenteritis seem to have a less favourable prognosis than lymphoplasmacytic gastritis. Canine mass-forming eosinophilic gastritis and feline GI eosinophilic sclerosing fibroplasia seem to have the best outcome in terms of clinical signs, resolution of eosinophilic infiltrations and prolonged survival times when treated with adjunctive prednisolone in contrast to sole surgical or antibiotic treatment.

Atrophic gastritis:
Diagnosis: Histology of endoscopic biopsy samples reveals loss of parietal cell mass and mucosal thickness with lymphoplasmacytic infiltration and possible mucous neck cell proliferation (mucous metaplasia).

Treatment and prognosis: To date there are no reports on the treatment and follow-up of patients with atrophic gastritis. Atrophic gastritis has not been shown to be associated with *Helicobacter* spp. infection and thus eradication attempts do not seem indicated. Since it is a chronic inflammatory condition, treatment measures can be tried as for lymphoplasmacytic gastritis to improve clinical signs. The usefulness of acid-reducing drugs is questionable.

Giant hypertrophic gastritis: Giant hypertrophic gastritis (GHG) is a rare, possibly inheritable, condition in dogs of different breeds, characterized by marked thickening of the gastric wall. It is not the same as Ménétrier disease in humans, which is non-inflammatory. The hypertrophic gastric mucosa appears cerebriform and the rugal folds protrude into the gastric lumen, affecting the fundus and body rather than the antrum (Figure 33.21). A possible neoplastic transformation to gastric carcinoma in dogs has been proposed.

Diagnosis: The physical examination and MDB are not diagnostic, with the exception of hypoalbuminaemia associated with GHG. Measuring the serum gastrin level aids differentiation of hypertrophic gastritis from gastrinoma, where the serum concentration would be >3–10 times the upper reference limit (≤27.8 ng/l). Antisecretory therapy with H_2-receptor antagonists and PPIs (e.g. omeprazole) also induces hypergastrinaemia, but for less than 2 weeks after cessation of treatment and at concentrations unlikely to confuse the diagnosis of gastrinoma.

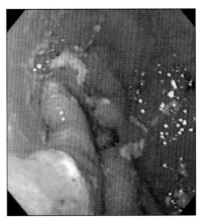

33.21 Endoscopic appearance of giant hypertrophic gastritis. Thickened, cerebriform rugae are present and do not flatten on insufflation.
(Courtesy of Edward J. Hall)

Abdominal ultrasonography can reveal thickening of the mucosal and/or muscular layer in the antrum and/or corpus, but gas in the lumen may impair visualization. Endoscopy allows visualization of the localization and extension of mucosal and rugal thickening, papillary proliferations and the degree of antral obstruction. Histology of endoscopic biopsy samples reveals a hypertrophic/hyperplastic mucosa that may or may not include secondary folds of muscularis mucosae and submucosa. However, malignant changes can be missed during endoscopic sampling. Surgical resection of the affected area delivers superior diagnostic and also therapeutic value.

Treatment and prognosis: Surgical resection of hypertrophic areas is considered curative. Early resection is advisable since GHG has been linked to gastric carcinoma. In cats, the possible association of *Ollulanus tricuspis* infection with GHG suggests adjunctive antiparasitic therapy.

Feline acquired pyloric stenosis: Acquired pyloric stenosis is associated with lymphoplasmacytic mucosal infiltration and fibrosis. It has recently been reported in cats with chronic vomiting and is characterized by pyloric narrowing to a median diameter of 7 mm (normal interquartile range 9–10 mm) (Freiche *et al.*, 2017; Lamoureux *et al.*, 2019).

Diagnosis: An endoscopic examination may reveal a decreased pyloric diameter when measured either with the open cups of the biopsy forceps or with interchangeable, biocompatible olives (4–12 mm diameter). Alternatively, the inability to pass an 8.8 mm tip diameter endoscope is suggestive of pyloric stenosis. Histology of endoscopic mucosal biopsy samples excludes malignancy and reveals non-specific chronic inflammation and fibrosis.

Treatment and prognosis: To date, no clinical trials have been undertaken to assess treatment modalities and responses. Due to the underlying non-specific mucosal inflammation, dietary measures and medication are advised as for lymphoplasmacytic gastritis. Feeding regimens should be adjusted to facilitate pyloric transit (soft rather than dry food, feeding small portions frequently). Antiemetic and acid-reducing drugs for supportive care depend on the severity of the clinical signs and the response to dietary adjustments. Possible surgical interventions include pyloroplasty and pylorectomy with gastroduodenostomy. For more information, see the *BSAVA Manual of Canine and Feline Abdominal Surgery*.

Idiopathic, chronic, non-inflammatory gastropathies

Non-neoplastic polyps

Non-malignant, pedunculated or sessile polyps (approximately 5–30 mm in size) are either hyperplastic (regenerative) or inflammatory (benign lymphoid) and occur in the pyloric antrum of older dogs (Figure 33.22). A hereditary predisposition has been proposed for the French Bulldog.

Diagnosis: Abdominal ultrasonography can reveal, and endoscopy with biopsy sample collection can confirm, the presence of benign polyps.

Treatment and prognosis: Polyps can be endoscopically removed via snare resection or submucosal dissection. There have been no reports of possible transformation of benign polyps into malignant tumours or their recurrence after removal.

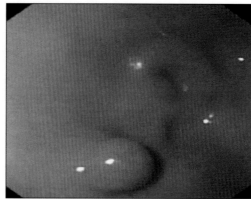

33.22 Endoscopic image of a pedunculated, non-malignant polyp near the pylorus of a dog.

Chronic hypertrophic pyloric gastropathy

Chronic hypertrophic pyloric gastropathy refers to a syndrome of pyloric obstruction in dogs due to hyperplasia of the antropyloric mucosa (Figure 33.23). Hypertrophy of the circular pyloric muscles is often a congenital anomaly in Boxers, Bulldogs and Boston Terriers. Adult forms mainly affect male brachycephalic small-breed dogs, often in combination with antritis.

Diagnosis: Diagnostic investigation is similar to that of GHG, including serum gastrin determination to differentiate from gastrinoma. The diagnosis is confirmed by anatomical localization and histology.

Treatment: Surgical resection of the affected tissue is the treatment of choice. For more information, see the *BSAVA Manual of Canine and Feline Abdominal Surgery*.

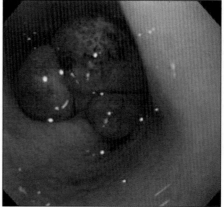

33.23 Endoscopic appearance of chronic hypertrophic pyloric gastropathy. (Courtesy of Edward J. Hall)

Gastric foreign bodies

Gastric foreign bodies are more common in dogs than in cats. The availability of endoscopy has greatly improved their diagnosis and treatment.

Diagnosis

The MDB is used to help estimate dehydration and to look for systemic effects, especially with metallic foreign bodies containing zinc (e.g. coins), as zinc intoxication can cause haemolytic anaemia and, potentially, kidney injury. Radiography is needed to verify and localize radiodense objects (Figure 33.24). Positive (barium sulphate) or negative (air) contrast studies help to reveal radiolucent material, if

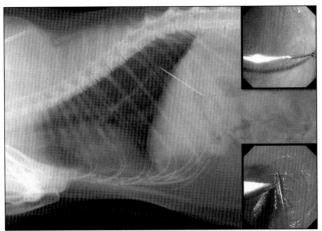

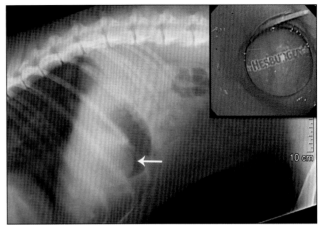

33.24 Lateral view of a radiopaque perforating foreign body (needle) in a cat, with endoscopic images of the gastric perforation and removal of the needle along with thread.

33.25 Lateral radiographic and endoscopic images of an intact rubber ball in the stomach of a dog (arrowed). Such foreign bodies lodged in the antrum usually require surgical removal.

abdominal ultrasonography or endoscopy are not available. Abdominal ultrasonography is especially helpful to rule in or exclude intestinal obstruction.

Endoscopy is the technique of choice when there is no evidence of intestinal involvement requiring surgery and the object is not too large to grasp and pull *per os*. If the stomach is filled with food, stabilizing the patient and delaying endoscopy to allow for gastric emptying is advised. However, foreign bodies of adequate size could be propelled into the intestine during the migrating motor complex between meals, and prokinetic antiemetics (e.g. metoclopramide) should definitely be avoided. After prolonged fasting periods, it is advisable to repeat radiographic imaging to verify that the object(s) has remained in the stomach before undertaking endoscopy. Metallic foreign bodies should be immediately removed, especially when they are believed to be zinc-based alloys or multiple magnets. Multiple magnetic foreign bodies pose a very high risk for GI perforation and lethal complications, as the GI wall can be compressed between two magnets attracting each other, causing ischaemic necrosis.

Treatment and prognosis

Gastric foreign bodies are best removed via endoscopy using foreign body grasping forceps, a wire or Roth basket or a snare, selected according to the shape and size of the object. A magnet can be placed on the skin over the stomach when searching for and retrieving metallic foreign bodies (i.e. those containing iron or nickel); this may be especially useful when the stomach is filled with food. When there is evidence of obstructing foreign bodies in both the stomach and small intestine, surgery should be performed immediately. Surgery is also indicated when the foreign body is clearly too large to be retrieved endoscopically or when attempted endoscopic retrieval is not successful within approximately 1 hour (Figure 33.25). Endoscopic removal of gastric foreign bodies has high success and low overall complication rates (e.g. no complications after discharge in 92% of cases in the authors' practice). Negative prognostic factors are dogs weighing <10 kg and foreign bodies present for more than 3 days.

Gastric ulceration

Gastric ulceration can be the result of any type of chronic gastritis, drug administration, abrasive/sharp foreign bodies or secondary to neoplastic infiltration.

Diagnosis

History and clinical signs: The history and clinical signs help determine the time course (acute versus chronic) and clinical severity (obvious versus occult bleeding, degree of anaemia) of the gastric ulceration.

Minimum database: The MDB may initially reveal regenerative anaemia with acute gastric bleeding, but continued low-grade, chronic bleeding leads to microcytic, hypochromic anaemia of iron deficiency, often associated with thrombocytosis. Eosinophilia in dogs may point towards hypoadrenocorticism, eosinophilic gastroenteritis, a paraneoplastic effect of lymphoma, mastocytosis or hypereosinophilic syndrome. Fever, leucocytosis with neutrophilia and left shift, and increased serum C-reactive protein are indicative of a deep ulcer and possible gastric perforation. Specific laboratory tests include coagulation tests, where an abnormal bleeding tendency or DIC is suspected (Figure 33.26), and serum gastrin concentration to diagnose gastrinoma.

Plain radiography: Gastric ulceration cannot be detected on plain radiographs, but any foreign body causing the ulceration is likely to be visible.

Contrast radiography: Obtaining radiographs using barium sulphate as a single- or double-contrast agent with the patient in different positions can help delineate mucosal defects when endoscopy is not available. The sensitivity of the single-contrast technique is 75%, and that of the double-contrast technique is 95%. Gastric ulcers appear as round, ovoid or linear collections of barium contrast medium. Lesions smaller than 5 mm may be missed. When

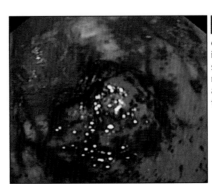

33.26 Endoscopic image of diffuse gastric bleeding in a dog with Evans syndrome (immune-mediated haemolytic anaemia and thrombocytopenia).

perforation is suspected, barium sulphate is contra-indicated as it may cause peritonitis; an iodine-based contrast medium should be used instead.

Ultrasonography: This imaging modality is used to help rule out other causes of abdominal pain, such as biliary and pancreatic disease. Mucosal defects, such as superficial and deep ulcers, appear as relatively depressed areas with increased echogenicity, and occasionally air tracking is visible in the tissues (see Chapter 3). Gastric wall layer changes may provide information about lesion depth and the risk or presence of perforation. Ultrasound-guided sampling of free abdominal fluid aids in diagnosing septic peritonitis associated with gastric perforation.

Endoscopy: Contemporaneous visual examination and biopsy sampling for histological classification of lesions (diffuse superficial, local benign or malignant ulcer) are advantages of gastroscopy. Multiple deep biopsy samples from ulcer margins are needed to maximize diagnostic yield. When anaesthesia must be avoided, capsule endoscopy may help to locate the source of gastric bleeding. Endoscopy is contraindicated when perforation has occurred, as this requires immediate surgical attention.

Treatment

Gastroprotective medication: This is the mainstay of treating gastric ulceration. It includes the use of histamine (H_2)-receptor antagonists (H_2-blockers), PPIs and sucralfate (see Chapter 28).

H_2-blockers: Ranitidine, nizatidine and famotidine can be used for short-term therapy (days to a few weeks), since the effect has been shown to diminish in dogs by day 14. The effect of intravenous ranitidine is dose dependent: 5 mg/kg increases gastric pH in dogs within 1 hour, but 2 mg/kg has no effect in dogs or cats. Famotidine increases gastric pH in dogs when given intravenously (0.5 mg/kg q12h) and in cats when given orally (0.88–1.26 mg/kg q12h).

Proton pump inhibitors: Omeprazole, esomeprazole, lansoprazole and pantoprazole are indicated for short- to longer-term (weeks to months) treatment of severe gastric ulcerative disorders, including gastrinoma. Suppression of gastric acid is achieved in dogs with intravenous pantoprazole (1 mg/kg) and intravenous or oral omeprazole (1 mg/kg), typically once daily. However, a recent case report indicates that twice daily administration may be needed in some cases to promote healing of peptic ulcers (Lane *et al.*, 2017). In cats, oral omeprazole (1.1–1.3 mg/kg) is effective only when given twice-daily. Discontinuation of prolonged acid suppression may lead to an acid rebound effect due to up-regulated H_2-receptors and hypergastrinaemia; tapering down the medication might prevent this effect.

Sucralfate: This adheres to mucosal defects, forming a protective coating. Since it must attach to the mucosa and it interferes with the absorption of other drugs, it needs to be given on an empty stomach 2 hours apart from other drugs.

Misoprostol: This synthetic prostaglandin E has been shown to prevent but not to heal NSAID-induced gastric ulcers. It also induces uterine contractions and may cause abortion.

Surgery: Surgical intervention is indicated for resection of severe chronic peptic ulcers (Figure 33.27) and gastrinomas, and for repairing gastric perforations. In humans, endoscopy is used to treat actively bleeding ulcers using adrenaline (epinephrine) injection, fibrin glue, thermal coagulation or endoscopic clips.

Prognosis

Most acute benign ulcers tend to heal or scar within days to weeks after removal of the inciting cause (e.g. cessation of NSAIDs; Figure 33.28) and starting gastroprotective treatment. Advanced chronic peptic ulcers may not respond to gastroprotective treatment alone, but after resection they have a favourable prognosis. For neoplastic ulcers, the overall prognosis is related to the degree of local extension and presence of metastasis.

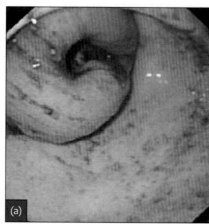
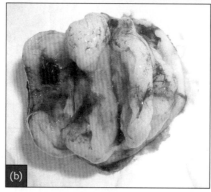

33.27 (a) Endoscopic image of a severe chronic peptic ulcer, which was (b) resected surgically.

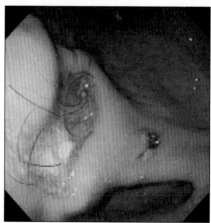

33.28 Ulcer on the lesser curvature following non-steroidal anti-inflammatory drug administration. Hair and debris are stuck in the ulcer; the fresh blood seen is from an adjacent biopsy site. (Reproduced from the *BSAVA Manual of Canine and Feline Endoscopy and Endosurgery*)

Neoplasia

Diagnosis

Physical examination: Very large gastric masses may be palpable, but typically the physical examination only reveals non-specific findings, such as weight loss and pale mucous membranes if the patient is anaemic. The correlation between the severity of vomiting and the extent of gastric wall changes seems to be rather low, as gastric carcinoma can also be subclinical. However, symptomatic dogs with gastric carcinoma tend to be older than 8 years, with a body condition score <4/9 (Seim-Wikse *et al.*, 2019).

Minimum database: Results of the MDB are non-specific and can include mild anaemia, mild neutrophilia and increased hepatic enzymes. Circulating lymphoblasts are occasionally found with GI lymphoma. Severe hypoalbuminaemia (<20 g/l) without hypoglobulinaemia, due to renal loss or hepatic insufficiency can occur in feline lymphoma. Hypercalcaemia is an uncommon finding in alimentary lymphoma. Serum C-reactive protein concentrations >25 mg/l and abnormally low serum folate concentrations have been found to be associated with gastric carcinoma in dogs (Seim-Wikse *et al.*, 2019).

Radiography: Plain radiographs are insensitive for identifying gastric masses. Sensitivity can be enhanced by contrast studies, but they are worthwhile only if computed tomography (CT) or endoscopy is not available.

Ultrasonography: This modality can reveal masses and abnormal mural thickness and layering. It can also detect infiltration or metastasis and allows fine-needle aspirates to be collected for cytology from the thickened gastric wall, regional lymph nodes, liver or other organs.

Computed tomography: If available, CT imaging allows evaluation of the gastric wall and can provide evidence of metastasis (e.g. involvement of lymph nodes). Using intragastric water (30 ml/kg) and intravenous iodine contrast medium (helical hydro-CT) improves wall imaging for evaluating the location and extent of lesions.

Endoscopy: This procedure allows visual assessment and biopsy of sessile polyps, masses, ulcers and diffuse changes. However, there may be inconspicuous changes in the mucosa, which are visible only with more advanced endoscopic imaging techniques. Chromoendoscopy, narrow-band imaging or similar technologies enable the detection of discrete mucosal changes for better direct sampling and increased diagnostic yield. Several, deep biopsy samples should be taken from the suspected area and from the rim but not the centre of ulcers. When anaesthesia must be avoided, capsule endoscopy may be helpful but lacks the opportunity for biopsy specimen collection.

Surgical biopsy: A full-thickness biopsy is indicated to reveal stromal tumours and to differentiate gastric neoplasia from severe benign chronic ulcers or hypertrophic gastritis/gastropathy.

Biopsy sample evaluation: Standard histology and immunohistochemistry are used for tumour differentiation.

- **Mesenchymal tumours** comprise smooth-muscle tumours (leiomyoma, leiomyosarcoma) positive for smooth muscle actin and/or desmin, and GISTs positive for CD117 and CD34.

- **Small cell lymphoma** is differentiated from severe lymphoplasmacytic inflammation by immunostaining for CD3 and CD79 in tissue samples obtained by endoscopy or, preferably, full-thickness biopsy. PCR for antigen receptor rearrangement (PARR) evaluation of biopsy samples can also be used to test for clonality.

Treatment and prognosis

Treatment of gastric tumours is mostly palliative and includes surgical removal and/or chemotherapy (see the *BSAVA Manual of Canine and Feline Oncology*). Decision-making is dependent on staging, as the prognosis is associated with the localization and invasiveness (local, metastatic) of the individual tumour.

Gastric adenocarcinoma:

Medical treatment: This may be indicated to postpone euthanasia in patients experiencing milder signs of gastric disease, or just prior to planned surgery; it is palliative and aimed at improving welfare and preventing complications. This includes protection from ulceration (PPIs, sucralfate) and analgesia. There are a few reports of chemotherapy alone or as adjuvant after surgical resection (e.g. carboplatin, doxorubicin), associated with survival times of weeks to months.

Minimally invasive techniques: Currently used in humans for the removal of selected pre-neoplastic or neoplastic mucosal lesions that have not yet invaded the underlying tissues (e.g. carcinoma *in situ*), these techniques are rarely available in veterinary practice. Both endoscopic mucosal resection and endoscopic submucosal dissection require an electrosurgical device and insufflation with carbon dioxide.

Surgical resection: Partial gastrectomy can be potentially curative (Figure 33.29), but extension and location of the tumour may preclude resection. Well delineated tumours (often diagnosed incidentally, such as sessile polypoid masses on the distal greater curvature of the gastric body or in the antrum), in the absence of known neoplastic invasion or regional metastasis, are best treated by surgical resection with wide margins and consideration of lymphadenectomy. The tumours should be resected with wide margins (1–2 cm) and lymphadenectomy should be considered. In humans, the removal of perigastric and more distal lymph nodes is recommended according to tumour grading and staging.

Prognosis: The prognosis for gastric adenocarcinoma varies according to the stage at diagnosis and location, and surgical resection is curative in only a few selected cases. Metastasis is present in 70–90% of cases at diagnosis and long-term survival time after resection has been

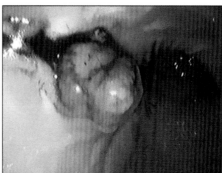

33.29 Endoscopic image of an adenocarcinoma *in situ* in a Tervuren (Belgian Shepherd Dog). Partial gastrectomy was curative, as confirmed by endoscopic biopsy 3 years after the intervention.

reported as poor (a few months) (Eisele *et al.*, 2010; Hugen *et al.*, 2017). Median survival time after extensive resection (pylorectomy with gastroduodenostomy) was only 33 days. Compromised function and welfare confer major ethical constraints in pets. Euthanasia should be considered in the face of escalating clinical signs, which commonly include anorexia due to severe pain.

Gastric lymphoma:
Medical treatment:

- **Lymphoblastic (large cell) lymphoma (LBL):** Treatment in dogs and cats can involve different combination chemotherapy protocols (including cyclophosphamide, doxorubicin, vincristine and prednisolone), but are prone to worse adverse effects (vomiting, diarrhoea, perforation) when there is severe intramural infiltration. The prognosis for LBL is poor: response to treatment is variable (50–70%) and mean survival time ranges between 3 and 6 months.
- **Small cell (lymphocytic) lymphoma (SCL):** In cats, SCL has a much less aggressive progression compared with LBL. It is more commonly located in the ileum and is associated with chronic weight loss and diarrhoea. The diagnosis can be challenging. Gastric infiltration is associated with hyporexia and emesis. SCL may respond well to medical treatment with chlorambucil and prednisolone, with a prognosis for a median survival time of 1.5–2 years with an excellent quality of life. Gastric lymphoma in cats is invariably B-cell in origin. SCL has recently been characterized as T-cell lymphoma in dogs, but diagnosed only in the small intestine (Couto *et al.*, 2018).

Surgical resection: Solitary gastric lymphomas tend to be B-cell in origin. Surgical removal of the mass is anecdotally reported to be curative.

Delayed gastric emptying and motility disorders

Pyloric stenosis

Pyloric stenosis can either be acquired, with hypertrophic gastritis/gastropathy, gastric neoplasia and feline pyloric stenosis, or be congenital, as in brachycephalic dog breeds. Congenital pyloric stenosis often manifests at weaning by projectile vomiting of food after introduction of more solid meals and non-responsiveness to medical therapy with antiemetics and gastroprotective drugs.

Diagnosis: Acquired pyloric stenosis is diagnosed as described for hypertrophic gastritis/gastropathy. In cases of congenital stenosis, abdominal ultrasonography of the pylorus shows gastric wall thickening or a mass effect, which can be confirmed by endoscopy and deep mucosal biopsy.

Treatment and prognosis: Medical treatment (antiemetics, gastroprotectants), in combination with dietary management, can be successful in cases of mild disease. Surgical removal of the hypertrophic tissue via pyloroplasty and submucosal resection or even pylorectomy with end-to-end gastroduodenostomy is curative.

Idiopathic motility disorders

Functional disorders causing delayed gastric emptying or duodenogastric reflux are difficult to confirm when mechanical, inflammatory or neoplastic disorders and critical illness have been ruled out. The term idiopathic motility disorder is used to describe all conditions for which the cause is currently unknown and that require symptomatic or supportive therapy due to the lack of knowledge regarding the cause.

Diagnosis: Mechanical, inflammatory and neoplastic disorders are ruled out by the diagnostic procedures mentioned above. Positive-contrast gastrography has been used to compare gastric emptying following different gastropexy procedures in dogs. Repeated contrast radiographs taken after the oral administration of liquid or food mixed with barium sulphate or barium-impregnated polyethylene spheres are more helpful in diagnosing mechanical than functional obstruction. The natural variations in gastric emptying times of barium sulphate mixed with food have been reported to be 4–16 hours for dogs and 4–17 hours for cats.

Suggested alternative diagnostic methods include fluoroscopic assessment of meal progression and real-time ultrasonographic evaluation, but these lack critical validation in diseased pets. Other non- or minimally invasive methods are rather sophisticated and limited to specialist institutions. They include radioactive methods, such as scintigraphy, or non-radioactive tracer studies using isotopes, such as carbon-13 in breath or blood tests to assess an increase of the labelled isotope after ingestion or SmartPill technology. These methods have been validated for reference values and medication studies in healthy dogs but lack clinical validation in diseased pets.

Treatment and prognosis: The treatment can only be supportive and its success is very variable. Multiple feeds of low-fat, highly digestible blended or liquid diets may be beneficial. GI prokinetics, such as metoclopramide, cisapride or prucalopride, can lead to some success. Low-dose erythromycin has also been advocated due to its motilin-like action, but increasing awareness of bacterial resistance development, especially with low-dose and long-term treatment, may preclude the use of the antibiotic for this indication.

Gastrointestinal pseudo-obstruction

This syndrome is rare in dogs and very rare in cats. A visceral myopathy (leiomyositis) or an even rarer visceral neuropathy can cause ileus with dilatation of intestinal loops that radiographically has the appearance of an intestinal obstruction. The condition can affect the stomach alone or be seen with intestinal involvement.

Diagnosis: GI pseudo-obstruction caused by leiomyositis is confirmed by ruling out mechanical obstruction and proving permanent GI ileus without megaoesophagus using radiography and abdominal ultrasonography. The histological examination of full-thickness biopsy samples allows the diagnosis intra vitam or post mortem.

Treatment and prognosis: There is currently no known treatment and the prognosis is grave. Almost all cases reported to date have not responded to supportive, prokinetic or immunosuppressive therapy, with the exception of one cat that was responsive to cisapride (Harvey *et al.*, 2005) and one dog that was responsive to steroids (Murtagh *et al.*, 2013). Other patients have either been diagnosed post mortem or euthanased after diagnosis and poor treatment response.

Dysautonomia

Diagnosis: Dysautonomia is suspected when the clinical signs, neurological deficits and imaging findings suggest that multiple organ systems are affected. A Schirmer tear test confirms decreased lacrimal secretion. Autonomic nervous system testing includes pilocarpine and physostigmine ocular response tests, subcutaneous injections of atropine and intradermal administration of histamine. A definitive diagnosis requires histology of autonomic ganglia.

Treatment and prognosis: There is currently no known specific treatment. Supportive care to improve GI motility includes metoclopramide (0.5–1 mg/kg q8h) or cisapride (1 mg/kg q8h). The prognosis for spontaneous recovery is grave. In cats, survival time is <30% and correlates negatively with the severity of the clinical signs.

Gastric dilatation-volvulus

Diagnosis:

Physical examination: The physical examination reveals dramatic tympanitic gastric distension. This sign may be less obvious in very deep-chested dogs due to the localization of much of the stomach within the ribcage. Severe cases present in lateral recumbency with tachypnoea and shock.

Minimum database: The MDB is non-specific. Haemoconcentration, hypokalaemia, azotaemia (pre-renal effects of shock) and increased hepatic enzymes are common findings.

Specific laboratory tests: Specific tests, such as blood pH gas and electrolyte analysis, are useful to tailor individual fluid therapy plans due to the large variety of possible imbalances. Thrombin and prothrombin times may initially be reduced (hypercoagulability), but later may be delayed with increased D-dimers and thrombocytopenia as signs of DIC. Increased plasma lactate and serum pepsinogen A are considered markers of poor prognosis (Suchodolski *et al.*, 2002; Israeli *et al.*, 2012). However, at the time of writing, serum pepsinogen A assay is not commercially available.

Radiography: A right lateral view is best for the confirmation of GDV. The gas-filled antrum is displaced craniodorsally to the larger round gastric body, resulting in the characteristic 'double bubble' or 'boxing glove' appearance (Figure 33.30). A single gas-filled image is a sign of gastric dilatation without volvulus, and may not require immediate surgery if the stomach can be decompressed.

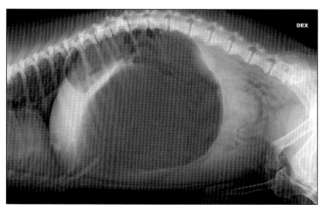

33.30 Typical 'boxing glove' radiographic appearance of gastric dilatation-volvulus in a Dachshund.

Abdominal ultrasonography: This may be useful before surgery to assess indicators of poorer prognosis, such as free fluid in the abdomen and splenic torsion. The examination is, however, hindered by intragastric gas.

Electrocardiography: This is performed repeatedly/continuously to detect and monitor cardiac arrhythmias, such as ventricular premature beats or ventricular tachycardia. These may be present at or develop within 72 hours after initial examination.

Treatment: GDV is a critical and, most often, surgical emergency. Initial patient stabilization is essential in terms of haemodynamic stability (shock, arrhythmia), pain relief, prevention of bacterial translocation and gastric decompression before starting surgery. Surgical treatment often involves exploratory laparotomy, resection of necrotic tissue (partial gastrectomy or invagination of necrotic regions, splenectomy), anatomical correction and gastropexy (for further information, see the *BSAVA Manual of Canine and Feline Abdominal Surgery* and the *BSAVA Manual of Canine and Feline Emergency and Critical Care*). There is strong evidence that after surgical correction a gastropexy should always be performed to prevent recurrence of gastric torsion.

Intravenous fluid therapy: This is fundamental and the jugular or both cephalic veins should be cannulated with large-bore catheters. Correction of hypovolaemia and imbalances of acid-base and electrolytes should be initiated before decompression, as reperfusion syndrome may occur. A balanced electrolyte solution, such as lactated Ringer's, should be administered at a rate of 60–90 ml/kg during the first hour or as boluses of 20 ml/kg at 15-minute intervals. Small-volume hypertonic solution (7% NaCl in 6% dextran at 5 ml/kg) over 5–10 minutes, followed by NaCl at 20 ml/kg/h, maintains better myocardial performance, heart rate and systemic vascular resistance, but needs adequate laboratory monitoring (Allen *et al.*, 1991).

Pain relief and sedation: This is required for orogastric tube placement and can be achieved by administering butorphanol (0.5 mg/kg i.v.) or oxymorphone (0.1 mg/kg i.v.) and diazepam (0.1 mg/kg slow i.v.).

Adjunctive therapy: This is aimed at controlling the complications of systemic inflammatory response syndrome, and includes a broad-spectrum antibiotic combination (e.g. a cephalosporin with enrofloxacin) to control bacterial translocation and endotoxaemia. Intravenous lidocaine helps combat ischaemia–reperfusion injury and cardiac arrhythmias. Intravenous corticosteroids (methylprednisolone succinate, dexamethasone) are often given to patients in septic shock. In humans, hydrocortisone correlates better with shock reversal, but controlled studies in dogs are lacking.

Decompression: Ideally, decompression should be performed under general anaesthesia, with a cuffed endotracheal tube to protect the airway, and it is better achieved in right lateral recumbency. In awake patients, an overtube protected with a cloth plus a soft muzzle around the nose and mandible can be used as a mouth gag. A lubricated orogastric tube, previously marked (with tape/permanent marker) for the distance between the nares and the last thoracic vertebra, is passed into the stomach to relieve gas accumulation. Tubes designed for horses (e.g. sturdy nasogastric tubes with a rounded tip) can be useful for larger dogs, but excessive force should not be applied.

When gastric intubation is initially not achieved, aseptic percutaneous aspiration may facilitate decompression. A large-gauge catheter is used as a trocar at the place of maximum tympanic distension to liberate some of the gas (usually just caudal to the last left rib); percussion may help avoid splenic laceration and proper immobilization is required.

If gastric lavage is required, a smaller-gauge tube may be passed alongside (or inside) the orogastric tube to deliver warmed fluids.

Prognosis: The mortality rate is high (reportedly 10–28%) despite appropriate medical and surgical treatment. The risk of death is higher in dogs with severe clinical signs, of advanced age or developing acute kidney injury and gastric ulceration. Monitoring is mandatory for assessing the response to treatment and adjusting infusion rates. In particular, the heart and respiratory rate, pulse, capillary refill time, mucous membrane colour and mentation should be evaluated. A multi-parameter monitor has proven beneficial to follow the electrocardiogram, blood pressure and SpO_2. Monitoring is essential to detect complications, as the prognosis worsens with progression towards a systemic inflammatory response and multiple organ dysfunction syndromes with cardiovascular, respiratory, GI, renal and coagulation dysfunction.

The recurrence rate in conservatively treated cases is up to 80%, but less than 5% of dogs treated with gastropexy present with recurrence of volvulus alongside the dilatation. Prognostic biomarkers include plasma lactate. Dogs with initial plasma lactate levels <4 mmol/l have better survival rates and fewer complication rates. Concentrations >6 mmol/l indicate that gastric necrosis is more likely and that greater expense may be incurred for treatment. Many dogs with persistent lactataemia (over 24–48 hours) do not survive. A reduction of plasma lactate of >40% after haemodynamic stabilization indicates improved survival times. The pre-surgical pepsinogen A concentration correlates with the severity of the gastric wall lesion and is a moderate outcome predictor, but the assay is not commercially available.

References and further reading

Allen DA, Schertel ER and Valentine AK (1991) Hypertonic saline/dextran resuscitation of dogs with experimentally induced gastric dilatation-volvulus shock. *American Journal of Veterinary Research* **52**, 92–96

Amorim I, Taulescu MA, Day MJ et al. (2016) Canine gastric pathology: a review. *Journal of Comparative Pathology* **154**, 9–37

Anacleto TP, Lopes LR, Andreollo NA et al. (2011) Studies of distribution and recurrence of *Helicobacter* spp. gastric mucosa of dogs after triple therapy. *Acta Cirúrgica Brasileira* **26**, 82–87

Balsa IM, Culp WT, Johnson EG et al. (2016) Efficacy of two radiologic-assisted prophylactic gastropexy techniques. *Veterinary Surgery* **45**, 464–470

Barnes J (2010) Digestive system. In: *Atlas of Feline Anatomy for Veterinarians, 2nd edn*, ed. LC Hudson and WP Hamilton, pp. 115–128. Teton New Media, Jackson

Bell JS (2014) Inherited and predisposing factors in the development of gastric dilatation volvulus in dogs. *Topics in Companion Animal Medicine* **29**, 60–63

Bersenas AM, Mathews KA, Allen DG and Conlon PD (2005) Effects of ranitidine, famotidine, pantoprazole, and omeprazole on intragastric pH in dogs. *American Journal of Veterinary Research* **66**, 425–331

Binvel M, Poujol L, Peyron C et al. (2018) Endoscopic and surgical removal of oesophageal and gastric fishhook foreign bodies in 33 animals. *Journal of Small Animal Practice* **59**, 45–49

Bruchim Y and Kelmer E (2014) Postoperative management of dogs with gastric dilatation and volvulus. *Topics in Companion Animal Medicine* **29**, 81–85

Connolly SL, Frank C, Thompson CA et al. (2012) Dual infection with *Pythium insidiosum* and *Blastomyces dermatitidis* in a dog. *Veterinary Clinical Pathology* **41**, 419–423

Couto KM, Moore PF, Zwingenberger AL et al. (2018) Clinical characteristics and outcome in dogs with small cell T-cell intestinal lymphoma. *Veterinary and Comparative Oncology* **16**, 337–343

Da Riz F, Laloy E, Benchekroun G and Freiche V (2018) Acquired pyloric stenosis in cats: a prospective study of 15 cats (2015–2017). Research communications of the 27th ECVIM-CA congress. St. Julian's, Malta, 2017. *Journal of Veterinary Internal Medicine* **32**, 525–609

Dobson J and Lascelles D (2011) *BSAVA Manual of Canine and Feline Oncology, 3rd edn*. BSAVA Publications, Gloucester

Donnelly E and Lewis D (2015) Gastric dilatation and volvulus. *Veterinary Focus* **25**, 33–38

Eisele J, McClaran JK, Runge JJ et al. (2010) Evaluation of risk factors for morbidity and mortality after pylorectomy and gastroduodenostomy in dogs. *Veterinary Surgery* **39**, 261–267

Evans EH and de Lahunta A (2013) Stomach. In: *Miller's Anatomy of the Dog, 4th edn*, ed. EH Evans and A de Lahunta, pp. 314–319. Elsevier Saunders, St. Louis

Fitzgerald E, Lam R and Drees R (2017b) Improving conspicuity of the canine gastrointestinal wall using dual phase contrast-enhanced computed tomography: a retrospective cross-sectional study. *Veterinary Radiology and Ultrasound* **58**, 151–162

Fitzgerald E, Barfield D, Lee KC and Lamb CR (2017a) Clinical findings and results of diagnostic imaging in 82 dogs with gastrointestinal ulceration. *Journal of Small Animal Practice* **58**, 211–218

Fox JG (2012) Gastric *Helicobacter* infections. In: *Infectious Diseases of the Dog and Cat, 4th edn*. ed. CE Greene, pp. 374–380. Elsevier, St. Louis

Freiche V, da Riz F, Faucher M et al. (2017) Presumed acquired pyloric stenosis in cats: epidemiologic, clinical, histopathological and endoscopic data. A retrospective study of 34 cases. Research communications of the 26th ECVIM-CA congress. Goteborg, Sweden, 8–10, 2016. *Journal of Veterinary Internal Medicine* **31**, 186–270

Garneau MS and McCarthy RJ (2015) Multiple magnetic gastrointestinal foreign bodies in a dog. *Journal of the American Veterinary Medical Association* **246**, 537–539

Gazzola KM and Nelson LL (2014) The relationship between gastrointestinal motility and gastric dilatation-volvulus in dogs. *Topics in Companion Animal Medicine* **29**, 64–66

Gianella P, Pfammatter NS and Burgener IA (2009) Oesophageal and gastric endoscopic foreign body removal: complications and follow-up of 102 dogs. *Journal of Small Animal Practice* **50**, 649–654

Gibbison B, López-López JA, Higgins JP et al. (2017) Corticosteroids in septic shock: a systematic review and network meta-analysis. *Critical Care* **21**, 78

Grooters AM and Foil CS (2012) Pythiosis. In: *Infectious Diseases of the Dog and Cat, 4th edn*, ed. CE Greene, pp. 677–681. Elsevier, St. Louis

Gualtieri M, Olivero D and Costa Devoti C (2015) Spontaneous linear gastric tears in a cat. *Journal of Small Animal Practice* **56**, 581–584

Hardy BT, Gentile-Solomon J and Solomon JA (2016) Multiple gastric erosions diagnosed by means of capsule endoscopy in a dog. *Journal of the American Veterinary Medical Association* **249**, 926–930

Harvey AM, Hall EJ, Day MJ et al. (2005) Chronic intestinal pseudo-obstruction in a cat caused by visceral myopathy. *Journal of Veterinary Internal Medicine* **19**, 11–114

Heilmann RM, Berghoff N, Grützner N et al. (2017) Effect of gastric acid-suppressive therapy and biological variation of serum gastrin concentrations in dogs with chronic enteropathies. *BMC Veterinary Research* **13**, 321

Henderson AK and Webster CRL (2006) Disruption of the gastric mucosal barrier in dogs. *Compendium on Continuing Education for the Practicing Veterinarian* **28**, 340–356

Hugen S, Thomas RE, German AJ et al. (2017) Gastric carcinoma in canines and humans, a review. *Veterinary and Comparative Oncology* **15**, 692–705

Husnik R, Fletcher JM, Gaschen L and Gaschen FP (2017) Validation of ultrasonography for assessment of gastric emptying time in healthy cats by radionuclide scintigraphy. *Journal of Veterinary Internal Medicine* **31**, 394–401

Ianiro G, Molina-Infante J and Gasbarrini A (2015) Gastric microbiota. *Helicobacter* **20(S1)**, 68–71

Israeli I, Steiner J, Segev G et al. (2012) Serum pepsinogen-A, canine pancreatic lipase immunoreactivity, and C-reactive protein as prognostic markers in dogs with gastric dilatation-volvulus. *Journal of Veterinary Internal Medicine* **26**, 920–928

Kim JS, Park SM and Kim BW (2015) Endoscopic management of peptic ulcer bleeding. *Clinical Endoscopy* **48**, 106–111

King L and Boag A (2018) *BSAVA Manual of Canine and Feline Emergency and Critical Care, 3rd edn*. BSAVA Publications, Gloucester

Kleinschmidt S, Harder J, Nolte I et al. (2010) Chronic inflammatory and non-inflammatory diseases of the gastrointestinal tract in cats: diagnostic advantages of full-thickness intestinal and extraintestinal biopsies. *Journal of Feline Medicine and Surgery* **12**, 97–103

Ko JJ and Mann FA (2014) Barium peritonitis in small animals. *Journal of Veterinary Medical Science* **76**, 621–628

Konstantinidis AO, Mylonakis ME, Psalla D et al. (2017) Pyloric obstruction due to massive eosinophilic infiltration in a young adult dog. *Canadian Veterinary Journal* **58**, 1164–1166

Lamoureux A, Benchekroun G, German AJ and Freiche V (2019) An endoscopic method for semi-quantitatively measuring internal pyloric diameter in healthy cats: a prospective study of 24 cases. *Research in Veterinary Science* **122**, 165–169

Lane MB, Larson JC, Stokes JE and Tolbert MK (2017) Continuous radiotelemetric monitoring of intragastric pH in a dog with peptic ulceration. *Journal of the American Veterinary Medical Association* **250**, 530–533

Lecoindre P, Bystricka M, Chevallier M and Peyron C (2012) Gastric carcinoma associated with Menetrier's-like disease in a West Highland white terrier. *Journal of Small Animal Practice* **53**, 714–718

Lee HC, Kim JH, Jee CH et al. (2014) A case of gastric adenocarcinoma in a Shih Tzu dog: successful treatment of early gastric cancer. *The Journal of Veterinary Medical Science* **76**, 1033–1038

Lhermette P and Sobel D (2008) *BSAVA Manual of Canine and Feline Endoscopy and Endosurgery.* BSAVA Publications, Gloucester

Linton M, Nimmo JS, Norris JM (2015) Feline gastrointestinal eosinophilic sclerosing fibroplasia: 13 cases and review of an emerging clinical entity. *Journal of Feline Medicine and Surgery* **17**, 392–404

Marolf AJ, Bachand AM, Sharber J and Twedt DC (2015) Comparison of endoscopy and sonography findings in dogs and cats with histologically confirmed gastric neoplasia. *Journal of Small Animal Practice* **56**, 339–344

McLeland SM, Lunn KF, Duncan CG et al. (2014) Relationship among serum creatinine, serum gastrin, calcium-phosphorus product, and uremic gastropathy in cats with chronic kidney disease. *Journal of Veterinary Internal Medicine* **28**, 827–837

Mooney E, Raw C and Hughes D (2014) Plasma lactate concentration as a prognostic biomarker in dogs with gastric dilation and volvulus. *Topics in Companion Animal Medicine* **29**, 71–76

Mordecai A, Sellon RK and Mealey KL (2011) Normal dogs treated with famotidine for 14 days have only transient increases in serum gastrin concentrations. *Journal of Veterinary Internal Medicine* **25**, 1248–1252

Munday JS, Aberdein D, Cullen GD and French AF (2012) Ménétrier disease and gastric adenocarcinoma in 3 Cairn terrier littermates. *Veterinary Pathology* **49**, 1028–1031

Murtagh K, Oldroyd L, Ressel L and Batchelor D (2013) Successful management of intestinal pseudo-obstruction in a dog. *Veterinary Record Case Reports* **1**, e000025

Neiger R, Robertson E and Stengel C (2013) Gastrointestinal endoscopy in the cat: diagnostics and therapeutics. *Journal of Feline Medicine and Surgery* **15**, 993–1005

Novellas R, Simpson KE, Gunn-Moore DA and Hammond GJ (2010) Imaging findings in 11 cats with feline dysautonomia. *Journal of Feline Medicine and Surgery* **12**, 584–591

Ogawa A, Mochiki E, Yanai M et al. (2012) Interdigestive migrating contractions are coregulated by ghrelin and motilin in conscious dogs. *American Journal of Physiology: Regulatory, Integrative and Comparative Physiology* **302**, R233–R241

Parente NL, Bari Olivier N, Refsal KR and Johnson CA (2014) Serum concentrations of gastrin after famotidine and omeprazole administration to dogs. *Journal of Veterinary Internal Medicine* **28**, 1465–1470

Park YH and Kim N (2015) Review of atrophic gastritis and intestinal metaplasia as a premalignant lesion of gastric cancer. *Journal of Cancer Prevention* **20**, 25–40

Pereira DI, Botton SA, Azevedo MI et al. (2013) Canine gastrointestinal pythiosis treatment by combined antifungal and immunotherapy and review of published studies. *Mycopathologia* **176**, 309–315

Péré-Védrenne C, Flahou B, Loke MF, Ménard A and Vadivelu J (2017) Other Helicobacters, gastric and gut microbiota. *Helicobacter* **22(S1)**, e12407

Pietra M, Zanoni RG, Peli A et al. (2016) Gastric inflammatory pseudotumour secondary to *Actinomyces hordeovulneris* infection in a cat. *Irish Veterinary Journal* **69**, 12

Pratt CL, Reineke EL and Drobatz KJ (2014) Sewing needle foreign body ingestion in dogs and cats: 65 cases (2000-2012). *Journal of the American Veterinary Medical Association* **245**, 302–308

Przywara JF, Abel SB, Peacock JT and Shott S (2014) Occurrence and recurrence of gastric dilatation with or without volvulus after incisional gastropexy. *Canadian Veterinary Journal* **55**, 981–984

Qvigstad G, Kolbjørnsen Ø, Skancke E and Waldum HL (2008) Gastric neuroendocrine carcinoma associated with atrophic gastritis in the Norwegian Lundehund. *Journal of Comparative Pathology* **139**, 194–201

Reagan KI, Marks SL, Pesavento PA et al. (2019) Successful management of 3 dogs with colonic pythiosis using itraconazole, terbinafine, and prednisone. *Journal of Veterinary Internal Medicine* **33**, 1434–1439

Sanderson JJ, Boysen SR, McMurray JM, Lee A and Stillion JR (2017) The effect of fasting on gastrointestinal motility in healthy dogs as assessed by sonography. *Journal of Veterinary Emergency and Critical Care* **27**, 645–650

Sattasathuchana P and Steiner JM (2014) Canine eosinophilic gastrointestinal disorders. *Animal Health Research Reviews* **15**, 76–86

Schmitz S, Götte B, Borsch C et al. (2014) Direct comparison of solid-phase gastric emptying times assessed by means of a carbon isotope-labeled sodium acetate breath test and technetium Tc 99m albumin colloid radioscintigraphy in healthy cats. *American Journal of Veterinary Research* **75**, 648–652

Seim-Wikse T, Skancke E, Nødtvedt A et al. (2019) Comparison of body condition score and other minimally invasive biomarkers between dogs with gastric carcinoma and dogs with chronic gastritis. *Journal of the American Veterinary Medical Association* **254**, 226–235

Sharman M, Bacci B, Simpson K and Mansfield C (2016) Comparison of *in vivo* confocal endomicroscopy with other diagnostic modalities to detect intracellular *Helicobacters*. *The Veterinary Journal* **213**, 78–83

Sharp CR and Rozanski EA (2014) Cardiovascular and systemic effects of gastric dilatation and volvulus in dogs. *Topics in Companion Animal Medicine* **29**, 67–70

Sihvo HK, Simola OT, Vainionpää MH and Syrjä PE (2011) Severe chronic multifocal intramural fibrosing and eosinophilic enteritis, with occasional intralesional bacteria, consistent with feline gastrointestinal eosinophilic sclerosing fibroplasia (FIESF). *Journal of the American Veterinary Medical Association* **238**, 585–587

Simpson KW (2017) Diseases of the stomach. In: *Textbook of Veterinary Internal Medicine, 8th edn* ed. SJ Ettinger, EC Feldman and E Côté, pp. 1495–1516. Elsevier, St. Louis

Sjaastad OV, Hove K and Sand O (2003) Stomach. In: *Physiology of Domestic Animals*, ed. OV Sjaastad, K Hove and O Sand, pp. 527–536. Scandinavian Veterinary Press, Oslo

Steiner JM, Berridge BR, Wojcieszyn J and Williams DA (2002) Cellular immunolocalization of gastric and pancreatic lipase in various tissues obtained from dogs. *American Journal of Veterinary Research* **63**, 722–727

Suchodolski JS, Steiner JM, Ruaux CG et al. (2002) Purification and partial characterization of canine pepsinogen A and B. *American Journal of Veterinary Research* **63**, 1585–1590

Sung JK (2016) Diagnosis and management of gastric dysplasia. *Korean Journal of Internal Medicine* **31**, 201–209

Šutalo S, Ruetten M, Hartnack S et al. (2015) The effect of orally administered ranitidine and once-daily or twice-daily orally administered omeprazole on intragastric pH in cats. *Journal of Veterinary Internal Medicine* **29**, 840–846

Syrcle JA, Gambino JM and Kimberlin WW (2013) Treatment of pyloric stenosis in a cat via pylorectomy and gastroduodenostomy (Billroth I procedure). *Journal of the American Veterinary Medical Association* **242**, 792–797

Taulescu MA, Valentine BA, Amorim I et al. (2014) Histopathological features of canine spontaneous non-neoplastic gastric polyps – a retrospective study of 15 cases. *Histology and Histopathology* **29**, 65–75

Taylor MA, Coop RL and Wall RL (2015) Parasites of dogs and cats. In: *Veterinary Parasitology, 4th edn*, ed. MA Taylor, RL Coop and RL Wall, pp. 599–677. Wiley-Blackwell, Hoboken

Terragni R, Vignoli M, Rossi F et al. (2012) Stomach wall evaluation using helical hydro-computed tomography. *Veterinary Radiology and Ultrasound* **53**, 402–405

Terragni R, Vignoli M, van Bree HJ et al. (2014) Diagnostic imaging and endoscopic finding in dogs and cats with gastric tumors: a review. *Schweizer Archiv Tierheilkunde* **156**, 569–576

Tolbert K, Bissett S, King A et al. (2011) Efficacy of oral famotidine and 2 omeprazole formulations for the control of intragastric pH in dogs. *Journal of Veterinary Internal Medicine* **25**, 47–54

Tolbert MK, Graham A, Odunayo A et al. (2017) Repeated famotidine administration results in a diminished effect on intragastric pH in dogs. *Journal of Veterinary Internal Medicine* **31**, 117–123

Tolbert MK, Odunayo A, Howell RS et al. (2015) Efficacy of intravenous administration of combined acid suppressants in healthy dogs. *Journal of Veterinary Internal Medicine* **29**, 556–560

Tsukamoto A, Ohno K, Tsukagoshi T et al. (2011) Real-time ultrasonographic evaluation of canine gastric motility in the postprandial state. *Journal of Veterinary Medical Science* **73**, 1133–1138

Uzal FA, Plattner BL and Hostetter J (2016) Stomach and abomasum. In: *Jubb, Kennedy, and Palmer's Pathology of Domestic Animals, 6th edn* vol. 2, ed. MG Maxie, pp. 44–59. Elsevier, St. Louis

van der Gaag I, van Niel MHF, Belshaw BE and Wolvekamp WTC (2011) Gastric granulomatous cryptococcosis mimicking gastric carcinoma in a dog. *Veterinary Quarterly* **13**, 185–190

Vaughn DP, Syrcle J and Cooley J (2014) Canine giant hypertrophic gastritis treated successfully with partial gastrectomy. *Journal of the American Animal Hospital Association* **50**, 62–66

Watson VE, Sycamore KF and Rissi DR (2016) Diffuse, invasive, undifferentiated gastric carcinoma in a dog. *Journal of the American Veterinary Medical Association* **248**, 893–895

Weingart C and Kohn B (2009) Zinc intoxication in a Yorkshire Terrier due to Euro cent ingestion. *Schweizer Archiv Tierheilkunde* **151**, 75–81

Weissman A, Penninck D, Webster C et al. (2013). Ultrasonographic and clinicopathological features of feline gastrointestinal eosinophilic sclerosing fibroplasia in four cats. *Journal of Feline Medicine and Surgery* **15**, 148–154

Whitehead K, Cortes Y and Eirmann L (2016) Gastrointestinal dysmotility disorders in critically ill dogs and cats. *Journal of Veterinary Emergency and Critical Care* **26**, 234–253

Willard MD (2012) Alimentary neoplasia in geriatric dogs and cats. *Veterinary Clinics of North America: Small Animal Practice* **42**, 693–706

William J and Niles J (2015) *BSAVA Manual of Canine and Feline Abdominal Surgery, 2nd edn*. BSAVA Publications, Gloucester

Wrigglesworth DJ, Bailey MQ, Colyer A and Hughes KR (2016) Pilot study to assess meal progression through the gastrointestinal tract of habituated dogs determined by fluoroscopic imaging without sedation or physical restraint. *Veterinary Radiology and Ultrasound* **57**, 565–571

Useful websites

American Association of Veterinary Parasitologists: http://www.aavp.org/

Small intestine: general

Edward J. Hall

The cardinal sign of small intestinal disease is diarrhoea, a significant increase in the frequency, fluidity or volume of faeces, but this can also be caused by disease either elsewhere in the gastrointestinal (GI) tract or in other organ systems (Figure 34.1). Conversely, diarrhoea is not always present in small intestinal disease, and there are many other signs of small intestinal dysfunction, although some are non-specific (Figure 34.2).

Primary gastrointestinal (GI) disease
• Diffuse GI disease (e.g. inflammation or lymphoma)
• Gastric disease
• Achlorhydria[a]
• Intestinal disease
• Diet-related (e.g. food poisoning, gluttony, sudden change of diet, toxins)
• Primary small intestinal disease
– Dietary
– Dysbiosis
– Infectious
– Inflammatory
– Neoplastic
– Toxic
• Primary large intestinal disease (see Chapter 35)
Non-GI disease
• Pancreatic disease (see Chapter 36)
• Exocrine pancreatic insufficiency[b]
• Pancreatitis (acute, chronic)
• Pancreatic carcinoma[b]
• APUDoma (gastrinoma causing Zollinger–Ellison syndrome)[a]
• Liver disease
• Portosystemic vascular anomalies
• Hepatocellular failure
• Intra-hepatic and extra-hepatic cholestasis
• Endocrine disease
• Typical hypoadrenocorticism[b]
• Atypical hypoadrenocorticism[b]
• Hyperthyroidism[c]
• Hypothyroidism[b]
• Renal disease
• Uraemia
• Nephrotic syndrome[b]
• Polysystemic infection
• Dogs: distemper, leptospirosis, infectious canine hepatitis
• Cats: feline infectious peritonitis, feline leukaemia virus, feline immunodeficiency virus
• Miscellaneous
• Toxaemias (e.g. pyometra, peritonitis)
• Portal hypertension and right-sided heart failure
• Autoimmune disease
• Metaplastic neoplasia
• Various toxins and drugs

34.1 Causes of diarrhoea. [a] Rare conditions. [b] Rare in cats only. [c] Rare in dogs only. APUDoma = amine precursor uptake and decarboxylation tumour.

Cardinal sign
• Diarrhoea – increase in the frequency, volume and fluidity of faeces
Other signs
• Vomiting
• Weight loss and/or failure to thrive/stunting
• Haematemesis
• Melaena
• Altered appetite
• Inappetence/dysorexia
• Anorexia
• Polyphagia
• Coprophagia
• Pica
• Abdominal discomfort/pain
• Protein-losing enteropathy
• Hypocalcaemic tetany
• Abdominal distension: ascites
• Peripheral oedema
• Hydrothorax
• Pulmonary thromboembolism
• Borborygmi and flatus
• Halitosis
• Dehydration
• Polydipsia (compensatory)
• Shock

34.2 Clinical signs of small intestinal disease.

Historically, chronic diarrhoea has been classified as 'small intestinal' or 'large intestinal' in origin, based on the nature of the diarrhoea and how the patient defecates (see Chapter 18), but 'mixed-intestinal diarrhoea' is seen in many chronic inflammatory enteropathies, as the disease tends to be diffuse. Differentiation by these signs is most useful in directing from where endoscopic intestinal biopsy samples should be taken. Significant weight loss and/or melaena indicate small intestinal disease, and haematochezia and tenesmus indicate large intestinal disease. However, studies have shown that ileal biopsies yield more diagnoses than duodenal biopsies in chronic inflammatory enteropathies, and feline alimentary lymphoma (Casamian-Sorrosal *et al.*, 2010; Procoli *et al.*, 2013; Scott *et al.*, 2011); therefore, both upper and lower GI endoscopy tend to be performed concurrently, as ileal biopsy is ideally required (see Chapter 4). Upper GI endoscopy alone is indicated more for chronic vomiting and suspected gastric disease. Colonoscopy without concurrent duodenoscopy is really indicated only if there is focal bleeding without diarrhoea (e.g. suspected neoplasia), or isolated colitis is suspected (e.g. granulomatous colitis in Boxers and French Bulldogs), or after cleaning the colon due to recurrent constipation (see Chapter 35).

Structure and function of the small intestine

The small intestine has competing functions of nutrient digestion/absorption whilst hosting a commensal microbiome, yet protecting the body from environmental threats and preventing enteric loss of protein-rich interstitial fluid. Consequently, it is the largest immunological organ in the body, in addition to its essential role in digestion and body fluid homeostasis.

Anatomy

The small intestine is divided into three segments: the duodenum proximally, then the jejunum, and finally the ileum. The duodenum starts at the pylorus and the ileum ends at the ileocolic valve (see Chapter 4). Blood is supplied by branches of the coeliac and cranial mesenteric arteries and drains to the liver via the portal vein. Lacteals in the villi drain via mesenteric lymphatics to the cisterna chyli and onwards to the thoracic duct. The autonomic innervation of the small intestine is from the vagus and splanchnic nerves.

The small intestine has a basic cross-sectional structure of serosa, muscularis (outer longitudinal and inner circular muscle layers), submucosa and mucosa around the lumen (Figure 34.3i–ii). The mucosal layer is the most important clinically, being responsible for secretory, absorptive and barrier functions. It varies in thickness along the small intestine, being thinner distally (see Chapter 3), and comprises an epithelium over the lamina propria, which contains components of the mucosal immune system. The mucosa is modified by gross folds and finger-like processes, the villi, covered by a layer of enterocytes bearing microvilli that increase their surface area many hundred-fold (Figure 34.3ii–iv). Crypt cells are the site of intestinal secretion and continually produce undifferentiated epithelial cells, which develop into enterocytes as they migrate from the crypt to the villus tip where, after approximately 3 days, they are shed.

Normal function

Differentiated enterocytes on the villi undertake digestion, absorption and transfer of simple nutrients and water from the lumen to the blood and lymphatics. Enzymes and carrier proteins are expressed on their luminal cell membrane, the microvillar membrane, also called the brush border because of its ultrastructural appearance. Glutamine derived from food is the major energy source for enterocytes, which explains the villus atrophy and reduced epithelial barrier and immune functions that occur during prolonged anorexia. Glutamine metabolism is also a major source of postprandial ammonia production, which can exacerbate hepatoencephalopathy in patients with portosystemic shunts (see Chapter 37b).

Digestion

Major dietary constituents (carbohydrates, proteins, triglycerides) are polymers that must be hydrolysed into simpler molecules to be transported across the mucosa. Digestion is largely achieved by bile salt emulsification and hydrolysis by pancreatic enzymes (see Chapter 36) in the optimal environment provided by the small intestinal lumen. Terminal hydrolysis of carbohydrates and proteins is performed by brush border enzymes.

Absorption

The products of carbohydrate and protein digestion (monosaccharides, amino acids and oligopeptides) and water-soluble vitamins are absorbed by active or facilitated carrier-mediated transport. The products of fat digestion (fatty acids) and fat-soluble vitamins (A, D, E and K) are absorbed by passive diffusion into lacteals. In health, net fluid absorption occurs. However, the water flux through the intestine is massive, and any net losses (i.e. increased secretion or decreased absorption) result in diarrhoea and potentially severe dehydration. Colonic water absorption is important as it can help compensate for mild net small intestinal losses, but diarrhoea will occur if its reserve capacity is overwhelmed (see Chapter 35).

Motility

Slow wave, segmental and peristaltic contractions of the small intestine are generated by the coordinated contraction of longitudinal and circular smooth muscle in response to spontaneous electrical activity: interstitial cells of Cajal are the pacemaker cells. Segmental contractions slow intestinal transit and ensure mixing and digestion of nutrients, whilst progressive peristalsis propels the ingesta onwards. The duration and pattern of contractile activity in the fed state is determined by the nature of the diet, with unabsorbed fats and fibre prolonging activity. The migrating motor complex is an 'intestinal housekeeper' wave induced during the fasted state by the hormone motilin, which clears debris from the GI tract. It can be replicated by low doses of erythromycin (see Chapter 33).

Small intestinal microbiome

The microbiome comprises bacteria, protozoa, fungi and viruses, and is an integral part of the healthy small intestine, helping the balance of the mucosal immune system and preventing invasion/colonization by pathogens. The healthy microbiome is relatively resistant to environmental changes, but can be modified, both positively (probiosis) and negatively (dysbiosis), by dietary changes and antibacterial use. Although the effects of antibacterial therapy on the microbiome are often clinically mild and self-limiting, persistent changes do occur, and so the indiscriminate use of antibiotics to treat diarrhoea should be avoided, especially as it may also enhance antibiotic resistance (see Chapter 29). In small intestinal disease, the diversity of the bacterial component of the microbiome is reduced and there is a shift to potentially harmful species, whilst the viral component (the virome) is diversified.

Gastrointestinal immune system

The gut-associated lymphoid tissue (GALT) consists of inductive and effector sites: inductive sites comprise Peyer's patches, isolated lymphoid follicles and the mesenteric lymph nodes; effector sites comprise the intestinal lamina propria and the epithelium. The lamina propria consists of a matrix of connective tissue with a mixed, but predominantly lymphoplasmacytic, immune cell component. An intraepithelial lymphocyte population also exists between enterocytes. The barrier function of the small intestinal epithelium and the GALT allow tolerance to harmless antigens such as commensal bacteria and food. Immune tolerance is driven by antigen-specific regulatory T-cells responding to particular elements of the microbiome. Conversely, the GALT is able to generate a protective (inflammatory) response against pathogens.

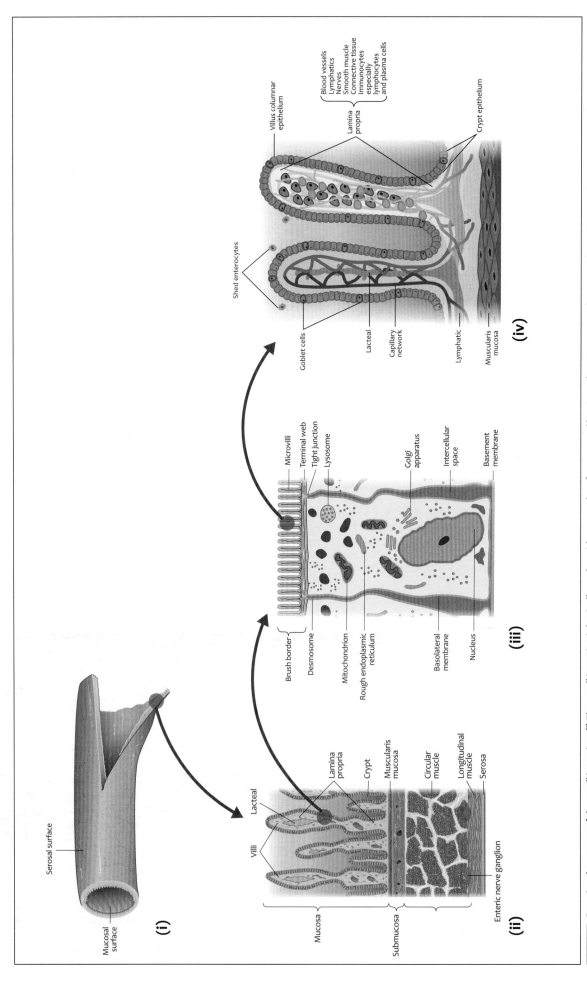

34.3 Functional anatomy of the small intestine. **(i)** The small intestine is basically a tube with a serosal surface covered by visceral peritoneum and an inner absorptive and digestive surface, the mucosa. **(ii)** Beneath the outer serosa, longitudinal and circular muscle layers produce peristaltic and segmental contractions for propelling and mixing the luminal contents coordinated by the enteric nervous system. The submucosa is rich in blood and lymphatic vessels. The mucosa comprises the thin muscularis mucosa, the lamina propria and the columnar epithelium; it is thrown into folds and is covered by finger-like villi to increase the digestive and absorptive surface area. **(iii)** The luminal membrane of the enterocyte is thrown into processes called microvilli, which increase the luminal surface area. Tight junctions between enterocytes maintain epithelial integrity. Absorbed nutrients are passed from the enterocyte into the intercellular space for distribution to the body. **(iv)** Enterocytes, which are shed from the villus tip and are continually replaced through division of crypt cells, are the site of nutrient digestion and absorption. Goblet cells secrete protective mucus. Water-soluble nutrients pass into the rich capillary network of the lamina propria, and fat is passed as chylomicrons into the lacteals. Immunocytes in the lamina propria are involved in maintaining tolerance to luminal antigens.

Pathophysiology

Considering the complex structure and function of the small intestine, it is not surprising that minor functional upsets occur, but they usually resolve spontaneously. Dietary indiscretion or infection can cause diarrhoea but most episodes are acute and self-limiting (Hubbard *et al.* 2007). Persistent perturbations of the microbiome (dysbiosis) and/or abnormal immune responses (inflammation), or neoplasia lead to chronic enteropathies.

Diarrhoea

Diarrhoea can be classified mechanistically as dysmotility, exudative, osmotic and secretory. These categories are not mutually exclusive, but most small intestinal diseases have a component of osmotic diarrhoea caused by malabsorption. Exudative diarrhoea is due to inflammation or neoplastic infiltration, and secretory diarrhea is caused by chemical or bacterial toxins. Primary motility abnormalities causing diarrhoea are rare: feline hyperthyroidism is a common secondary cause.

Malabsorption

Failure to assimilate food is sometimes classified as either a primary failure to digest (maldigestion, for example, due to exocrine pancreatic insufficiency (EPI)) or a primary failure to absorb (malabsorption). However, such a distinction is misleading, because failure to digest inevitably leads to failure to absorb. It is more logical to consider malabsorption to be the defective absorption of a dietary constituent resulting from interference with the digestive and/or absorptive processing of that molecule. The site of the primary abnormality causing malabsorption may be found in the luminal, mucosal or transport phases of digestion (Figure 34.4).

The clinical manifestations of malabsorption are diarrhoea, weight loss and altered appetite. The reserve capacity of the distal small intestine and colon may prevent overt diarrhoea despite significant malabsorption and weight loss. Polyphagia, coprophagia and pica are a result of the lack of nutrient uptake (see Chapter 7), but anorexia may occur if an underlying neoplastic or severe inflammatory condition is present (see Chapter 8).

Mechanism		Examples
Premucosal (luminal) phase		
Dysmotility	Rapid intestinal transit	Hyperthyroidism
Defective substrate hydrolysis	Enzyme inactivation	Gastric hypersecretion
	Lack of pancreatic enzymes	Exocrine pancreatic insufficiency
	Impaired release of cholecystokinin and secretin	Impairment of pancreatic secretion due to severe small intestinal disease
	Fat maldigestion • Decreased bile salt delivery • Increased bile salt loss • Bile salt deconjugation • Fatty acid hydroxylation	• Cholestatic liver disease, biliary obstruction • Ileal disease • Bacterial overgrowth • Bacterial overgrowth
Cobalamin malabsorption	Intrinsic factor deficiency	Exocrine pancreatic insufficiency
	Cobalamin receptor deficiency	Inherited selective cobalamin deficiency (Imerslund–Gräsbeck syndrome)
	Competition for cobalamin	Bacterial overgrowth
Mucosal phase		
Brush border enzyme deficiency	Congenital	Trehalase (cats) Aminopeptidase N (Beagle)
	Acquired	Relative lactase deficiency in cats
Brush border transport protein deficiency	Congenital/inherited	Inherited selective cobalamin deficiency
	Acquired	Folate and cobalamin malabsorption secondary to diffuse small intestinal disease
Enterocyte defects	Enterocyte processing abnormality	Dirlotapide administration
	Reduction in surface area	Villus atrophy
	Immature enterocytes	Increased enterocyte turnover
Mucosal inflammation		Idiopathic chronic inflammatory enteropathies
Postmucosal (transport) phase		
Lymphatic obstruction	Primary	Lymphangiectasia
	Secondary	Obstruction caused by neoplasia, infection or inflammation
Vascular compromise	Vasculitis	Infection, immune-mediated
	Portal vein thrombosis	Hypercoagulable states
	Portal hypertension	Hepatopathy, right-sided heart failure, cardiac tamponade

34.4 Pathophysiological mechanisms of malabsorption of which several may exist concurrently.

Polydipsia (to be distinguished from compensatory drinking) is an unusual and peculiar manifestation of excessive appetite. Animals with malabsorption are often systemically healthy, but they lose weight despite an increased appetite: only when the patient is severely malnourished or develops hypoproteinaemia (and consequent ascites) does it appear unwell.

Melaena

The presence of dark, tarry, oxidized blood in faeces is called melaena, and it reflects either generalized bleeding, swallowed blood (oral, nasal or respiratory) or localized GI bleeding proximal to the large intestine (see Chapter 20). Small intestinal ulceration and bleeding is seen with non-steroidal anti-inflammatory drug-induced duodenal ulcers, severe inflammatory (often eosinophilic) disease, alimentary lymphoma and solid tumours (carcinoma, leiomyoma/leiomyosarcoma, GI stromal tumour).

Protein-losing enteropathy

When small intestinal disease is severe enough for protein leakage into the gut lumen to exceed plasma protein synthesis, hypoproteinaemia develops (see Chapter 34c). Clinical signs associated with protein-losing enteropathy (PLE) include weight loss, vomiting and fluid accumulation but, confusingly, diarrhoea is not invariably present. Thromboembolism secondary to hypoproteinaemia is a feature of some cases of PLE, as these patients are hypercoagulable in part due to loss of antithrombin. Emaciation is common, with extreme muscle wasting in some patients. Other physical examination findings may include emaciation, thickened intestines, melaena, hydrothorax, oedema, ascites and hypocalcaemic tetany. Non-intestinal diseases causing ascites through portal hypertension usually present with ascites before diarrhoea develops. Hypoproteinaemia and ascites associated with small intestinal disease are much less common in cats than in dogs, and when they occur, they are most often related to alimentary lymphoma.

Diagnostic approach

The first step in a patient with diarrhoea is to eliminate extra-intestinal diseases by the history, physical examination findings and minimum database before investigating primary GI disease. The diagnostic approach to acute and chronic diarrhoea due to primary GI disease is detailed in Chapters 17 and 18, respectively, and the diagnostic features of specific small intestinal diseases are given in Chapter 34c. Yet, many cases of acute diarrhoea involve the whole GI tract and only require supportive and symptomatic treatment; a definitive diagnosis may be needed only if they are life-threatening, and/or are potentially infective to other animals, and/or represent a zoonotic risk. If significant hypovolaemia or dehydration is present, fluid and electrolyte deficits must be addressed simultaneously with any diagnostic effort.

The history, breed susceptibility and physical examination are crucial steps in the diagnostic process, and in some cases may be all that is required when investigating primary GI disease. A rectal examination should be performed to confirm diarrhoea, identify any unreported melaena and obtain samples for faecal examination (see Chapter 2) and rectal cytology (see Chapter 6). Preliminary investigations should also include collection of baseline data through haematology, serum biochemistry and urinalysis. Diagnostic imaging may be indicated, especially if a disease requiring surgical intervention is suspected from the history and/or physical examination findings (see Chapter 3).

Early in the investigation of chronic diarrhoea, exclusion of EPI in dogs by the canine trypsin-like immunoreactivity test (see Chapter 36) and hyperthyroidism in older cats by measuring serum thyroxine concentration is important. The availability of assays for faecal biomarkers of small intestinal damage/inflammation (e.g. faecal alpha$_1$-proteinase inhibitor, faecal calprotectin) is geographically restricted (see Chapter 2), but measurement of serum folate and cobalamin concentration as indirect tests of intestinal function are widely available. This is important clinically because their malabsorption may help determine the site and severity of the small intestinal disease, and supplementation is indicated whenever a deficiency is detected (see Chapter 27). Hypocobalaminaemia can cause metabolic changes leading to anorexia, and, as a healthy small intestine itself needs these vitamins to function normally, deficiencies may lead to suboptimal response to other, more specific treatments.

Folate monoglutamate is absorbed in the proximal small intestine by a passive carrier-mediated mechanism after enzymatic digestion of dietary folate polyglutamate (Figure 34.5a). The absorption of cobalamin is more complex, with most being absorbed in the ileum by an active carrier-mediated process after liberation from food and eventual binding by intrinsic factor (Figure 34.5b). Dogs, and cats in particular, have less ability to sustain adequate cobalamin status in the face of malabsorption than humans do; deficiencies can develop within weeks to months. Cats also lack the binding protein transcobalamin I, and lose cobalamin rapidly through enterohepatic recycling. Thus, severe cobalamin malabsorption can deplete cobalamin stores in cats within 4–6 weeks.

While not always conclusive, direct inspection of the small intestine by endoscopy or surgery as well as histological examination of biopsy samples may be required for a definitive diagnosis and specific management of chronic enteropathies (see Chapters 4 and 6).

However, empirical treatment trials with fenbendazole and then a diet are indicated in clinically well patients that are still eating (see Chapter 27). When commencing a diet trial, a decision has to be made as to what type of diet should be used. The answer largely depends on the patient's dietary history, but there is confusion as to whether it should be an exclusion (elimination), a limited-ingredient novel protein or a hydrolysed diet. A 'hypoallergenic' diet is an unsuitable term, as it is not clear whether it means there is a reduced number of antigenic molecules or a reduced variety of antigens in the diet, and further confusion occurs because it is also a tradename of a hydrolysed diet. For similar reasons, a 'limited antigen' diet is an imprecise term that should be avoided.

The term exclusion (elimination) diet is used, perhaps illogically, to indicate that the patient is being trialled with a completely novel diet and not simply that a single constituent is excluded. A 'single novel protein' exclusion diet theoretically contains just a single protein source, although the term 'limited ingredient novel protein diet' is preferred as the carbohydrate source may also contain protein. Such diets are typically 'gluten-free', indicating that they do not contain wheat protein (gliadins), nor the closely related proteins in rye (secalins), barley (hordeins) and sometimes also oats (avenins). The proteins in rice (oryzeins) and maize/corn (zeins) are immunologically

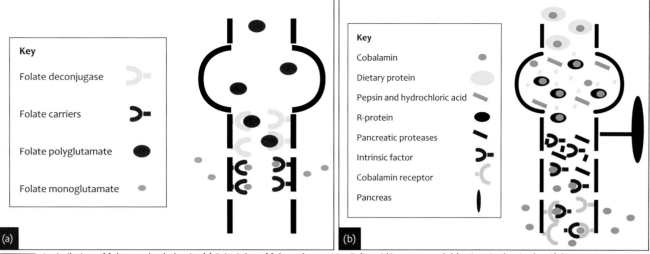

34.5 Assimilation of folate and cobalamin. (a) Principles of folate absorption. Folic acid is a water-soluble vitamin that is plentiful in most commercial pet foods. However, dietary folic acid is present as folate polyglutamate, which cannot be readily absorbed. In the proximal small intestine, folate polyglutamate is converted by brush border folate deconjugase to folate monoglutamate, which is then absorbed by specific folate carriers located exclusively in the proximal small intestine. (b) Principles of cobalamin absorption. Cobalamin is also a water-soluble vitamin that is plentiful in most commercial dog and cat foods. Dietary cobalamin is bound to dietary protein and cannot be absorbed in this form. In the stomach, digestion of dietary protein is initiated by pepsin and hydrochloric acid, and cobalamin is released. Free cobalamin is immediately bound by R-proteins (haptocorrins) present in saliva and gastric secretions, thereby once again rendering the vitamin unabsorbable. In the small intestine, R-proteins are digested by pancreatic proteases and the liberated cobalamin is bound by intrinsic factor, of which approximately 90% is secreted by the pancreas in the dog, and 99% in the cat. Finally, cobalamin–intrinsic factor complexes are absorbed by specific receptors in the ileum. Note that a very small proportion of oral cobalamin is absorbed directly, and large daily doses can be used to supplement cobalamin deficiency.

distinct from gliadins and these cereals can be used as carbohydrate sources. Alternatively, cereals can be totally avoided by using potato or tapioca starch. A hydrolysed veterinary diet is often a better choice for a diet trial, as the previous dietary history is not relevant. However, they are not always palatable, and in both hydrolysed and limited ingredient novel protein diets, some may contain undeclared proteins (Ricci *et al.*, 2018). Therefore, a patient should ideally fail trials with at least two hydrolysed diets and limited-ingredient novel protein diet before concluding that it does not have a food-responsive enteropathy.

After a diet trial, an antibacterial trial might be considered in patients with suspected dysbiosis, although empirical use of antibiotics is not encouraged. It has been suggested that in cats a high protein/low carbohydrate diet may have a beneficial effect on the microbiome. Only when a patient has failed a properly conducted diet trial, or when there are criteria of concern (Figure 34.6), is small intestinal biopsy indicated. However, in cases where biopsy is not possible due to financial constraints or patient factors, empirical corticosteroids may be considered.

- Anorexia
- Hypocobalaminaemia or hypofolataemia
- Severe weight loss
- Hypoproteinaemia (protein-losing enteropathy)
- Abnormal findings on imaging
- Melaena due to small intestinal bleeding

34.6 Criteria of concern in chronic enteropathies suggesting intestinal biopsy may be helpful.

References and further reading

Casamian-Sorrosal D, Willard MD, Murray JK *et al.* (2010) Comparison of histopathologic findings in biopsies from the duodenum and ileum of dogs with enteropathy. *Journal of Veterinary Internal Medicine* **24**, 80–83

Hubbard K, Skelly BJ, McKelvie J and Wood JLN (2007) Risk of vomiting and diarrhoea in dogs. *Veterinary Record* **161**, 755–757

Procoli F, Motskuela PF, Keyte SV *et al.* (2013) Comparison of histopathologic findings in duodenal and ileal endoscopic biopsies in dogs with chronic small intestinal enteropathies. *Journal of Veterinary Internal Medicine* **27**, 268–274

Ricci R, Conficoni D, Morelli G *et al.* (2018) Undeclared animal species in dry and wet novel and hydrolyzed protein diets for dogs and cats detected by microarray analysis. *BMC Veterinary Research* **14**, 209

Scott KD, Zoran DL, Mansell J *et al.* (2011) Utility of endoscopic biopsies of the duodenum and ileum for diagnosis of inflammatory bowel disease and small cell lymphoma in cats. *Journal of Veterinary Internal Medicine* **25**, 1253–1257

Small intestine: acute disease

Andrea Boari

Presentation of canine and feline patients with sudden-onset anorexia, vomiting and/or diarrhoea due to gastrointestinal (GI) upset is very common. These presenting clinical signs are discussed in detail in Chapters 8, 14 and 17. While the causative factors of acute GI disease are often unknown and many conditions are self-limiting with simple supportive care, that is not always the case, and consideration should be given to potential causes that require active intervention for successful resolution.

Self-limiting enteritis

Diet-induced acute enteritis

Acute, self-limiting small intestinal disorders in dogs and cats are most commonly food-associated. Puppies and older dogs with scavenging habits are at major risk of developing acute enteritis because of ingestion of inappropriate foods or foreign bodies. Usually, dietary indiscretion is the result of pets getting into garbage and eating bones, spoiled or otherwise unsuitable foods, plants and insects. Furthermore, the digestive tract may be upset by ingestion of a large volume of any food, or by abrupt changes in the type of food provided, resulting in the acute onset of clinical signs.

Food poisoning in these circumstances is generally attributed to microbial contamination and potential toxins, either incorporated at the time of manufacture (e.g. benzoic acid or propylene glycol) or produced during microbial spoilage. Enterotoxigenic strains of bacteria, including *Escherichia coli*, *Staphylococcus pseudintermedius*, *Salmonella* spp., and *Clostridium* spp., can contaminate food, and raw food diets are particularly likely to be a source of such potentially pathogenic bacterial infections. Several mycotoxins have been identified in commercial foods, with cereal grains and their byproducts most commonly incriminated. Indeed, as it is common practice to use multiple grain sources in animal diets, the risk of exposure to several mycotoxins increases with diet complexity.

Deoxynivalenol (DON, 'vomitoxin'), a trichothecene mycotoxin produced by *Fusarium* spp., frequently occurs in cereal grains and has been associated with animal food poisoning. DON compromises several intestinal functions, including digestion, absorption, permeability and immunity, and can cause anorexia, vomiting, bloody diarrhoea and leucopenia. In addition, accidental ingestion of some drugs (e.g. non-steroidal anti-inflammatory drugs) and insecticides

or pesticides, as well as antibacterial soaps and other cleaning agents can cause acute diarrhoea and vomiting.

Diagnosis

In the majority of cases, there is usually a clear association between the ingestion of a particular substance or food and the onset of clinical signs. Historical information may establish a definitive or presumptive diagnosis, but the exact cause may not be determined. Recent dietary changes (including provision of food intended for humans), treats, food storage and dietary supplements should be investigated.

Treatment

Supportive therapy should be based on clinical signs, i.e. antiemetics (e.g. maropitant at 1 mg/kg s.c. or i.v. q24h, metoclopramide at 0.3 mg/kg s.c. q8–12h) and antacid therapy (e.g. ranitidine at 2 mg/kg s.c. q12h). Dehydration and electrolyte imbalances should be rectified. Subcutaneous fluids are adequate only in cases of mild dehydration, but are not ideal, and are not generally recommended; dextrose-containing fluids should never be used subcutaneously. Oral rehydration fluids may suffice in animals with mild dehydration (i.e. less than 8%) if the patient is not vomiting. However, in most situations, fluids should be administered intravenously, or via an intraosseous route if venous access is not immediately achievable. Withdrawal of food could be detrimental and should be reserved only for those patients with severe vomiting. Very young and small animals can become hypoglycaemic due to their limited reserves and may benefit from intravenous glucose administration. Small and frequent feedings of highly digestible foods may limit and neutralize gastric acid secretion, thereby helping to decrease abdominal discomfort.

Prognosis

Recovery is usually uneventful with supportive care and the prognosis is usually excellent.

Acute haemorrhagic diarrhoea syndrome in dogs

Acute haemorrhagic diarrhoea syndrome (AHDS), previously known as haemorrhagic gastroenteritis or HGE, is an idiopathic disease characterized by acute-onset vomiting, anorexia and lethargy, progressing to severe haemorrhagic diarrhoea in dogs. Different aetiologies have been discussed, including an intestinal type 1 hypersensitivity reaction to food components and bacterial endotoxin or enterotoxigenic clostridial strains (*Clostridium perfringens* enterotoxin and *Clostridium difficile* toxins A and B). Recently, the pore-forming netF toxin, a type A toxin produced by *C. perfringens* has been suggested as responsible for the necrotizing lesions in the intestines of a significant proportion of dogs with AHDS (Sindern *et al.*, 2019). AHDS occurs more commonly in young to middle-aged small-breed dogs and during the winter. Miniature and small breeds (Yorkshire Terrier, Miniature Pinscher, Maltese and Miniature Schnauzer) are predisposed (Mortier *et al.*, 2015).

Clinical signs

Clinical signs include acute-onset vomiting, haematemesis and haemorrhagic diarrhoea. Other clinical signs include obtundation, abdominal discomfort, anorexia and lethargy; fever is unusual. Clinical assessment of the severity of the disease and the outcome in dogs with AHDS can be performed by means of the AHDS index score (Figure 34.7): this includes clinical parameters such as activity, appetite, vomiting, faecal consistency and dehydration, which is often severe and can lead to marked or severe haemoconcentration (Mortier *et al.*, 2015). Hypothermia and tachycardia are most likely related to hypovolaemia and the subsequent decreased peripheral perfusion.

Leucocyte counts are sometimes increased in dogs with AHDS, with increased monocytes and neutrophils but reduced lymphocytes and eosinophils. Mild to moderate increases in band neutrophils are sometimes observed and probably reflect the extensive mucosal damage and inflammation associated with mucosal necrosis and neutrophilic infiltration. Thrombocytosis is also commonly observed: this is most likely related to adrenaline (epinephrine) release secondary to stress and/or hypovolaemia, which leads to splenic contraction and the release of platelets (Mortier *et al.*, 2015).

Enteric protein loss leads to a normal to low serum albumin concentration, despite severe dehydration, and is often pronounced after effective fluid therapy. Pre-renal azotaemia is surprisingly rare in these patients, but increases in serum alanine aminotransferase (ALT) activity are common and most likely reflect transient hepatic injury secondary to hypoxia and absorption of toxins from the intestine. A low venous pH and bicarbonate concentration and an increased lactate concentration, as a consequence of poor tissue perfusion in hypovolaemic patients, are also common (Mortier *et al.*, 2015).

Diagnosis

A presumptive diagnosis of AHDS is made upon observation of characteristic acute clinical signs and the exclusion of other diseases known to cause haemorrhagic diarrhoea, such as pancreatitis and hypoadrenocorticism. These conditions can usually be eliminated by considering the history and findings on physical examination, complete blood count, serum biochemistry, coagulation times, diagnostic imaging and faecal examination. The absence of leucopenia and marked haemoconcentration can help distinguish AHDS from parvovirus infection, but pancreatitis and hypoadrenocorticism still need to be ruled out. Traditionally, a packed cell volume (PCV) ≥60% has been used as a hallmark of AHDS. However, in a recent study, the haematocrit exceeded 60% only in 31% of affected dogs, and was within the normal range in 52% of cases (Mortier *et al.*, 2015).

Treatment

A rapid clinical improvement is normally seen with symptomatic therapy, and the disease is considered self-limiting. However, if not treated promptly the disease can progress to hypovolaemic shock and death. The initial therapy should be aimed at correcting dehydration. This can be achieved using intravenous crystalloid fluid therapy, which in severely affected individuals should be aggressive. The administration of colloids may be required in some cases. Symptomatic antiemetic and analgesic therapy may be considered, but antacid therapy is now thought not to be useful. Once the patient's appetite has been restored, a highly digestible GI diet is probably desirable for a few days while intestinal recovery takes place.

The value of antimicrobial therapy in patients with AHDS is still controversial. Studies have suggested that in the absence of evidence of life-threatening systemic inflammatory response syndrome (SIRS)/sepsis (i.e. tachypnoea, tachycardia, leucocytosis or leucopenia, and fever or hypothermia), antibiotics provide no benefit for the treatment of canine AHDS, and their administration merely increases the risk of inducing antibiotic resistance and enteric dysbiosis (Unterer *et al.*, 2011).

Prognosis

The prognosis for most dogs with AHDS is good, but if sepsis or severe hypoproteinaemia develop the prognosis is more guarded.

Parameter	AHDS index score			
	0	1	2	3
Activity	Normal	Mildly reduced	Moderately reduced	Severely reduced
Appetite	Normal	Mildly reduced	Moderately reduced	Severely reduced
Vomiting (times/day)	0	1	2–3	>3
Faecal consistency	Normal	Slightly soft	Very soft	Watery diarrhoea
Defecation (times/day)	1	2–3	4–5	>5
Dehydration (%)	0	<5	5–10	>10
Total AHDS score	0–3	4–5	6–8	≥9
Clinical significance of disease	Clinically insignificant	Mild AHDS	Moderate AHDS	Severe AHDS

34.7 Criteria for assessment of canine acute haemorrhagic diarrhoea syndrome (AHDS). (Data from Mortier *et al.*, 2015)

Infectious enteritis

Canine and feline infectious gastroenteritis is one of the most common reasons for presentation to a veterinary clinic and hospitalization. It can be challenging for the clinician to determine the causative agent responsible for the diarrhoea due to the diverse array of pathogenic agents that could be responsible. These agents include viruses (in particular, parvovirus and coronavirus), bacteria (*Clostridium* spp., *E. coli*, *Campylobacter* spp. and *Salmonella*) and parasites (including protozoa), or a combination thereof. Infectious and parasitic agents are considered common in animals that are young, immunologically naive or immunocompromised, housed in large numbers or housed in unsanitary conditions.

Viral infections

Several canine and feline viral infections can cause enteritis as an important component of the clinical syndrome (e.g. canine and feline parvovirus, canine and feline coronavirus, feline leukaemia virus, feline immunodeficiency virus, canine distemper virus). Other viruses with a lower prevalence have also been associated with enteric disease, including canine adenovirus type 1, rotaviruses, reovirus, caliciviruses (such as norovirus and sapovirus), torovirus-like agent and circovirus (Dowgier *et al.*, 2017).

Canine strains of bocavirus have been associated with enteritis in puppies, and a fatal infection has been seen with a novel strain of canine bocavirus type 2. A fatal outbreak of AHDS in kennel dogs has been reported recently, associated with a calicivirus with sequence homology to a vesivirus (Renshaw *et al.*, 2018). Many other novel enteric viruses, such as kobuvirus, sakobuvirus and astrovirus, have been identified but their pathogenic role remains to be elucidated.

Canine and feline parvovirus

Canine parvovirus (CPV) and feline panleukopenia virus (FPV) are considered highly contagious agents of acute GI diseases in young, unvaccinated or incompletely vaccinated pets. CPV-2, which is closely related to FPV, was first described in 1978 and has subsequently mutated into CPV-2a, CPV-2b and, lately, CPV-2c. All genetic variants coexist worldwide with a globally different distribution in frequency and genetic variability.

The transmission of parvoviruses occurs by direct contact with an infected animal or its faeces, via contaminated fomites, or even as a result of contact with contaminated rodents and insects. It is important to remember that virus shedding can continue for approximately 14 days, even after resolution of all clinical signs. Similarly, animals with subclinical infections or mild transient signs also shed virus and pose risks to other animals that come into contact with them or their environment.

CPV recognizes the intestinal crypts and lymphoid organs as target tissues for viral replication, but the virus can spread to all tissues, including the brain. After penetration through the oronasal route, the virus replicates in the gastroenteric-associated lymphoid tissues and is disseminated by infected leucocytes to the germinal epithelium of the crypts of the small intestine, causing diarrhoea. Infection of leucocytes, mainly circulating and tissue-associated lymphocytes, causes leucopenia (lymphopenia often associated with neutropenia) with white blood cell (WBC) counts dropping below 2×10^9 cells/litre of blood.

However, total WBC counts may be within the normal ranges consequent to co-infection by opportunistic bacteria. *In utero* infection in CPV-naive bitches can cause foetal death or perinatal mortality. In 2–5-week-old seronegative puppies, CPV is also able to replicate in cardiac cells, inducing a fatal myocarditis, and in the brain cells, causing necrotizing vasculitis and encephalomalacia. However, these forms are rarely observed since protection is provided by maternally derived antibodies (MDA).

Most puppies and kittens are protected by MDA in the first week of life, but generally will have decreased MDA by 6–12 weeks to a level that allows active immunization (Day *et al.*, 2016). Thus, CPV almost exclusively affects puppies between the ages of approximately 6 weeks and 6 months; most adult dogs are immune. In cats, CPV causes a very severe gastroenteritis both in kittens over 3 or 4 weeks of age and in adult cats. There is evidence that some dog breeds are more susceptible to infection, with Rottweilers, American Pit Bull Terriers, Dobermanns, English Springer Spaniels, German Shepherd Dogs and Labrador Retrievers being at increased risk. Other factors that may exacerbate the severity of clinical signs include concurrent viral, bacterial and parasitic infections, unsanitary housing and overcrowding, as well as stressful environmental conditions. No breed susceptibility to FPV has been recognized in cats.

Clinical signs: The incubation period from the time of exposure to the onset of clinical disease ranges from 4 days in experimental studies from 1–2 weeks in spontaneous outbreaks, although 5–7 days is most typical. The earliest clinical signs are fever, lethargy and appetite loss; these are then followed by diarrhoea and vomiting in both CPV and FPV cases. Vomiting can become very severe and frequent. Diarrhoea is often absent for the first 24–48 hours of illness, but then may be yellow, mucoid or haemorrhagic.

In young cats, peracute FPV can cause death within 12 hours following the onset of lethargy, due to severe septic shock, dehydration and hypothermia. In these cases, vomiting and diarrhoea can be minimal or even absent. Abdominal pain secondary to acute gastroenteritis may be evident on palpation. Intestinal intussusception, ileus and GI motility alterations are recognized complications of CPV infection.

Transient or prolonged neutropenia, mainly due to damage to bone marrow progenitors and partially due to an overwhelming demand in the gut, makes canine and feline patients susceptible to serious bacterial infection (e.g. *E. coli*, *Clostridium* spp., *Salmonella* spp., *Campylobacter* spp.). An abnormally permeable intestinal tract allows increased bacterial translocation across the mucosa, with increased risk of sepsis. Massive fluid, electrolyte and protein losses through the GI tract may result in severe dehydration, hypokalaemia and hypovolaemic shock. Clinical signs associated with impaired tissue perfusion may be evident, including changes in mentation, tachycardia, tachypnoea, weak pulses, hypotension, prolonged capillary refill times, cool extremities and low rectal temperature.

Respiratory abnormalities, such as tachypnoea, dyspnoea and increased respiratory sounds, may be observed secondary to SIRS or concurrent pulmonary infections. Natural FPV infection, or use of a live FPV vaccine in a pregnant queen, can cause cerebellar hypoplasia in kittens when they are exposed *in utero* or in the early neonatal period.

The ultimate cause of death in patients with CPV or FPV infection is endotoxaemia, septicaemia and shock.

Diagnosis: The first suspicion of CPV or FPV infection is often based on the history and characteristic clinical signs. The typical signalment (young and unvaccinated or inadequately vaccinated animals) and signs of lethargy, anorexia, vomiting and diarrhoea associated with fever, dehydration and dilated fluid- and gas-filled intestinal loops (identified during abdominal palpation), as well as leucopenia, strongly suggest parvoviral disease. In many cases, further diagnostic tests are not performed and a presumptive diagnosis of parvoviral infection is made and the patients treated accordingly.

Definitive diagnostic tests include detection of CPV in the faeces, serology (seldom used) and post-mortem examination with histopathology. An enzyme-linked immunosorbent assay to detect CPV-2 in faeces is the best readily available in-house test to detect CPV-2a, CPV-2b and CPV-2c, but test sensitivity is <100% (see Chapter 2). Viral particles are shed in the faeces transiently, particularly very early or late in the course of the disease, and faecal antibodies may bind to viral particles, making them difficult to detect. False-negative results certainly occur, but the accuracy of positive test results is not disputed. In both dogs and cats, weak false-positive results may occur 4–8 days after vaccination with a modified-live vaccine, secondary to faecal shedding of vaccine virus. A faecal polymerase chain reaction (PCR) test is recommended in cases suggestive of CPV or FPV in the face of a negative faecal antigen test. In addition, faecal flotation should be routinely performed in all suspected cases to rule out concomitant parasitic infection.

Diagnostic imaging findings are not specific for CPV infection, but are useful to help eliminate other causes of vomiting and diarrhoea, such as intestinal obstruction. However, abdominal radiography often reveals a dilated small intestinal ileus that is sometimes difficult to differentiate from intestinal obstruction. Abdominal ultrasonographic findings may include altered wall layering of the duodenum and jejunum, with hyperechoic mucosal speckling and undulation of the luminal–mucosal interface, thinning of the duodenal and jejunal mucosa without a significant decrease in overall wall thickness, and generalized hypomotility to immobility, with a fluid-filled lumen. Intussusception is both an important complication and a differential diagnosis for canine parvoviral enteritis that is usually readily detectable on ultrasonography.

A definitive diagnosis can be established during post-mortem examination, using parvovirus antigen tests on faecal samples and/or intestinal mucosal scrapes. Histopathological evidence of characteristic parvovirus enteritis is considered the gold standard for confirming the diagnosis.

Treatment: Patients with parvovirus enteritis need to be isolated for the duration of the virus shedding period. In addition, exposed asymptomatic animals should be quarantined, strict biocontainment measures should be in place and environmental decontamination using an effective disinfectant (common household sodium hypochlorite bleach, at 1:30 dilution, left in contact for at least 10 minutes) should be instigated (Greene and Decaro, 2012).

Treatment of individual patients focuses on supporting effective circulating volume, controlling secondary bacterial infections and preserving the GI tract. Fluid and electrolyte therapy is crucial and typically combined with antibiotics. Canine parvoviral enteritis is a potentially life-treating condition and it is very important to monitor the patient's status carefully. Frequent physical examinations should be performed to evaluate hydration status, alertness and the severity of vomiting and diarrhoea. Bodyweight, PCV, WBC count and serum protein, glucose and potassium concentrations should be monitored and treatment adjusted accordingly.

Colloid administration (see Chapter 27) may be indicated in patients with hypoalbuminaemia (<20 g/l), especially if peripheral oedema and/or effusion in third spaces develop. Fresh frozen plasma containing active clotting factors and serum proteinase inhibitors may be helpful in dogs with abnormal coagulation profiles or SIRS. Antibodies contained in plasma have been presumed to be beneficial, but there is no proof that this is the case, and administration of a single dose of immune plasma soon after the onset of CPV enteritis in dogs has not been effective in ameliorating clinical signs, reducing viraemia or hastening haematological recovery. Ideally, packed red blood cells should be given to dogs that become anaemic through GI bleeding, and display signs of decreased tissue oxygenation; whole blood can be used if packed cells are not available.

Antibiotic therapy is required if there is evidence of infection (i.e. sepsis) or an increased risk of infection (i.e. severe neutropenia). Parenteral administration of an antibiotic combination with a broad aerobic and anaerobic spectrum is recommended in patients with signs of sepsis. Suitable combinations include an aminoglycoside or fluoroquinolone with a beta-lactam penicillin (co-amoxiclav, ampicillin/sulbactam) or first-generation cephalosporin. Aminoglycosides should only be used in well hydrated dogs and when renal perfusion is no longer compromised. Fluoroquinolones may cause cartilage abnormalities in large-breed, rapidly growing puppies.

Concurrent parasitism may be an aggravating factor leading to a worse prognosis, and empirical administration of anthelmintic therapy is appropriate.

Severe vomiting complicates therapy, and antiemetic drugs such as maropitant (1 mg/kg s.c. or slow i.v. q24h) or ondansetron (0.5 mg/kg i.v. loading dose followed by 0.5 mg/kg/h constant rate infusion (CRI) for 6 hours or 0.5–1 mg/kg orally q12–24h) may be useful. Metoclopramide (1–2 mg/kg/day CRI) often enhances the efficacy of antiemetic therapy. Inhibition of gastric acid secretion may be useful in vomiting dogs with secondary oesophagitis (omeprazole or pantoprazole at a dose of 1 mg/kg i.v. q12–24h).

Once vomiting stops, patients may be offered water. If there is no further vomiting, then enteral nutrition should be encouraged. Evidence indicates that early enteral nutrition promotes improved barrier function, which limits endotoxin absorption and bacterial translocation. In addition, compared with dogs that are given food only when cessation of vomiting has been confirmed, early enteral nutritional therapy has been shown to promote earlier clinical improvement and weight gain.

An easily digestible, low-fat diet should be fed because the villus structure and intestinal function will require several days to recover. Voluntary ingestion of food may be promoted by the administration of the ghrelin receptor agonist capromorelin (see Chapter 27). If the dog refuses to eat, administration of an enteral liquid diet via a naso-oesophageal tube may facilitate intestinal recovery. Parenteral nutrition can be life-saving for patients unable to meet their nutritional requirements.

Pain management is important, and synthetic opioids (i.e. methadone at 0.1–0.5 mg/kg i.m. or 0.1–0.3 mg/kg i.v. q4h; buprenorphine at 0.01–0.02 mg/kg i.v., i.m. s.c. q6–8h;

butorphanol at 0.1–0.2 mg/kg s.c., i.m. or i.v. q4–6h; trama-dol at 2–5 mg/kg orally q8h or 2 mg/kg i.v.) can alleviate abdominal pain. With higher doses or long-term opioid use, increased GI sphincter tone and reduced peristalsis and intestinal fluid secretion may lead to constipation and worsen ileus; sedation may also occur.

Recombinant feline interferon ω (rFeIFN-ω) has proved promising as an adjuvant treatment. In a study of 94 dogs with naturally occurring CPV enteritis, the severity of the clinical signs and the mortality rate were significantly reduced in those animals treated with rFeIFN-ω (2.5 mIU/kg i.v. q24h for 3 days) compared with those dogs given a placebo (De Mari et al., 2003). In another experimental study, rFeIFN-ω (2.5 mIU/kg i.v. q24h for 3 days) was simi-larly effective (Martin et al., 2002). Currently, the limited commercial availability and the particularly high cost in many countries prohibit rFeIFN-ω from being regularly used in a clinical setting.

In a recent study, the efficacy of recombinant canine granulocyte-colony stimulating factor (rcG-CSF) was assessed in a clinical trial (Armenise et al., 2019). A positive haematological effect (increased leucocyte counts, marked stimulation of lymphocytes and monocytes; neutrophil counts did not improve as quickly as lymphocytes and monocytes), together with a shorter duration of hospitaliza-tion and a zero mortality rate, were seen in dogs treated with rcG-CSF compared with those animals that were not.

In addition, another recent study demonstrated that faecal microbial transplantation in conjunction with stand-ard treatment resulted in a more rapid clinical recovery and a decreased duration of hospitalization in surviving puppies with CPV compared with puppies treated with the standard therapy alone (Pereira et al., 2018).

Prior to discharge or contact with other dogs, patients that have recovered from CPV infection should be bathed to ensure that any virus present on their coats is removed.

Prognosis: Typically, the prognosis is guarded to poor; however, puppies that survive the first 3–4 days usually make a full recovery within a week. With adequate sup-portive care, 70% of dogs will recover and develop long-term immunity. The prognosis is poorer in very young kittens (<8 weeks of age) and patients with leucopenia, thrombocytopenia, hypoalbuminaemia or hypokalaemia.

Prevention: To prevent and control CPV, vaccination with a modified-live vaccine is recommended (see the World Small Animal Veterinary Association (WSAVA) Vaccination Guidelines). CPV can remain in the environment for an extended period of time, thus cages and equipment should be thoroughly disinfected (see above). Vaccination is advisable in all cats, in order to provide a solid, long-lasting immunity (see WSAVA Vaccination Guidelines).

Animal shelters

The following policy has been recommended in the USA for vaccination of dogs and cats on admission to an animal shelter:

'All dogs and cats 4 weeks of age and older should receive a vaccine containing modified-live parvovirus on intake, regardless of intake status (stray, owner surrender, rabies quarantine, cruelty case, pregnant, lactating, injured, ill). A delay of even a day can signifi-cantly increase the risk of infection. All puppies and kittens should be re-vaccinated every 2 weeks whilst in the shelter until they are 5 months old because of the potential for MDAs to interfere with vaccination efficacy.'

Canine coronaviral enteritis

Canine enteric coronavirus (CCoV) is a common infection of dogs, particularly those housed in large groups (e.g. kennels, shelters, breeding facilities). CCoV is an alpha-coronavirus and two distinct serotypes (types I and II) have been identified. CCoV replicates in the cytoplasm of mature enterocytes on the villi, while those in the intestinal crypts are spared. The loss of mature villous enterocytes causes atrophy of the intestinal villi, an increase in mitotic activity of the crypt epithelium and a net expansion of the pool of immature enterocytes. These changes in small intestinal morphology cause a loss of normal digestive and absorptive function, leading to diarrhoea and dehydration.

While CCoV traditionally causes only mild GI clinical signs, there are increasing reports of lethal CCoV infec-tions in dogs, with evidence of both GI and systemic viral dissemination (Decaro et al., 2013). Thus, CCoV is now considered to be an emerging infectious disease of dogs. Novel recombinant variants of CCoV have been found con-taining spike protein N-terminal domains that are closely related to those of feline and porcine strains (i.e. pantropic CCoV-IIa). The increase in pathogenicity reported in dogs and the emergence of novel CCoVs can be attributed to the high level of recombination within the spike gene that can occur during infection by more than one CCoV type in the same host.

CCoV is spread primarily by the faecal–oral route via a contaminated environment; however, it is unclear whether transmission by other routes (including aerosol) can occur. CCoV generally causes a mild, but highly contagious, enteritis in young dogs, most commonly <12 weeks of age. Concurrent infection with infectious agents such as CPV is thought to potentiate CCoV-associated illness. Older dogs can be infected but appear less likely to develop clinical signs of disease.

The duration of faecal shedding in infected dogs is normally 6–9 days, but can be longer in some animals.

Clinical signs: The clinical signs range from loose faeces to severe watery diarrhoea, as well as vomiting. Morbidity and mortality are largely determined by the age of the animal at the onset of infection, the level and type of pathogen expo-sure, concurrent infection(s) and the degree of passive maternal immunity. Recently, an increasing number of infec-tions with highly virulent CCoVs have been reported in puppies without apparent co-infections worldwide, although not yet in the UK (Buonavoglia et al., 2006; Licitra et al., 2014). In the case of pantropic CCoV-IIa viruses, infection results in a fatal multisystemic illness, with clinical signs mimicking severe CPV infection, including high fever, haem-orrhagic gastroenteritis, neurological signs and leucopenia.

Diagnosis: A definitive diagnosis of CCoV-induced disease is currently difficult to achieve and, therefore, not com-monly undertaken. While rarely available, electron micro-scopic evaluation of faecal samples allows direct visualization of viral particles. Virus isolation can be achieved for CCoV-II viruses, but not for CCoV-I viruses; however, this is also not commonly available. The definitive test is post-mortem identification of viral antigen by immu-nofluorescence or immunohistochemical staining of tissue sections. The most useful ante-mortem tests are highly sensitive real-time PCR-based assays. A common PCR test can reliably detect alpha-coronaviruses and more specific PCR tests can be employed to further characterize the viral serotype or genotype. However, due to the highly variable nature of CCoV genomes, novel variants may be missed with this approach. Serological tests are of limited use, since they can only confirm exposure to CCoV and cannot currently discriminate between infecting CCoV serotypes or genotypes.

Treatment: The treatment for CCoV is primarily supportive and involves fluid therapy and antiemetics. The role of antibiotics in the treatment of CCoV infection has not been assessed, but they are probably not helpful in most cases. There are no antiviral drugs available for the treatment of CCoV infections.

Prognosis: The prognosis is usually good.

Prevention: Several inactivated and modified-live virus vaccines are available, but to date it is considered that vaccination provides only partial protection.

Feline coronavirus

Feline enteric coronavirus (FECoV) is ubiquitous in the cat population. Infection in adults is often asymptomatic, whereas kittens may have a mild transient diarrhoea that may be associated with weight loss. Asymptomatic cats shed FECoV in faeces. The prognosis for a full recovery is excellent.

The enteric virus may also mutate to feline infectious peritonitis (FIP) virus, but neither isolation of FECoV from faeces by PCR nor serological evidence of FECoV infection are proof of FIP. An unusual manifestation of FIP infection is isolated mural intestinal lesions. The clinical signs associated with this condition include chronic diarrhoea and vomiting, and cats often have a palpable mass in the colon or at the ileocaecocolic junction. Affected intestine is markedly thickened and nodular, with multifocal pyogranulomas extending through the intestinal wall.

Bacterial infections

Although bacterial infections are considered an uncommon cause of small intestinal disease in dogs and cats, various bacteria can affect the small intestine, including *Campylobacter jejuni*, *Salmonella enterica*, *Clostridium* spp., and adherent-invasive *E. coli* (AIEC) in Boxers and French Bulldogs. *E. coli*, notably enterotoxigenic (ETEC), enteropathogenic (EPEC) and enterohaemorrhagic (EHEC) strains, are associated with canine GI disease, particularly in young puppies (Beutin, 1999). In addition, since all of these agents can cause acute or chronic enterocolitis in humans, bacterial enteric infection in animals can represent a public health concern.

The severity of illness (if any) in infected dogs and cats has not been established, but is generally considered to be mild and self-limiting in the absence of host immunosuppression, but probably varies with the type and quantity of microorganism involved. For example, *C. jejuni* is considered to cause usually self-limiting illness in dogs younger than 6 months old, living in crowded conditions such as kennels, whereas, in cats, clinical signs of campylobacteriosis are poorly documented.

Salmonella spp. may cause acute diarrhoea, sepsis and sudden death, especially in very young or geriatric dogs and cats and patients receiving immunosuppressive drugs. Feeding contaminated raw foods may be a contributing factor. Pneumonia can also be associated with acute *Salmonella* enteritis. Other bacteria, such as sporulating *C. perfringens* producing toxins have been associated with acute, bloody, self-limiting diarrhoea in dogs.

Diagnosis

Culture, PCR testing and toxin detection in faeces can be used to identify the bacterial agents responsible for small intestinal disease. However, it should be remembered that a positive result does not confirm the diagnosis, as healthy dogs and cats may shed the same bacteria at a similar frequency to that of patients with diarrhoea. A negative result is more helpful, ruling out the likely transmission of infection from animals to humans.

Treatment

Most cases are considered to be self-limiting and respond to conservative management with fluid therapy and temporary dietary modification. Antibiotics are commonly administered but their use is appropriate only in patients with signs of sepsis (see Chapter 29).

Parasitic infections

Dogs and cats may be infected by several endoparasites, including helminths and protozoa (i.e. coccidia, *Giardia*).

Helminths

Hookworms (*Ancylostoma caninum*, *Ancylostoma tubaeforme*, *Uncinaria stenocephala*) can cause enteritis in dogs and cats. Whipworms (*Trichuris vulpis*) typically cause more chronic colitis-like signs. Roundworms (e.g. *Toxocara canis*, *Toxocara cati*, *Toxascaris leonina*) less commonly cause clinical signs, and tapeworms (e.g. *Dipylidium caninum*) are rarely associated with any clinical signs in dogs or cats.

Roundworms are found frequently in dogs and cats, predominantly in those animals aged <1 year, and a large number of worms may cause an intestinal blockage or induce an intussusception. Hookworms inhabit the small intestine and feed by grasping the intestinal mucosa with their mouthparts and damaging the surface to obtain nutrients. Severe lactogenic-transmitted hookworm infection can lead to significant anaemia, bloody diarrhoea and death in young puppies.

Diagnosis: The diagnosis is based on identifying eggs in faeces using a flotation technique (see Chapter 2).

Treatment: As puppies can become heavily infected with *T. canis* either *in utero* or in the neonatal period, and this may cause serious illness before diagnosis is possible by faecal examination, they should be treated with appropriate anthelmintics at 2 weeks of age, continuing at fortnightly intervals until 2 weeks after weaning, and then at monthly intervals until 6 months of age. In kittens, prenatal infection does not occur and fortnightly treatment can begin at 3 weeks of age, continuing until 2 weeks after weaning, and then at monthly intervals for 6 months. Nursing bitches and queens should be treated concurrently with the first treatment of their offspring as they may have a patent infection.

It is generally recommended that dogs and cats be treated with an anthelmintic at least four times a year. Alternatively, faecal examinations can be performed at suitable intervals and treatment instigated as required (see the European Scientific Counsel Companion Animal Parasite (ESCCAP) and the Companion Animal Parasite Council (CAPC) guidelines).

Protozoa

A wide range of intestinal protozoa commonly infect dogs and cats, and younger animals are more typically affected.

Older animals tend to be immune following previous exposure. Infections are often asymptomatic and usually self-limiting; however, severe clinical signs can occur and can be related to co-infection with other pathogens. Dogs and cats living in kennels/catteries, animal shelters or in crowded conditions with poor sanitation may have a higher risk of acquiring protozoal infections (e.g. *Giardia*, *Cryptosporidium* and *Cystoisospora*).

Diagnosis: The diagnosis is difficult and often requires repeated sampling and molecular typing. Due to intermittent shedding, negative findings on faecal examination cannot rule out infection.

Treatment: The treatment is often complicated due to the lack of effective drugs or the need for 'off-label' use of existing drugs. Fenbendazole is authorized for the treatment of giardiasis in dogs in most European countries and can be recommended for use in cats (50 mg/kg orally q24h for 5 days). The treatment can be repeated if evidence of infection persists. Alternatively, a combination product containing febantel, pyrantel and praziquantel can be administered at the standard oral deworming dose (15.0 mg/kg febantel, 14.4 mg/kg pyrantel, 5.0 mg/kg praziquantel) once daily for 3 days for giardiasis.

Conditions requiring surgical intervention

Acute small intestinal conditions that require surgical intervention include obstruction due to the ingestion of foreign bodies, incarceration of a bowel loop in hernias and the development of an intussusception.

- Common foreign bodies in dogs include peach stones, corn cobs and toys. In cats, linear foreign bodies are more common and may anchor around the base of the tongue, pylorus or even at more distal sites.
- Intussusception is the invagination of one intestinal segment (intussusceptum) into the lumen of an adjacent segment (intussuscipiens). Intussusception occurs more commonly in dogs and may be located anywhere along the small intestine; however, ileocolic and jejunojejunal intussusceptions are seen most frequently.
- Intestinal volvulus is a rare but peracute emergency that requires immediate surgery after cardiovascular stabilization. The prognosis is very guarded.

Younger animals are more likely to develop an intussusception following enteritis (e.g. due to parasitism, viral or bacterial infection, dietary indiscretion or change, foreign body or mass) or systemic illness. Intussusceptions have also been reported following abdominal surgery and environmental changes, but in most cases the cause is unknown. One study comparing intussusceptions in dogs and cats revealed that cats with intussusceptions are more likely to be older than dogs and to have underlying neoplasms, while dogs are more likely to have inflammatory disease.

Clinical signs

The clinical signs of intestinal obstruction vary with the site, duration and completeness of obstruction, the degree of distension, the presence of peritonitis and whether there is concurrent systemic sepsis. Complete upper intestinal obstruction is associated with persistent and severe vomiting of large volumes, together with marked intestinal fluid and electrolyte loss. The major cause of mortality from upper small intestinal obstruction is severe hypovolaemia with electrolyte disturbances. Without treatment, dogs with high, complete obstructions usually die within 3–4 days.

With distal small intestinal obstructions (distal jejunum, ileum or ileocaecal junction), clinical signs are less severe and include anorexia and intermittent vomiting of small volumes of material that may have a faecal-like appearance. Defecation may be absent or decreased in frequency and the faeces are occasionally bloody. Diarrhoea is more common in animals with partial obstruction, and it may be attributed to the combined osmotic effects of unabsorbed substances in the intestinal lumen and to the secretory activity of enterocytes.

Intestinal obstruction is a painful condition, due to intestinal dilatation, mechanical trauma, ischaemia and bacterial toxin absorption, although some affected animals do not demonstrate much discomfort. With complete intraluminal obstruction, the intestine orad to the lesion distends with gas and fluid. Secretions from the salivary, biliary, gastric, intestinal and pancreatic glands are normally reabsorbed in the lower jejunum and ileum; however, in cases of obstruction, this absorption is reduced because of lymphatic and venous congestion, increased intraluminal osmolality and decreased enterocyte turnover rate.

Most linear foreign bodies do not obstruct the intestine themselves, but rather gathering and pleating of the intestine around the foreign body causes partial to complete obstruction. Continued peristalsis may cause the foreign body to penetrate the mucosa and lacerate the mesenteric border of the intestine, leading to peritonitis. Some animals with linear foreign bodies may have concurrent intussusceptions.

Diagnosis

A diagnosis of intestinal foreign body obstruction or intussusception can frequently be made based on the history and physical examination alone. Abdominal palpation may permit localization of pain to a specific region of the intestine, or it may be more generalized (especially when peritonitis is present). In many cases, a foreign body can be directly palpated, as can plication or bunching of the intestines, which may indicate the presence of a linear foreign body. Intussusceptions can often be palpated as firm, frequently painful, tubular structures that cannot be indented with digital pressure, thus differentiating them from faeces.

Laboratory findings

A minimum database helps to characterize the fluid losses and inflammation. Abnormal laboratory findings may include dehydration, stress leucograms, anaemia, and electrolyte and acid–base abnormalities.

Imaging

Radiography: A radiographic diagnosis of intestinal obstruction is based on signs including gastric and intestinal dilatation by gas and/or fluid, abnormal shape of the intestinal loops, the presence of foreign material and the 'gravel' sign (i.e. the accumulation of radiodense particulate matter proximal to the obstruction). Of these, localized dilatation of the intestine is considered to be the key radiographic sign. The length of dilated intestine and degree of dilatation observed radiographically may vary depending on the site, duration and completeness of the obstruction. Linear foreign bodies often have a specific and pathognomonic radiographic appearance of one or more loops of small intestine bunched or pleated together, giving a wrinkled appearance (Figure 34.8).

The published criterion for normal intestinal diameter in the dog is the ratio of the maximal small intestinal external diameter (SI_{max}) and the height of the L5 vertebral body ($SI_{max}/L5$). This ratio should not exceed 1.6 in normal dogs. A ratio higher than 1.6 indicates distension and a ratio greater than 2 indicates a high probability of obstruction.

Contrast radiography: Contrast radiography can assist in the diagnosis, as it may delineate foreign bodies, reveal luminal filling defects or demonstrate delayed transit time or the displacement of intestinal loops. In general, however, radiographic contrast studies are infrequently undertaken for this purpose because they are impractical in an emergency situation and often do not provide more information than plain radiography.

Ultrasonography: An ultrasonographic examination can be highly specific for the diagnosis of intestinal obstruction. It allows measurement of intestinal wall thickness, assessment of wall stratification and intestinal mobility, and evaluation of adjacent structures, such as lymph nodes and the peritoneum. All foreign bodies have a characteristic appearance – a well defined hyperechoic, hyperreflective acoustic interface with distal acoustic shadowing (see Figure 34.8c). Intestinal dilatation caused by mechanical obstruction is readily detected (jejunal serosal-to-serosal diameter of at least 1.5 cm). The ultrasonographic appearance of an intussusception is best characterized on a transverse view, which reveals the wall layers as a multilayered series of concentric rings or a target-like lesion (Figure 34.9).

Endoscopy

Endoscopy rarely diagnoses intestinal foreign bodies that have not already been detected by radiography or ultrasonography. However, endoscopy is useful for identifying

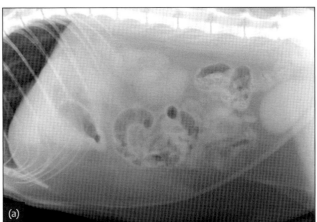
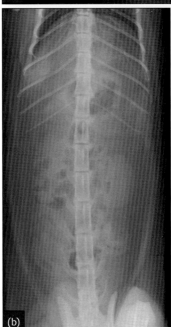
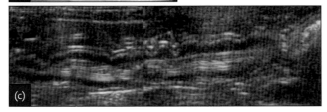

34.8 (a) Right lateral and (b) ventrodorsal views of an 8-year-old male neutered Domestic Shorthaired cat. Gathering of the small intestine is visible in the mid-abdomen. (c) A linear foreign body was detected on ultrasonography as parallel hyperechoic lines within the small intestinal lumen.
(Courtesy of Professor M Vignoli, VTH Teramo University)

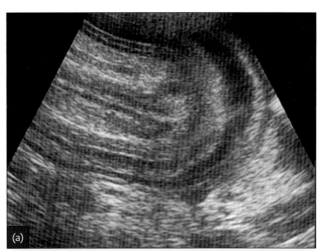
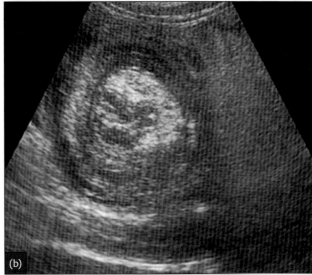

34.9 Ultrasonograms of the abdomen of a dog with a surgically confirmed intestinal intussusception. (a) The longitudinal view shows a double intestinal wall, typical of an intestinal loop containing another intestinal loop. (b) On the transverse view, the hyperechoic mesenteric fat containing hypoechoic vessels is visible.
(Courtesy of Professor M Vignoli, VTH Teramo University)

and removing gastric and high duodenal foreign bodies. In addition, endoscopy may be useful for detecting and/or removing linear foreign bodies lodged at the pylorus.

Treatment

Some foreign bodies will successfully pass through the intestine without requiring therapy. In patients with acute clinical signs, failure to radiographically demonstrate foreign body movement within the intestine over an 8-hour period or failure to pass the object within approximately 36 hours are indications for surgery. If abdominal pain, fever, vomiting or lethargy are apparent, surgical intervention should not be delayed.

Although endoscopic retrieval may be successful in some cases of gastric foreign bodies, it is rarely possible to remove foreign material from the small intestine. Small intestinal obstructions are best removed via laparotomy and enterotomy. Intussusceptions should be managed surgically, even if they can be manually reduced, as recurrence is common. Examination of biopsy specimens obtained from the intestine at the time of surgical correction may help identify the cause of the intussusception.

Hydration, electrolyte and acid–base abnormalities should be corrected prior to surgery, if possible. Antibiotic therapy is essential because of the probability of systemic sepsis and the risk of contamination during surgery (see Chapter 5). Analgesia should be provided, if necessary, to control postoperative pain. If no vomiting occurs, water can be offered 8–12 hours following surgery and food can be provided 12–24 hours later.

References and further reading

Armenise A, Trerotoli P, Cirone F et al. (2019) Use of recombinant canine granulocyte-colony stimulating factor to increase leukocyte count in dogs naturally infected by canine parvovirus. Veterinary Microbiology **231**, 177–182

Beutin L (1999) Escherichia coli as a pathogen in dogs and cats. Veterinary Research **30**, 285–298

Buonavoglia C, Decaro N, Martella V et al. (2006) Canine coronavirus highly pathogenic for dogs. Emerging Infectious Diseases **12**, 492–494

Caddy SL (2018) New virus associated with canine gastroenteritis. The Veterinary Journal **232**, 57–64

Cave N (2013) Adverse food reactions. In: Canine and Feline Gastroenterology, ed. RJ Washabau and MJ Day, pp. 398–408. Saunders, St. Louis

Ciasca TC, David FH and Lamb CR (2013) Does measurement of small intestinal diameter increase diagnostic accuracy of radiography in dogs with suspected intestinal obstruction? Veterinary Radiology and Ultrasound **54**, 207–211

Day MJ, Horzinek MC, Schultz RD and Squires RA (2016) Guidelines for the vaccination of dogs and cats. Journal of Small Animal Practice **57**, E1–E45

Decaro N, Cordonnier N, Demeter Z et al. (2013) European surveillance for pantropic canine coronavirus. Journal of Clinical Microbiology **51**, 83–88

De Mari K, Maynard L, Eun HM and Lebreux B (2003) Treatment of canine parvoviral enteritis with interferon-omega in a placebo-controlled field trial. Veterinary Record **152**, 105–108

Dowgier G, Lorusso E, Decaro N et al. (2017) A molecular survey for selected viral enteropathogens revealed a limited role of canine circovirus in the development of canine acute gastroenteritis. Veterinary Microbiology **204**, 54–58

Finck C, D'Anjou MA, Alexander K et al. (2014) Radiographic diagnosis of mechanical obstruction in dogs based on relative small intestinal external diameters. Veterinary Radiology and Ultrasound **55**, 472–479

Garcia DA, Froes TR, Vilani RG et al. (2011) Ultrasonography of small intestinal obstructions: a contemporary approach. Journal of Small Animal Practice **52**, 484–490

Greene CE and Decaro N (2012) Canine viral enteritis. In: Infectious Diseases of the Dog and Cat, 4th edn, ed. CE Greene, pp 67–80. Elsevier, St. Louis

Hartmann K (2017) Coronavirus infections (canine and feline), including feline infectious peritonitis. In: Textbook of Veterinary Internal Medicine, 8th edn, ed. SJ Ettinger, EC Feldman and E Cote., pp. 983–991. Elsevier, St. Louis

Hobday MM, Pachtinger GE, Drobatz KJ and Syring RS (2014) Linear versus non-linear gastrointestinal foreign bodies in 499 dogs: clinical presentation, management and short-term outcome. Journal of Small Animal Practice **55**, 560–565

Leisewitz AL (2017) Canine and feline parvovirus infection. In: Textbook of Veterinary Internal Medicine, 8th edn, ed. SJ Ettinger, EC Feldman and E Cote pp. 991–996. Elsevier, St. Louis

Levien AS and Baines SJ (2011) Histological examination of the intestine from dogs and cats with intussusception. Journal of Small Animal Practice **52**, 599–606

Licitra BN, Whittaker GR, Dubovi EJ and Duhamel GE (2014) Genotypic characterization of canine coronavirus associated with fatal canine neonatal enteritis in the United States. Journal of Clinical Microbiology **52**, 4230–4238

Martin V, Najbar W, Guegue S et al. (2002) Treatment of canine parvoviral enteritis with interferon-omega in a placebo-controlled challenge trial. Veterinary Microbiology **89**, 115–127

Mortier F, Strohmeyer K, Hartmann K and Unterer S (2015) Acute haemorrhagic diarrhoea syndrome in dogs: 108 cases. Veterinary Record **176**, 627

Pereira GQ, Gomes LA, Santos IS et al. (2018) Fecal microbiota transplantation in puppies with canine parvovirus infection. Journal of Veterinary Internal Medicine **32**, 707–711

Radlinsky MG (2013) Surgery of the digestive system. In: Small Animal Surgery, 4th edn, ed. TW Fossum, pp. 516–542. Elsevier, St. Louis

Renshaw RW, Griffing J, Weisman J et al. (2018) Characterization of a vesivirus associated with an outbreak of acute hemorrhagic gastroenteritis in domestic dogs. Journal of Clinical Microbiology **56**, e01951–17

Shanaman MM, Schwarz T, Gal A and O'Brien RT (2013) Comparison between survey radiography, B-mode ultrasonography, contrast-enhanced ultrasonography and contrast-enhanced multi-detector computed tomography findings in dogs with acute abdominal signs. Veterinary Radiology and Ultrasound **54**, 591–604

Sharma A, Thompson MS, Scrivani PV et al. (2011) Comparison of radiography and ultrasonography for diagnosing small intestinal mechanical obstruction in vomiting dogs. Veterinary Radiology and Ultrasound **52**, 248–255

Sindern N, Suchodolski JS, Leutenegger CM et al. (2019) Prevalence of Clostridium perfringens netE and netF toxin genes in the feces of dogs with acute hemorrhagic diarrhea syndrome. Journal of Veterinary Internal Medicine **33**, 100–105

Unterer S, Lechner E, Mueller RS et al. (2015) Prospective study of bacteraemia in acute haemorrhagic diarrhoea syndrome in dogs. Veterinary Record **176**, 309

Unterer S, Strohmeyer K, Kruse BD et al. (2011) Treatment of aseptic dogs with hemorrhagic gastroenteritis with amoxicillin/clavulanic acid: a prospective blinded study. Journal of Veterinary Internal Medicine **25**, 973–979

Washabau RJ (2013) Diseases of the gastrointestinal tract. In: Canine and Feline Gastroenterology, 1st edn, ed. RJ Washabau and MJ Day, pp. 699–706. Saunders, St. Louis

Useful websites

Companion Animal Parasite Council (CAPC) – Parasite guidelines: https://capcvet.org/guidelines/

European Scientific Counsel Companion Animal Parasites (ESCCAP) – Worm control in dogs and cats: www.esccap.org/page/GL1+Worm+Control+in+Dogs+and+Cats/25/#.XTbpq-hKg2w

University of Florida – Canine and feline parvovirus in animal shelters: https://sheltermedicine.vetmed.ufl.edu/files/2017/01/Canine-and-feline-parvovirus-in-shelters.2018.pdf

World Small Animal Veterinary Association (WSAVA) – Vaccination guidelines: www.wsava.org/Guidelines/Vaccination-Guidelines

Small intestine: chronic disease

Alison Ridyard

The major clinical manifestations of chronic small intestinal disease, namely diarrhoea, vomiting and weight loss, reflect perturbations in the digestive and absorptive function of the small intestine and its resident bacterial population.

Infectious diseases

Although numerous infectious agents, including bacterial enteropathogens, viruses, protozoa, helminths and, rarely, fungal organisms, have the capacity to cause diarrhoea in dogs and cats, in the context of chronic, infectious small intestinal disease of most concern is parasitic infections. Enteric viruses typically cause acute clinical signs (see Chapter 34b), with the notable exception of when feline enteric coronavirus mutates to feline infectious peritonitis virus, and the clinical significance of culturing an enteric bacterial pathogen, particularly in dogs with chronic diarrhoea, is the subject of much ongoing debate.

With advances in diagnostic tests, such as the introduction of multiplex polymerase chain reaction (PCR) tests, there is an increasing awareness that co-infection with multiple enteropathogens is not uncommon in dogs and cats with chronic diarrhoea. The difficulty that the clinician faces is deciding which, if any, of the potential pathogens identified is clinically relevant, as a positive test result does not prove causality.

Bacteria

Typically, enteric pathogens such as *Campylobacter jejuni*, *Salmonella* spp., *Clostridium perfringens* and *Clostridium difficile* are associated with acute, and often self-limiting, diarrhoea. Their role in chronic diarrhoea remains controversial, primarily as the organisms and/or associated toxin(s) are frequently detected in the faeces of non-diarrhoeic individuals. Causality is difficult to prove as in individuals with another primary gastrointestinal (GI) disease (e.g. intestinal inflammation or neoplasia), colonization may be secondary to alteration of local immune defences. Given the zoonotic potential of *Campylobacter* and *Salmonella* spp., it is probably prudent to recognize these as possible contributory factors in a diarrhoeic dog or cat, particularly in a household where there are immunocompromised people, but still to search for an underlying cause. Failure of clinical signs to resolve following treatment should prompt further assessment for an underlying disease or co-infection. For a more detailed description of these infections, see Chapter 34b.

Protozoa

Giardia species

These flagellated protozoan parasites are found on the surface of enterocytes in the small intestine, particularly in the duodenum of dogs and the ileum of cats, where they are thought to cause clinical signs by a number of pathological mechanisms, including the production of enterotoxins, alteration of enterocyte function, induction of intestinal inflammation, disruption of the normal enteric flora (dysbiosis) and by disturbing intestinal motility. Infection occurs following ingestion of oocysts and, as with other protozoan parasites, potential sources of infection include contaminated water and food, mutual grooming of infected individuals and ingestion of infected prey species.

Although the different species of *Giardia* are morphologically indistinguishable, genetic analysis has identified a number of genotypes and has challenged the widely held perception that *Giardia* has minimal host specificity.

Giardia infection may cause small intestinal diarrhoea, which can have a mucoid component and, as a consequence of fat maldigestion, steatorrhoea may be reported. In some cases, weight loss occurs as a consequence of maldigestion and malabsorption. It is probable that different genotypes have differing pathogenic potential and that host factors and co-infection with other protozoa play a role in determining whether an infected individual develops clinical signs. Consequently, subclinical infection is probably the rule in dogs and cats, and when clinical signs are present the possibility of an alternative concurrent cause should always be considered, particularly when a cycle of treatment does not resolve the clinical signs.

There are several methods of diagnosing *Giardia* infection, including detection of oocysts by zinc sulphate faecal flotation, immunofluorescence antigen testing of faeces (which can also be used to detect *Cryptosporidium*), faecal antigen enzyme-linked immunosorbent assay (ELISA) (SNAP®) tests and faecal PCR tests, which have become available more recently. Consideration should be given to the strengths and limitations of each assay (see Chapter 2). Analysis of several faecal samples over a 3- to 5-day period may increase the chances of detecting infections.

Current recommendations for the treatment of *Giardia* infection include the use of fenbendazole (50 mg/kg orally q24h for 5 days) or metronidazole (25 mg/kg orally q12h for 5–7 days). Treatment with a combination of febantel, pyrantel and praziquantel has also been reported, although it is not licensed for this purpose in the UK. The primary aim of treatment is to control diarrhoea, as eradication of infection can be difficult. Re-infection occurs frequently and attempts at environmental decontamination may be necessary. In this instance, treatment of in-contact animals should be considered, particularly if they are found to be positive on faecal antigen testing.

Coccidia

Cystoisospora *species:* Infection with this coccidial protozoan, formerly called *Isospora*, is caused by ingestion of sporulated oocysts from environment, or by ingestion of paratenic hosts. Replication takes place in enterocytes and infection results in direct damage to the intestinal epithelium.

Clinical signs are uncommon in adult dogs and cats and usually occur only when large numbers of cysts are ingested, or when the patient is immunocompromised, or where co-infection is present. Typically, signs consist of acute vomiting, abdominal discomfort and watery diarrhoea (sometimes containing fresh blood). Subclinical or persistent infection can be responsible for recurrent bouts of GI disease. Where coccidial infection is associated with chronic diarrhoea, the presence of an underlying disease or immunosuppression should be suspected.

Diagnosis is made by identification of *Cystisospora* oocysts in faeces (faecal flotation) during an acute episode and, as clinical signs may precede shedding of oocysts, evaluation of more than one faecal sample may increase the chances of diagnosis.

Most infections do not require treatment. However, treatment may be useful in shortening the duration of clinical signs and in reducing the environmental contamination. Treatment of in-contact animals may be prudent where heavy infections have been documented. Treatment options include trimethoprim/sulphonamide (15–30 mg/kg orally q12–24h for 5 days) or sulfadimethoxine (50–60 mg/kg orally q24h for 5–20 days). Oral amprolium and toltrazuril are also considered to be effective treatments (and preventatives). Although toltrazuril is licensed in the EU for treating coccidiosis in dogs, neither drug is licensed for use in dogs and cats in the UK.

Cryptosporidium *species:* *Cryptosporidium* is an uncommon cause of small intestinal diarrhoea in dogs and cats. Infection occurs following ingestion of environmental oocysts or paratenic hosts. *Cryptosporidium* replicates within enterocytes, and clinical signs are attributable to damage to intestinal microvilli and intestinal epithelial cells, villus atrophy and lymphoplasmacytic inflammation. Autoinfection is common, with some thin-walled oocysts rupturing within the intestinal tract, releasing sporozoites and thus amplifying infection.

Clinical signs tend to be seen in young or immunocompromised animals, although more commonly infection is subclinical. Co-infection with other protozoal parasites is common and where co-infection occurs, clinical signs are more likely.

Diagnosis can be made by demonstration of oocysts using faecal flotation techniques, although immunofluorescence assay and PCR-based diagnostic tests are likely to be more sensitive.

Treatment of *Cryptosporidium* infection can be problematic and, although numerous antimicrobial agents have been used, none are consistently effective at eliminating the infection. Options include tylosin and azithromycin. Treatment of co-infection(s) and addressing the underlying immune compromise may contribute to a positive outcome.

Helminths

Whipworms (*Trichuris vulpis*) are parasites of the large intestine (see Chapter 35), while hookworms, roundworms and tapeworms tend to be found in the small intestine. With the exception of hookworms, helminths are rarely the cause of significant disease, except in puppies and kittens. However, many have zoonotic potential, and regular anthelmintic treatment is recommended.

Hookworms

There are three species of hookworm of clinical relevance in the UK and northern Europe, namely *Uncinaria stenocephala* (dog and cat) and, very uncommonly, *Ancylostoma caninum* (dog) and *Ancylostoma tubaeforme* (cat). *A. caninum* is not reported in the UK, and is more common in southern Europe, Africa and the Americas.

Hookworms have a direct life cycle, and infection occurs via ingestion of infective L3 larvae in the environment, ingestion of larvae during nursing (transmammary infection: dogs only) or ingestion of paratenic hosts (e.g. rodents); the infective larvae of *Uncinaria* can also penetrate the skin. Adult hookworms inhabit the small intestine where, in addition to causing blood loss (by ingestion), they can cause ulceration of the small intestine, blunting of the microvilli and eosinophilic infiltration of the intestinal mucosa.

Clinical infections are uncommon in adult dogs, but heavy worm burdens in puppies and kittens can cause clinically significant disease. Severe anaemia can occur as a direct result of blood loss, especially where concurrent flea infestation is present. With chronic infections, in addition to chronic iron deficiency anaemia, infected individuals may develop small intestinal diarrhoea, melaena and weight loss; poor hair coat and pica may also be reported. Interdigital skin lesions (pruritus, erythema and papules) may be noted where transcutaneous infection has occurred.

Diagnosis is made by detection of hookworm eggs on faecal flotation. Fenbendazole, milbemycin oxime, moxidectin and pyrantel are all licensed in the UK for the treatment of hookworms. Decontamination of the environment is recommended for the prevention of reinfection, in addition to anthelmintic prophylaxis.

Ascarids (roundworms)

Infection with *Toxocara* spp. (*T. canis* and *T. cati*) is common and *Toxascaris leonina* (dog and cat) infection has been reported. Infection occurs following the ingestion of embryonated eggs or other vertebrate hosts. The adult nematodes inhabit the small intestine, and infection can cause vomiting and small intestinal diarrhoea, a pot-bellied appearance and failure to thrive, particularly in puppies and kittens. With very heavy worm burdens, a protein-losing enteropathy (PLE) can develop.

Diagnosis is made by detection of nematode eggs on faecal flotation. Fenbendazole, milbemycin oxime, moxidectin and pyrantel are all licensed in the UK for treatment of roundworms. Decontamination of the environment is recommended for the prevention of reinfection, in addition to anthelmintic prophylaxis.

Cestodes (tapeworms)

Dipylidium caninum and *Taenia* spp. are the most commonly encountered cestodes in cats and dogs, respectively. *Echinococcus multilocularis* and *Echinococcus granulosa* are found in dogs, and, although the adult worms inhabit the small intestine, they rarely cause clinical signs. *E. granulosa* causes hydatid disease in sheep and humans, while *E. multilocularis* is a very serious zoonotic concern among dog and fox populations, but is not yet present in the UK.

Diagnosis is by demonstration of eggs on faecal flotation. Praziquantel is licensed for the treatment of all three genera of tapeworms in the UK. Fenbendazole has some efficacy against *Taenia* spp. and *D. caninum*. Flea treatment and prevention should be instituted where *D. caninum* is diagnosed.

Chronic enteropathies

A number of chronic enteropathies, characterized by persistent or recurrent GI signs, are recognized in both dogs and cats. Most commonly, these patients have inflammatory changes within the intestinal mucosa and as such come under the umbrella terms of 'inflammatory bowel disease' (IBD) or 'chronic inflammatory enteropathy'. However, in some instances there is minimal intestinal inflammation and, in these cases, clinical signs may be a consequence of true dietary intolerance (e.g. the gluten-sensitive enteropathy in Irish Setters), intestinal dysbiosis (see later) or secondary to intestinal dysmotility (see later).

Inflammatory enteropathies

Chronic inflammatory enteropathies are characterized by persistent or recurrent GI signs in combination with idiopathic inflammation affecting any part of the GI tract. Traditionally, they have been classified according to the predominant inflammatory cell type and anatomical location. Lymphoplasmacytic enteritis is seen most frequently, followed by eosinophilic enteritis; the granulomatous and neutrophilic forms occur less commonly. Historically, these histopathological variations were grouped together under the umbrella term of IBD, although it is not known whether they are variations of the same problem and, histologically, they do not resemble IBD in humans. Furthermore, cases can be classified by their response to therapy (e.g. food-responsive enteropathy (FRE), antibiotic-responsive diarrhoea). Therefore, when using the term IBD in veterinary gastroenterology, it probably should be restricted to idiopathic inflammation that only responds to immunosuppression, and it is safer to use the broader term of chronic inflammatory enteropathy.

The aetiopathogenesis of chronic inflammatory enteropathies remains incompletely understood, although it is likely that immunological, environmental and genetic factors contribute to the development of inflammation. Alterations in intestinal epithelial barrier function, polymorphisms in toll-like receptor and cytokine genes, and intestinal dysbiosis have all been implicated in the pathogenesis of the inflammation. In some cases, response to dietary modification and/or manipulation of the intestinal microbiome supports the concept that chronic inflammatory enteropathy occurs as a result of an inappropriate immunological response to bacterial and/or food-derived luminal antigens. Where neutrophilic and granulomatous changes occur, an undiagnosed infectious disease has to be considered.

A number of breed-specific inflammatory enteropathies have been described in the dog, including Basenji enteropathy and a familial PLE and protein-losing nephropathy (PLN) in Soft Coated Wheaten Terriers (see later).

Clinical presentation

Idiopathic chronic inflammatory enteropathies typically occur in middle-aged dogs and cats and, although any breed can be affected, there appear to be some breed predispositions: German Shepherd Dogs, Shar Peis and Siamese cats in particular appear to be predisposed. Clinical signs reflect the region of the intestinal tract that is affected by inflammation and include vomiting, diarrhoea and weight loss. Haematemesis and melaena are seen uncommonly. These conditions may be associated with GI protein loss and the syndrome of PLE (see later). Although a variety of extra-intestinal clinical signs (e.g. arthritis) have been reported in humans with IBD, these are not commonly recognized in dogs and cats. There are few distinguishing clinical features of the different forms of chronic inflammatory enteropathy, although dogs and cats with food-responsive enteropathies tend to be younger and have milder clinical signs. It should be noted that clinical signs may wax and wane.

Diagnosis

Laboratory abnormalities: By definition, idiopathic chronic inflammatory enteropathy is a diagnosis of exclusion, and therefore the investigation should be designed to rule out known causes of chronic vomiting, diarrhoea and weight loss. Faecal analysis, routine haematological and serum biochemical analysis, assessment of exocrine pancreatic function and diagnostic imaging are not only useful in this respect, but also provide information regarding the clinical status of the patient and severity of the disease. Ultimately, a definitive diagnosis requires demonstration of typical histopathological changes.

Haematology: Haematological abnormalities associated with the inflammation are often non-specific. Eosinophilia may be suggestive of occult parasitic disease or dietary hypersensitivity, and in cats may be suggestive of eosinophilic enteritis, but can be seen as a paraneoplastic effect of alimentary lymphoma. Thrombocytopenia or thrombocytosis may be seen, although they may not be clinically significant. Anaemia can be seen either as a result of chronic inflammatory disease or as a consequence of chronic blood loss.

Biochemistry: Serum biochemical analysis is used to exclude significant extra-intestinal disease, which may have GI manifestations. Reactive increases in serum liver enzyme activities (alanine aminotransferase and alkaline phosphatase) are often seen in dogs with chronic enteropathy. In cats, the presence of GI signs and increased liver enzyme activities may reflect the syndrome of 'triaditis', a combination of feline lymphoplasmacytic enteritis, pancreatitis and cholangitis (see Chapter 37). A reduction in serum protein concentrations occurs in some dogs (and rarely in cats) before the development of overt clinical signs of hypoproteinaemia such as ascites, and this has negative prognostic implications as well as providing a useful marker for monitoring response to therapy.

A subnormal serum cobalamin concentration is seen relatively commonly in intestinal inflammatory enteropathies and, as this is likely to contribute to ongoing GI dysfunction, it provides a useful therapeutic target. Hypocobalaminaemia is also a negative prognostic indicator in some studies. A subnormal serum folate concentration is less frequently found, although, when decreased, it may reflect severe intestinal disease. Increased activity of serum pancreatic lipase may provide evidence of concurrent pancreatopathy and may indicate a poorer prognosis.

Diagnostic imaging: Although radiography may be useful to rule out conditions such as chronic gastric foreign body or intussusception that may result in chronic vomiting, diarrhoea and/or weight loss, its usefulness in the investigation of dogs with chronic inflammatory enteropathies, in general, is limited, and it has been largely superseded by abdominal ultrasonography (see Chapter 3). Not only does ultrasonography enable thorough evaluation of the intra-abdominal extra-GI structures, but it may also aid in the differentiation of a chronic inflammatory enteropathy from neoplastic conditions of the GI tract. For example, although increased intestinal wall thickness may be associated with both inflammatory disease and neoplasia, loss of intestinal wall layering is highly predictive of intestinal neoplasia. Ultrasonography also has a role in indicating the most appropriate method of obtaining intestinal biopsy samples (i.e. endoscopy *versus* coeliotomy).

Ultrasonographic changes associated with chronic inflammatory enteropathy include increased intestinal wall thickness and the presence of hyperechoic speckles within the intestinal mucosa. In the cat, thickening of the muscularis layer (Figure 34.10) can be a feature, but may also be seen with intestinal small cell lymphoma (Zwingenberger *et al.*, 2010; Daniaux *et al.*, 2014). Hyperechoic mucosal striations are associated with lacteal dilatation and frequently associated with inflammatory disease and with lymphangiectasia (Gaschen *et al.*, 2008) and PLE (Figure 34.11). However, the absence of ultrasonographic findings does not preclude significant intestinal pathology.

Endoscopy: Chronic inflammatory enteropathies are often associated with gross abnormalities of the GI mucosa. Increased granularity (Figure 34.12) and friability of the duodenal mucosa is often observed with or without ulceration. Dilated lacteals may be grossly visible (Figure 34.13). Endoscopic evaluation enables localization of abnormalities and targeted collection of pinch biopsy samples from mucosal lesions in the duodenum and ileum. Potential disadvantages include limited ability to evaluate the jejunum and the superficial nature of the biopsy samples. Full-thickness intestinal biopsy samples may provide additional information, but collection is associated with higher morbidity.

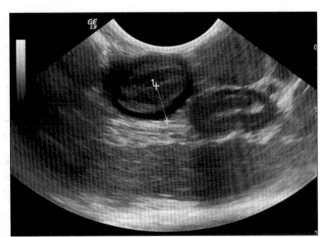

34.10 Thickening of the intestinal wall in a 12-year-old Domestic Shorthaired cat presented for the investigation of chronic diarrhoea and weight loss of 6 months' duration. Note the prominent muscularis, which can be seen with both inflammatory diseases and intestinal lymphoma. Histopathology of duodenal and ileal mucosal biopsy samples was compatible with moderate to severe intestinal inflammation. Final diagnosis: lymphoplasmacytic enteritis.

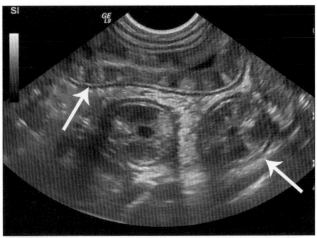

34.11 Ultrasonographic changes in the intestinal mucosa of an 18-month-old English Bulldog presented for the investigation of severe weight loss and chronic diarrhoea. Note the hyperechoic mucosal striations (arrowed), which are highly suggestive of intestinal lymphangiectasia. Milky fluid may be seen oozing when intestinal biopsy samples are taken. Histopathology revealed severe intestinal lymphangiectasia with mild neutrophilic inflammation. Final diagnosis: primary intestinal lymphangiectasia causing protein-losing enteropathy. (Courtesy of Gerard McLauchlan, Small Animal Medicine Department, University of Glasgow)

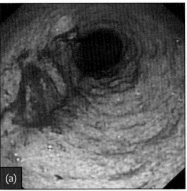

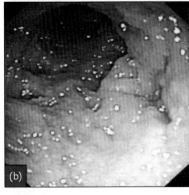

34.12 Endoscopic changes in the duodenum of dogs with chronic inflammatory enteropathies. (a) Hyperaemia, ulceration and mucosal friability are visible. (b) The duodenal mucosa is very irregular and the individual villi cannot be appreciated.

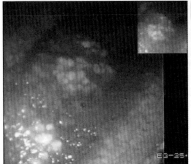

34.13 Endoscopic changes in the duodenum characteristic of lymphangiectasia with the white spots being dilated lacteals.

Histological abnormalities: Histological evaluation of the intestinal mucosa is required for a definitive diagnosis of chronic inflammatory enteropathy and the World Small Animal Veterinary Association GI Standardization Group guidelines have assisted in standardizing the interpretation of intestinal biopsy samples. In addition to infiltration of the intestinal mucosa with inflammatory cells, chronic inflammation is associated with architectural abnormalities, such as villus atrophy, glandular distortion and/or necrosis, and mucosal epithelial changes, such as ulceration.

Lymphoplasmacytic inflammation can be difficult to differentiate from enteropathy-associated T-cell lymphoma, particularly in cats. However, immunohistochemical (IHC) markers are now often employed to help differentiate these two conditions. If IHC fails to provide a definitive diagnosis, PCR-based analysis of lymphocyte antigen-receptor rearrangements (PARR) can be used to demonstrate clonality, indicative of alimentary lymphoma (Kiupel *et al.*, 2011). However, the specificity of PARR analysis of intestinal biopsy samples has been questioned by a recent finding of clonality in endoscopic biopsy samples from clinically healthy cats that had long-term follow-up showing they did not go on to develop alimentary lymphoma (Marsilio *et al.*, 2019).

Treatment and prognosis

Strategies for the management of inflammatory enteropathies include dietary modification, manipulation of the intestinal microbiome and immunosuppressive treatment. The therapeutic approach adopted should take into account the severity of the clinical presentation and, where negative prognostic indicators such as a high disease activity score (see below), hypoalbuminaemia and hypocobalaminaemia are present, combined therapy is indicated from the outset. Objective evaluation of therapeutic interventions can be achieved by assessment of disease activity indices.

Dietary modification: This is usually recommended as the first step in the management of chronic inflammatory enteropathies. This is due in part to the fact that over 50% of cases show a clinical response to dietary changes alone, even though there may be histopathological evidence of ongoing inflammation at follow-up biopsy. Retrospectively, these cases are classed as having 'food-responsive enteropathy'. Dietary management involves changing to a restricted-antigen or 'elimination' diet, or feeding one of the hydrolysed-protein diets available commercially. Restricted-antigen diets are generally limited to a single protein and carbohydrate source and although selection of a novel protein source is recommended, the selection is often empirical, based on commercially available products. Home-cooked diets may be useful in some cases but should be formulated by a board-certified veterinary nutritionist to ensure it is complete and balanced for long-term feeding. Reduction in the fat content of the diet may be beneficial in dogs as fat maldigestion and malabsorption may contribute to diarrhoea but is clearly not helpful in cats. Although at least a 3-week and up to 10-week diet trial has been recommended, in reality most dogs and cats with food-responsive vomiting and diarrhoea will respond to dietary modification in a shorter time frame, and often within 2 weeks. Subsequent dietary challenge may support a diagnosis of dietary hypersensitivity, although few owners consent to this process.

Antibiotics: Where dietary modification is unsuccessful at resolving the clinical signs, the options are to prescribe a trial course of antibiotics or to move on to an immunosuppressive therapy. The rationale for an antibiotic trial reflects current thoughts on the pathogenesis of chronic enteropathy and the possibility of secondary small intestinal dysbiosis (SID) (see later), although the public health concern of empirical antibiotic usage should be considered. In this scenario, antibiotic-responsive diarrhoea (ARD) generally improves within a few days of starting treatment. Interestingly, clinical improvement does not appear to be related to quantitative changes in total bacterial flora, and is more likely to be related to qualitative changes in the intestinal microbiome. Prebiotics (e.g. fructo-oligosaccharides) and probiotics may have a role as an adjunctive therapy for management of chronic enteropathy, particularly where secondary SID is suspected, but there are few data documenting their efficacy.

Immunosuppressive therapy: Immunosuppression is necessary in cases where dietary modification and antibiotic therapy, either alone or in combination, have failed to control clinical signs, or where the clinical status of the patient dictates a more aggressive approach to treatment. Glucocorticoids, typically prednisolone, are generally used as the first-line treatment. The recommended doses are 1–2 mg/kg orally q24h in dogs, and 2–4 mg/kg orally q24h in cats. In certain situations (e.g. in hypoproteinaemic patients or where GI ulceration has been documented), it may be prudent to start prednisolone at a lower than is recommended dosage and to titrate upwards. Alternative immunosuppressive agents may be a safer first-line treatment in diabetic patients.

Where severe signs of GI disease are present (i.e. frequent vomiting or severe malabsorption), parenteral glucocorticoids may be indicated initially, but oral prednisolone is preferred for long-term treatment. In those dogs where prednisolone causes unacceptable side effects, the locally acting glucocorticoid budesonide has been used, although the doses are, at best, empirical. Due to its high first-pass metabolism, clinical side effects are minimal, although suppression of the hypothalamic–pituitary–adrenal axis and canine steroid hepatopathy are still observed.

In cases that appear refractory to glucocorticoid therapy, adjunctive immunosuppressive therapy should be considered. Options include azathioprine, ciclosporin and chlorambucil. The combination of prednisolone (2 mg/kg orally q24h) and chlorambucil (4–6 mg/m^2 orally q24h) has been shown to improve outcome compared with a prednisolone/azathioprine combination in dogs with PLE. In refractory cases, treatment with ciclosporin may be effective in some individuals.

When hypocobalaminaemia is documented, lifelong parenteral or oral supplementation is indicated (see Chapter 27).

Monitoring treatment by disease activity index: Evaluation of the clinical severity of the enteropathy using clinical scoring systems or indices (Figure 34.14) has greatly improved the ability to make objective decisions about response to treatment, particularly when more than one clinician is involved in case management.

In essence, the severity of a number of prominent GI signs associated with chronic inflammatory enteropathy is assessed, a cumulative disease activity score or index (AI) is calculated and disease activity is classified as clinically insignificant (score of 0–3), mild (4–5), moderate (6–8) or severe (>9). Subsequent scoring of patients is then used to assess the efficacy of treatment and to more objectively inform alterations to treatment regimens. Reassessment

Characteristic	Score			
	0	1	2	3
Attitude/activity	Normal	Slight decrease	Moderate decrease	Severe decrease
Appetite	Normal	Slight decrease	Moderate decrease	Severe decrease
Vomiting	None	Mild (once/week)	Moderate (2–3/week)	Severe (>3/week)
Faecal consistency	Normal	Slightly soft faeces or faecal blood and/or mucus	Very soft faeces	Watery diarrhoea
Defecation frequency	Normal	Slight increase (2–3/day)	Moderate increase (4–5/day)	Severe increase (>5/day)
Weight loss	None	Mild (<5%)	Moderate (5–10%)	Severe (>10%)
Serum albumin	>20 g/l	15–19.9 g/l	12–14.9 g/l	<12 g/l
Ascites and peripheral oedema	None	Mild ascites or peripheral oedema	Moderate ascites or peripheral oedema	Severe ascites/pleural effusion and peripheral oedema
Pruritus	None	Occasional episodes of itching	Regular episodes but stops when asleep	Dog regularly wakes up due to itching
Total score	0–3 Clinically insignificant disease 4–5 Mild intestinal inflammation 6–8 Moderate intestinal inflammation >9 Severe intestinal inflammation			

34.14 Assessment of severity of canine chronic inflammatory enteropathies. The canine inflammatory bowel disease activity index (CIBDAI, adapted from Jergens *et al.*, 2003) uses six clinical parameters to generate a disease activity score. The canine chronic enteropathy activity index (CCEAI, adapted from Allenspach *et al.*, 2007) includes three additional parameters.

every 2 weeks is recommended initially, with the expectation that a decrease in the AI category will be documented. In the absence of significant improvement, an adjunctive or alternative treatment strategy should be implemented.

Breed-specific enteropathies

Basenji enteropathy: An immunoproliferative enteropathy is seen in Basenji dogs, resulting in a progressive and ultimately fatal wasting disorder associated with chronic small intestinal diarrhoea, anorexia and vomiting. Affected dogs may develop PLE, although sometimes with hyper- rather than hypoglobulinaemia. On histopathology, in addition to mononuclear infiltrates in the intestinal mucosa, these dogs also develop varying degrees of gastric hypertrophy, lymphoplasmacytic gastritis and gastric mucosal atrophy. These dogs may have concurrent PLN.

Familial PLE and PLN in Soft Coated Wheaten Terriers: A familial predisposition for PLE and PLN is seen in the Soft Coated Wheaten Terrier. Individuals may have PLE or PLN or a combination of both. The mutation responsible for the PLN has been identified (it encodes the glomerular protein nephrin), but it is not associated with the PLE. The clinical and laboratory presentation of PLE in this breed is typical of that seen in other breeds, with the majority of affected dogs presenting with small intestinal diarrhoea with or without vomiting, weight loss, ascites and pleural effusion. Histopathology reveals lymphoplasmacytic enteritis with or without lymphangiectasia, and in a significant number of cases transmural lymphangitis also occurs. There appears to be a female predisposition and dogs that present with PLE tend to be younger than those presenting with PLN.

PLE in Yorkshire Terriers: A PLE syndrome has been reported in Yorkshire Terriers. Typically, dogs present with a combination of small intestinal diarrhoea, vomiting, muscle tremors and seizures, with or without uni- or bicavitary effusions (transudates). Ionized hypocalcaemia has been reported in some of these dogs. Histopathology in these cases is distinct in that, in addition to lymphoplasmacytic inflammation and secondary lymphangiectasia, the majority also have a neutrophilic component

to the mucosal inflammation and distinct crypt lesions, where crypts are distended with amorphous material and cellular debris (crypt abscesses).

PLE in Norwegian Lundehunds: Almost all Lundehunds will exhibit weight loss and diarrhoea associated with lymphangiectasia and lymphoplasmacytic inflammation. This usually progresses to cause panhypoproteinaemia and eventually becomes refractory to all treatments. Atrophic gastritis and gastric carcinoma are also unusually common in this breed (see Chapter 33).

Gluten-sensitive enteropathy (GSE) in Irish Setters: A familial enteropathy affecting young Irish Setters, GSE causes poor appetite, failure to gain weight and chronic diarrhoea. Gluten sensitivity can be ameliorated by exclusion of dietary cereals from weaning and, in affected dogs, feeding a gluten-free diet can obviate clinical signs. GSE may occur sporadically in all breeds.

Small intestinal dysbiosis

SID is a collective term for quantitative and/or qualitative abnormalities in the small intestinal microbiome that are probably associated with many enteropathies, including clinical entities that respond to antibiotics, historically referred to as:

- Small intestinal bacterial overgrowth (SIBO)
- Antibiotic-responsive diarrhoea (ARD)
- Tylosin-responsive diarrhoea (TRD).

Idiopathic chronic inflammatory enteropathies may also be associated with SID and, in particular, a shift towards decreased diversity and an increased proportion of Enterobacteriaceae. What is not clear is whether dysbiosis is the cause or the effect of the intestinal inflammation.

The GI tract contains a vast number of microorganisms, which collectively form the intestinal microbiome. This complex but integrated community of organisms, composed predominantly of symbiotic and commensal bacteria, has a range of functions, including generation of short-chain fatty acids, vitamin synthesis, regulation of local and systemic immune responses, maintenance of intestinal barrier function and competitive exclusion of pathogens. Bacterial number and diversity increases along the length of the GI tract, with intrinsic mechanism influencing the number and composition of the microbial flora in each region. For instance, gastric acid destroys many bacteria before they leave the stomach; biliary and pancreatic secretions limit bacterial growth; the intestinal mucus layer traps bacteria; and the ileocolic valve limits retrograde movement of bacteria from the colon to the ileum. Alteration to any one of these homeostatic mechanisms has the potential to alter the composition of the small intestinal microbiome.

SID has been implicated in the development of a spectrum of clinical disorders, including chronic diarrhoea syndromes and inflammatory disorders of the GI tract. Damage to brush border enzymes, deconjugation of bile acids and bacterial hydroxylation of fatty acids contribute to the development of diarrhoea due to maldigestion, fat malabsorption and increased colonic secretion, respectively.

Secondary SID can occur as a consequence of any disorder that interferes with the mechanisms controlling the small intestinal microbial populations (Figure 34.15). Primary or idiopathic SID is also reported in dogs. The original reports of primary SID in dogs, previously referred to as SIBO, described a syndrome of idiopathic chronic diarrhoea where small intestinal bacterial numbers met the diagnostic criteria for SIBO in humans, and where there were no or minimal histopathological lesions visible on light microscopy. More recently, the term ARD has been adopted to describe a syndrome of chronic idiopathic diarrhoea that responds clinically to antibiotics; in some cases, ARD may be due to primary intestinal dysbiosis. Some dogs with ARD have histopathological evidence of intestinal mucosal inflammation and abnormal host–bacterial interactions may be responsible for the clinical presentation rather than the dysbiosis *per se*.

Anatomical alterations
• Intestinal obstruction
• Redundant loop of intestine
• Intestinal adhesions
• Intestinal stricture or neoplasia
Decreased gastric acid secretion
• Proton pump inhibitors
• H$_2$-blockers
• Atrophic gastritis
Primary gastrointestinal, hepatic or pancreatic diseases
• Chronic inflammatory enteropathy
• Chronic liver disease
• Chronic pancreatitis
• Exocrine pancreatic insufficiency
Motility disorders
• Hypothyroidism
• Gastroparesis
• Postoperative ileus
• Opioid treatment

34.15 Conditions that have the potential to result in small intestinal dysbiosis.

Clinical presentation

In addition to chronic diarrhoea, dogs with SID may also have signs of maldigestion and malabsorption, namely weight loss and failure to thrive. Vomiting, borborygmi and changes in appetite (particularly polyphagia, coprophagia and/or scavenging) are also reported. Previous improvement with antibiotic therapy followed by relapse may assist in differentiating SID/ARD from other chronic enteropathies.

ARD typically affects young large-breed dogs, including German Shepherd Dogs, but has also been reported in laboratory Beagles. Clinical signs completely resolve with antibiotic therapy but relapse when antibiotic therapy is withdrawn. A syndrome of TRD has been reported in dogs from Scandinavia, which, although reported more commonly in middle-aged dogs, likely reflects a similar disease process.

Diagnosis

Although it is widely accepted that SID exists as a clinical entity in dogs, demonstrating its presence is far from straightforward. Classical criteria based on direct aerobic and anaerobic bacteriological culture of duodenal or jejunal juice are outdated (most enteric microbes are not culturable) and impractical. Indirect methods of diagnosis used in humans, such as breath tests and assay of serum unconjugated and primary/secondary bile acids, have had limited evaluation in veterinary medicine because of practical constraints (technical complexity and expense), appear to lack diagnostic sensitivity and specificity in dogs and, importantly, do not appear to be predictive of a clinical response to antibiotic therapy. Observation of high serum folate (produced by bacteria) and/or low serum cobalamin (utilized by intestinal bacteria) in dogs fed normal diets may provide indirect evidence of SID, albeit with limited sensitivity and specificity.

When animals with chronic diarrhoea fail to respond to a diet trial and appropriate supplementation with folate and/or cobalamin, primary SID may be suspected if the diarrhoea responds to antibiotics and relapses once they are withdrawn, particularly if the patient is a young German Shepherd Dog or another large-breed dog.

Treatment

Where SID occurs as a secondary disorder, the focus should be on treatment of the underlying condition, as when this is achieved, therapy for secondary SID may be unnecessary.

If a diet trial fails and idiopathic SID/ARD is likely, it can be managed with oral antibacterials: metronidazole (10 mg/kg q8–12h), oxytetracycline (10–20 mg/kg q8h) and tylosin (5–25 mg/kg q12–24h) are all reasonable choices of antibiotic. A minimum of 4–6 weeks of treatment is recommended.

Response to treatment, particularly in dogs with TRD, usually occurs within a few days of starting the antibiotics. Where there is a minimal response after 2 weeks, the diagnosis should be reviewed or an alternative antibiotic administered. On stopping the antibiotics, the time to relapse is variable, with some dogs being free of clinical signs for several weeks. Given the definition of ARD, a significant proportion of dogs will require long-term or intermittent treatment with antibiotics to control clinical signs. Low-dose tylosin (5 mg/kg q24h) has been shown to be as effective as higher doses for the management of relapses.

Adjunctive therapy with a low-fat diet has been proposed, although there is little evidence to support this recommendation. Where hypocobalaminaemia is documented, parenteral or oral supplementation is indicated.

Small intestinal neoplasia

A number of different tumour types can be found in the small intestine, including epithelial (carcinoma and adenocarcinoma), mesenchymal (leiomyoma/leiomyosarcoma,

GI stromal cell tumours) and haemopoietic (alimentary lymphoma, intestinal histiocytic sarcoma, intestinal mast cell tumour, extramedullary plasmacytoma). Neuroendocrine (carcinoid) tumours are also reported.

Intestinal neoplasia can be associated with a number of clinical signs, including the cardinal signs of small intestinal disease, namely diarrhoea, weight loss, vomiting, anorexia and melaena. Tumours may also result in intestinal obstruction and/or perforation and can be associated with paraneoplastic disorders such as hyperviscosity (plasmacytoma) and hypereosinophilic syndromes (mast cell tumour) and, rarely, nephrogenic diabetes insipidus or hypoglycaemia (leiomyoma/sarcoma).

Alimentary lymphoma

Alimentary lymphoma is the most common small intestinal neoplasm in both dogs and cats. It typically affects middle-aged to older individuals and results in a syndrome of malabsorption and weight loss. It can be classified based on histological grade as low-grade (LGAL), intermediate-grade (IGAL) or high-grade (HGAL), and/or according to immunophenotype (T-cell or B-cell) and morphological features (small cell, lymphocytic, lymphoblastic or large granular, Mott cell).

LGAL, which is usually a T-cell lymphoma, is synonymous with the terms well differentiated lymphocytic lymphoma, small cell lymphoma, epitheliotropic T-cell lymphoma and type 2 enteropathy-associated T-cell lymphoma. IGAL and HGAL, which may be a T- or B-cell phenotype, are typically lymphoblastic lymphomas. Large granular lymphocytic lymphoma (LGLL), which accounts for a small percentage of feline alimentary lymphoma, is typically T-cell in origin and has a variable histological grade. It is worth noting that, although the association between feline leukaemia virus (FeLV) infection and feline lymphoma is well established, the majority of cats with intestinal lymphoma are FeLV negative, at least on FeLV antigen testing.

Clinical presentation: Clinical signs of intestinal lymphoma typically include chronic vomiting, diarrhoea, weight loss and anorexia, although in cats weight loss and anorexia may be the only overt signs of disease. In addition to poor body condition, physical examination may reveal the presence of thickened loops of intestine or a palpable abdominal mass. The clinical presentation may be indistinguishable from that associated with other chronic enteropathies.

Diagnosis: Haematological and serum biochemical changes are generally non-specific. Anaemia is seen relatively frequently in cats with alimentary lymphoma, and hypoproteinaemia due to PLE is quite common in dogs. In cats, eosinophilia is occasionally seen as a paraneoplastic syndrome due to the release of interleukin-5.

The ultrasonographic appearance of alimentary lymphoma is variable and in a proportion of cases, there are no visible changes. Possible findings include nodular lesions (either focal or multifocal), diffuse thickening of the intestine, loss of wall layering and regional lymphadenopathy (more commonly associated with IGAL/HGAL). Concurrent hepatic and splenic involvement may be evident. LGAL in the cat tends to result in thickening of the muscularis, particularly of the jejunum and ileum, and although these changes are not pathognomonic for LGAL as chronic inflammatory enteropathy can result in similar changes, the presence of concurrent lymphadenopathy is more suggestive of lymphoma (see Chapter 3).

Diagnosis is based on cytological or histopathological assessment of affected tissue. Although their sensitivities and specificities are somewhat controversial, IHN, PARR or the recently developed histology-guided mass spectrometry (HGMS) may be helpful in differentiating alimentary small cell lymphoma from chronic inflammatory enteropathy.

Treatment and prognosis: In dogs, alimentary lymphoma is generally high-grade and has a very guarded to poor prognosis. CHOP-based (cyclophosphamide, doxorubicin, vincristine and prednisolone) chemotherapy protocols are generally recommended, although short-term remission may also be seen with less intensive protocols. IGAL/HGAL also carry a guarded to poor prognosis in cats.

In contrast, the prognosis for feline LGAL is reasonable. Response rates of 46–96% are reported with prednisolone/chlorambucil combinations, and in cats that respond to treatment median survival times are in the region of 2 years. In addition, this oral treatment protocol tends to be well tolerated.

Protein-losing enteropathy

The term PLE describes a syndrome where there is abnormal loss of protein into the GI tract, resulting in hypoalbuminaemia. Protein losses may be due to increased intestinal permeability, lymphatic obstruction, dysfunction resulting in lymphangiectasia (leakage of protein-rich lymph into the intestinal lumen), or as a consequence of mucosal ulceration and/or erosion.

Diseases causing PLE

In dogs, PLE is most often seen as a clinical manifestation of severe chronic inflammatory enteropathy, alimentary lymphoma or intestinal lymphangiectasia. Less commonly, it occurs secondary to GI ulceration and neoplasia, intestinal parasitic and fungal infections (e.g. histoplasmosis, pythiosis, trichuriasis, *Ancylostoma* infection), chronic intussusception, intestinal crypt lesions, hypoadrenocorticism and portal hypertension (e.g. secondary to right-sided heart failure or constrictive pericarditis). It should be noted that PLE is an uncommon manifestation of intestinal disease in the cat. There are a number of breed-specific enteropathies where PLE is a common feature, such as familial PLE and PLN in Soft Coated Wheaten Terriers, and a PLE syndrome in Yorkshire Terriers. Primary intestinal lymphangiectasia has been proposed as the cause of the familial PLE seen in the Norwegian Lundehund.

Inflammatory enteropathies: Idiopathic chronic inflammatory enteropathies are described above. Although typically associated with vomiting, diarrhoea and/or weight loss, a subset of dogs will also develop PLE. This is likely to be due to the combination of increased intestinal permeability and secondary lymphangiectasia.

Alimentary lymphoma: PLE is observed commonly in dogs with intestinal lymphoma and it is likely that increased intestinal epithelial permeability or ulceration leads to protein loss (see earlier).

Intestinal lymphangiectasia: Intestinal lymphangiectasia is characterized by dilatation and 'ballooning' of the lacteals in the intestinal mucosa, resulting in oedema within the lamina propria, and loss of protein-rich lymphatic fluid into the intestinal lumen. Intestinal lymphangiectasia can occur, rarely, as a primary congenital developmental disorder and has been reported in a number of breeds, including the Norwegian Lundehund. More commonly, it occurs as an acquired disorder secondary to occlusion of lymphatic outflow (e.g. due to primary lymphangitis or an inflammatory or neoplastic process within the intestinal mucosa). Theoretically, conditions causing an increase in hydrostatic pressure in the lymphatics draining the GI tract, such as right-sided congestive heart failure or constrictive pericarditis, have the potential to cause intestinal lymphangiectasia. This may be accompanied by intestinal lymphangitis and discrete lipogranulomas within the intestinal submucosa and/or mesenteric lymphatics. As these lipogranulomas enlarge they may contribute to the obstructive process.

Clinical presentation

Dogs with PLE typically present with a history of chronic relapsing GI signs and one or more of the clinical manifestations of hypoalbuminaemia, namely ascites, peripheral oedema and/or pleural effusion. It should be noted that a small number of dogs with PLE do not have a history of typical GI signs but exhibit weight loss and, rarely, the initial presentation may reflect one of the potential complications of PLE, such as thromboembolic disease (Figure 34.16) or seizures secondary to hypocalcaemia.

Physical examination typically reflects chronic GI disease, with signs of malabsorption (weight loss, poor body condition and muscle wasting) with or without abdominal distension due to ascites (see Chapter 24), peripheral oedema (particularly affecting the distal limbs and the scrotum in male dogs) and/or tachypnoea/dyspnoea due to pleural effusion. An abdominal mass may be palpable where intestinal neoplasia exists or, very rarely, where large mesenteric lipogranulomas have developed.

Diagnosis

A diagnosis of PLE is based on the typical clinical presentation and exclusion of other causes of hypoalbuminaemia, specifically PLN (by measurement of urine protein:creatinine ratio) and liver failure (by the presence of other signs and/or measurement of dynamic bile acid concentrations).

Laboratory abnormalities: Typical clinicopathological abnormalities associated with PLE include panhypoproteinaemia (low albumin and globulin), although it should be remembered that the absence of hypoglobulinaemia does not preclude a diagnosis of PLE. Furthermore, it is the hypoalbuminaemia that contributes most to the decrease in colloid osmotic pressure and the development of ascites. Where intestinal lymphangiectasia is present, lymphopenia and hypocholesterolaemia may also be found. Hypocalcaemia is frequently noted and, while this may merely reflect hypoalbuminaemia, in some cases serum ionized calcium is also low, likely reflecting hypovitaminosis D or secondary hypoparathyroidism due to hypomagnesaemia. Serum cobalamin and folate may also be decreased.

Measurement of faecal alpha$_1$-proteinase inhibitor, which has a similar molecular weight to albumin, has been advocated as a method of confirming PLE (and can reveal enteric protein loss before hypoalbuminaemia develops), but as this assay is currently unavailable outside the USA and, as fresh faeces must be frozen and shipped on ice, it is rarely used in other countries. Having established that PLE is the cause of hypoalbuminaemia, further evaluation should be focused on establishing the cause of the PLE.

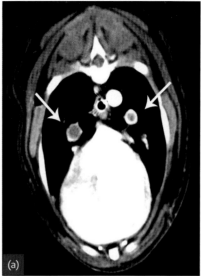

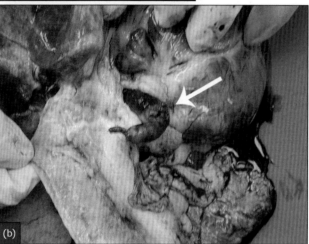

34.16 (a) Computed tomography angiogram of a dog with respiratory complications associated with protein-losing enteropathy (PLE). Note the filling defects in the main caudal lobar arteries (arrowed), consistent with pulmonary thromboembolism. (b) Post-mortem examination revealing a large thrombus in the pulmonary artery (arrowed) of a dog that died from thromboembolic complications of PLE secondary to chronic inflammatory enteropathy.
(b, Reproduced with permission of Linda Morrison, Department of Veterinary Pathology, University of Edinburgh)

Diagnostic imaging: Imaging findings are likely to reflect the underlying cause and consequences of PLE. Thoracic imaging (radiography, computed tomography (CT) and/or echocardiography) may reveal pleural effusion with or without pulmonary thromboembolism (TE) (see Figure 34.16) and/or a thoracic cause of portal hypertension. Abdominal ultrasonography is likely to be more informative than abdominal radiography in detecting underlying intestinal disease, and may reveal an anatomical cause of PLE, such as chronic intussusception or intestinal neoplasia (see Chapter 3). Hyperechoic mucosal striations are suggestive of PLE and lymphangiectasia (see Figure 34.12). The absence of ultrasonographic findings does not, however, preclude significant intestinal pathology resulting in PLE.

Histology: Histopathological assessment of the GI tract is frequently required to obtain a definitive diagnosis. Consideration should be given to the most appropriate method of obtaining intestinal biopsy samples; if an endoscopic approach is taken, attempts should be made to obtain both duodenal and ileal biopsy specimens to maximize the chances of obtaining a diagnosis.

Treatment

Treatment is aimed at management of the underlying disease process. Where PLE is secondary to a chronic inflammatory enteropathy, early intervention with immunosuppressive therapy is generally indicated. As stated previously, the combination of prednisolone (2 mg/kg orally q24h) and chlorambucil (4–6 mg/m² orally q24h) has been shown to improve outcome compared with a prednisolone/azathioprine combination.

Dietary recommendations are similar to those for the management of chronic inflammatory enteropathies. Although PLE infrequently occurs secondary to food-responsive diarrhoea, marked improvement in clinical signs can be seen within a few days of changing to a hydrolysed protein diet (e.g. while waiting for intestinal biopsy results) and, in these cases, immunosuppressive therapy may not be required. Ideally, diets should be low in fat, particularly where intestinal lymphangiectasia is present. When hypocobalaminaemia is documented, parenteral or oral supplementation is indicated.

The optimal treatment protocol for primary intestinal lymphangiectasia is poorly defined, largely due to the rarity of the condition. Dietary management is the mainstay of treatment in humans with this condition, with restriction of long-chain triglycerides in the diet and supplementation with medium-chain triglycerides (MCTs), which are absorbed directly into the portal venous circulation and thus avoid lacteal engorgement and dilation. Although the benefit of MCTs (derived from coconut oil) has been questioned in dogs, in part as they appear to be absorbed by the lymphatic route and partly because the neat product may be unpalatable, they are worth considering in refractory cases and are added to some commercial GI diets. Glucocorticoids (1 mg/kg q24h) are also recommended due to the perception that leakage from lymphatics may result in inflammation (lymphangitis) and contribute to the formation of lipogranulomas.

Complications

TE is recognized as a complication of PLE in the dog, where it is postulated that intestinal loss of antithrombin results in hypercoagulability. In reality, the aetiopathogenesis is likely to be more complex. Although the frequency of thromboembolic complications is unknown, the presence of respiratory compromise or exercise intolerance should raise suspicion for pulmonary TE, particularly in the absence of pleural effusion. Diagnosis of pulmonary TE can be confirmed by CT angiography (see Figure 34.16). Aortic TE and thrombosis of the mesenteric, splenic and portal vessels have also been infrequently reported. Currently, there is no reliable method of predicting thromboembolic events.

Managing complications: In severely hypoalbuminaemic patients, where there are concerns that extravascular fluid accumulation is causing intestinal mucosal oedema, administration of synthetic colloids (hydroxyethyl starches) or 25% human albumin solutions can be considered. However, at the recommended doses of 10–20 ml/kg q24h synthetic colloids are of limited clinical benefit. In addition, there are significant safety concerns with both products; hydroxyethyl starches have been withdrawn from human medicine due to concerns regarding their effects on renal function, and the administration of 25% human albumin solutions can cause severe life-threatening acute and delayed hypersensitivity reactions and thus are recommended only during the perioperative period when the patient is anaesthetized for intestinal biopsy.

Parenteral nutritional support can be of short-term benefit in improving serum albumin concentrations in some cases, although administration is not without risk and thromboembolic and metabolic complications have been reported.

Specific risk factors for the development of TE have not been established in dogs with PLE, but where there is a high index of suspicion or where TE is demonstrated, anticoagulant and/or thromboprophylactic therapy with ultra-low-dose aspirin or clopidogrel should be considered.

Where clinical signs of hypocalcaemia and hypomagnesaemia are present, parenteral supplementation is indicated. It is currently unclear whether parenteral or oral vitamin D administration will improve outcomes in individuals where deficiency is documented.

The prognosis for dogs with PLE secondary to idiopathic inflammation is very guarded and hypoalbuminaemia is consistently cited as a negative prognostic indicator in these cases.

Functional intestinal diseases

In many cases of chronic GI disease in dogs, an aetiological agent cannot be identified nor a histological diagnosis reached. While this may reflect a failure to find the cause (e.g. occult infection), in some cases it is likely to represent a functional disorder where there may be biochemical or neuromuscular GI abnormalities.

Irritable bowel syndrome

Well defined in human patients, this nebulous condition in dogs has been associated with recurrent bouts of vomiting, diarrhoea and abdominal discomfort, interspersed between periods of normality and with no evidence of GI bleeding. Symptomatic therapy includes empirical dietary modification, antispasmodics (hyoscine, mebeverine, peppermint oil) and anxiolytics (diazepam, chlordiazepoxide).

Dysautonomia

Aetiology: Dysautonomia is a sporadic idiopathic condition that results in a progressive clinical disease of the autonomic nervous system. Dysfunction or failure of the sympathetic and parasympathetic nervous systems is due to chromatolytic degeneration of the autonomic nervous ganglia (see Chapter 32).

Clinical presentation: Commonly reported clinical findings due to widespread degeneration of neurons include lethargy, anorexia, dysphagia, xerostomia, regurgitation or vomiting, constipation, dilated unresponsive pupils, prolapsed nictitating membranes, dry mucous membranes, reduced lacrimation, bradycardia (fixed heart rate), megaoesophagus, absent or reduced anal tone and distended urinary bladder.

Diagnosis: A clinical diagnosis is made in most cases based on anamnestic and clinical findings. Autonomic nervous system function tests that can be performed in practice comprise the Schirmer tear test, local administration of diluted pilocarpine ophthalmic solution and atropine and histamine response tests. Definitive diagnosis is based upon demonstration of characteristic histological lesions in the autonomic ganglia.

Treatment: No definitive therapy is currently available. Supportive care comprises increased frequency of feedings for megaoesophagus (see Chapter 32), artificial tears, expressing the urinary bladder, acid blockers, antibiotics and prokinetics (cisapride). Gastrostomy tube feeding may bridge the gap until neurological recovery occurs in some animals.

Prognosis: Dysautonomia typically carries a grave prognosis, and recovery rates are lower in dogs than in cats. In a study of 40 cats, complete resolution occurred in about 25% of affected cats and partial recovery was noted in some cats.

Visceral myopathy and chronic intestinal pseudo-obstruction

In this rare condition, reported almost exclusively in dogs, there is typically histological evidence of smooth muscle inflammation (leiomyositis) and fibrosis and, therefore, the diagnosis is missed if full-thickness biopsy samples are not taken. The radiographic appearance is of dilated intestinal loops consistent with intestinal obstruction, but without any true physical obstruction, hence the term pseudo-obstruction. Contrast radiographic studies demonstrate delayed gastric emptying and very slow intestinal transit. Thus, any patient undergoing an exploratory laparotomy for a suspected obstruction that is found to have diffuse gastrointestinal dilatation should have surgical biopsy samples collected. Vomiting, diarrhoea and weight loss occur and the prognosis is very poor. Symptomatic treatment with prokinetics such as cisapride may help, and one case has been reported as responding to steroids. While visceral myopathy is rare, a visceral neuropathy due to mesenteric ganglionitis is extremely rare but can also cause chronic intestinal pseudo-obstruction.

References and further reading

Allenspach K, Culverwell C and Chan D (2016) Long-term outcome in dogs with chronic enteropathies: 203 cases. *Veterinary Record* **178**, 368

Allenspach K, Wieland B, Gröne A and Gaschen F (2007) Chronic enteropathies in dogs: evaluation of risk factors for negative outcome. *Journal of Veterinary Internal Medicine* **21**, 700–708

Baez JL, Hendrick MJ, Walker LM and Washabau RJ (1999) Radiographic, ultrasonographic, and endoscopic findings in cats with inflammatory bowel disease of the stomach and small intestine: 33 cases (1990–1997). *Journal of the American Veterinary Medical Association* **215**, 349–354

Barrs VR and Beatty JA (2012a) Feline alimentary lymphoma: 1. Classification, risk factors, clinical signs and non-invasive diagnostics. *Journal of Feline Medicine and Surgery* **14**, 182–190

Barrs VR and Beatty JA (2012b) Feline alimentary lymphoma: 2. Further diagnostics, therapy and prognosis. *Journal of Feline Medicine and Surgery* **14**, 191–201

Carrasco V, Rodríguez-Bertos A, Rodríguez-Franco F et al. (2015) Distinguishing intestinal lymphoma from inflammatory bowel disease in canine duodenal endoscopic biopsy samples. *Veterinary Pathology* **52**, 668–675

Craven M, Simpson JW, Ridyard AE and Chandler ML (2004) Canine inflammatory bowel disease: retrospective analysis of diagnosis and outcome in 80 cases (1995–2002). *Journal of Small Animal Practice* **45**, 336–342

Dandrieux JR, Noble PJ, Scase TJ et al. (2013) Comparison of a chlorambucil-prednisolone combination with an azathioprine-prednisolone combination for treatment of chronic enteropathy with concurrent protein-losing enteropathy in dogs: 27 cases (2007–2010). *Journal of the American Veterinary Medical Association* **15**, 1705–1714

Daniaux LA, Laurenson MP, Marks SL et al. (2014) Ultrasonographic thickening of the muscularis propria in feline small intestinal small cell T-cell lymphoma and inflammatory bowel disease. *Journal of Feline Medicine and Surgery* **16**, 89–98

Dossin O and Lavoué R (2011) Protein-losing enteropathies in dogs. *Veterinary Clinics of North America: Small Animal Practice* **41**, 399–418

Gaschen L, Kircher P, Stüssi A et al. (2008) Comparison of ultrasonographic findings with clinical activity index (CIBDAI) and diagnosis in dogs with chronic enteropathies. *Veterinary Radiology and Ultrasound* **49**, 56–64

German AJ, Day MJ, Ruaux CG et al. (2003) Comparison of direct and indirect tests for small intestinal bacterial overgrowth and antibiotic-responsive diarrhea in dogs. *Journal of Veterinary Internal Medicine* **17**, 33–43

Goodwin LV, Goggs R, Chan DL and Allenspach K (2011) Hypercoagulability in dogs with protein-losing enteropathy. *Journal of Veterinary Internal Medicine* **25**, 273–277

Gow AG, Else R, Evans H et al. (2011) Hypovitaminosis D in dogs with inflammatory bowel disease and hypoalbuminaemia. *Journal of Small Animal Practice* **52**, 411–418

Gruffydd-Jones T, Addie D, Belák S et al. (2013) Giardiasis in cats: ABCD guidelines on prevention and management. *Journal of Feline Medicine and Surgery* **15**, 650–652

Jergens AE (2012) Feline idiopathic inflammatory bowel disease: what we know and what remains to be unravelled. *Journal of Feline Medicine and Surgery* **14**, 445–458

Jergens AE, Schreiner CA, Frank DE et al. (2003) A scoring index for disease activity in canine inflammatory bowel disease. *Journal of Veterinary Internal Medicine* **17**, 291–297

Kathrani A, House A, Catchpole B et al. (2011) Breed-independent toll-like receptor 5 polymorphisms show association with canine inflammatory bowel disease. *Tissue Antigens* **78**, 94–101

Kilpinen S, Spillmann T and Westermarck E (2014) Efficacy of two low-dose oral tylosin regimens in controlling the relapse of diarrhea in dogs with tylosin-responsive diarrhea: a prospective, single-blinded, two-arm parallel, clinical field trial. *Acta Veterinaria Scandinavica* **56**, 43

Kimmel SE, Waddell LS and Michel KE (2000) Hypomagnesemia and hypocalcemia associated with protein-losing enteropathy in Yorkshire Terriers: five cases (1992–1998). *Journal of the American Veterinary Medical Association* **217**, 703–706

Kiupel M, Smedley RC, Pfent C, et al. (2011) Diagnostic algorithm to differentiate lymphoma from intestinal inflammation in feline small intestinal biopsy samples. *Veterinary Pathology* **48**, 212–222

Littman MP, Dambach DM, Vaden SL and Giger U (2000) Familial protein-losing enteropathy and protein-losing nephropathy in Soft Coated Wheaten Terriers: 222 cases (1983–1997). *Journal of Veterinary Internal Medicine* **14**, 68–80

Loyd KA, Cocayne CG, Cridland JM and Hause WR (2016) Retrospective evaluation of the administration of 25% human albumin to dogs with protein-losing enteropathy: 21 cases (2003–2013). *Journal of Veterinary Emergency and Critical Care* **26**, 587–592

MacLachlan NJ, Breitschwerdt EB, Chambers JM et al. (1988) Gastroenteritis of Basenji dogs. *Veterinary Pathology* **25**, 36–41

Marsilio S, Ackermann MR, Lidbury JA et al. (2019)). Results of histopathology, immunochemistry, and molecular clonality testing of small intestinal biopsy specimens from clinially healthy client-owned cats. *Journal of Veterinary Internal Medicine* **33**, 551–558

Paris JK, Wills S, Balzer HJ et al. (2014) Enteropathogen co-infection in UK cats with diarrhoea. *BMC Veterinary Research* **10**, 13

Procoli F, Mötsküla PF, Keyte SV et al. (2013) Comparison of histopathologic findings in duodenal and ileal endoscopic biopsies in dogs with chronic small intestinal enteropathies. *Journal of Veterinary Internal Medicine* **27**, 268–274

Rudorf H, van Schaik G, O'Brien RT et al. (2005) Ultrasonographic evaluation of the thickness of the small intestinal wall in dogs with inflammatory bowel disease. *Journal of Small Animal Practice* **46**, 322–326

Rutgers HC, Batt RM, Elwood CM and Lamport A (1995) Small intestinal bacterial overgrowth in dogs with chronic intestinal disease. *Journal of the American Veterinary Medical Association* **206**, 187–193

Simmerson SM, Armstrong PJ, Wünschmann A et al. (2014) Clinical features, intestinal histopathology, and outcome in protein-losing enteropathy in Yorkshire Terrier dogs. *Journal of Veterinary Internal Medicine* **28**, 331–337

Suchodolski JS (2016) Diagnosis and interpretation of intestinal dysbiosis in dogs and cats. *The Veterinary Journal* **215**, 30–37

Toresson L, Steiner JM, Suchodolski JS and Spillmann T (2016) Oral cobalamin supplementation in dogs with chronic enteropathies and hypocobalaminemia. *Journal of Veterinary Internal Medicine* **30**, 101–107.

Washabau RJ, Day MJ, Willard MD et al. (2010) Endoscopic, biopsy, and histopathologic guidelines for the evaluation of gastrointestinal inflammation in companion animals. *Journal of Veterinary Internal Medicine* **24**, 10–26

Westermarck E, Skrzypczak T, Harmoinen J et al. (2005) Tylosin-responsive chronic diarrhea in dogs. *Journal of Veterinary Internal Medicine* **19**, 177–186

Whitehead J, Quimby J and Bayliss D (2015) Seizures associated with hypocalcemia in a Yorkshire Terrier with protein-losing enteropathy. *Journal of the American Animal Hospital Association* **51**, 380–384

Willard MD, Helman G, Fradkin JM et al. (2000) Intestinal crypt lesions associated with protein-losing enteropathy in the dog. *Journal of Veterinary Internal Medicine* **14**, 298–307

Zwingenberger AL, Marks SL, Baker TW and Moore PF (2010) Ultrasonographic evaluation of the muscularis propria in cats with diffuse small intestinal lymphoma or inflammatory bowel disease. *Journal of Veterinary Internal Medicine* **24**, 289–292

Chapter 35

Colon and rectum

Aarti Kathrani

Anatomy and function of the large intestine

Grossly, the large intestine comprises the caecum, colon and rectum. The caecum in dogs and cats is comparatively small and is in fact a diverticulum of the proximal colon. Therefore, in dogs and cats, the ileum communicates directly with the colon via an ileocolic sphincter, which is separate from the caececolic orifice. Anatomically, the colon comprises the ascending, transverse and descending colon. Functionally, the ascending and transverse sections form the proximal colon and the descending section the distal colon. The rectum begins at the entrance to the pelvic canal. Microscopically, the colon is similar to the small intestine and consists of four layers: mucosa, submucosa, muscularis and serosa; however, the colon lacks villi, has fewer microvilli and contains more mucus-secreting goblet cells than the small intestine.

The proximal colon absorbs water and electrolytes, and the distal colon is involved in storage and coordinated evacuation of faeces. Other functions of the colon include mucus production, immune surveillance, microbial fermentation and motility. Depending on which specific function is affected, large intestinal diarrhoea or constipation may be seen. For example, decreased fluid absorption and increased mucus production in chronic colitis may lead to diarrhoea, whereas decreased colonic motility in idiopathic feline megacolon may lead to constipation.

Diagnostic tests

Dogs and cats with large intestinal disease may present with constipation or large intestinal diarrhoea, which is characterized by urgency and increased frequency of small-volume mucoid and/or bloody diarrhoea with tenesmus (see Chapter 23). A thorough history should include questions regarding the diet, travel, environment, husbandry, comorbidities, medications, vaccination and deworming schedule, and signs in in-contact animals. Typically, animals with large intestinal disease are normal on physical examination; however, abnormalities may be appreciated with certain diseases (Figure 35.1). Rectal examination is mandatory in all dogs and cats presenting with large intestinal disease to assess for abnormalities (Figure 35.2); however, this may have to be performed under sedation or anaesthesia, depending on the temperament and size (i.e. cats and small dogs) of the animal.

Physical examination finding	Possible causes
Reduced body condition score	• Concurrent small intestinal chronic enteropathy (CE) • Small intestinal lymphoma • Granulomatous colitis • Advanced colonic neoplasia • Owner restricting food intake
Pyrexia	• Concurrent small intestinal CE • Colonic neoplasia • Caecal or colonic perforation • Fungal or bacterial infection
Abdominal pain	• Concurrent small intestinal CE • Colonic neoplasia • Foreign body • Caecal or colonic perforation
Abdominal mass	• Colonic neoplasia • Granulomatous colitis • Intussusception (caecocolic, ileocolic) • Pythiosis • Prostatomegaly
Small intestinal thickening	• Concurrent small intestinal CE • Small intestinal lymphoma
Mesenteric lymphadenopathy	• Concurrent small intestinal CE • Small intestinal lymphoma • Disseminated fungal disease
Hepatosplenomegaly	• Lymphoma • Disseminated fungal disease
Uveitis	• Lymphoma • Protothecosis • Feline infectious peritonitis
Perineal changes	• Perineal hernia • Anal furunculosis • Anal sac abscess
Autonomic neuropathy	• Dysautonomia
Hindlimb paresis	• Neurological disease
Hindlimb lameness	• Orthopaedic disease

35.1 Abnormalities that may be present on physical examination in dogs and cats presenting with large intestinal diarrhoea or constipation.

- Anal furunculosis
- Anal sac abscess
- Anal sac impaction
- Anal sac neoplasia
- Perineal hernia
- Prostatic neoplasia
- Prostatitis
- Prostatomegaly/prostatic hyperplasia
- Rectal mass
- Rectal mucosal irregularity
- Rectal polyp
- Rectal stricture

35.2 Possible digital rectal examination findings in dogs and cats with large intestinal disease.

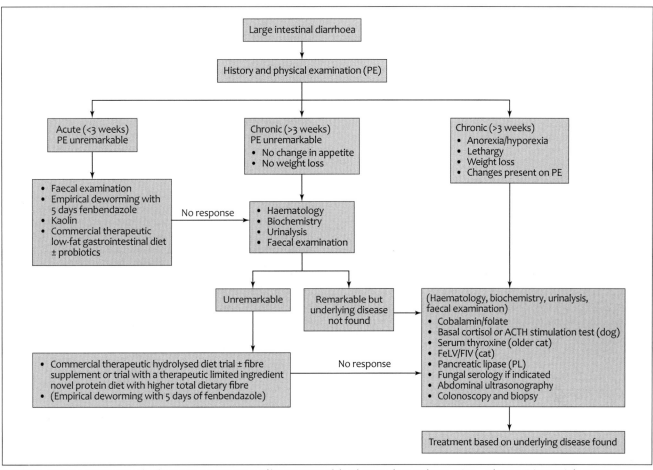

Large intestinal diarrhoea

↓

History and physical examination (PE)

Acute (<3 weeks)
PE unremarkable

Chronic (>3 weeks)
PE unremarkable
• No change in appetite
• No weight loss

Chronic (>3 weeks)
• Anorexia/hyperexia
• Lethargy
• Weight loss
• Changes present on PE

- Faecal examination
- Empirical deworming with 5 days fenbendazole
- Kaolin
- Commercial therapeutic low-fat gastrointestinal diet ± probiotics

No response →

- Haematology
- Biochemistry
- Urinalysis
- Faecal examination

Unremarkable

Remarkable but underlying disease not found

(Haematology, biochemistry, urinalysis, faecal examination)
- Cobalamin/folate
- Basal cortisol or ACTH stimulation test (dog)
- Serum thyroxine (older cat)
- FeLV/FIV (cat)
- Pancreatic lipase (PL)
- Fungal serology if indicated
- Abdominal ultrasonography
- Colonoscopy and biopsy

- Commercial therapeutic hydrolysed diet trial ± fibre supplement or trial with a therapeutic limited ingredient novel protein diet with higher total dietary fibre
- (Empirical deworming with 5 days of fenbendazole)

No response →

Treatment based on underlying disease found

35.3 Rational approach to the diagnostic investigation of large intestinal diarrhoea in dogs and cats. ACTH = adrenocorticotropic hormone; FeLV = feline leukaemia virus; FIV = feline immunodeficiency virus.

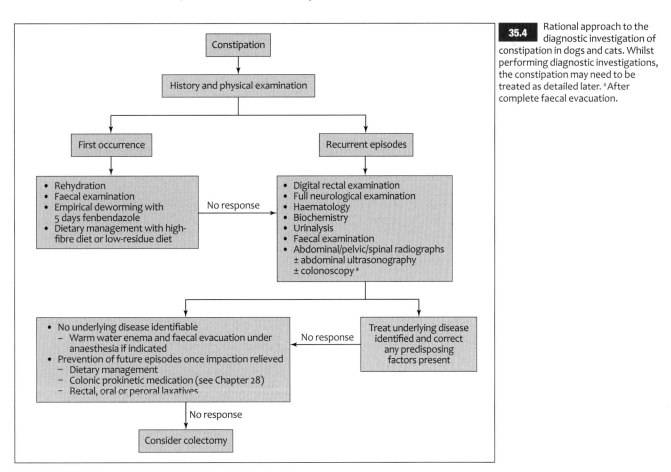

Constipation

↓

History and physical examination

First occurrence

Recurrent episodes

- Rehydration
- Faecal examination
- Empirical deworming with 5 days fenbendazole
- Dietary management with high-fibre diet or low-residue diet

No response →

- Digital rectal examination
- Full neurological examination
- Haematology
- Biochemistry
- Urinalysis
- Faecal examination
- Abdominal/pelvic/spinal radiographs ± abdominal ultrasonography ± colonoscopy [a]

- No underlying disease identifiable
  – Warm water enema and faecal evacuation under anaesthesia if indicated
- Prevention of future episodes once impaction relieved
  – Dietary management
  – Colonic prokinetic medication (see Chapter 28)
  – Rectal, oral or peroral laxatives

← No response

Treat underlying disease identified and correct any predisposing factors present

↓ No response

Consider colectomy

35.4 Rational approach to the diagnostic investigation of constipation in dogs and cats. Whilst performing diagnostic investigations, the constipation may need to be treated as detailed later. [a] After complete faecal evacuation.

Rectal examination allows assessment of the faeces and may provide samples for examination and rectal scrape cytology (see Chapter 6), but subsequent diagnostic investigations are guided by the history and physical examination (Figures 35.3 and 35.4). Haematology, biochemistry and urinalysis help to rule out systemic or metabolic disease (see Chapter 1). Measurement of serum cobalamin and folate concentrations allows assessment for concurrent small intestinal disease, serum trypsin-like immunoreactivity for exocrine pancreatic insufficiency, and serum pancreatic lipase for pancreatitis. Testing for feline leukaemia virus and feline immunodeficiency virus for all cats, and serum thyroxine for older cats with diarrhoea and younger cats with constipation, is recommended. Faecal examination may consist of cytology, wet mount, zinc sulphate flotation, culture and polymerase chain reaction (PCR) (see Chapter 2). Fungal serology is required for animals with a relevant travel history if rectal cytology is negative but suspicion remains. Diagnostic imaging includes survey radiographs, abdominal ultrasonography or computed tomography (see Chapter 3). Flexible colonoscopy with collection of mucosal biopsy specimens may be warranted if a definitive diagnosis has not been reached (see Figure 35.3 and Chapters 4 and 6).

Diseases of the colon

Acute colitis

Acute colitis is defined as the sudden onset of large intestinal diarrhoea and is a common complaint in many dogs presenting to veterinary practices. Although there are many potential causes, such as dietary indiscretion, bacterial and/or their toxins, protozoa, viruses, helminths and trauma (e.g. ingestion of bones, toys or sand), the underlying cause is rarely diagnosed. Most cases are self-limiting or readily respond to symptomatic treatment, consisting of fluid therapy, dietary management, kaolin-based antidiarrhoeal medication and/or probiotics. Dietary management consists of feeding small and frequent amounts of a commercial low-fat gastrointestinal diet. Kaolin-based antidiarrhoeal medication may help to bind bacterial toxins and firm up the faeces. Antibiotics are usually avoided in cases of undetermined aetiology due to their potential effect on the microbiota and the concern for antibiotic resistance. Instead, a probiotic could be considered. Acute colitis generally carries a good prognosis due to its self-limiting nature and favourable response to symptomatic treatment; however, those that fail to respond become cases of chronic colitis (see below).

Infectious colitis

The infectious agents listed below primarily affect the colon and, therefore, large intestinal disease is a prominent feature of infection.

Helminths

Trematodes: Heterobilharzia americana is a fluke that causes schistosomiasis in dogs, resulting in chronic large intestinal diarrhoea and haematochezia (see Chapter 21). Dogs may also present with clinical signs due to hypercalcaemia. Canine infection is restricted to the southeastern and Gulf Coast regions of the USA. Diagnosis is by the identification of eggs on faecal smear or flotation,

or by histopathology of the liver or intestine. An enzyme-linked immunosorbent assay (ELISA) is available for occult infections. Treatment is with fenbendazole and praziquantel. Prognosis is good for acute cases, but guarded to poor for chronic cases due to liver cirrhosis.

Nematodes: Trichuris vulpis is a whipworm and a common cause of large intestinal disease in dogs worldwide (although uncommon in the UK) and rare in cats. Clinical signs can be acute, chronic or intermittent and consist of large intestinal diarrhoea and haematochezia, although abdominal pain, vomiting, hyporexia and weight loss may be seen in some dogs. Caecal inversion has been infrequently reported secondary to whipworm infection. Dogs with severe infection may have eosinophilia, anaemia and hypoalbuminaemia. Decreased serum sodium and increased potassium may also be present; however, these dogs have a normal adrenocorticotropic hormone stimulation response test. Diagnosis is by the identification of characteristic eggs on faecal flotation. As the eggs can be shed intermittently, all dogs with large intestinal diarrhoea should receive empirical deworming treatment, and especially prior to colonoscopy. Treatment options include fenbendazole, pyrantel, febantel, moxidectin and milbemycin oxime, and should be repeated after 3 weeks and 3 months due to the long pre-patent period. Prognosis is excellent.

Bacteria

Many of the bacterial organisms discussed below can be isolated from the faeces of healthy animals and, therefore, isolation does not prove causation; many specialists are highly sceptical regarding the pathogenity of these bacteria. Hence, diagnosis is presumptive and individualized based on:

- Signalment (young, old, debilitated)
- Housing (overcrowded, breeding facility, shelter, hospitalized, signs in in-contact animals)
- Husbandry (feeding of raw food or undercooked meat)
- Medical history (vaccination, medications such as antibiotics or immunosuppressives, comorbidities)
- Clinical signs (haematochezia, pyrexia)
- Laboratory results (leucopenia, leucocytosis, hypoglycaemia, leucocytosis on rectal scrape cytology)
- Positive faecal culture or presence of toxins for relevant bacteria and elimination of other causes.

Clostridium difficile is a nosocomial pathogen in humans and can cause fatal pseudomembranous colitis in hospitalized patients receiving antibiotics. Up to 40% of both healthy dogs and cats are culture positive, with most of these isolates containing toxin genes, although toxins are more frequent in dogs with diarrhoea (Riley et al., 1991; Struble et al., 1994; Madewell et al., 1999). Dogs with suspected infection can have signs consistent with small and/or large intestinal signs. Metronidazole is the treatment of choice.

Clostridium perfringens has been implicated in the aetiology of canine acute colitis and acute haemorrhagic diarrhoea syndrome; however, it can be isolated in up to 80% of healthy dogs (Weese et al., 2001; Marks et al., 2002). Immunoassays are available to detect the C. perfringens enterotoxin (CPE) protein by ELISA, or the CPE gene by PCR. However, as CPE can also be isolated in approximately 15% of healthy dogs (Meer and Songer, 1997), it is currently unclear if C. perfringens is actually a cause of canine colitis. *C. perfringens* is susceptible to metronidazole, amoxicillin, erythromycin and tylosin. However, some patients with large intestinal diarrhoea and isolation of *C. perfringens* respond to a high-fibre diet in the absence of antibiotics.

Enterohaemorrhagic *Escherichia coli* (EHEC) has an affinity for the large intestine, causing haemorrhagic diarrhoea. Diagnosis is based on the demonstration of the Shiga-like toxin protein (ELISA) or gene (PCR) in faeces or isolates cultured from the faeces. However, isolation rates may range up to 15% and 5% in healthy dogs and cats, respectively (Abaas *et al.*, 1989; Prada *et al.*, 1991; Beutin *et al.*, 1993; Turk *et al.*, 1998; Bentancor *et al.*, 2007). Although EHEC O157:H7 has been isolated from the faeces of healthy dogs, it has been associated with some cases of 'Alabama rot' described in Greyhounds in the USA.

Enteropathogenic *E. coli* (EPEC) can damage the large intestine by causing attaching and effacing lesions. Infected dogs are typically less than 1 year of age and have concurrent infections with other agents that cause diarrhoea (Drolet *et al.*, 1994; Turk *et al.*, 1998). Fatal infection has been described in a 2-month-old kitten and an adult cat (Pospischill *et al.*, 1987). Diagnosis is by documentation of the attaching and effacing lesion on histopathology and the absence of Shiga-like toxin. Treatment involves supportive care with the use of co-amoxiclav, enrofloxacin or first- or second-generation cephalosporin antibiotics.

Campylobacter spp. can be cultured from the faeces of up to 90% of healthy dogs and cats and, therefore, it is currently unclear if they are definitively pathogenic. However, dogs and cats with suspected *Campylobacter* infection are typically puppies and kittens, animals that are stressed, living in unsanitary conditions or have concurrent disease. The diarrhoea ranges from mildly soft faeces to bloody mucoid or watery diarrhoea. Vomiting, hyporexia, pyrexia and leucocytosis may also be present. Diagnosis is based on positive culture and PCR for speciation. The optimal antibiotic choice is erythromycin.

Salmonella typhimurium can cause enterocolitis in dogs and cats, although infection is thought to be uncommon. Isolation rates are in the range of 1–36% and 1–18% in healthy dogs and cats, respectively, which is similar to rates in diarrhoeic dogs and cats. Higher isolation rates may be seen in animals fed raw or improperly cooked meat or in those hunting wild birds (Joffe and Schlesinger, 2002). Rates of infection are higher in animals that are young, debilitated and those in overcrowded environments with poor sanitation. Clinical signs include watery or mucoid diarrhoea, vomiting, pyrexia, dehydration and hyporexia. Rarely, salmonellosis may progress to a fatal bacteraemia or endotoxaemia. Diagnosis is based on positive culture and treatment is with fluid therapy and supportive care. Antibiotics (chloramphenicol, amoxicillin, trimethoprim/sulphonamide and enrofloxacin) are indicated when there is evidence of bacteraemia and endotoxaemia (pyrexia, neutropenia, hypoglycaemia). Post-treatment cultures should be performed to confirm eradication, and pet owners should be informed of the zoonotic risk.

Yersinia enterocolitica may cause acute or chronic haemorrhagic diarrhoea but can be isolated from the faeces of healthy dogs and cats. Therefore, diagnosis requires a positive culture with elimination of other causes. Effective antibiotic options include tetracyclines, trimethoprim/sulphonamide and cephalosporins.

Protozoa

Balantidium coli is an infectious agent of pigs and non-human primates, and rarely causes ulcerative colonic lesions in dogs, resulting in chronic haemorrhagic colitis. Dogs are frequently co-infected with *T. vulpis*. Diagnosis is by the identification of protozoa or eggs in faecal smears or zinc sulphate flotation. Treatment of concurrent helminth infection may be enough to be curative in some cases. Tetracycline and metronidazole are effective treatment options in humans.

Entamoeba histolytica is the cause of amoebic dysentery in humans. Infection in dogs and cats is rare and occurs following the ingestion of food or water contaminated by human faeces containing cysts. Diagnosis is by the identification of trophozoites or cysts on faecal smear or zinc sulphate flotation. Treatment is with metronidazole.

Tritrichomonas foetus primarily colonizes the large intestine of cats and causes chronic colitis with foul-smelling faeces with mucus and fresh blood, an oedematous and painful anus and faecal incontinence. Infection is most common in young, pedigree cats in overcrowded environments or in multi-cat households. Infected cats should be tested for underlying feline leukaemia virus and feline immunodeficiency virus. PCR of faeces is the most sensitive diagnostic test and mucoid/bloody faeces or colonic washes provide the best samples (see Chapter 2). False-negatives may be seen with antibiotic use in the past 7 days or when formed faeces are submitted for PCR testing. Treatment is with ronidazole. Although neurological signs have been reported with this drug, they resolve on discontinuation of therapy. The disease has a fair long-term prognosis for spontaneous resolution, as when left untreated, 88% of cats had spontaneous resolution of diarrhoea within 2 years. However, spontaneous resolution does not equate to full recovery, as 57% of these cats remained *T. foetus* PCR positive when tested 2–5 years after diagnosis (Foster *et al.*, 2004). Therefore, recrudescence may occur and may be more likely with travel, stress or diet change.

Pentatrichomonas hominis is often non-pathogenic but has been associated with colitis in dogs, and rarely cats. *P. hominis* is reportedly responsive to metronidazole treatment.

Fungi

Histoplasma capsulatum is a dimorphic fungus which occurs along the Ohio, Mississippi and Missouri river valleys in the USA. Infection occurs following inhalation and may result in pulmonary disease or disseminate to other organs including the colon. Large intestinal diarrhoea is common in dogs and cats with disseminated disease, and dogs may also show pyrexia, anorexia, vomiting and weight loss. The small intestine may also be affected and protein-losing enteropathy may develop. Diagnosis is by identification of the organism on cytological smears of rectal scrapings, lymph node aspirates or cytology brush samples obtained via endoscopy, or histopathology of tissue samples. Treatment is with itraconazole for at least 4–6 months. The prognosis depends on disease dissemination but is generally fair to good.

Oomycetes

Pythium insidiosum, the causative agent of pythiosis is endemic to the Gulf Coast of the USA, but the disease has been diagnosed in other parts of the USA. The organism has a predilection for the skin and gastrointestinal tract. Dogs with gastrointestinal pythiosis can have weight loss, vomiting, diarrhoea and haematochezia. A palpable abdominal mass is usually present and, although the upper gastrointestinal tract is most commonly affected, the colon can also be affected. Diagnosis is by the identification of organisms on intestinal histopathology using special stains. However, PCR on biopsy specimens or ELISA serology are available for diagnosis. Treatment of choice is radical surgical excision followed by itraconazole and terbinafine. As most dogs present late in the course of infection, the prognosis is guarded to grave. However, a recent case series of 3 dogs with colonic pythiosis were successfully managed with itraconalzole, terbinafine, and prednisone (Reagan KL et al., 2019).

Algae

Prototheca zopfii can cause gastrointestinal and disseminated disease in dogs. The algae live in animal waste and sewage-contaminated food, soil and water. Primary colonic infection is followed by dissemination to other tissues, and most dogs have signs of intermittent or persistent bloody diarrhoea. As ocular and neurological signs can accompany signs of colitis, distemper should be considered as a differential diagnosis. Diagnosis is by cytology of rectal scrapes or histopathology of affected tissue; culture can also be performed. Treatment is with varying combinations of amphotericin B and itraconazole; however, outcome is invariably fatal.

Viruses

Feline infectious peritonitis as a primary manifestation of colonic disease is uncommon in cats. Clinical signs may include diarrhoea or constipation, and physical examination may reveal a palpable mass in the colon or the ileocaecocolic junction. Diagnosis is supported by pyogranulomatous inflammation on histopathology and confirmed by the demonstration of intralesional feline coronavirus using immunohistochemistry. Prognosis is poor due to the multisystemic effects of the virus.

Idiopathic chronic colitis

Colonic inflammation (ICC) can affect the small intestine, large intestine or both, although isolated cases of colonic ICC are uncommon. The exact aetiology of ICC is unknown; however, it is hypothesized to involve the interplay of four key components:

- Genetic susceptibility
- Environmental risk factors
- Intestinal dysbiosis
- Altered gastrointestinal mucosal immune response (see Chapter 34).

ICC occurs more commonly in middle-aged dogs and cats. Prevalence in certain breeds has not yet been demonstrated, whereas purebreed cats are more susceptible. Dogs and cats with colonic ICC typically present with chronic large intestinal signs and generally the physical examination is unremarkable. However, abdominal palpation and rectal examination may reveal colonic or rectal mucosal thickening, respectively. Diagnostic investigation includes haematology, biochemistry and urinalysis to rule out systemic causes, measurement of serum cobalamin and folate concentrations to assess for concurrent small intestinal involvement, basal cortisol to rule out atypical hypoadrenocorticism (dogs), total thyroxine (cats above 8 years of age), faecal parasitology and/or culture, PCR for

T. foetus (cats), a course of fenbendazole for occult parasites and abdominal ultrasonography. Most animals with colonic ICC have unremarkable findings on abdominal ultrasound although some may have lymphadenopathy or colonic wall thickening; fine-needle aspirates of any lesions should be considered. If diagnostic investigations have not revealed an underlying cause at this stage, then either a trial with a commerical therapeutic hydrolysed diet with or without a prebiotic fibre supplment should be considered, or a trial with a commercial therapeutic limited-ingredient novel protein diet with higher total dietary fibre. Prebiotic fibres are a source of short chain fatty acids and therefore help to maintain mucosal health

Most dogs and cats that respond to diet will do so within 2 weeks. If there is no response to different diet trials, the clinical signs are severe at the onset or changes are seen on abdominal ultrasonography, then colonoscopy and collection of biopsy samples should be considered. Histopathology may reveal lymphoplasmacytic colitis, eosinophilic colitis, neutrophilic colitis or mixed inflammation. Unfortunately, at this time there is no information regarding response of the different histological types to treatment. However, neutrophilic inflammation may warrant fluorescence *in situ* hybridization (FISH) testing, to assess for invasive *Campylobacter* spp., which may necessitate the use of antimicrobial treatment (Maunder et al., 2016). For those cases of lymphoplasmacytic or eosinophilic colitis that have failed to respond to dietary management, sulfasalazine may be considered. Sulfasalazine exerts its anti-inflammatory effects directly on the colonic mucosa by inhibiting prostaglandin and leukotriene synthesis. The main adverse effect of this medication is keratoconjunctivitis sicca and, therefore, regular Schirmer tear tests should be performed. Corticosteroids may be used in dogs that fail to respond to sulfasalazine or in cats as a first line, as they may not be as tolerant of sulfasalazine. If cats fail to respond to corticosteroids, chlorambucil can be added, and in dogs, chlorambucil, ciclosporin or azathioprine can be considered. The prognosis for colonic ICC depends on the initial response to treatment and the severity of clinical signs. Young dogs with predominantly large intestinal signs respond more favourably to diet alone, whereas older dogs with severe disease that require corticosteroids have a poorer prognosis (Allenspach et al., 2007).

Granulomatous colitis

Granulomatous colitis, formerly known as histiocytic ulcerative colitis, is associated with adherent and invasive E. coli (AIEC) infection. This disease occurs predominantly in young (<2 years) Boxers and French Bulldogs, although it has been reported to occur in other breeds, such as Mastiffs, Alaskan Malamutes and English Bulldogs, and in one cat. The disease is usually exclusive to the large intestine with signs of severe chronic large intestinal inflammation. The diagnostic investigations are similar to those for dogs with colonic ICC and consist of haematology, biochemistry, urinalysis, faecal examination and abdominal ultrasonography. Abdominal ultrasonography may reveal a thickened colonic mucosa, although many dogs have unremarkable scans. Colonoscopy and biopsy are required for definitive diagnosis, and the accumulation of large amounts of periodic acid–Schiff (PAS)-positive macrophages on histopathology is considered pathognomonic for the disease. FISH performed on the biopsy samples reveals the presence of AIEC. Therefore, PAS staining and FISH remain the best ways to confirm the diagnosis. Treatment is with enrofloxacin or marbofloxacin for 6–10 weeks.

Neoplasia

Adenocarcinoma (ACA) and lymphoma are the most common neoplasms of the large intestine.

Adenocarcinoma

ACA is most common in the canine descending colon and rectum and may lead to mechanical obstruction. Metastasis of large intestinal ACA to distant sites is uncommon in dogs. Feline ACA can occur in the descending colon and ileocolic region, although exclusively ileal ACAs are more common. As the tumours tend to be more proximal in cats, haematochezia rather than mechanical obstruction is more likely. Approximately 60–80% of canine rectal ACAs are apparent on physical examination, and more than 50% of affected cats have colonic masses apparent on abdominal palpation (Paoloni *et al.*, 2002). However, abdominal ultrasonography can be used to help localize any tumours. Colonoscopy with biopsy is recommended for definitive diagnosis. Complete surgical excision is the treatment of choice for canine focal ACA; however, the prognosis is generally guarded to poor. Treatment of feline colonic ACA is with wide surgical excision, as there is a higher rate of local metastasis and systemic chemotherapy, with or without non-steroidal anti-inflammatory medication. The median survival time for cats with colonic ACA treated by subtotal colectomy with adjuvant carboplatin was reported as 269 days in one study (Arteaga *et al.*, 2012).

Lymphoma

Lymphoma generally affects the small intestine with or without involvement of the large intestine, and can cause a range of signs including anorexia, vomiting, diarrhoea, melaena (see Chapter 20), haematochezia, weight loss and, in cats, a palpable mass. Diagnosis can be made with cytology of fine-needle aspirates of mesenteric lymph nodes, thickened intestinal wall or peritoneal fluid; however, histology may be needed for definitive diagnosis. Lymphoma confined exclusively to the rectum in dogs responds well to combination chemotherapy (Van den Steen *et al.*, 2012). Unfortunately, all other forms of canine alimentary large cell lymphoma respond very poorly to chemotherapy or by tumour lysis result in intestinal perforation and septic peritonitis. Most cases of colonic lymphoma in cats are B-cell in origin and are treated with combination chemotherapy.

Polyps

Polyps may occur in the descending colon and rectum of adult dogs, with Miniature Daschunds being over-represented. Signs may include formed faeces with fresh blood or clots. Diagnosis may be made by rectal examination or colonoscopy. Submucosal resection of the base of the polyp's stalk is needed for cure. Polyps should always be submitted for histopathological assessment, which may reveal a benign polyp, inflammatory polyp, adenoma or carcinoma *in situ*.

Constipation/obstipation/feline idiopathic megacolon

Constipation is defined as infrequent or difficult evacuation of faeces, whereas obstipation is defined as intractable constipation that requires intervention. Signs include

tenesmus, dyschezia (see Chapters 22 and 23) and abdominal pain, and chronically affected animals may exhibit weight loss, hyporexia, vomiting and lethargy. There are many causes (Figure 35.5) and megacolon is usually the end stage of colonic dysfunction regardless of the aetiology. The majority of cases are idiopathic, orthopaedic or neurological in origin. The diagnosis is based on a relevant history, followed by physical examination, where constipation or obstipation are readily apparent on abdominal palpation. A complete neurological examination should be performed, as well as a careful digital rectal examination, performed under sedation or general anaesthesia in cats. If the cause is not apparent on physical examination, then haematology, biochemistry and urinalysis should be performed to screen for metabolic diseases. Abdominal radiographs to characterize the severity of colonic impaction, as well as to identify the underlying cause, should be considered. Extraluminal mass lesions should be further evaluated by abdominal ultrasonography and intraluminal lesions by colonoscopy after thorough faecal evacuation.

- Neuromuscular dysfunction
  - Idiopathic megacolon
  - Lumbosacral disease (cauda equina syndrome, sacral spinal cord deformities (Manx cat))
  - Hypogastric or pelvic nerve disorders (traumatic injury, malignancy, dysautonomia)
  - Submucosal or myenteric plexus neuropathy (dysautonomia, ageing)
  - Irritable bowel syndrome?
- Mechanical obstruction
  - Intraluminal (foreign material ingestion (e.g. gravel, stones, bones, hair), neoplasia, rectal diverticula, perineal hernia, anorectal stricture)
  - Intramucosal (neoplasia)
  - Extraluminal (pelvic fracture, neoplasia, prostatic disease)
- Orthopaedic
  - Pelvic fracture
  - Arthritis
- Inflammation
  - Anal furunculosis
  - Proctitis
  - Anal sac disease
  - Anorectal foreign body
  - Perianal bite wounds
- Metabolic
  - Dehydration
  - Hypokalaemia
  - Hypercalcaemia
- Endocrine
  - Hypothyroidism
  - Secondary nutritional hyperparathyroidism
- Obesity
- Environmental/behavioural
  - Soiled litter tray
  - Not enough litter trays in multi-cat household
  - Inactivity
  - Hospitalization
  - Stress
  - Fear
  - Change in environment
- Pharmacological
  - Opioids
  - Atropine
  - Anticholinergics
  - Barium sulphate
  - Diuretics
  - Phenothiazines
  - Beta-agonists
  - Iron supplements
  - Antihistamines
  - Sucralfate

35.5 Causes of constipation in dogs and cats.

Medical management consists of treatment of the underlying disease where possible and/or a combination of dietary modification, oral or suppository laxatives and colonic prokinetic medication. For patients with chronic constipation that still have some level of colonic motility, insoluble or mixed fibre may help. The motility patterns of patients with obstipation are completely abolished and, therefore, in these patients, non-fermentable fibre-enhanced foods should not be used as these may worsen their signs; in these cases, a highly digestible, low-residue diet with a high energy density should be used to markedly reduce faecal mass. If the animal is overweight, a weight-reduction programme should be considered.

Rectal suppository laxatives may contain emollient (e.g. dioctyl sodium sulfosuccinate (DSS)), lubricant (e.g. glycerol) or stimulant (e.g. bysacodyl) laxatives. Their use requires a compliant pet and owner; however, they may be effective as a first-line treatment, or in prevention of recurrence. Oral laxatives include emollient (e.g. DSS), lubricant (e.g. liquid paraffin, petroleum jelly), hyperosmotic (e.g. lactulose) or stimulant (e.g. bisacodyl). Administration of polyethylene glycol solution by infusion through a nasogastric tube for 24–48 hours can be remarkably effective in even severely obstipated cats with idiopathic megacolon (see below), precluding the need for warm water enemas and manual extraction under general anaesthesia. Once impacted faeces have been removed, prevention is attempted by dietary management, colonic prokinetic medication such as cisapride, and oral or rectal laxatives. Cats that are refractory to medical management require subtotal colectomy (see the *BSAVA Manual of Canine and Feline Abdominal Surgery*). Cats can have a favourable prognosis after colectomy, particularly if the ileocolic valve is preserved, although diarrhoea can occur for weeks to months afterwards in some cats.

Feline idiopathic megacolon is most commonly diagnosed in middle-aged male Domestic Shorthaired, Domestic Longhaired or Siamese cats. The aetiology is unknown, but affected cats have permanent loss of colonic motility. Medical therapy for constipation described above may be effective initially, but most cats eventually require colectomy.

Miscellaneous

Intussusception

Ileocolic intussusception is the most common type and is most likely to cause an obstruction. Predisposing factors include intestinal parasites, viral enteritis, foreign body and, in older animals, tumours. The intussusception may be palpable or visible on imaging and, in extreme cases, may pass through the anus. Treatment is by surgery. Caecocolic intussusception (caecal inversion) is less common and largely exclusive to dogs. Signs consist of fresh blood and clots mixed with formed faeces. The intussusception may be palpable or visible on imaging, although colonoscopy is needed for definitive diagnosis. Treatment is by typhlectomy.

Irritable bowel syndrome

Irritable bowel syndrome (IBS) is an idiopathic functional gastrointestinal disorder in humans. The cardinal symptoms include abdominal pain and constipation, diarrhoea, or both. Currently, it is unknown if dogs and cats experience IBS. Diagnosis of IBS would require consistent clinical signs

and exclusion of other known causes of gastrointestinal disease, including ICC. Treatment of presumptive IBS in dogs and cats is likely to be similar to that in humans, which includes lifestyle changes, dietary intervention and symptomatic management. Reducing stress and increasing physical activity are important in managing the disease. Diets with increased digestibility or higher fibre content may be needed to manage clinical signs. Medications such as analgesia, anxiolytics and prokinetics may help to alleviate signs. Probiotics may also help in selected cases.

References and further reading

Abaas S, Franklin A, Kuhn I *et al.* (1989) Cytotoxin activity on Vero cells among *Escherichia coli* strains associated with diarrhea in cats. *American Journal of Veterinary Research* **50**, 1294–1296

Allenspach K, Wieland B, Grone A and Gaschen F (2007) Chronic enteropathies in dogs: evaluation of risk factors for negative outcome. *Journal of Veterinary Internal Medicine* **21**, 700–708

Arteaga TA, McKnight J and Bergman PJ (2012) A review of 18 cases of feline colonic adenocarcinoma treated with subtotal colectomies and adjuvant carboplatin. *Journal of the American Animal Hospital Association* **48**, 399–404

Bentancor A, Rumi MV, Gentilini MV *et al.* (2007) Shiga toxin-producing and attaching and effacing *Escherichia coli* in cats and dogs in a high hemolytic uremic syndrome incidence region in Argentina. *FEMS Microbiology Letters* **267**, 251–256

Beutin L, Geier D, Steinruck H *et al.* (1993) Prevalence and some properties of verotoxin (Shiga-like toxin)-producing *Escherichia coli* in seven different species of healthy domestic animals. *Journal of Clinical Microbiology* **31**, 2483–2488

Borriello SP, Honour P, Turner T and Barclay F (1983) Household pets as a potential reservoir for *Clostridium difficile* infection. *Journal of Clinical Pathology* **36**, 84–87

Drolet R, Fairbrother JM, Harel J and Helie P (1994) Attaching and effacing and enterotoxigenic *Escherichia coli* associated with enteric colibacillosis in the dog. *Canadian Journal of Veterinary Research* **58**, 87–92

Foster DM, Gookin JL, Poore MF *et al.* (2004) Outcome of cats with diarrhea and *Tritrichomonas foetus* infection. *Journal of the American Veterinary Medical Association* **225**, 888–892

Joffe DJ and Schlesinger DP (2002) Preliminary assessment of the risk of *Salmonella* infection in dogs fed raw chicken diets. *Canadian Veterinary Journal* **43**, 441–442

Madewell BR, Bea JK, Kraegel SA *et al.* (1999) *Clostridium difficile*: a survey of fecal carriage in cats in a veterinary medical teaching hospital. *Journal of Veterinary Diagnostic Investigation* **11**, 50–54

Marks SL, Kather EJ, Kass PH and Melli AC (2002) Genotypic and phenotypic characterization of *Clostridium perfringens* and *Clostridium difficile* in diarrheic and healthy dogs. *Journal of Veterinary Internal Medicine* **16**, 533–540

Maunder CL, Reynolds ZF, Peacock L *et al.* (2016) *Campylobacter* species and neutrophilic inflammatory bowel disease in cats. *Journal of Veterinary Internal Medicine* **30**, 996–1001

Meer RR and Songer JG (1997) Multiplex polymerase chain reaction assay for genotyping *Clostridium perfringens*. *American Journal of Veterinary Research* **58**, 702–705

Paoloni MC, Penninck DG and Moore AS (2002) Ultrasonographic and clinicopathologic findings in 21 dogs with intestinal adenocarcinoma. *Veterinary Radiology and Ultrasound* **43**, 562–567

Pospischil A, Mainil JG, Baljer G and Moon HW (1987) Attaching and effacing bacteria in the intestines of calves and cats with diarrhea. *Veterinary Pathology* **24**, 330–334

Prada J, Baljer G, De Rycke J *et al.* (1991) Characteristics of alpha-hemolytic strains of *Escherichia coli* isolated from dogs with gastroenteritis. *Veterinary Microbiology* **29**, 59–73

Reagan KL, Marks SL, Pesavento PAJ *et al.* (2019) Successful management of 3 dogs with colonic pythiosis using itraconazole, terbinafine, and prednisone. *Journal of Veterinary Internal Medicine* **33**, 1434–1439

Riley TV, Adams JE, O'Neill GL and Bowman RA (1991) Gastrointestinal carriage of *Clostridium difficile* in cats and dogs attending veterinary clinics. *Epidemiology and Infection* **107**, 659–665

Struble AL, Tang YJ, Kass PH *et al.* (1994) Fecal shedding of *Clostridium difficile* in dogs: a period prevalence survey in a veterinary medical teaching hospital. *Journal of Veterinary Diagnostic Investigation* **6**, 342–347

Turk J, Maddox C, Fales W *et al.* (1998) Examination for heat-labile, heat-stable, and Shiga-like toxins and for the *eaeA* gene in *Escherichia coli* isolates obtained from dogs dying with diarrhea: 122 cases (1992–1996). *Journal of the American Veterinary Medical Association* **212**, 1735–1736

Van den Steen N, Berlato D, Polton G *et al.* (2012) Rectal lymphoma in 11 dogs: a retrospective study. *Journal of Small Animal Practice* **53**, 586–591

Weese JS, Staempfli HR, Prescott JF *et al.* (2001) The roles of *Clostridium difficile* and enterotoxigenic *Clostridium perfringens* in diarrhea in dogs. *Journal of Veterinary Internal Medicine* **15**, 374–378

Williams J and Niles J (2015) *BSAVA Manual of Canine and Feline Abdominal Surgery, 2nd edn.* BSAVA Publications, Gloucester

Chapter 36

Exocrine pancreas

David A. Williams

Secretion of digestive enzymes is the major function of the exocrine pancreas. Normally, the pancreas very effectively protects itself against autodigestion by several mechanisms, including synthesis, storage and secretion of potentially damaging enzymes as inactive zymogens, which are normally only activated after secretion into the small intestinal lumen. The pancreas also produces an enzyme inhibitor, pancreatic secretory trypsin inhibitor (PSTI), which protects it against the harmful effects of trace amounts of intrapancreatic enzyme activation. However, when these protective mechanisms are disrupted pancreatitis can develop. This can range from an acute, severe, life-threatening condition to a chronic process that may remain subclinical until approximately 90% of the exocrine tissue has been destroyed, when exocrine pancreatic insufficiency (EPI) may develop because of inadequate digestive enzyme secretion (Figure 36.1).

Enzymes secreted as inactive zymogens	
Trypsinogen	Trypsin
Chymotrypsinogen	Chymotrypsin
Proelastase	Elastase
Procarboxypeptidase	Carboxypeptidase
Prophospholipase A₂	Phospholipase A₂
Coenzyme	
Procolipase	Colipase
Enzymes	
α-Amylase	
Pancreatic lipase	
Inhibitor	
Antibacterial factors	
• Various antimicrobial peptides	
Pancreatic secretory trypsin inhibitor	

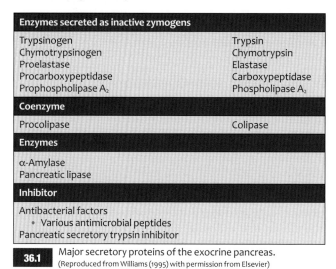

36.1 Major secretory proteins of the exocrine pancreas. (Reproduced from Williams (1995) with permission from Elsevier)

Anatomy, biochemistry and physiology

The pancreas of dogs and cats consists primarily of right and left lobes closely associated with the duodenum and stomach, respectively, with a small central body adjacent to the portal vein where the lobes join (Figure 36.2). While there is individual variation, in dogs there are generally two ducts, one of which opens adjacent to the common bile duct on the major duodenal papilla, the other on the minor

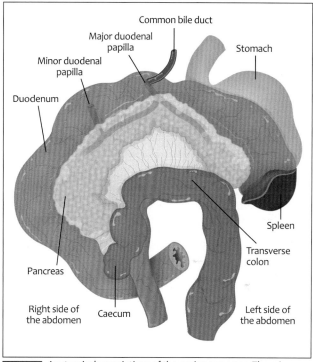

36.2 Anatomical associations of the canine pancreas. There is major variation between individual dogs in the anatomy and degree of anastomosis of the two subdivisions of the duct system.

duodenal papilla a few centimetres distal to the major duodenal papilla. The duct systems usually intercommunicate within the gland. In some dogs, only the duct opening on the minor duodenal papilla is present. In the majority of cats, only a single duct is present and it fuses with the bile duct before opening on the major duodenal papilla.

The pancreatic acinar cells secrete the digestive enzymes into the branching duct system, the proximal lining of which secretes bicarbonate-rich fluid and intrinsic factor. The endocrine pancreatic tissue in the islets of Langerhans accounts for only 1–2% of the pancreas.

Nervous and hormonal mechanisms mediate the secretion of digestive enzymes in response to a meal, and in dogs and cats the endocrine mechanisms are probably of particular importance. Secretin and cholecystokinin are released into the blood from the proximal small intestine when acidified partly digested food is emptied from the stomach into the duodenum, and they stimulate the secretion of bicarbonate-rich and enzyme-rich components of pancreatic juice, respectively. Traces of pancreatic enzymes are present in the blood of normal, healthy animals, and assays for these enzymes in serum or plasma are clinically useful in the diagnosis of pancreatic disease.

Nodular hyperplasia

Nodular pancreatic hyperplasia occurs quite frequently in older cats and dogs. Disseminated small nodules can be found throughout the exocrine portion of the pancreas. Pancreatic nodular hyperplasia can be differentiated from pancreatic adenomas by the absence of a capsule. Nodular hyperplasia does not lead to functional changes, does not cause any clinical signs, and is usually diagnosed incidentally at necropsy.

Pancreatitis

Acute pancreatitis refers to inflammation of the pancreas with a sudden onset and little or no permanent pathological change after recovery. Chronic pancreatitis is a continuing inflammatory disease characterized by irreversible morphological change (fibrosis and atrophy), and it may lead to permanent impairment of function. Both acute and chronic pancreatitis may be further subdivided based on aetiology, which is unfortunately usually unknown, and severity.

Complications of both types may include fluid accumulations around the inflamed pancreas:

- **Pseudocyst** (a collection of sterile pancreatic juice enclosed by fibrous or granulation tissue)
- **Localized necrosis**
- **Infected necrosis** (very rare) from which bacteria can be cultured
- **Pancreatic abscess** (a circumscribed collection of pus, usually in proximity to the pancreas, containing little or no pancreatic necrosis).

When examined at exploratory laparotomy or post mortem, an affected pancreas is often oedematous, swollen and soft, and there may be fibrinous adhesions to adjacent organs. Serosanguinous fluid may be free in the abdomen. Severely affected areas of pancreas may be liquefied, and pseudocysts may have formed. Haemorrhages may be present in the omentum and in the pancreas, and there are often chalky areas of abdominal fat necrosis (Figure 36.3). Histologically, there is extensive multifocal infiltration by neutrophils and varying degrees of haemorrhage, necrosis, oedema and vessel thrombosis.

If an initial acute episode of pancreatitis is not fatal, there may be complete resolution or, alternatively, the inflammatory process may smoulder continuously but asymptomatically. Extensive destruction of pancreatic tissue may reduce the gland to a few distorted lobules adjacent to where the ducts enter the duodenum (Figure 36.4) before clinical signs of EPI become evident.

While acute necrotizing pancreatitis similar to that seen in dogs does occur in cats, a histologically distinct suppurative form has been described. However, chronic mild interstitial pancreatitis characterized by inflammation of interstitial tissue, often associated with the ducts, is the type of pancreatic inflammation most commonly reported in cats. This latter type of pancreatitis is usually accompanied by subnormal serum cobalamin or other evidence of idiopathic chronic enteritis and also, much less commonly, by cholangitis in a syndrome that has been termed 'triaditis'.

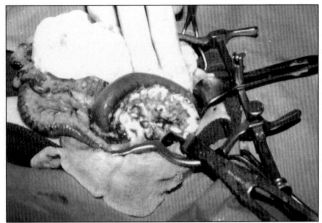

36.3 Acute pancreatitis in a cat. The pancreas is swollen and oedematous, and areas of haemorrhage and chalky fat necrosis are visible in the pancreatic parenchyma and adjacent mesentery.
(Courtesy of Dr Steve Holloway)

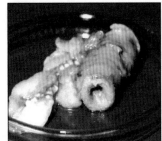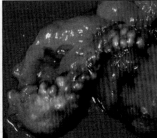

36.4 Chronic pancreatitis observed at post-mortem examination of an old dog with a prior history of several bouts of severe acute pancreatitis. Acinar cells were restricted to a few residual nodular areas of relatively normal-looking tissue adjacent to a segment of duodenum. The pancreatic pathology was not associated with any clinical signs in the 2-year period between the bouts of pancreatitis and subsequent euthanasia for an unrelated reason; during this time, serum trypsin-like immunoreactivity had fluctuated at subnormal concentrations between 2.8–3.9 μg/l, but fell short of the 2.5 μg/l value considered diagnostic for exocrine pancreatic insufficiency.

Aetiology and pathophysiology

It is generally believed that pancreatitis develops when there is activation of digestive enzymes within the gland, triggering the release of numerous inflammatory mediators and free radicals that are also important in the progression of pancreatitis. Plasma α-macroglobulins and α_1-proteinase inhibitor are both vital in protecting against the otherwise fatal effects of proteolytic enzymes in the vascular space. Once these defences are overwhelmed, affected animals may die rapidly from disseminated intravascular coagulation and shock, as the free proteases activate the kinin, coagulation, fibrinolytic and complement cascade systems (Figure 36.5).

The inciting cause of pancreatitis in dogs and cats is usually unknown, but the following potential causes and risk factors should be considered.

Severity	Acute pancreatitis	Chronic pancreatitis
Mild	No multisystem failure; uncomplicated recovery	Minimal morphological change; subclinical loss of exocrine function
Severe	Multisystem failure; complications (e.g. pseudocyst, abscess)	Severe morphological damage; clinical exocrine pancreatic insufficiency or diabetes mellitus

36.5 Classification of pancreatitis.
(Reproduced from Williams (1995) with permission from Elsevier)

Nutrition

It has been reported that pancreatitis is more prevalent in obese dogs, but it is commonly seen in many dogs and cats of normal or low bodyweight. Low protein/high fat content diets may induce pancreatitis, and pancreatitis is more severe when induced in dogs fed a high fat content diet and less severe when induced in lean dogs. There are anecdotal reports that spontaneous pancreatitis in dogs often develops following a fatty meal. Malnutrition has also been reported to cause pancreatic inflammation in human patients, and pancreatitis can follow re-feeding after a prolonged fast. Diets containing unbalanced concentrations of amino acids may also induce pancreatitis in dogs and cats.

Hypertriglyceridaemia

Hyperlipidaemia, often grossly apparent, is common in dogs with acute pancreatitis and may develop from abdominal fat necrosis, or may be a cause of the disease in some cases. The high prevalence of pancreatitis observed in Miniature Schnauzers may be related to the idiopathic hypertriglyceridaemia that is so common in that breed. There does not seem to be any relationship between lipid abnormalities and pancreatitis in cats.

Hereditary factors

Hereditary pancreatitis is well documented in human beings, and several contributory mutations of trypsinogen and PSTI have been identified. Variants of these molecules have also been reported in dogs, but their clinical significance is not yet clear. However, Miniature Schnauzers, Yorkshire Terriers and other terriers, Boxers, Cocker Spaniels and other spaniels are among the breeds often said to be over-represented.

Drugs, toxins and hypercalcaemia

More than 50 drugs and drug classes have been implicated as a cause of pancreatitis in human beings, although absolute proof of a causal relationship is often lacking. Suspect drugs that are also commonly used in veterinary medicine include L-asparaginase, azathioprine, phenobarbital, furosemide, potassium bromide, salicylates, sulphonamides, tetracyclines, thiazide diuretics and vinca alkaloids. Contrary to former belief, corticosteroids are generally now not thought to be a risk factor for inducing pancreatitis, although subclinical pancreatitis may be more common in dogs with spontaneous hyperadrenocorticism than previously thought.

Hyperstimulation of pancreatic secretion by cholinesterase inhibitor insecticides, cholinergic agonists, scorpion venom and both spontaneous and iatrogenic hypercalcaemia may induce pancreatitis. Zinc toxicosis has also been reported to cause pancreatitis in dogs.

Pancreatic ischaemia and hypoxia

Experimental and clinical reports have indicated that ischaemia is very important in the pathogenesis of acute pancreatitis, either as a primary cause or as an exacerbating influence. Pancreatic ischaemia may develop during shock, severe acute anaemia (e.g. post haemolysis) or dehydration (e.g. post high small intestinal obstruction), secondary to hypotension during general anaesthesia, or during temporary occlusion of venous outflow during surgical manipulation in the cranial abdomen; this may explain some instances of postoperative pancreatitis when areas remote from the pancreas have undergone surgery.

Pancreatic trauma, duct obstruction and duodenal/biliary reflux

Surgical manipulation and blunt abdominal trauma are potential causes of pancreatitis but reports of pancreatitis following such insults are rare. Pancreatitis following pancreatic biopsy is extremely rare, and is also uncommon following resection of pancreatic neoplasms. Experimental obstruction of the pancreatic ducts produces only atrophy and fibrosis, although inflammation and oedema may also develop when pancreatic secretion is stimulated. Reflux of duodenal juice or bile through a compromised papilla is probably rare but could exacerbate pancreatitis. Clinical conditions that may uncommonly lead to partial or complete obstruction of the pancreatic ducts include biliary calculi, sphincter spasm, oedema of the duct or duodenal wall, neoplastic conditions, parasites, trauma, duodenal foreign bodies and surgical interference. Congenital anomalies of the pancreatic duct system may predispose to pancreatitis in humans, and similar mechanisms may occur in the dog but have not been documented.

Miscellaneous aetiologies

Viral, mycoplasma, and parasitic infections may be associated with pancreatitis, although this is usually recognized as part of a more generalized disease process. Pancreatitis has been recognized as a potential complication of babesiosis and idiopathic immune-mediated haemolytic anaemia, perhaps as a consequence of anaemia and haemagglutination causing pancreatic ischaemia. There is little evidence that bacterial infection plays a role in the development of pancreatitis in dogs or cats, but concomitant bacterial infection does increase the severity of experimental pancreatitis. Pancreatitis may occur in association with end-stage renal failure, but this is rare; it is likely that renal failure secondary to acute pancreatitis is encountered more frequently. Acute pancreatitis has been observed in patients with liver disease, perhaps reflecting vascular compromise secondary to coagulation abnormalities, accumulation of toxins (endotoxins, bile acids) secondary to impaired liver function, response to a common initial cause, or reaction to drugs given in an attempt to manage the hepatic failure. Finally, immune-mediated mechanisms that respond to glucocorticoid therapy have been incriminated in some patients with pancreatitis, and autoimmune disease causing chronic pancreatitis in Cocker Spaniels has been postulated.

Diagnosis
History and clinical signs

Dogs and cats with acute pancreatitis are usually presented because of lethargy, anorexia and vomiting; diarrhoea develops in some patients. Severe acute disease may be associated with shock and collapse, while other cases may have a history of less dramatic signs extending over several weeks. Signs of pain may be elicited by abdominal palpation. A cranial abdominal mass is palpable in some cases and occasionally there is mild ascites. Most affected animals are mildly to moderately dehydrated and febrile. Uncommon systemic complications of pancreatitis that may be apparent on physical examination include jaundice, respiratory distress, bleeding disorders and cardiac arrhythmias. While patients of any age may develop pancreatitis, affected animals are usually middle-aged or older. Severity varies widely and, in some patients, pancreatitis is subclinical. Pancreatitis should be suspected in any cat that stops eating and is not behaving normally, even if only for a day or two, if no other obvious explanation is apparent.

Diagnostic imaging

Definitive radiographic evidence of pancreatitis is rarely seen, the most common finding being a somewhat subjective loss of visceral detail ('ground glass appearance') in the cranial abdomen (see Chapter 3). However, abdominal radiographs may provide evidence to rule in or rule out alternative diagnoses. Classical abnormalities reported with pancreatitis include:

- Increased density
- Diminished contrast and granularity in the right cranial abdomen
- Displacement of the stomach to the left
- Widening of the angle between the pyloric antrum and the proximal duodenum
- Displacement of the descending duodenum to the right
- Presence of a mass medial to the descending duodenum
- Static gas pattern in or thickened walls of the descending duodenum
- Static gas pattern in or caudal displacement of the transverse colon
- Gastric distension suggestive of gastric outflow obstruction
- Delayed passage of barium through the stomach and duodenum, with corrugation of the duodenal wall indicating abnormal peristalsis.

Abdominal ultrasonography is highly specific for pancreatitis when stringent criteria are applied, with a sensitivity of up to approximately 70% in dogs and 30% in cats. Enlargement of the pancreas and/or localized peritoneal effusion, pain on applying pressure with the probe and changes in echogenicity are supportive observations. Decreased echogenicity indicates pancreatic necrosis, which is often associated with hyperechogenicity in the peripancreatic region. Hyperechogenicity of the pancreatic parenchyma itself indicates pancreatic fibrosis and can be seen in cases of chronic pancreatitis. Pancreatic duct dilatation has also been reported. Serial examinations are particularly useful for identification and management of pancreatic complications, such as pancreatic pseudocyst or abscess associated with cystic masses.

Laboratory tests

Results of a complete blood count, serum biochemical profile and urinalysis are non-specific and highly variable, reflecting the variation in disease severity and duration. Anaemia, haemoconcentration, leucocytosis, azotaemia (usually pre-renal), increased liver enzyme activities (especially alkaline phosphatase) and hyperbilirubinaemia, hyper- or hypoglycaemia, hypoalbuminaemia, hypertriglyceridaemia, hypercholesterolaemia, hypokalaemia, hypochloraemia and hyponatraemia have all been reported. Hypocalcaemia is commonly associated with hypoalbuminaemia, and low ionized calcium in cats has been reported to be a poor prognostic finding.

The advent of sensitive and specific immunoassays for canine and feline pancreatic lipases (cPL and fPL, respectively) has greatly facilitated the accurate diagnosis of pancreatitis in these species. These species-specific assays detect only digestive lipases made by the acinar cells of the pancreas and are generally held to be the most specific and sensitive tests for pancreatitis. Pancreatic lipase testing is available as a quantitative ELISA from IDEXX reference laboratories (Spec PL) and a quantitative in-hospital format (SNAP® PL) that indicates normal or above normal serum concentrations. A negative SNAP® test result makes pancreatitis very unlikely; it is recommended that a positive test result is followed up by a quantitative Spec PL determination to confirm and determine the magnitude of the increased serum concentration. Serum trypsin-like immunoreactivity (cTLI and fTLI) assays similarly detect pancreas-specific trypsinogen, but the latter has a very short half-life and is excreted by renal filtration, and these assays are both less sensitive and less specific for diagnosis of pancreatitis than PL assays. Classical catalytic assays for serum amylase and lipase activities lack both sensitivity and specificity and are not recommended. Recently, newer catalytic assays for the measurement of serum lipase activity have been marketed with claims that they have comparative diagnostic utility to the measurement of serum PL concentration. While these assays utilize substrates other than the traditional 1,2 diglyceride, such as triolein or 1,2-o-dilauryl-rac-glycero glutaric acid-(6' methyl resorufin)-ester (DGGR), neither of these substrates is specific for the measurement of pancreatic lipase and both assays detect other lipases that do not originate from the exocrine pancreas. If increased lipase activities are found using a catalytic assay, then a follow-up immunoassay of cPL or fPL is warranted. Caution should be exercised when utilizing commercial laboratories claiming to offer reliable immunoassays for cPL and fPL that those methods have been adequately validated; results from some laboratories are simply not reliable, and some recently introduced in-house assays have been shown to have poor reproducibility. Finally, it should also be noted that while not species-specific, catalytic assays are also often subject to interference from lipaemia, haemolysis and icterus, whereas immunoassays are not. Evaluation of the entire clinical picture in patients with increased serum PL, particularly if supported by ultrasonographic pancreatic abnormalities, will in many instances give a high degree of confidence in the diagnosis. If gross or histopathological confirmation of the diagnosis is required, or the possibility of other abdominal disease needs to be eliminated, it is important to ensure that the cardiovascular, fluid and electrolyte status is stable prior to general anaesthesia and surgical exploration of the abdomen.

Treatment

The treatment of acute pancreatitis involves correction and maintenance of fluid and electrolyte balances, while the underlying inciting cause, if known, is rectified. The traditional wisdom of withholding food to 'rest' the pancreas is now discounted unless vomiting is intractable, and in anorexic patients, particularly cats, enteral tube feeding is considered desirable to maintain enteric mucosal integrity and, in cats, to prevent hepatic lipidosis.

Many mild cases of pancreatitis are self-limiting and spontaneously improve after 1 or 2 days of basic supportive therapy. Other patients require aggressive fluid therapy over several days to maintain hydration and electrolyte balance. Care should be taken to avoid both hypokalaemia and pre-renal azotaemia, and, in rare cases, calcium supplementation may be needed to treat signs of hypocalcaemia.

Analgesic therapy should be given to provide relief of pain, even if obvious signs of pain are not apparent. Options include pethidine (meperidine) hydrochloride, buprenorphine, fentanyl, morphine, lidocaine or bupivicaine, which may be administered orally, subcutaneously, transdermally, by constant rate intravenous infusion or by epidural or intraperitoneal injection, either alone or in combination depending upon local availability, convenience and expense. Non-steroidal anti-inflammatory drugs are probably best avoided, since some have been implicated as causes of pancreatitis and they are less potent than the drugs mentioned above. Any hyperglycaemia is often mild and transient but, in some cases, diabetes mellitus may develop and require treatment with insulin. Respiratory distress, neurological problems, cardiovascular abnormalities, bleeding disorders, and acute kidney injury are all poor prognostic indicators. Attempts should be made to manage these complications by appropriate supportive measures (see the *BSAVA Manual of Canine and Feline Emergency and Critical Care*).

Antiemetic treatment with maropitant is often helpful and may have additional benefits of providing some analgesia and reducing nausea; this may be particularly important for cats, in which restoring appetite to avoid other complications, such as hepatic lipidosis, is so important. Other or additional antiemetics (5-HT$_3$ antagonists (ondansetron), dopamine antagonists (metoclopramide)) are sometimes required to reduce intractable vomiting in dogs. Gastric and upper intestinal ileus can be profound, and impaired gastric emptying may exacerbate abdominal discomfort. Prokinetics (metaclopramide, erythromycin, cisapride and ranitidine) and aspiration of gastric contents via nasogastric tube are helpful in some patients with distended stomachs.

Transfusion of plasma or whole blood to replace α-macroglobulins may be life-saving in patients with severe disease and has the additional benefit of helping to maintain plasma albumin and oncotic pressure. Albumin is probably beneficial in pancreatitis because of its oncotic properties which not only help maintain blood volume and prevent pancreatic ischaemia, but also limit pancreatic oedema formation. While less expensive, other colloids will expand plasma volume but may aggravate bleeding tendencies and contain no protease inhibitor. Hypertonic saline–dextran 70 combinations may help maintain cardiac function without massive fluid administration and minimize the risk of pulmonary oedema. Hyperoncotic ultra-high molecular weight dextran solutions have been shown to reduce trypsinogen activation, prevent acinar necrosis and lower mortality in experimental pancreatitis, perhaps by promoting pancreatic microcirculation (for further information regarding colloid use, including potential serious adverse effects, see Chapter 27).

In contrast to human beings, cats and dogs with pancreatitis rarely have infectious complications, and prophylactic antibiotic therapy would appear to be of minimal benefit. For cases in which infectious complications are identified, therapy should be based on culture and sensitivity testing; trimethoprim/sulphonamide, enrofloxacin, ciprofloxacin, metronidazole, clindamycin and cefotaxime penetrate well into the canine pancreas.

Historically, caution has been recommended regarding administration of corticosteroids to severely ill animals with pancreatitis, since they may impair removal of activated pancreatic enzymes from the blood and also induce a prothrombotic state. However, a recent study of 65 dogs with acute pancreatitis provided evidence that initial treatment with prednisolone at 1 mg/kg/day resulted in earlier reductions in plasma C-reactive protein concentration and earlier improvement of clinical signs compared to a control group that did not receive the drug. There was no difference in mortality during hospitalization between the groups, but at 1 month following diagnosis, survival was 89% in the treated group, but only 59% in the control group. These preliminary findings of improved outcome

and no adverse effects will hopefully be extended in future studies but would seem to support routine administration of prednisolone to canine patients with acute pancreatitis.

Nasogastric suctioning of gastric secretions and use of antacids, H$_2$-receptor blockers or proton pump inhibitors have been recommended in order to indirectly inhibit pancreatic secretion and mitigate any gastric irritation; however, none of these methods has been consistently shown to be effective and their value has largely been discounted. Attempts to 'rest' the pancreas using direct inhibitors of secretion, such as atropine, acetazolamide, glucagon and calcitonin, have not proved to be effective. Indeed, secretin, the hormone that naturally stimulates pancreatic secretion, was beneficial in a rat model of pancreatitis when given at a high dose intravenously.

Somatostatin and its analogues (e.g. octreotide) may reduce complications and improve survival in human patients but there is insufficient evidence to recommend their routine use in cats and dogs. Infusion of dopamine at a dose that stimulates both dopaminergic and β-adrenergic receptors (5 μg/kg/min i.v.) is helpful in reducing severity and progression of some feline models of pancreatitis; it is thought that the beneficial effect of dopamine is related to the reduction of microvascular permeability rather than to the promotion of pancreatic blood flow.

Administration of a variety of naturally occurring and synthetic enzyme inhibitors with selective actions against individual pancreatic digestive enzymes, as well as free-radical scavengers, such as selenium, has shown promise in experimental studies, but their value remains to be demonstrated in clinical trials. Other novel approaches to ameliorate local and systemic inflammatory responses include experimental drugs that modify cytokine expression and neutrophil activity. Such approaches hold promise to reduce severity of complications and enhance recovery.

The use of peritoneal dialysis to remove toxic material accumulated in the peritoneal cavity is beneficial experimentally and is thought by many to be useful in human patients, and so may be of value in some veterinary patients with peritoneal effusions. Certainly, in those patients in which acute pancreatitis is confirmed at exploratory laparotomy, removal of as much free fluid as possible followed by abdominal lavage is advisable. Reports of surgical intervention to resect or debride and drain affected areas are not favourable, although in one report of six dogs with fibrotic biliary obstructive masses, cholecystoduodenostomy was followed by recovery. However, many patients that develop obstructive jaundice in association with acute pancreatitis recover spontaneously over 2 or 3 weeks with conventional supportive care alone.

Small amounts of water should be offered after the patient has stopped vomiting. If there is no recurrence of clinical signs, food may be gradually reintroduced. The diet should have a high carbohydrate content (rice, pasta, potatoes or low-fat commercial food), since protein and fat are more potent stimulants of pancreatic secretion and may perhaps be more likely to promote a relapse. If there is continued improvement, gradual transition to a low fat content maintenance diet is recommended. Another period of supportive care should be instituted if signs of pancreatitis recur. While the prognosis is poor for those patients that repeatedly refuse or cannot tolerate food, enteral feeding by tube may be beneficial. Total parenteral nutrition has been carried out in patients that do not tolerate enteral feeding, but this is complex and expensive, and reported outcomes are very poor.

Treatment of complications

Utilization of ultrasonographic imaging has contributed to increased recognition of pancreatic masses as complications in patients with pancreatitis.

Pancreatic pseudocysts: These have been described in dogs and cats. Clinical signs are those associated with pancreatitis and the significance of such lesions is unclear. On abdominal ultrasonography, a cystic structure in close proximity to the pancreas can be identified. Transabdominal ultrasound-guided aspiration of the pseudocyst is relatively safe and should be attempted for diagnostic and therapeutic purposes. Fluid from pancreatic pseudocysts is of low cellularity and is not inflammatory in nature. Pancreatic pseudocysts can be treated medically or surgically. Medical management of pancreatic pseudocysts involves ultrasound-guided percutaneous aspiration and close monitoring of the size of the pseudocyst. Surgical correction can involve extirpation of the pseudocyst, external drainage or internal drainage; internal drainage is the preferred method in human patients. Surgical intervention should be considered in cases in which clinical signs persist and the size of the pseudocyst does not decrease significantly over time.

Pancreatic abscess: This is a less common potential complication of pancreatitis, and bacterial infection is only rarely present. Associated clinical signs and laboratory abnormalities are non-specific and overlap with those of pancreatitis, but may include vomiting, lethergy, abdominal pain, anorexia, fever, diarrhoea and dehydration. In some patients, a mass in the cranial abdomen can be identified upon abdominal palpation. Surgical drainage combined with aggressive antimicrobial therapy is the treatment of choice in human patients with pancreatic abscess. However, in one report only five of nine dogs survived the immediate postsurgical period. Thus, given the mixed results, risks, difficulties and expense associated with anaesthesia, surgery and postoperative care, surgical intervention is best avoided unless there is clear evidence of an enlarging mass and/or sepsis in a patient that is not responding well to medical therapy. Antimicrobial therapy is of questionable value unless an organism is identified upon bacterial culture.

Long-term therapy

In many patients with a single episode of pancreatitis, the only long-term management recommended is to avoid feeding high-fat meals. In other patients, repeated bouts of pancreatitis occur, and feeding a fat-restricted diet permanently should be considered. In some patients hypertriglyceridaemia may need to be controlled pharmacologically if dietary therapy fails to normalize triglyceride concentrations. Despite all efforts, some animals, especially cats, experience recurrent clinical signs with laboratory evidence of ongoing chronic (or recurrent acute) disease. Trial therapy with a corticosteroid (oral prednisolone at an initial dose of 1 mg/kg q12–24h for 1 week in cats, tapering to 0.5 mg/kg every other day as needed) is warranted. Equivalent strategies in dogs are also effective in some cases. Adverse responses are rare and if ineffective after a month or so, the trial can be discontinued.

Some reports have indicated that oral pancreatic enzyme supplements decrease the abdominal pain and discomfort that accompanies chronic pancreatitis in human beings. There is no evidence that they are of similar value in dogs or cats, but a trial period of enzyme therapy may be warranted in individuals with chronic signs and other evidence of pancreatitis that have not responded to other treatments, including corticosteroids.

Prognosis

Pancreatitis is unpredictable and varies widely in severity, and it is difficult to give a prognosis even when a diagnosis is definitively established. Life-threatening signs accompanying acute pancreatitis are sometimes followed by death despite aggressive supportive measures, but some dogs recover fully following an isolated severe episode. In other cases, relatively mild pancreatitis persists despite all therapy and the patient either dies from an acute, severe exacerbation of the disease, or is euthanased because of failure to recover or long-term cost. It should be emphasized, though, that most patients with pancreatitis, given supportive care, recover spontaneously after a single episode and do well in the long term as long as potential precipitating causes are avoided.

Exocrine pancreatic insufficiency

Progressive loss of pancreatic acinar cells ultimately leads to malabsorption due to inadequate production of digestive enzymes. The functional reserve of the pancreas is considerable, however, and signs of EPI do not occur until most of the exocrine tissue has been lost. Although pancreatic enzymes perform essential digestive functions, alternative pathways of digestion for some nutrients do exist. Following experimental exclusion of pancreatic secretion from the intestine, dogs can still absorb up to 63% of ingested protein and 84% of ingested fat. This residual enzyme activity probably originates from gastric lipases and pepsins, from intestinal mucosal esterases and peptidases and, in young animals, from bile salt-activated lipase in milk. Nonetheless, when exocrine pancreatic function is severely impaired, these alternative routes of digestion are inadequate, and clinical signs of malabsorption occur. Feline EPI is much less common than EPI in dogs, but increased utilization of a reliable test for fTLI has shown the disease to be more prevalent than previously realized.

Aetiology
Pancreatic acinar atrophy

Spontaneous development of pancreatic acinar atrophy (PAA) in previously healthy adult animals appears to be surprisingly common in dogs and is the most common cause of EPI (Figure 36.6). Similar conditions occur sporadically in other species, including cats.

Recent studies have revealed that in German Shepherd Dogs and Rough Collies PAA is preceded by subclinical lymphocytic pancreatitis that leads to acinar cell destruction. Smouldering subclinical EPI is occasionally identified by observation or by measurement of mildly to moderately subnormal serum cTLI in dogs with lymphocytic pancreatitis that has not yet progressed to frank PAA. What triggers this inflammatory process is not known; however, since islet cells are spared, these patients do not develop diabetes mellitus.

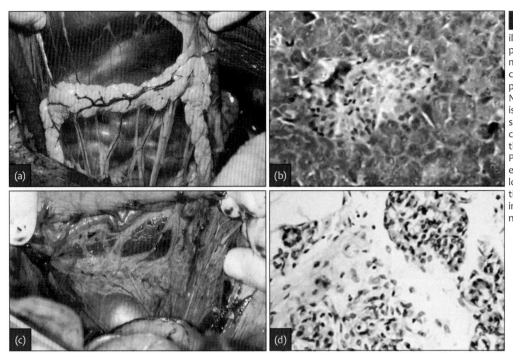

36.6 (a) Gross and (b) microscopic images illustrating normal canine pancreas. (c) Gross and (d) microscopic images illustrating canine pancreas affected by pancreatic acinar atrophy (PAA). Normal pancreas contains small islands of endocrine tissue that secrete hormones, surrounded by copious amounts of exocrine tissue that secretes digestive enzymes. In PAA, the exocrine cells have essentially disappeared, leaving a loose collection of endocrine tissue, so while digestion is severely impaired, diabetes mellitus does not develop.

Chronic pancreatitis

While chronic pancreatitis resulting in progressive destruction of pancreatic tissue is a common cause of EPI in human beings and cats, this is a relatively rare cause of EPI in dogs. Animals with EPI and coexistent diabetes mellitus probably have chronic pancreatitis, since pancreatic inflammation is likely to damage both endocrine and exocrine tissue, in contrast to the selective acinar cell damage in PAA.

Hypoplasia/aplasia and congenital abnormalities

Deficiencies of individual pancreatic digestive enzymes or of intestinal enteropeptidase have not been well documented in dogs or cats, but probably occur very rarely. A familial congenital absence of acinar cells, but not islet cells, has been described in English Setters. Occasionally, young dogs, especially Greyhounds, are seen to have signs of EPI and sometimes diabetes mellitus from a very early age, and congenital pancreatic hypoplasia or aplasia may be the underlying cause.

Miscellaneous causes

EPI has been reported as a complication of proximal duodenal resection and cholecystoduodenostomy in cats, reflecting the absence of dual pancreatic ducts in this species, with blockage of pancreatic secretion occurring because of damage to the major duodenal papilla. Blockage of the ducts by flukes may also lead to EPI in cats (see below). Total pancreatectomy will of course also lead to EPI.

Pathophysiology

Nutrient malabsorption in canine EPI does not arise simply because of failure of intraluminal digestion. Morphological changes in the small intestine of some dogs with EPI have been reported, and studies of naturally occurring and experimental EPI in several species have revealed abnormal activities of mucosal enzymes and impaired function, indicated by abnormal transport of sugars, amino acids and fatty acids. Absence of the trophic influence of pancreatic

secretions, lack of pancreatic bacteriocidal secretions leading to small intestinal dysbiosis, and endocrine and nutritional factors may all contribute to this pathology.

Small intestinal mucosa

EPI in several species is associated with reduced degradation of exposed brush border proteins, such as maltase and sucrase, because of decreased pancreatic protease activity within the gut lumen. It has been suggested that accumulation of these brush border membrane proteins may interfere with normal absorption.

Small intestinal microbiota

Small intestinal dysbiosis is common in both untreated and treated dogs with EPI. Depending on the quantity and species of bacteria present, there may be diverse pathophysiological alterations associated with variable clinical signs. Histological changes are rare but may include partial villous atrophy and inflammation (Figure 36.7). However, both intraluminal and mucosal changes may lead to nutrient malabsorption, which can be severe.

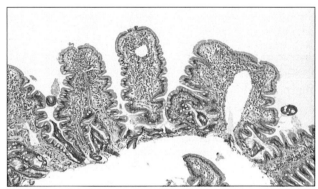

36.7 Partial villous atrophy in a jejunal biopsy specimen from a dog with exocrine pancreatic insufficiency due to pancreatic acinar atrophy. Villi are short and stumpy with a broadened plateau at the extrusion zone, and there is evidence of folding or fusion of villi.
(Reproduced from Williams *et al.* (1987) with permission from the *Journal of the American Veterinary Medical Association*)

Pancreatic regulatory peptides and glucose intolerance

Histopathological examination of pancreatic samples from dogs with PAA reveals almost total atrophy of acinar tissue but plentiful, albeit highly disorganized, islet tissue containing many insulin-, glucagon-, somatostatin- and pancreatic polypeptide-immunoreactive cells. Clinically significant endocrine changes, such as diabetes, are therefore very rare, unless the EPI is secondary to inflammatory destruction of islet cells in end-stage chronic pancreatitis.

Nutritional status

Some patients with EPI suffer from malabsorption for a considerable period before a diagnosis is made. Thus, the clinical and pathophysiological features associated with EPI may in some instances be due to malnutrition rather than EPI *per se*. Malnutrition in rats impairs the capacity to maintain protective mucosal mucin content, and accelerates the development of brush border enzyme abnormalities associated with intestinal dysbiosis.

Mildly to severely subnormal serum cobalamin concentrations are commonly observed in dogs and cats with EPI, and if not present at the time of diagnosis, will almost certainly develop after 1–2 years of treatment. Effective treatment with pancreatic enzymes rarely prevents the development of hypocobalaminaemia and does not rectify it. Deficiencies of pancreatic proteases, pancreatic intrinsic factor and microbial competition for cobalamin could all contribute to cobalamin malabsorption. Intestinal dysfunction due to persistent cobalamin deficiency may be a contributory factor in those patients with EPI and a suboptimal response to enzyme replacement therapy. Cobalamin deficiency might also be responsible for the anorexia reported in some patients with EPI.

Serum tocopherol (vitamin E) concentrations are often severely subnormal in EPI and do not increase in response to treatment, perhaps because treatment does not return fat absorption to normal or because dysbiosis persists. Tocopherol deficiency may cause insidious pathological changes in erythrocyte membranes, smooth muscle, the central nervous system, skeletal muscle and retina.

Subnormal serum concentrations of retinol (vitamin A) have also been observed in dogs with EPI, but no associated signs of deficiency have been reported. However, recent evidence implicating the importance of retinol in modulating immune function suggests that more attention should be given to retinol status in EPI. Vitamin K-responsive coagulopathy does develop in rare patients with EPI, and is seen more often in cats than dogs. There are no data to suggest that vitamin D deficiency is ever encountered in canine or feline EPI.

Diagnosis
History

Dogs and cats with EPI usually have a history of weight loss in the face of a normal or increased appetite. Polyphagia is often severe and owners may complain that dogs ravenously devour all food offered to them and scavenge from waste bins yet, in contrast, some dogs have periods of inappetence. Coprophagia and pica are also common in dogs. Water intake may also increase in some dogs, and in those with chronic pancreatitis causing concurrent diabetes mellitus there may be polydipsia and polyuria. Diarrhoea often accompanies EPI, but can be very variable in character. Most owners report frequent

passage of large volumes of semi-formed faeces, although some patients have intermittent or continuous explosive watery diarrhoea, while in other instances diarrhoea is infrequent and is not considered a problem. Any diarrhoea generally improves or resolves in response to fasting. Feeding a highly digestible 'gastrointestinal' diet or other dietary changes may also decrease or eliminate diarrhoea. There may be a history of vomiting and, commonly, there is marked borborygmus and flatulence, sometimes with episodes of apparent abdominal discomfort. PAA is prevalent in young German Shepherd Dogs, and thus EPI is often initially suspected because of the age and breed of the affected dog. It must be emphasized, however, that even in young German Shepherd Dogs small intestinal disease is more prevalent than EPI and that PAA may occur in a wide variety of breeds at any age. Similarly, most cats with polyphagia, weight loss and diarrhoea are ultimately diagnosed as having small intestinal disease associated with severe cobalamin deficiency; these cases are clinically indistinguishable from those with EPI without appropriate diagnostic testing. Interestingly, it has been reported that more cats with EPI present with anorexia (46%) than with polyphagia (42%).

Clinical signs

Mild to marked weight loss is usually seen in association with EPI in both cats and dogs. Some dogs are very emaciated at presentation, with severe muscle wasting and no palpable body fat and, in extreme cases, dogs may be physically weak due to loss of muscle mass. The hair coat is often in poor condition and some animals may give off a foul odour because of soiling of the coat with fatty faecal material and the passage of excessive flatus. Cats with EPI may exhibit a greasy, wet-looking and generally unkempt hair coat, especially in the perineal region, which may, in part, reflect severe cobalamin deficiency (Figure 36.8).

Laboratory diagnosis

The history and clinical signs of EPI do not distinguish the condition from other causes of malabsorption (see Chapter 34), and while replacement therapy with oral pancreatic enzymes is generally successful, response to treatment is not a reliable diagnostic approach.

In PAA, extreme atrophy of the pancreas is readily observed on gross inspection at either exploratory laparotomy or laparoscopy. In chronic pancreatitis it may be impossible to gauge accurately the amount of residual exocrine pancreatic tissue because of severe adhesions and fibrosis. However, these procedures involve unnecessary anaesthetic and surgical risks, and their use for diagnostic purposes cannot be recommended, given the availability of reliable non-invasive tests.

Routine laboratory test results are generally not helpful in establishing the diagnosis of EPI. Serum alanine aminotransferase activities are sometimes mildly to moderately increased, probably reflecting a non-specific secondary hepatopathy; this usually resolves completely following successful therapy for EPI. Other routine serum biochemical test results are unremarkable, except that triglycerides and cholesterol may be reduced, especially in malnourished patients. Serum protein concentrations are usually normal even when patients are severely malnourished. Lymphopenia and eosinophilia are not uncommon but other laboratory abnormalities should be considered as evidence for additional, or alternative, underlying disorders.

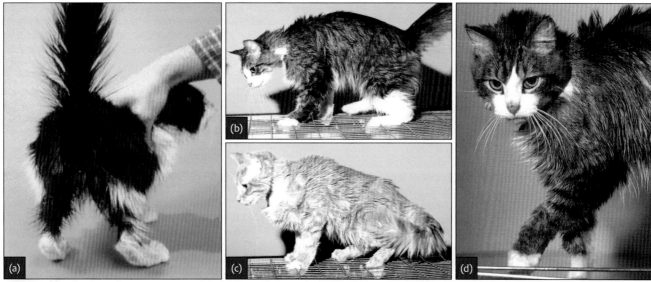

36.8 (a) Unkempt and wet appearance of the haircoat of a cat with exocrine pancreatic insufficiency. This may reflect simple greasy soiling (especially around the perineal region) and/or changes secondary to the severe cobalamin deficiency that is commonly seen in affected cats. (b–d) These three cats show the wet-looking, unkempt hair coat due to cobalamin deficiency.
(Courtesy of Dr Jim Morris)

Canine serum amylase, isoamylases, lipase and phospholipase A_2 activities are normal or minimally reduced in EPI, indicating that non-pancreatic sources of these enzyme activities are clearly present in dogs and cats. The most reliable and widely used test currently available is assay of serum TLI.

Serum trypsin-like immunoreactivity

Trypsinogen is synthesized exclusively by the acinar cells of the pancreas, and measurement of the serum concentration of this zymogen by species-specific immunoassay provides a good indirect index of exocrine pancreatic functional mass in dogs and cats. Serum TLI concentration is both highly sensitive and specific for the diagnosis of EPI, since concentrations are dramatically reduced compared with those in normal animals and those with small intestinal disease (Figure 36.9). Marked reductions in serum TLI (to <2 µg/l in dogs or 8 µg/l in cats) may even precede signs of weight loss or diarrhoea. Utilization of this test is simple in that analysis of a single serum sample obtained after food has been withheld for several hours is all that is required. Serum TLI is very stable and samples can therefore be mailed to an appropriate laboratory for analysis. It is important to remember that there is no cross-reactivity between canine and feline TLI, and that serum fTLI values in normal cats, as well as in cats with EPI, are greater than those in dogs. At the time of writing, reliable assay of serum fTLI is only available from the Gastrointestinal Laboratory at Texas A&M University (http://vetmed.tamu.edu/gilab), but many commercial laboratories will forward samples for analysis internationally, as can individual veterinary surgeons (veterinarians), given the stability of serum TLI even when shipped without refrigeration. Results of fTLI tests run in-house at other laboratories are rarely reliable, and the author is aware of numerous false-positive and false-negative results. With regard to cTLI assays, the situation is better because nearly all laboratories worldwide use a highly reliable automated chemiluminescent method (Immulite, Siemens). While other tests for EPI have been used historically, many give significant proportions of false-negative and false-positive results and their use even as crude 'screening'

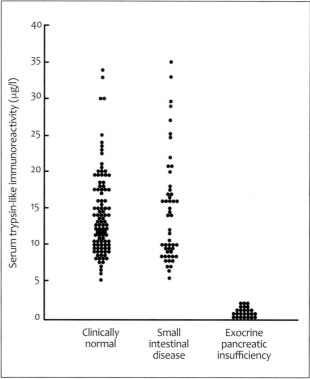

36.9 Serum trypsin-like immunoreactivity in 100 healthy dogs, 50 dogs with small intestinal disease and 25 dogs with exocrine pancreatic insufficiency.
(Reproduced from Williams and Batt (1988) with permission from the *Journal of the American Veterinary Medical Association*)

tests is not recommended. When EPI is suspected in cats or dogs, serum TLI should be assayed. Serum cPL and fPL are not very helpful since, while assays are readily available, some normal dogs have serum concentrations below the lower limit of the assay, and, in both cats and dogs, inflammation of residual pancreas can lead to slightly increased values despite the reduced pancreatic mass; observation of markedly increased serum fPL or cPL does make EPI highly improbable. However, only serum TLI, perhaps because of its very short half-life, accurately reflects the severely reduced pancreatic mass in EPI.

Treatment

Enzyme replacement

Most dogs and cats with EPI can be successfully managed by supplementing each meal with pancreatic enzymes present in commercially available dried pancreatic extracts; generic products are available to purchase online, they are relatively inexpensive and can be shipped internationally to many countries (e.g. www.enzymediane.com). Numerous formulations of these extracts are available (tablets, capsules, powders, granules) and their enzyme contents and bioavailabilities vary. Some preparations are enteric-coated to reduce enzyme inactivation by exposure to gastric acid and pepsins; while this has been shown to be effective for some formulations, some enteric coatings, and tablets in particular, may not be adequately broken down to release active enzymes in the proximal small intestine, leading to treatment failure. Suppliers of enteric-coated preparations should be able to provide data demonstrating that their products are at least as clinically effective and cost-effective as untreated dried pancreatic extract or raw pancreas.

Addition of approximately two teaspoons of powdered porcine or bovine pancreatic extract per 20 kg bodyweight to each meal is generally an effective starting dose. The extract should be mixed with a maintenance food immediately prior to feeding. Two meals a day are usually sufficient to promote weight gain. In uncomplicated cases, diarrhoea, polyphagia and coprophagia often resolve within 4–5 days, but bodyweight may take several weeks or even months to return to normal. It is important to feed more than the calculated requirement of the patient's ideal bodyweight to optimize weight gain. However, bodyweight and body condition should be monitored regularly, as daily calories may need to be increased further to ensure optimal body condition is reached.

As soon as clinical improvement is apparent, owners can determine a minimum effective dose of enzyme supplement that prevents return of clinical signs. This varies slightly between batches of extract and from patient to patient, probably reflecting individual variation in extrapancreatic digestive reserve. Most affected dogs require at least one teaspoonful of pancreatic extract per meal, but lower doses will be adequate in cats and small dogs. One meal per day is sufficient in some dogs, while others continue to require two. If available, fresh chopped raw ox, pig, sheep or other species' pancreas (100–150 g per 20 kg bodyweight), obtained from animals certified as healthy following appropriate post-mortem inspection, may be an inexpensive alternative to dried extract. Fresh pancreas can be stored frozen at −20°C for at least 3 months without loss of enzyme activity.

Measures to increase the effectiveness of enzyme supplementation

While administration of pancreatic enzymes with food is generally successful, only a small proportion of the administered enzymes is delivered functionally intact to the small intestine, and fat absorption does not return to normal. With the exception of some enteric-coated preparations, efforts to increase the effectiveness of enzyme supplementation by pre-incubation of enzymes with food prior to feeding, supplementation with bile salts and neutralization or inhibition of secretion of gastric acid have not proved effective. New preparations containing acid-resistant fungal or gastric lipases may one day prove to be effective and economical. Such new preparations are unlikely to help in the management of patients with suboptimal weight gain, since they rarely improve after increasing the dose of enzymes over that recommended above, suggesting that factors other than enzyme delivery to the small intestine are involved.

Dietary modification

Fat absorption does not return to normal despite appropriate enzyme therapy. Patients appear to compensate by eating slightly more than usual and, as with any individual, it is necessary to regulate the amount of food given in order to maintain ideal bodyweight. In order to overcome residual digestive deficits, the feeding of a highly digestible, low-fibre diet may be beneficial. Some types of dietary fibre impair pancreatic enzyme activity *in vitro* and high-fibre diets probably should be avoided. Low-fat diets merely impair caloric uptake and should not be fed. A non-blinded clinical study found that owners considered that their dogs generally did better (reduced flatulence and borborygmi, decreased faecal volume and frequency of defecation) when fed a commercial highly digestible diet compared with previously fed home-cooked or regular maintenance diets, but there was no difference in appetite, drinking, colour or consistency of faeces, or in coprophagy. Results of experimental studies to evaluate highly digestible diets have shown consistent reductions in faecal weight, but have not shown consistent benefit with regard to fat digestibility. Highly digestible commercial therapeutic gastrointestinal diets, particularly if they contain readily hydrolysed protein and medium-chain triglycerides, may be of value in promoting caloric uptake in those dogs with EPI that do not regain normal bodyweight.

Vitamin supplementation

Dogs and cats with EPI may have severely subnormal concentrations of serum cobalamin and tocopherol (vitamin E). Serum concentrations of these vitamins rarely normalize without supplementation, and may even decrease following otherwise effective treatment with oral pancreatic enzymes. Clinical signs associated with naturally occurring deficiencies of these vitamins in dogs and cats have not been well documented, but intestinal mucosal changes, myopathy, myelopathy and other abnormalities of nervous tissue have been reported in other species. This is especially important with regard to cobalamin in cats. In the author's experience, supplementation with large oral doses of tocopherol (5–25 IU/kg bodyweight given orally q24h with food for 1 month) is effective in returning serum vitamin E concentrations to normal. Cobalamin may be given parenterally (250–1000 μg s.c. once a week for several weeks) or orally (250–1000 μg daily for 1 month) to normalize serum concentrations. Long-term monitoring of serum cobalamin concentration, especially in cats, is recommended. Lifelong supplementation is required using either daily oral or periodic (usually monthly for dogs and every 2 weeks for cats) cobalamin to prevent relapse of hypocobalaminaemia.

Malabsorption of retinol (vitamin A) has also been demonstrated in association with EPI, as has vitamin K- responsive coagulopathy. Successful enzyme supplementation does not correct or prevent these deficiencies. Routine supplementation with these vitamins without evidence of clinical deficiency (bleeding in the case of vitamin K) is currently not recommended and may be harmful in excess. Given new findings regarding immunological and other functions of retinol, cautious supplementation after appropriate testing may be recommended in the future.

It should be noted that doses of individual vitamins in multivitamin preparations are usually insufficient to normalize serum concentrations when there is malabsorption, and that parenteral or very high oral doses may be required for adequate supplementation to rectify and prevent recurrence of specific deficiencies.

Antibiotic therapy

Dogs with EPI commonly have small intestinal dysbiosis, but in most cases this is a subclinical abnormality and affected individuals respond very well to treatment with oral enzyme replacement alone, even though the dysbiosis often persists. Altered intestinal microbiota can cause malabsorption and diarrhoea, however, and in those individuals that do not respond to oral enzyme supplementation alone, dietary or antibiotic therapy to change the microbiome may be of value. Changing the fermentable component of the diet by reducing some carbohydrates and/or addition of prebiotics, such as fructo-oligosaccharides, inulin (chicory root extract) or aleurone, may be all that is required; many commercially available diets now contain defined amounts of such prebiotics. If no effective diet or supplement can be found, oral tylosin or oxytetracycline may be effective in improving the clinical response in some of these patients; some clinicians prefer to administer tylosin for 4–6 weeks prior to starting what may be a lengthy search for an optimal diet, and sometimes this does lead to resolution of clinical signs after cessation of antibiotic therapy. However, long-term dietary change is probably preferable to long-term antibacterial administration, if a suitable diet can be found. Probiotics may also be helpful in some patients. Unfortunately, there is currently no way to predict what is likely to be effective, and so individualized trial and error testing for between 2 and 4 weeks with each treatment is required. This can be quite time-consuming and frustrating for owners, and online support groups (e.g. www.epi4dogs.com) may be helpful in finding a solution. Chronic small intestinal dysbiosis may cause mucosal damage that is only partially reversible, and this may explain why some animals fail to return to normal bodyweight and suffer from intermittent recurrences of other gastrointestinal signs.

Glucocorticoid therapy

In those few patients that respond poorly to the above treatments, oral prednisolone (or prednisone) at an initial dosage of 1–2 mg/kg q12h for 7–14 days may be beneficial. This may be due to resolution of coexisting lymphoplasmacytic gastroenteritis or other effects of glucocorticoids on the gastrointestinal tract. Long-term glucocorticoid administration is generally unnecessary.

Prognosis

The underlying pathological process leading to EPI is generally irreversible and lifelong treatment is required. It is particularly important to recognize that feline patients often require other therapies in addition to enzyme replacement, most notably cobalamin supplementation. Given the expense of treatment, it is reasonable in some cases to either repeat a serum TLI assay or withdraw enzyme supplementation for a trial period every 6 months or so and observe the patient for recurrence of clinical signs. Pancreatic acinar tissue does have some capacity to regenerate, and very rarely following either pancreatitis

or subtotal PAA, residual acinar tissue might regenerate sufficiently to normalize digestive function; apparent recoveries from clinically significant enzyme deficiency have been reported. However, in almost all cases treatment will be required for life but, providing owners are willing to accept the cost of enzyme replacement, the prognosis is generally good. Some patients may fail to regain normal bodyweight but these animals usually have either marked improvement or total resolution of diarrhoea and polyphagia, and are quite happy pets. A high prevalence of mesenteric torsion and gastric dilatation-volvulus has been reported in German Shepherd Dogs and Rough Collies with PAA in Finland, but this has not been documented elsewhere.

Treatment of patients with diabetes mellitus and EPI due to chronic pancreatitis is likely to be more troublesome and expensive. Diabetes mellitus secondary to chronic pancreatitis is potentially more difficult to regulate than simple diabetes in view of probable coexisting derangements in the secretion of glucagon and somatostatin. Moreover, anorexia and vomiting due to residual pancreatitis may further complicate treatment of diabetes mellitus. Paradoxically, the diabetes mellitus of some of these patients, especially cats, may be more easily managed with concurrent treatment with oral prednisolone, often at a dose as low as 0.5 mg/kg every other day; this may help moderate pancreatic inflammation or modulate a concurrent enteropathy.

Exocrine pancreatic neoplasia

Pancreatic adenomas are benign tumours, which are usually singular and can be differentiated from pancreatic nodular hyperplasia by the presence of a capsule. Pancreatic adenocarcinoma is the more common neoplastic condition of the exocrine pancreas in the dog and cat, but occurs rather infrequently in both species. Adenocarcinomas usually originate from the duct system, but can also originate from acinar tissue. A few cases of pancreatic sarcomas (i.e. spindle cell sarcoma and lymphosarcoma) have been reported. Whether these tumours are primary neoplastic lesions of the exocrine pancreas, metastatic lesions from tumours of other organs or a localized lesion of a multicentric neoplasm is open to question.

Aetiology and pathogenesis

The aetiology of neoplastic conditions of the exocrine pancreas is unknown. Benign neoplastic lesions can lead to displacement of cranial abdominal organs. However, these changes are subclinical in most cases and the diagnosis is often made as an incidental finding at postmortem examination. In very few cases, a benign growth can obstruct the pancreatic duct and cause secondary atrophy of the remaining exocrine pancreas, leading to EPI. Adenocarcinomas can also cause displacement of cranial abdominal organs and obstruction of the pancreatic duct. In addition, adenocarcinomas can be associated with tumour necrosis and resulting pancreatic inflammation, when the tumour outgrows its vascular supply or interferes with blood flow to otherwise healthy pancreatic acinar tissue, mimicking spontaneous, idiopathic pancreatitis. Pancreatic adenocarcinomas can also spread to neighbouring or distant organs.

Clinical signs and diagnosis

The presentation of patients with exocrine pancreatic neoplasia is non-specific and clinical signs observed are often those of chronic pancreatitis, including vomiting, anorexia, diarrhoea, or chronic weight loss. Multifocal necrotizing steatitis, particularly affecting subcutaneous fat, has been described in a few dogs that were ultimately diagnosed with pancreatic adenocarcinoma. Clinical signs related to metastatic lesions, such as lameness, bone pain or dyspnoea, have also been reported in some cases of pancreatic adenocarcinoma. Several cases of paraneoplastic alopecia have been reported in cats with pancreatic adenocarcinoma, and this has been termed 'shiny skin disease'. The reported alopecia consists of generalized alopecia of the ventrum, limbs and face in most cases, or diffuse zones of alopecia in other cats (Figure 36.10).

Neutrophilia, anaemia, hypokalaemia, bilirubinaemia, azotaemia, hyperglycaemia and increases in hepatic enzyme activities have all been reported in affected patients, but results of routine blood tests may be unremarkable. Increases in hepatic enzyme activities and serum bilirubin concentration are identified most commonly. Hyperglycaemia, when present, is related to concurrent destruction of pancreatic beta cells. Some dogs with pancreatic adenocarcinoma have extremely high serum lipase activities that reach as high as 25 times the upper limit of the reference range. Hypercalcaemia due to pseudohyperparathyroidism secondary to pancreatic adenocarcinoma has been described, and it is likely that other paraneoplastic sydromes occur sporadically.

Radiographic findings are also non-specific in most cases. Abnormal findings include decreased contrast in the cranial abdomen, suggesting peritoneal effusion into this area, transposition of the spleen caudally and shadowing in the pyloric region. In some cases, abdominal radiographs can suggest the presence of a mass in the cranial abdomen. In most cases, a soft tissue mass can be identified by abdominal ultrasonography in the region of the pancreas. However, in many if not most cases, a pancreatic origin of the mass cannot be conclusively established. Similarly, neoplastic lesions of neighbouring organs may be falsely presumed to be of pancreatic origin. In addition, patients with severe pancreatitis may show an ultrasonographic mass effect in the area of the pancreas that can be confused with a pancreatic adenocarcinoma. If peritoneal effusion is identified on abdominal ultrasonography, a sample should be aspirated and evaluated cytologically, although pancreatic neoplastic cells are not routinely identified on cytological examination because they do not readily exfoliate. Fine-needle aspiration under ultrasound guidance can be attempted when suspicious masses are identified and has been reported to be successful in approximately 25% of all cases. The low success rate of fine-needle aspiration is probably due to the poor exfoliation of pancreatic adenocarcinoma cells. In other cases, carcinoma cells can be identified, but the origin of the cells cannot be determined conclusively. Ultrasound-guided biopsy with histopathological evaluation of biopsy specimens has been reported infrequently, but is increasingly utilized with few adverse effects and successful diagnosis. In many cases, the diagnosis is made at exploratory laparotomy or definitively at post-mortem examination.

Therapy and prognosis

Pancreatic adenomas are benign and theoretically do not need to be treated, unless they cause clinical signs. However, since the final diagnosis of pancreatic adenocarcinoma is often made at exploratory laparotomy, a partial pancreatectomy should be performed even in cases of suspected pancreatic adenoma where the prognosis is excellent (see Chapter 5).

Pancreatic adenocarcinomas often present at a late stage of the disease; metastatic disease is usually present at the time of diagnosis. The most common sites of metastatic disease are the liver, abdominal and thoracic lymph nodes, mesentery, intestines and the lungs, but various other sites have also been reported. In those few cases when gross metastatic lesions are not identified at the time of diagnosis, surgical resection of the tumour may be attempted, but owners should be forewarned that clean surgical margins are only rarely achieved. Total pancreatectomy and pancreaticoduodenectomy, although theoretically possible, have not been described in dogs or cats with spontaneous disease. Extrapolation from human patients suggests high morbidity and mortality for these procedures. Chemotherapy or radiation therapies have shown little success in human or veterinary patients with pancreatic adenocarcinomas. Overall, the prognosis for dogs and cats with pancreatic adenocarcinoma is grave.

Pancreatic parasites

These have not been reported in UK cats.

Eurytrema procyonis

The pancreatic fluke of cats can be found in the pancreatic ductular system of foxes, raccoons and cats. Little is known about the life cycle of this parasite, but it can lead to thickening of the pancreatic duct system and fibrosis. Even though a significant decrease of exocrine pancreatic secretion has been shown to occur in affected animals, cats presenting with clinical signs of EPI secondary to infestation with this parasite are extremely rare. The diagnosis can be made by detection in fresh faeces of characteristic dicrocoeliid eggs (average size 34 μm x 50 μm) with a single operculum during routine faecal flotation. Fenbendazole at a dose of 30 mg/kg orally q24h for 6 consecutive days has been recommended for therapy.

36.10 Paraneoplastic alopecia in a cat with pancreatic adenocarcinoma.

(Courtesy of Dr Robert Kennis)

Amphimerus pseudofelineus

The hepatic fluke of the cat, *Amphimerus pseudofelineus*, can also infest the pancreas and can lead to pancreatitis. Infection with this parasite has been reported in cats from Illinois, Iowa, Louisiana, Maryland, Nebraska, Ohio, Texas and Virginia in the USA. The life cycle of this parasite is unknown, but it is presumed to be similar to that of other Opisthorchiidae, with molluscs serving as first and fresh-water fish as second intermediate hosts. Diagnosis can be made on faecal examination with formalin-ethyl acetate sedimentation by identification of yellow-brown eggs of approximately 16 µm x 31 µm with a single operculum. Eggs are destroyed during routine faecal flotation and infestation will be missed in those cases. Treatment with praziquantel at 40 mg/kg q24h for 3 consecutive days has been reported to be effective.

Pancreatic bladder

A pancreatic bladder is an abnormal extension of the pancreatic duct. Pancreatic bladders can be congenital or acquired, and have been described in several cats presented with signs compatible with biliary duct obstruction. Surgical reconstruction may be of benefit in cases with clinical signs attributable to this abnormality.

References and further reading

Armstrong PJ and Williams DA (2012) Pancreatitis in cats. *Topics in Companion Animal Medicine* **27**, 140–147

Clark LA and Cox ML (2012) Current status of genetic studies of exocrine pancreatic insufficiency in dogs. *Topics in Companion Animal Medicine* **27**, 109–112

German AJ (2012) Exocrine pancreatic insufficiency in the dog: breed associations, nutritional considerations, and long-term outcome. *Topics in Companion Animal Medicine* **27**, 104–108

Kennedy OC and Williams DA (2012) Exocrine pancreatic insufficiency in dogs and cats: online support for veterinarians and owners. *Topics in Companion Animal Medicine* **27**, 117–122

King L and Boag A (2018) *BSAVA Manual of Canine and Feline Emergency and Critical Care, 3rd edn.* BSAVA Publications, Gloucester

Mansfield C (2012) Acute pancreatitis in dogs: advances in understanding, diagnostics, and treatment. *Topics in Companion Animal Medicine* **27**, 123–132

Okanishi H, Nagate T, Nakane S and Wateri T (2019) Comparison of initial treatment with and without corticosteroids for suspected acute pancreatitis in dogs. *Journal of Small Animal Practice* **160**, 298–304

Steiner JM (2012) Exocrine pancreatic insufficiency in the cat. *Topics in Companion Animal Medicine* **27**, 113–116

Watson P (2012) Chronic pancreatitis in dogs. *Topics in Companion Animal Medicine* **27**, 133–139

Westermarck E and Wiberg M (2012) Exocrine pancreatic insufficiency in the dog: historical background, diagnosis, and treatment. *Topics in Companion Animal Medicine* **27**, 96–103

Williams DA, Batt RM and McLean L (1987) Bacterial overgrowth in the duodenum of dogs with exocrine pancreatic insufficiency. *Journal of the American Veterinary Medical Association* **191**, 201–206

Williams DA and Batt RM (1988) Sensitivity and specificity of radioimmunoassay of serum trypsin-like immunoreactivity for the diagnosis of canine exocrine pancreatic insufficiency. *Journal of the American Veterinary Medical Association* **192**, 195–201

Williams DA (1995) Exocrine pancreatic disease. In: *Textbook of Veterinary Internal Medicine, 4th edn*, eds. SJ Ettinger and EC Feldman, pp. 1345–1367. WB Saunders, Philadelphia

Williams DA (2012) Introduction: exocrine pancreatic insufficiency and pancreatitis. *Topics in Companion Animal Medicine* **27**, 95

Xenoulis PG, Levinski MD, Suchodolski JS and Steiner JM (2011) Serum triglyceride concentrations in Miniature Schnauzers with and without a history of probable pancreatitis. *Journal of Veterinary Internal Medicine* **25**, 20–25

Xenoulis PG, Zoran DL, Fosgate GT, Suchodolski JS and Steiner JM (2016) Feline exocrine pancreatic insufficiency: a retrospective study of 150 cases. *Journal of Veterinary Internal Medicine* **30**, 1790–1797

Zoia A and Drigo M (2017) Association between pancreatitis and immune-mediated hemolytic anemia in cats: a cross-sectional study. *Journal of Comparative Pathology* **156**, 384–388

Liver: hepatocellular and biliary tract disorders

Penny Watson

Structure and function

The liver lies in the cranial abdomen, between the diaphragm and the stomach, and is made up of six lobes and a gall bladder (Figure 37.1). The gall bladder is linked to the duodenum via a common bile duct, with a slightly different anatomical arrangement in cats and dogs (Figure 37.2). The lateral parts of the right and left liver lobes are seen on lateral abdominal radiographs in dogs and cats as the caudoventral edge of the liver shadow under the costal arch (see Chapter 3).

The liver effectively has two afferent blood supplies:

- The hepatic artery, which brings 25–30% of the afferent blood and 50% of the oxygen used by the liver
- The hepatic portal vein, which carries the other 70–75% of the afferent blood supply and 50% of hepatic oxygen requirements, bringing all the blood draining from the stomach, intestines (except the rectum), pancreas and spleen into the liver.

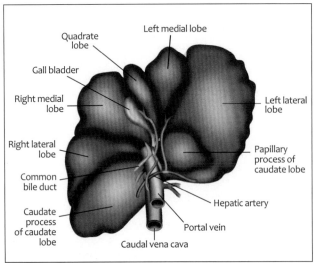

37.1 Anatomy of the liver with portal blood supply. The right branch of the portal vein supplies the right lateral lobe and caudate process of the caudate lobe (right division). The left branch divides further, with a central branch supplying the right medial and quadrate lobes (central division) and the left branch supplying the left medial and lateral lobes and the papillary process of the caudate lobe (left division).

(Reproduced from the BSAVA Manual of Canine and Feline Abdominal Surgery, 2nd edn)

All of the afferent blood arriving in both the portal vein and hepatic artery then passes into the hepatic sinusoids, mixes and flows in close proximity to the hepatocytes towards the hepatic veins. Most of the metabolic and detoxifying functions of the liver occur during the passage of blood along the sinusoids. The hepatocytes are divided into functional 'zones', with zone 1 being nearest to the portal triad (comprising the hepatic portal vein, hepatic artery and bile duct branch), zone 3 being nearest the hepatic vein and zone 2 being in the middle. Hepatocytes in each zone are exposed to different concentrations of oxygen, hormones, metabolites and other substances, and their functions are correspondingly different in each location (Figure 37.3). They also vary in their sensitivity to various pathological processes: for example, zone 3 hepatocytes are most susceptible to hypoxia.

Bile is made in the hepatocytes in zone 3 and flows in small canaliculi in the opposite direction to blood. Bile is composed of bilirubin, cholesterol and bile acids (cholic and chenodeoxycholic acid, conjugated with glycine or taurine in dogs and solely with taurine in cats) together with water and bicarbonate; it is also rich in immunoglobulin A (IgA). Bile flow is directly related to the excretion of bile acids into the canaliculi, which provides an osmotic gradient pulling water with it. The gall bladder acts as a storage organ for bile, but is not essential for bile excretion and function (as is demonstrated in dogs and cats which have had cholecystectomies). In healthy dogs and cats, less than half of the bile produced is stored in the gall bladder; the rest bypasses the gall bladder and is transported directly via the common bile duct into the duodenum. The gall bladder concentrates the bile and also produces mucin, which gives the bile its viscoelastic properties. Gall bladder contraction and bile release into the small intestine are stimulated by the hormone cholecystokinin, which is released by endocrine cells in the duodenum in response to an increase in luminal fat and amino acids. It is important to note that the gall bladder does not empty completely after eating; in dogs only about a third of gall bladder bile is expelled during a meal. The gall bladder also contracts intermittently during fasting in response to the hormone motilin, at the same time, at least in dogs, as the migrating motility complexes.

The liver has an astounding array of functions, many of which are disrupted in liver disease. In the normal liver, all of the portal blood from the splanchnic bed is filtered, which allows the 'first pass' metabolism of food, hormones, drugs and toxins, and the removal of the

Category	Cats	Dogs	Significance
Anatomy	Bile duct usually joins the single pancreatic duct just before entering the small intestine at major duodenal papilla	Most dogs have two pancreatic ducts and neither joins the bile duct. The smaller pancreatic duct opens adjacent to the bile duct on the major duodenal papilla	Choleliths and masses at the papilla will block both bile and pancreatic ducts in cats but not dogs. Bile reflux into the pancreatic duct is more likely in cats
Metabolism of drugs and toxins	Relative deficiency of hepatic detoxifying enzymes, increasing susceptibility to toxicity	No deficiency of enzymes, but breed variability (e.g. Dobermanns show impaired detoxification of potentiated sulphonamides)	Cats are more susceptible to hepatotoxins than dogs
Clinical pathology	Cats do not have a steroid-induced isoenzyme of ALP. All liver enzymes have very short half-lives	Dogs do have a steroid-induced isoenzyme of ALP. Liver enzymes have long half-lives	Steroids (endogenous or exogenous) increase serum ALP activity in dogs but not in cats. Repeat blood tests to monitor liver enzyme activities should be less frequent in dogs than cats
Metabolism of dietary components	High dietary protein requirements and metabolism, and inability to down-regulate if deficient. Dietary requirements for taurine and arginine	Lower dietary protein requirement compared with cats, and ability to down-regulate if needed. Lower arginine requirement than cats and no dietary taurine requirement	Cats rapidly develop protein-calorie malnutrition when fed a protein-restricted diet
Hepatic diseases	Diseases of the biliary tract and lipidosis most common. Significant fibrosis and cirrhosis are uncommon	Parenchymal diseases most common. Fibrosis and cirrhosis common. Clinically significant primary hepatic lipidosis is not recognized	Very different spectrum of disease presentations, differential diagnoses, investigations and treatment

37.2 Differences between cats and dogs in liver structure, function and disease. ALP = alkaline phosphatase.

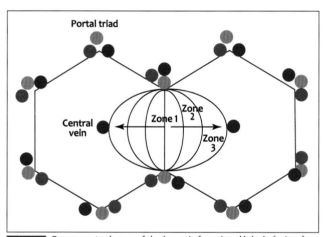

37.3 Rappaport scheme of the hepatic functional lobule (acinus), organized according to biochemical considerations. This is centred on a line connecting two portal triads and describes functional zones radiating from the triad to the central vein. For example, zone 1 cells are responsible for protein synthesis, urea and cholesterol production, gluconeogenesis, bile formation and β-oxidation of fatty acids; zone 2 cells also produce albumin and are actively involved in glycolysis and pigment formation; and zone 3 cells are the major site of liponeogenesis, ketogenesis and drug metabolism. Zone 3 hepatocytes, being furthest from the hepatic artery and hepatic portal veins, also have the lowest oxygen supply and are therefore most likely to suffer hypoxic damage. Arrows show the direction of blood flow. The portal triad comprises one or more branches of the bile duct (green), hepatic artery (red), and hepatic portal vein (violet). (Reproduced from Watson (2014) with permission from Mosby)

products of digestion for metabolism. There are some important functional differences between dogs and cats, which are highlighted in Figure 37.2.

The functions of the liver can be summarized as follows:

- Detoxification and excretion: including ammonia and drug detoxification, and bilirubin, cholesterol and copper excretion
- Metabolism and storage: including glucose and fat metabolism and storage, and protein metabolism
- Synthesis: including synthesis of albumin; the sole source of anticoagulant factors and all coagulation factors with the exception of factor VIII, which is not only

produced by endothelial cells within the liver but also by endothelial cells elsewhere; apoproteins for triglyceride transport and all globulins except immunoglobulins

- Immunological functions: clearance of bacteria and gut-derived antigens by Kupffer cells (which comprise 90% of total body macrophages); IgA in bile; complement and interleukin metabolism
- Haematological functions: haematopoiesis in utero and extramedullary haematopoiesis in times of need, such as severe anaemia; breakdown of senescent red blood cells and iron homeostasis
- Digestive functions: synthesis, storage and secretion of bile acids for emulsification of fats in the small intestine.

It is important to remember that the liver is very closely related, both structurally and functionally, to the pancreas and small intestine, and that diseases of one of these organs often affect the others. This is well documented in cats, but is also recognized in dogs. Diet, drugs and toxins ingested orally might also have a profound effect on the liver (probably more often than is realized), as everything in the portal blood, including pancreatic venous drainage, passes through the liver prior to entering the systemic circulation, unless there is portosystemic shunting.

Pathophysiology of hepatobiliary disease

The pathophysiology of hepatobiliary disease in dogs and cats reflects disruption of the functions listed above, together with the local and systemic effects of hepatobiliary inflammation, biliary stasis and (particularly in dogs) the development of portal hypertension. As noted in Figure 37.2, there is a marked difference in the types of liver disease seen in dogs and cats: dogs suffer more often from parenchymal liver disease and are much more likely to develop progressive hepatic fibrosis, cirrhosis and portal hypertension; these are rare in cats. Cats more often suffer from primary biliary tract disease, and hepatic lipidosis is a clinically significant disease in this species, but not in dogs.

Functional plasticity and regenerative capacity

It is important to remember that the liver has tremendous functional and structural reserve and also a great regenerative capacity, given the right environment. The functional zonation, as described in Figure 37.3, is flexible, such that if hepatocytes in one zone are damaged, others can adapt to take over their function. However, this functional adaptation takes time and, therefore, acute hepatic failure will result in clinical signs after loss of less liver mass than chronic hepatic disease; with the latter, the hepatocytes have time to adapt and take over the functions of damaged cells and, therefore, clinical signs usually do not develop until at least 70% of the hepatic functional mass has been lost. The liver also has a tremendous ability to regenerate, provided the animal is not starved and the damage is not too severe or ongoing.

Fibrosis

Progressive fibrosis is common in canine chronic liver disease but uncommon in cats. Fibrosis represents a 'final common pathway' for a variety of insults and is analogous to the wound-healing response in other tissues. It is, therefore, fundamentally a dynamic process, and can eventually lead to cirrhosis with marked loss of liver function and portal hypertension. Preventing this progression is a goal of treatment of canine chronic liver disease. However, to date there is no effective antifibrotic drug and the most effective way to reduce hepatic fibrosis is to remove the underlying cause.

Collagen is secreted by hepatic stellate cells (also known as Ito cells), which are located in the extracellular space of Disse, between the sinusoidal endothelial cells and the hepatocytes. In the normal liver, stellate cells are the major storage sites of vitamin A. They synthesize extracellular matrix components, matrix metalloproteinases, cytokines and growth factors, and are stimulated in a number of ways: indirectly via the release of cytokines from inflammatory cells, particularly neutrophils, lymphocytes, platelets and necrotic hepatocytes, or directly by toxins and oxidant stress. In chronic hepatic injury they undergo a major phenotypic transformation to collagen-secreting, proliferating activated myofibrocytes, which lose their usual content of vitamin A, become contractile and secrete high-density matrix and collagen. Cirrhotic liver contains approximately six times more extracellular matrix than normal liver. Changes in activation and inhibition of zinc-dependent matrix metalloproteinases are also important to the balance between fibrogenesis and hepatic recovery, and the stellate cells are intimately involved in these changes. Their contractile nature when activated contributes to the pathogenesis of intra-hepatic portal hypertension by altering sinusoidal tone and blood flow. In addition to being activated, stellate cells are stimulated to proliferate and migrate to points of injury. This can be obvious in liver biopsy samples from dogs with early chronic liver disease, where an increase in the number of stellate cells can often be noted histologically before any obvious fibrosis. This has to be considered an ominous sign, signalling impending fibrosis.

Early fibrosis in the hepatic connective tissue does not initially disrupt the hepatic architecture. This tends to progress to involve more of the liver and to bridge between the portal tracts, developing into cirrhosis, which is defined by the presence of progressive bridging fibrosis, inflammation and nodular regeneration. Traditionally, it has been believed that 'early' fibrosis is potentially reversible, whereas more chronic, bridging fibrosis and cirrhosis are not reversible. However, recent work in humans has indicated that even cirrhosis may be reversible if the underlying cause is removed, graphically illustrating that hepatic fibrosis is a dynamic process. Effective reversal of cirrhosis has not yet been conclusively documented in dogs.

Portal hypertension

Portal hypertension is common in dogs but rare in cats. It describes a sustained increase in pressure in the portal vein which is usually caused by an increase in resistance to flow through the hepatic vessels and sinusoids. This can occur in acute diseases, such as feline hepatic lipidosis, due to hepatocyte swelling obstructing sinusoids or in more chronic diseases, such as canine chronic hepatitis (CH), due to fibrosis and remodelling together with the direct contractile effects of activated stellate cells. A thrombus in the portal vein is a less common cause of portal hypertension. Portal hypertension can also develop as a result of chronic hepatic congestion with right-sided heart failure, cardiac tamponade or obstruction of the hepatic vein or terminal caudal vena cava. A few typical clinical signs develops as portal pressure rises:

- Development of ascites, as hydrostatic pressure rises in the splanchnic bed (the mechanisms are described in more detail in Chapter 24). The ascites in portal hypertension is worsened by activation of the renin-angiotensin-aldosterone system (RAAS) as a result of splanchnic pooling of blood reducing systemic blood pressure. RAAS activation leads to further renal sodium and water retention, thus worsening ascites. Consequently, aldosterone antagonists are often the most effective diuretics to use in the ascites of liver disease
- Gastrointestinal (GI) wall congestion and oedema followed by ulceration, or at least a high risk of ulceration with any additional trigger factor (such as steroid therapy)
- GI ulcers may cause haematemesis and melaena, and the blood released into the gut acts as a 'high-protein meal' and may trigger a worsening of encephalopathy. The potentially serious consequences of GI ulceration underlie the importance of avoiding, where possible, potential triggers such as steroids in the therapy of liver disease and treating ulcers aggressively if they occur
- Development of acquired portosystemic shunts (PSS). These typically develop in chronic liver disease in dogs, but are very rare in cats. Acquired PSS develop with sustained portal hypertension with portal pressure consistently higher than the pressure in the caudal vena cava. Multiple embryonic vessels open up as 'escape valves' between the portal vein and caudal vena cava. These acquired shunting vessels are often recognized grossly at surgery as a fine network of small vessels near the right kidney. They perform an important protective role, protecting the hepatocytes and gut wall from the worst effects of sustained portal hypertension, and attempts at ligation are absolutely contraindicated.

Biliary stasis

Biliary stasis occurs as a result of intra-hepatic or extra-hepatic biliary obstruction, or both, and results in jaundice (for more details about the production and excretion of bilirubin see Chapter 25 and the *BSAVA Manual of Canine and Feline Clinical Pathology*). Intra-hepatic biliary stasis occurs due to impaired hepatic uptake of bilirubin, conjugation or excretion into bile and is typically seen with hepatic disorders in which severe intra-hepatic cholestasis develops, such as acute inflammatory liver diseases and lipidosis. Jaundice is less common in canine CH until a late stage in the disease where it is a negative prognostic indicator. Post-hepatic jaundice is due to interruption of flow in the extra-hepatic bile ducts. The most common causes are acute pancreatitis or an acute flare-up of chronic pancreatitis, but it may also occur with choleliths, which are uncommon in dogs and cats, biliary or pancreatic neoplasia, gall bladder mucocoele, biliary tract infection or rupture of the biliary tract. With complete obstruction of the bile duct, such as by a migrating intestinal foreign body, faeces are pale grey and acholic due to the absence of stercobilin, but this is a very uncommon occurrence.

Bile is a potent detergent, so it is very damaging to hepatocytes. Leakage of bile back into the liver as a result of intra- or extra-hepatic cholestasis therefore results in damage to hepatocytes and both increased hepatocellular and cholestatic enzymes. Bile is also a potent oxidative toxin in the liver, damaging mitochondrial membranes and disrupting oxidation.

Diagnosis of hepatobiliary disease

Animals being investigated for liver disease usually fall into one of two groups depending on the questions posed:

- The animal has clinical signs – could it be liver disease?
- The animal has increased serum activities of liver enzymes on routine blood testing but no relevant clinical signs – are these important? Is the liver problem primary or secondary? Is further investigation warranted?

In either situation, a further question is whether or not to perform a liver biopsy, and it is important to realize that the majority of diseases of the liver cannot be diagnosed without a liver biopsy. The results of clinical examination, blood tests and diagnostic imaging can be suggestive of disease, but without a biopsy it is impossible to be sure. The exceptions are gall bladder mucocoele and congenital vascular anomalies, which may be diagnosed on the basis of imaging without biopsy (see later), and biliary tract infections, which can be diagnosed on bile culture (see later). It is also important to remember that secondary hepatopathies are a much more common cause of increased liver enzyme activities in dogs than primary liver disease, whereas they are less common in cats. Increased serum activities of liver enzymes are notoriously non-specific and it is a mistake to assume that a dog with increased activities has hepatitis unless further investigations are undertaken. The most common causes of secondary hepatopathies in dogs and cats are outlined in Figure 37.4. Secondary hepatopathies usually resolve when the underlying cause is treated. However, in a few cases, a secondary hepatopathy can develop into a more serious 'primary' liver problem. An example would be chronic cardiac cirrhosis in dogs, which sometimes develops after chronic passive congestion as a result of right-sided heart failure.

It is important to recognize whether the hepatopathy is secondary as early as possible to avoid unnecessary

- Right-sided congestive heart failure, including pericardial effusion and heartworm
- Hypoxia
  - Immune-mediated haemolytic anaemia
  - Shock
- Glucocorticoids
  - Most significant in dogs. Cause a marked increase in alkaline phosphatase activity with mild increases in alanine aminotransferase and aspartate aminotransferase activities and bile acids
  - Endogenous (hyperadrenocorticism)
  - Exogenous
- Diabetes mellitus
- Hyperlipidaemia (e.g. Miniature Schnauzers)
- Hyperthyroidism (cats)
- Hypothyroidism (dogs)
- Non-hepatic inflammatory disease
  - Toxaemia
  - Sepsis
  - Gastrointestinal disease
  - Pancreatitis
  - Dental disease (particularly cats)
- Drug-induced (e.g. phenobarbital)
- Metastatic neoplasia

37.4 Common causes of secondary hepatopathies in dogs and cats.

hepatic investigations (such as liver biopsies), which might take time and money away from diagnosing and treating the true disease. This differentiation is usually achieved through careful interpretation of the history, physical examination, clinicopathological tests and diagnostic imaging.

History and clinical signs

The clinical signs in canine and feline liver disease are often mild and non-specific. Waxing and waning anorexia and GI signs are the most common. More specific, but less common, signs include jaundice, ascites and hepatic encephalopathy (HE) with congenital or acquired PSS, although even these signs have other potential causes. Clinical signs are particularly non-specific in cats and the situation is further complicated in this species by the high incidence of concurrent chronic enteropathy and/or pancreatitis, which present with very similar signs. The severity of the clinical signs seen in liver disease depends on the speed with which the disease develops, the amount of functional liver tissue damaged and the degree of portal hypertension that develops. As described, the liver has tremendous structural and functional reserve. If disease develops slowly, not only can liver tissue regenerate, but also zonal adaptation can occur such that new zones of hepatocytes can take over the function of damaged cells, limiting clinical signs. However, if the damage is acute, there is no time for this adaptation to occur. For example, hyperammonaemia and HE will develop very quickly in acute disease but more slowly in chronic disease. Therefore, animals with very extensive chronic liver disease may show no clinical signs at all or very subtle signs until the end-stage (Figure 37.5). Typical clinical signs of acute and chronic liver disease are listed in Figures 37.6 and 37.7.

Body condition, muscle condition, mucous membrane colour, any ascites and abdominal organ abnormalities should be carefully assessed, and the animal should be checked for evidence of coagulopathy (petechiae and/or ecchymoses), particularly in acute disease. In dogs, chronic primary liver disease (other than neoplasia) is usually associated with a smaller than normal liver, which will only be appreciated on diagnostic imaging and not on clinical examination. The liver is often not palpable in both

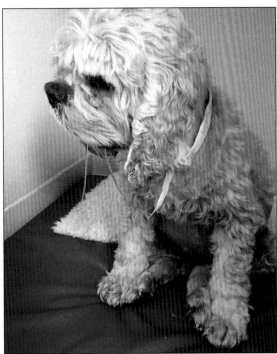

37.5 Ptyalism, as demonstrated by this American Cocker Spaniel, can be a sign of nausea or hepatic encephalopathy in chronic liver disease.

Acute onset of:
- Anorexia
- Hepatic encephalopathy: depression progressing to seizures and/or coma
- Vomiting
- Polydipsia
- Dehydration
- Jaundice (more marked/earlier if periportal lesion)
- Fever
- Cranial abdominal pain (some but not all cases)
- Coagulopathy, petechiae ± haematemesis/melaena
- Ascites and splenomegaly due to portal hypertension (less common but poor prognostic indicator)
- Acute kidney injury is a severe complication in some cases; both pre-renal and intrinsic renal components

37.6 Typical clinical signs of acute fulminating hepatitis in dogs and cats.

- Vomiting and/or diarrhoea
- Occasionally haematemesis and melaena
- Inappetence
- Weight loss
- Polydipsia, polyuria and poorly concentrated urine
- Ascites
- Jaundice
- Hepatic encephalopathy: depression; excitement; ptyalism (especially cats); pacing, fitting or coma (uncommon)
- Bleeding diatheses (uncommon but serious: suggests large loss of liver mass)

37.7 Typical clinical signs of chronic liver disease in dogs and cats. (Often no clinical signs until >70% loss of hepatic mass.)

normal and abnormal dogs and cats because of its position within the rib cage. Palpable hepatomegaly is often indistinguishable from splenomegaly without diagnostic imaging and hence the term 'hepatosplenomegaly' is typically used. However, a significant number of cats with chronic liver disease (e.g. cholangitis, lipidosis) have palpable hepatomegaly. Pain on cranial abdominal palpation may be found in acute liver disease, but is uncommon in chronic disease in either species, although it may be elicited in some dogs. It might also reflect concurrent pancreatitis or upper GI disease.

Clinicopathological changes

Blood tests to assess liver enzyme activities and liver function are usually the next (and simplest) step in the investigation of the suspected hepatic case. Carefully chosen blood tests should also help in differentiating primary from secondary disease, and in assessing liver function. A detailed discussion of clinical pathology is beyond the scope of this text and the reader is referred to the *BSAVA Manual of Canine and Feline Clinical Pathology.*

It is important to remember that clinical pathology is only a part of the diagnostic investigations of the liver case and is most important in guiding further tests (imaging and biopsy). It is never possible to make a diagnosis of liver disease on the basis of blood tests alone, and it is often not even possible to differentiate primary from secondary hepatopathies, although the pattern of changes found, combined with the history and clinical findings, often helps towards this differentiation. It is also a mistake to think that serum liver enzyme activities are tests of liver function, or that blood results generally give prognostic information – the degree of increase of liver enzyme activities in serum is not related to the degree of liver damage or function, and it is not helpful prognostically.

Liver enzymes in cats have shorter half-lives than in dogs and even mildly increased serum activities are significant. In dogs, mild, relatively transient increases are not uncommon as a reaction to other diseases. However, persistent significant increases for weeks, particularly of hepatocellular enzymes (alanine aminotransferase (ALT) or aspartate aminotransferase (AST)) in a dog, or either hepatocellular or biliary enzymes in a cat, should stimulate further investigations. The clinician should be particularly alert to increased serum liver enzyme activities in asymptomatic individuals in a 'high-risk' group, such as persistently increased ALT in a Dobermann or Cocker Spaniel, or increased alkaline phosphatase (ALP) in an obese, anorexic cat. In contrast, persistent mild to moderate increased activities of ALP are not uncommon in old dogs and, if hepatocellular enzyme activities are normal, these animals should not have a liver biopsy before other causes are ruled out. It is important to remember that dogs have a steroid-induced isoenzyme of ALP. In many cases, increased ALP activity in dogs is a result of a hepatopathy secondary to other diseases, such as chronic pancreatitis or hyperadrenocorticism, or may be the result of benign nodular hyperplasia, a clinically insignificant ageing change. Increased activities of ALP are usually more significant in cats because of the enzyme's short half-life and the lack of a steroid-induced isoenzyme in this species.

Increased serum bilirubin concentration is only recognized in a subset of liver diseases, but is more specific for the liver once pre-hepatic causes (haemolysis) have been ruled out. Further investigations are then necessary, particularly diagnostic imaging, to differentiate hepatic from post-hepatic causes. Cholestasis also causes increased concentrations of the other components of bile (i.e. bile acids and cholesterol). It is, therefore, important to realize that increased bile acids in a dog or cat with biliary stasis will give no indication of liver function or portosystemic shunting, but just indicate cholestasis.

Anaemia is not uncommon in chronic liver disease and may be due to iron chelation by the liver, anaemia of chronic disease, or blood loss into the gut due to portal hypertension. The anaemia may, therefore, be mild to severe and normocytic, microcytic or macrocytic, depending on the cause and chronicity. There may be a neutrophilic leucocytosis in inflammatory liver diseases and biliary tract infections. Thrombocytopenia may occur in portal hypertension with splenic sequestration, but is most often due to disseminated intravascular coagulation and thus is a poor prognostic indicator.

Non-specific indicators of reduced liver function include reduced serum concentrations of urea, total protein and albumin, and prolonged coagulation times (partial thromboplastin time, activated partial thromboplastin time). Coagulation times are commonly prolonged in cats with biliary tract disease, particularly if they have concurrent pancreatic disease and small intestinal malabsorption, presumably due to vitamin K deficiency. Prolonged coagulation times are much less common in dogs with liver disease and are a poor prognostic indicator in this species, suggesting marked loss of liver function or disseminated intravascular coagulation. Other poor prognostic indicators in canine CH are low albumin and globulin concentrations.

In addition to blood samples, a urine sample provides useful information in the animal with suspected liver disease. Animals with chronic liver disease often have poorly concentrated urine. In addition, urate crystals or stones may be seen due to reduced purine metabolism, particularly in animals with congenital or acquired PSS. However, urate crystals are not pathognomonic for liver disease and can be found in some normal dogs and cats and as an inherited condition in some dogs such as Dalmatians.

If ascites is present, a sample of the fluid should be taken and analysed for cell count, protein level and cytology, as this can give useful information. The details of analysis of ascitic fluid are given in Chapter 24.

Diagnostic imaging

The next investigation, after blood tests, should be diagnostic imaging. Ultrasonography is particularly helpful, although radiographs may also identify or rule out other diseases (for more details see Chapter 3). Abdominal radiographs are generally unhelpful in an animal with ascites because the fluid obscures all details, although ultrasonography is more rewarding, since the fluid separates the organs and enhances their visibility.

In the animal without ascites, abdominal radiographs may give a crude indication of liver size. In general, dogs and cats with acute liver disease have normal to enlarged livers, dogs with chronic liver disease and PSS have small livers, and cats with chronic liver disease have normal to enlarged livers. However, normal dogs (particularly deep-chested breeds) may have apparent microhepatica on radiographs, and dogs with PSS or chronic liver disease may have an apparently normal-sized liver on radiographs. Abdominal radiographs may also identify focal hepatic enlargement associated with a hepatic tumour, and rare, radiopaque gall stones. If neoplasia is suspected, right and left lateral thoracic radiographs should also be taken to check for metastases. Radiographs may also indicate more generalized disease in other organs; for example, there may be concurrent splenomegaly and/or lymphadenopathy in lymphoma, mast cell tumours or histiocytic neoplasia.

Ultrasonography, in the hands of an experienced operator, is an extremely useful tool in the diagnostic investigations of the liver case, as it allows assessment of the structure of the hepatic parenchyma, gall bladder and biliary tract, portal vein branches and other organs, and ultrasound-guided collection of samples of abdominal fluid and bile, and biopsies of the liver. Laparoscopy and laparotomy allow direct visualization of the external appearance of the organ, but ultrasonography is still a useful adjunct to these investigations as it allows visualization of the internal structure and lesions hidden within the parenchyma. The liver is relatively straightforward to examine with ultrasonography, and the increasing availability of peripatetic ultrasonographers should put this within the reach of most primary care practices.

Ultrasonography allows assessment of the size and structure of the gall bladder, common bile duct and biliary tree. If the common bile duct is grossly dilated, the area distal to it, including the pancreas and proximal duodenum, should be carefully examined for any neoplastic or inflammatory mass, or another lesion causing an obstruction. The hepatic parenchyma can be examined for focal or diffuse changes in echogenicity. Focal changes may indicate neoplasia but it is important not to over-interpret ultrasonographic findings and to remember that ultrasonography cannot give a histological diagnosis: such focal changes may equally well represent patchy extramedullary haematopoiesis, patchy lipid or glycogen infiltrate or benign nodular hyperplasia in older dogs. A biopsy is essential to rule these out and diagnose neoplasia – an animal should never be euthanased on the basis of ultrasonographic appearance of a lesion alone.

Diffuse changes in hepatic echogenicity are common. They may represent metabolic changes, such as hepatic glycogen accumulation in hyperadrenocorticism or fat in diabetes mellitus or primary hepatic lipidosis. Changes in other primary liver diseases are variable. There is often a diffuse increase in echogenicity in cirrhosis with a reduction in visualization of vessels. The spleen may appear congested in these cases due to portal hypertension. However, occasionally the liver looks ultrasonographically normal in advanced cirrhosis. Lymphoma classically results in a hypoechoic appearance of the liver, as well as the spleen, but may also result in a hyperechoic or normal-appearing liver, and so neither cirrhosis nor hepatic lymphoma can be ruled out on the basis of a normal-appearing liver on ultrasonography.

Other imaging modalities used less often in the diagnostic investigations of liver disease include scintigraphy, computed tomography (CT) and magnetic resonance imaging (MRI). CT and MRI are used extensively in humans, particularly in the assessment of biliary tract and vascular disease, but their use in small animals is limited. They are used most commonly in the investigation of vascular anomalies.

Fine-needle aspiration

Hepatic fine-needle aspirates are frequently taken but are rarely helpful in the diagnosis of liver disease. The results can be misleading and should always be viewed with some suspicion. Cytology of fine-needle aspirates is not helpful with diffuse inflammatory diseases, but it may be diagnostic in focal tumours, hepatic lymphoma and hepatic lipidosis. Ultrasound guidance is preferable and allows the fine-needle aspirates to be taken from the area of interest, avoiding blood vessels and the biliary tract. Fine-needle aspiration (FNA) of bile from the gall bladder is possible if undertaken with care under ultrasound guidance, or at laparotomy or laparoscopy. It is the most reliable way of diagnosing biliary tract infections in dogs and cats, and the fluid obtained should be submitted for culture and sensitivity testing, as well as cytology.

Liver biopsy

The next, and arguably most important, step in the diagnostic investigation of a liver case is liver biopsy. It is impossible in most cases to make a definitive diagnosis of disease and to make logical decisions about management without a liver biopsy. For example, finding a small, diffusely hyperechoic liver in an animal with ascites may suggest cirrhosis, but it is impossible to be sure without a biopsy. In particular, steroid, immunosuppressive or copper chelation therapies should never be used without histological confirmation of an indication because of the risk of side effects with inappropriate use. Without a biopsy, therapy of liver disease in dogs and cats will be at best non-specific or counterproductive, and at worst dangerous.

Platelet counts and coagulation times should be checked prior to performing a biopsy. A whole-blood clotting time in a glass tube is usually a sufficient clinical test of coagulation time. If coagulation times are significantly prolonged, vitamin K therapy q12h prior to biopsy can help, particularly in cats. In fact, coagulopathies are so common in cats with chronic liver disease that many veterinary surgeons (veterinarians) routinely administer 0.5–1.0 mg/kg vitamin K_1 s.c. q12h for three doses prior to biopsy. If coagulation times are prolonged in dogs, a plasma transfusion should be given prior to biopsy to replenish clotting factors temporarily. However, prolonged coagulation times in dogs are a poor prognostic indicator, particularly in CH, and in these cases it would be wise to delay biopsy for a few days in case of imminent marked clinical deterioration.

Biopsy samples may be taken at laparotomy or laparoscopy or under ultrasound guidance (see Chapters 4 and 5). The American College of Veterinary Internal Medicine (ACVIM) Consensus Group on diagnosis and management of canine CH recommends laparoscopy as the method of choice for obtaining liver biopsy samples, or laparotomy if facilities for laparoscopy are unavailable (Webster et al., 2019). Laparotomy is more invasive than ultrasound-guided biopsy, but it allows examination of other abdominal organs (such as the pancreas and small intestine) and observation of the liver with guided biopsy. The risk of serious haemorrhage is smaller than with Tru-Cut® biopsies, as any haemorrhage can be seen and dealt with at the time of surgery. The biopsy samples obtained are generally bigger and more diagnostic, with the proviso that focal lesions deep in the parenchyma may be missed if ultrasonography has not been used as well. If one part of the liver looks normal and another part abnormal, biopsy samples should be taken from both areas, as it is not uncommon for the apparently 'normal' part to be the diseased area! Laparoscopy is less invasive than laparotomy and has similar advantages in terms of biopsy size.

Ultrasound-guided, transcutaneous Tru-Cut® biopsies are less invasive than laparotomy or laparoscopy, can be performed under heavy sedation or general anaesthesia and are better than no biopsy at all. However, the samples obtained are often too small and non-representative, and have been shown to be misleading in about 50% of cases of canine chronic liver disease. Multiple biopsy samples should be taken with as large a Tru-Cut® needle as possible to maximize the chances of obtaining diagnostic samples. The animal should be monitored carefully for haemor-rhage afterwards (preferably hospitalized overnight), which, although uncommon, can develop unnoticed in these animals and be life-threatening. Semi-automated biopsy guns should be avoided in cats because fatalities have been reported when these were used (Proot and Rothuizen, 2006).

Liver biopsy samples should be sent for histology and bacterial culture. If copper storage disease is suspected, a piece of fresh tissue may be retained to send for quantitative copper estimation, although copper can be measured in formalin-fixed tissue. Ideally, bile aspirates should also be taken from the gall bladder under ultrasound guidance, or at laparotomy or laparoscopy, for cytology and culture.

Interpretation of the biopsy sample and extrapolating this to treatment recommendations can be a problem. The clinician should have a good understanding of the pathophysiology and treatment of liver disease to allow interpretation of the biopsy findings, and should not just read the 'bottom line' (final diagnosis). Preferably, a pathologist who is interested in small animal liver disease should be employed, and often the clinician will gain more information by discussing the results on the phone with the pathologist. The pathological description of liver disease in dogs and cats has been standardized by the World Small Animal Veterinary Association (WSAVA) (Rothuizen et al., 2006).

Hepatobiliary diseases

Liver diseases in dogs and cats can be classified as inflammatory and non-inflammatory and as hepatocellular, vascular or biliary, although many diseases will, in fact, affect the liver parenchyma, biliary tract and vasculature. For example, canine chronic hepatitis is primarily a parenchymal disease, but progressive fibrosis can cause intra-hepatic biliary stasis and, eventually, also acquired portosystemic shunting as a result of portal hypertension. The most common causes of canine and feline hepatobiliary disease are listed in Figures 37.8 and 37.9. It is very important to remember that, particularly in dogs, secondary hepatopathies are much more common than primary liver disease (see Figure 37.4).

- Secondary hepatopathy (see Figure 37.4)
- Chronic hepatitis
- Copper storage disease
- Acute toxic hepatitis
- Acute infectious hepatitis (e.g. leptospirosis or canine adenovirus type 1)
- Congenital vascular disorders
- Extra-hepatic biliary obstruction (mass, cholelith or inflammation of the pancreas or duodenum)
- Gall bladder mucocoele
- Bacterial cholangitis
- Metastatic neoplasia
- Primary neoplasia (hepatocellular is more common than biliary)
- Chronic infectious causes (e.g. *Bartonella*, systemic fungal disease)

37.8 Commonest causes of liver disease in dogs in approximate order of frequency.

- Chronic cholangitis
- Acute (suppurative/bacterial) cholangitis
- Feline hepatic lipidosis
- Feline infectious peritonitis-associated hepatitis
- Secondary hepatopathy (see Figure 37.4)
- Toxic hepatopathy
- Liver fluke (in parts of the USA; not in the UK)
- Extra-hepatic biliary obstruction (mass, cholelith or inflammation in the pancreas or duodenum, or spasm of the sphincter of Oddi)
- Congenital vascular disorders
- Metastatic neoplasia
- Primary neoplasia (biliary tract neoplasia is more common than hepatocellular)
- Hepatic involvement in other systemic infections (e.g. toxoplasmosis)
- Copper storage disease (rare)
- Amyloidosis

37.9 Commonest causes of liver disease in cats in approximate order of frequency.

Dogs with increased serum liver enzyme activities are four times more likely to have secondary than primary liver disease (Watson *et al.*, 2010). Therefore, clinicians should carefully rule out other causes, such as endocrine disease, as much as possible in dogs before undertaking liver biopsies. Secondary liver disease is less common in cats, but has recently been reported in 20% of feline liver biopsies (Bayton *et al.*, 2018).

Primary biliary tract diseases occur in both dogs and cats but are reported much more commonly in cats. Affected animals usually present with jaundice and increased liver enzymes, and differentiation of pre-hepatic, hepatic and post-hepatic causes of jaundice is important in all cases. Finding a normal or only mildly reduced packed cell volume rules out pre-hepatic (haemolytic) jaundice. Diagnostic imaging, particularly ultrasonography, is very helpful in diagnosing extra-hepatic biliary obstruction or gall bladder mucocoele, and cytology and culture of a bile aspirate is the most sensitive means of diagnosing suppurative (infectious) cholangitis and cholecystitis in dogs and cats. Definitive diagnosis of chronic cholangitis requires a liver biopsy.

Inflammatory hepatocellular disease

Canine chronic hepatitis

Definition, breed predispositions and potential aetiology: CH is the most common liver disease in dogs and, in many cases, the cause is unknown. In contrast, CH is very rarely reported in cats: the only well documented feline cases in the literature are copper-associated and these are rare. Whilst copper storage disease is much more common in dogs than cats (see below), the majority of causes of canine CH remain idiopathic. However, it is important to maintain an open mind and rule out chronic infectious and toxic causes as much as possible. Increasing use of more sensitive diagnostic techniques shows a higher prevalence of chronic bacterial infections in dogs with idiopathic hepatitis than previously recognized, including chronic leptospirosis (McCallum *et al.*, 2019).

Canine CH can only be definitively diagnosed with a liver biopsy. The clinical signs and clinicopathological and imaging findings are all non-specific. Histologically, CH is defined as the presence of hepatocellular apoptosis or necrosis with a variable mononuclear or mixed inflammatory cell infiltrate, regeneration and fibrosis (Rothuizen *et al.*, 2006; Webster *et al.*, 2019). Typically, the inflammation affects zone 1 of the hepatic acinus (portal area), although this may not always be the case. Fibrosis tends to progress to cirrhosis, but not inevitably. Cirrhosis describes progressive bridging fibrosis, inflammation and nodular regeneration, which has classically been considered to be end-stage and irreversible.

It is very important to realize that CH can be caused by more than one aetiological agent, but can then appear the same clinically, on clinical pathology and on liver biopsy. A lymphoplasmacytic infiltrate is not pathognomonic for immune-mediated disease and some dogs may have chronic infectious or toxic causes of disease, and so steroid therapy is not always appropriate. Copper can build up in the liver, either as a primary aetiological cause or secondary to reduced clearance (see below for more details). However, any copper in the liver is potentially damaging so should be addressed with therapy.

Idiopathic CH can affect any breed or crossbreed of dog. However, there are some clearly defined increased breed prevalences. Historically, a study in Sweden identified Labrador Retrievers, English and American Cocker Spaniels,

West Highland White Terriers, Scottish Terriers and Dobermanns as having increased prevalence of disease, with Labrador Retrievers showing a strong female predisposition and American and English Cocker Spaniels showing a strong male predisposition (Andersson and Sevelius, 1991). A more recent study in the UK also identified Labrador Retrievers, American and English Cocker Spaniels and Dobermanns as having increased risk of disease. In addition, Dalmatians, English Springer Spaniels, Samoyeds, Cairn Terriers and Great Danes had an increased risk of CH, compared with the wider population of insured dogs. Female Dalmatians, Dobermanns, English Cocker Spaniels, English Springer Spaniels and Labrador Retrievers, and male American Cocker Spaniels appeared to be over-represented. Median age for all breeds with CH was 8 years, but Dobermanns and English Springer Spaniels were significantly younger than Labrador Retrievers, English Cocker Spaniels and Cairn Terriers (Bexfield *et al.*, 2012a).

The increased prevalence in certain breeds suggests there may be breed-related aetiologies, which are currently largely unknown. The limited literature available suggests a potential immune-mediated aetiology in some Dobermanns, English Springer Spaniels and potentially Cocker Spaniels. In addition, copper has been implicated in some Dobermanns, a proportion of Labrador Retrievers and Dalmatians. The cause of disease in Skye Terriers has recently been questioned, and it is possible that these dogs suffer from a congenital ductal plate developmental defect rather than a primary hepatitis.

Granulomatous hepatitis, where there is a prominent infiltration of macrophages, is a particular form of CH, which may be associated with bacterial or fungal infection, including chronic hepatic *Leptospira* infection, or copper build-up (McCallum *et al.*, 2019). This histological finding should prompt a search for bacterial or fungal disease including special histological stains and consideration of molecular techniques, such as fluorescence *in situ* hybridization.

A particular form of chronic hepatitis, called 'lobular dissecting hepatitis', has been described with a characteristic histological appearance of distinctive fibrotic dissection of lobular parenchyma into individual and small groups of hepatocytes. It has been reported in young dogs of a number of breeds, including Standard Poodles, and also in a number of littermates. Its cause remains unknown and it may, indeed, have a number of causes mimicking CH in older dogs. Lobular dissecting hepatitis is probably a response of the juvenile liver to a variety of insults rather than a diagnosis in itself. Infectious aetiologies have been suggested, although not proven, and the age of onset and histological appearance resemble atypical leptospiral infection in dogs.

Diagnosis:

History and clinical signs: Dogs with CH typically present with non-specific clinical signs which are initially low grade. Many dogs with quite advanced disease may have no clinical signs at all and increased liver enzyme activities may be picked up on blood screens. It is important to remember that the large reserve capacity of the liver means that dogs with CH will not show signs until late in the disease. Further investigations of a dog with increased serum liver enzyme activities should not be unduly delayed, while the clinician waits for the dog to show signs.

The most common presenting signs are vomiting, diarrhoea, anorexia and polydipsia/polyuria. Jaundice and/or ascites occur in some cases at presentation and develop later in others, but not in all cases. HE is uncommon until end-stage disease. The presence of ascites and HE strongly suggests the development of portal hypertension and acquired PSS (see Pathophysiology section earlier). Affected dogs also usually have some degree of protein-calorie malnutrition due to chronic compromise of liver metabolism together with anorexia and GI signs. They are often overtly thin. They may be lethargic, but are often surprisingly bright considering the severity of their disease.

Clinicopathological findings: Most dogs with CH have increases of serum liver enzyme activities with a mixed hepatocellular and hepatobiliary pattern. Moderate increases of ALP and ALT are common. Increases in bilirubin concentration are less common. However, unlike other breeds, English Springer Spaniels with CH often present with jaundice. Persistent increases of ALT, particularly in a breed predisposed to CH, are the most suspicious marker of hepatocellular disease and should lead to early hepatic biopsy. However, it is important to remember that increases in hepatocellular enzyme activity are not specific for primary liver disease. In addition, in more end-stage CH and cirrhosis, liver enzyme activities may be only mildly increased or even return to normal. In end-stage disease, other function tests are abnormal and a very abnormal bile acid stimulation test would be expected. If both liver enzymes and bile acid stimulation tests are normal, it is very unlikely that the dog has CH.

Diagnostic imaging: Dogs with CH often have a small, hyperechoic liver on radiographs and ultrasonography, although the liver may also look normal ultrasonographically. There may be ascites and ultrasonography may reveal evidence of multiple acquired shunts in those cases in which they have developed. Splenomegaly may also be documented due to splenic congestion.

It is important to note that all these findings are supportive of a diagnosis of CH, but none are specific: for example, it is possible to have increased liver enzyme activities and bile acids, ascites and a small liver in a dog with idiopathic non-cirrhotic portal hypertension (also known as portal vein hypoplasia) (see Chapter 37b). Without a biopsy, these cases may be presumptively diagnosed as having cirrhosis and a poor prognosis, whereas idiopathic portal hypertension carries a better prognosis as the disease is non-progressive.

Liver biopsy: This is indicated as the next step in the diagnostic investigation of the dog with suspected CH, after checking coagulation times and platelets. Wedge biopsies by laparoscopy or laparotomy are preferred (see Chapters 4 and 5). A biopsy not only allows confirmation of diagnosis, but also allows assessment for any potential cause or contributing factor, such as primary or secondary copper build-up or evidence of toxic or infectious causes. Without a biopsy, diagnosis is only presumptive and treatment of the dog can only be supportive. Specific therapies with potential side effects, such as steroids, immunosuppressives and copper chelators, should never be used without histological confirmation of disease.

Treatment: Treatment of canine CH is largely supportive and non-specific unless an underlying cause can be identified. Specific treatments are reserved for dogs with copper storage disease or significant secondary hepatic copper build-up, where chelators and a low-copper diet are indicated (see below) and for dogs with strongly suspected autoimmune disease, where immunosuppressive doses of steroids or ciclosporin are indicated. Clinicians should not be afraid to discuss the histological findings with a pathologist to help optimize treatment.

Autoimmune disease may be suspected in a dog with a marked lymphoplasmacytic inflammation with no other apparent cause, although the clinician should remember that other aetiologies, such as chronic leptospiral or viral infections, can appear similar. There is currently no test available to definitively diagnose autoimmune hepatitis in dogs. However, autoimmunity is suspected in a subset of Dobermanns without increased hepatic copper (Dyggve et al., 2010; Dyggve et al., 2017), in some Cocker Spaniels and also in English Springer Spaniels (Bexfield et al., 2012b). In these cases, and only after confirmation by liver biopsy, steroids can be given at 1–2 mg/kg/day initially, reducing gradually. Owners should be warned of possible side effects, including increased risk of ascites and GI ulceration in dogs with portal hypertension. Ciclosporin has been reported as an effective alternative in dogs with suspected immune-mediated CH to avoid these side effects (Ullal et al., 2019) The dose used is 5 mg/kg initially twice a day, tapering to once a day (Webster et al., 2019).

Other dogs with idiopathic CH should be given non-specific dietary and drug treatments aiming to support liver function, treat clinical signs and provide antioxidant activity, until understanding of the aetiology of their disease improves. Dietary management involves the use of a palatable, high-quality, digestible diet. Dogs with hepatitis are often partially anorexic and the priority is encouraging them to eat. Commercial therapeutic liver diets, which are copper- and protein-restricted, are not necessary unless the dog has increased hepatic copper or signs of protein intolerance such as HE or urate urolithiasis. Dogs with CH may be cachexic and the priority in these dogs is to avoid negative nitrogen balance and feed sufficient high-quality protein using a digestible, palatable diet such as those designed for GI disease.

Oxidant damage is particularly severe in cases with biliary stasis or toxic hepatopathies, but any dog with CH may benefit from supplementation with antioxidants. S-Adenosylmethionine (SAMe) at approximately 20 mg/kg orally q24h and vitamin E (400 IU orally daily for a 30 kg dog) are usually supplemented, and silymarin (milk thistle) is also often used. The choleretic ursodeoxycholic acid is indicated in dogs with evidence of cholestasis at a dose of 10–15 mg/kg/day split in to two doses 12 hours apart. This drug is not licensed for use in animals, but has been used safely many times. It not only encourages bile flow, but also is a relatively non-toxic hydrophilic bile acid, which displaces toxic hydrophobic bile acids.

There are no clearly effective antifibrotic drugs for dogs with CH. The most effective antifibrotic treatment is to remove the underlying cause of the disease, which is often not possible in dogs as the cause is unknown. Colchicine has been used in some cases, but the evidence for its use is unconvincing and it often causes anorexia as a side effect. It is not licensed for dogs and should not be used in cats. The author does not recommend its use. Spironolactone has been shown to have an antifibrotic effect in rats with liver disease and is licensed for use in dogs (although indicated for cardiac disease and not liver disease). It is indicated as the first-choice diuretic in dogs with ascites of liver disease because of the pathophysiology of fluid build-up in liver disease (see earlier). It can be supplemented with additional furosemide in cases with marked ascites. Needle drainage of the abdominal fluid is to be avoided in dogs with liver disease, as it tends to result in a precipitous drop in the concentration of serum albumin, which the compromised liver cannot easily replace.

Other supportive care indicated in some dogs with CH includes anti-ulcer medication (omeprazole or ranitidine) if there is evidence of GI ulceration, antibiotics if bacterial infection is suspected, and antiemetics for vomiting.

Prognosis: The prognosis for dogs with CH is very variable. Some dogs have stable disease, doing well for years with supportive care, whereas others deteriorate rapidly. Both ascites and jaundice have been shown to be negative prognostic indicators in dogs, but it is important to remember this is on a population basis, and some individual dogs with ascites or jaundice can do well (Raffan *et al.*, 2009; Gomez Selgas *et al.*, 2014). English Springer Spaniels with CH in the UK were reported to have a short life expectancy with a median survival time of 189 days (Bexfield *et al.*, 2011), although, anecdotally, the authors of that study are now seeing much longer survival times in Springer Spaniels treated with steroids.

Copper storage disease and copper-associated liver disease in dogs

Definitions and pathophysiology: It is relatively common to find increased hepatic copper concentrations in dogs with CH. In some cases, this may be a primary copper storage disease and in others it may be secondary to reduced biliary excretion. There is an ongoing debate amongst veterinary hepatologists and pathologists about differentiating primary from secondary copper accumulation in the livers of dogs but, to a large extent, the differentiation is academic and not practical. Copper accumulation is potentially pathogenic regardless of whether it is primary or secondary. Copper is an oxidant toxin in the liver and not only results in hepatocyte necrosis itself, but also increases the susceptibility of the liver to other insults such as non-steroidal toxicity. Therefore, it is wise to administer chelators to any dog with significant copper build-up in the liver.

The difficulty in differentiating primary and secondary copper accumulation likely reflects the fact that this is an interaction between genes and the environment (i.e. genetic susceptibility, dietary copper concentrations and other insults). Some dog breeds, such as Bedlington Terriers, have a fairly clear-cut genetic predisposition to copper storage disease which means that they can only tolerate small amounts of copper in their diet. Other breeds or individual dogs may have a number of differences in genes encoding for copper storage and transport which make them less able to clear excess copper than others. When combined with a higher dietary copper concentration and/or biliary stasis reducing copper clearance, these dogs would be more susceptible to damaging hepatic copper accumulation. There is accumulating evidence that high concentrations of readily available copper in commercial canine diets may be contributing to hepatic copper accumulation in dogs. One early study showed that Beagles were very resistant to accumulating copper with biliary obstruction: much more so than humans. To show increased hepatic copper in that study, dogs needed to be copper loaded via their food and/or have an additional problem with excretion (Azumi, 1982).

The Bedlington Terrier has the best described breed-related copper storage disease (Figure 37.10). It is clearly a primary copper storage disease and is distinguished from secondary 'copper-associated' hepatopathies by distinctive features:

- Affected dogs show progressive pathological accumulation of copper in their hepatocytes, starting in

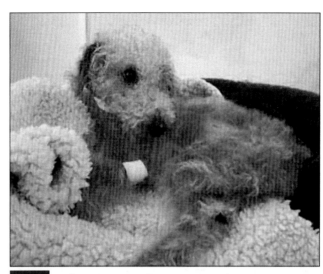

37.10 Bedlington Terrier with copper storage disease.

zone 3 (perivenous). This is distinct from secondary copper accumulation, which occurs in zone 1 (periportal)
- The severity of the hepatitis in affected dogs correlates with the copper concentration in the liver: the higher the copper, the more severe the damage
- There is co-localization of inflammation (typically histiocytic) and copper
- Copper builds up progressively throughout life (unless there is a dietary or drug intervention to stop it)
- The build-up of copper precedes the development of liver disease rather than developing secondary to it.

The Bedlington Terrier disease is believed to be inherited as an autosomal recessive trait and, at one time, up to 60% of Bedlington Terriers in some countries were affected. The prevalence has been reduced with selective breeding. The disease is confined to the liver, and there appears to be a specific defect in hepatic biliary copper excretion, probably in transport from the hepatocytes to the biliary tract. Studies have identified at least one genetic defect associated with the disease, a deletion in the *COMMD1* (previously *MURR1*) gene (Van de Sluis *et al.*, 2002), which codes for a protein of unknown function. However, Bedlington Terriers with copper storage disease but without a *COMMD1* deletion have been reported in the USA, UK and Australia (Coronado *et al.*, 2003; Hyun *et al.*, 2004; Haywood, 2006), suggesting that there are additional mutations involved in the breed. One of these has recently been identified in homozygous *COMMD1*-negative Bedlington Terriers in the UK where a mutation has been found in the *ABCA12* gene, which encodes for an ATP-binding cassette – a divalent metal transporter protein (Haywood *et al.*, 2016). Recommendations for screening of Bedlington Terriers for copper storage disease are summarized in Figure 37.11.

Proposed copper-associated hepatitis has also been reported in a number of other breeds, including Dalmatians (in the USA and Canada) (Webb *et al.*, 2002), Labrador Retrievers (in the USA and the Netherlands) and some Dobermanns (in the Netherlands), although individual members of all these breeds have also been reported with CH without copper accumulation. In addition, copper storage disease has been suspected but not extensively investigated in West Highland White Terriers. In one study in the Netherlands of several dog breeds, hepatitis was ascribed to copper storage disease in 36% and was idiopathic (and not copper-associated) in 64% of 101 dogs

37.11 Recommendations for screening Bedlington Terriers for copper storage disease. PCR = polymerase chain reaction; RNA = ribonucleic acid.

studied with acute and chronic liver disease (Poldervaart *et al.*, 2009). It is also possible for seemingly normal dogs without a recognized copper storage disease to develop copper-associated CH if fed a diet very high in copper, such as dry calf feed (Van den Ingh *et al.*, 2007).

Increased liver copper was also reported in Skye Terriers with CH, but this was proposed to be secondary rather than a primary cause of disease, and recent work suggests Skye Terriers may have a congenital ductal plate abnormality.

Diagnosis:

History and clinical signs: The severity of clinical signs in affected dogs depends on the speed of build-up of copper in the liver and exposure to other stresses. Most commonly, dogs present with very similar signs to dogs with idiopathic CH (see previous section). In a small number of cases with rapid build-up of copper with or without an additional stress, acute fulminant hepatic necrosis can develop with no previous signs. This is usually seen in young to middle-aged dogs, when it is often accompanied by acute haemolytic anaemia due to the rapid release of copper into the circulation.

Clinical pathology and diagnostic imaging: Dogs with the chronic form of copper storage disease will present with the same clinicopathological and diagnostic imaging changes as dogs with CH (see above). If a Bedlington Terrier, Dalmatian or other high-risk breed has persistent increases in ALT activity, even with no clinical signs, this is suspicious of copper storage disease and a liver biopsy is indicated. However, copper storage disease can occur in any breed or crossbreed and there is no non-invasive way of diagnosing it, so this is a strong reason for biopsy, as it allows the most effective treatment.

Dogs presenting at the more acute end of the spectrum with acute hepatic necrosis and haemolysis will have marked increases in liver enzyme activities together with anaemia and haemoglobinuria.

Liver biopsy: Definitive diagnosis relies on some form of liver biopsy and staining the samples obtained for copper

with rhodanine or rubeanic acid (Figure 37.12). Histology allows assessment of the localization of copper (zone 1 or 3) and association with inflammation. Qualitative scoring systems for copper estimation have been published (Hoffmann *et al.* 2006), correlating the amount of staining on slides to likely copper concentrations in the liver, and these are most accurate when using a digital slide scanner (Center *et al.*, 2013). A more quantitative method of analysis relies on measuring copper concentrations on large (minimum 15 mg) fresh liver biopsy samples.

The timing of liver biopsy is also important. For screening in susceptible breeds such as Bedlington Terriers, it is recommended that samples are not taken before 1 year of age, to allow time for sufficient copper build-up. Conversely, biopsy samples taken from older dogs with significant CH and remodelling may be misleading because areas of nodular regeneration will have lower copper concentrations, or because dietary copper intake has been restricted.

Interpretation of quantitative and qualitative measurements of copper in liver biopsy samples is detailed in Figure 37.13.

Treatment: This depends on the degree of copper build-up and severity of disease, and is summarized in Figure 37.13. Dogs with CH associated with copper accumulation should have non-specific and supportive care as detailed in the section above on chronic idiopathic hepatitis.

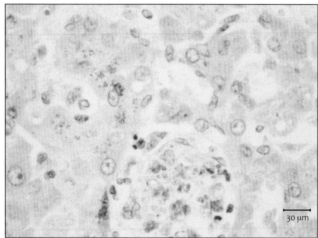

37.12 Histological section of canine liver stained for copper with rhodanine stain. Note the pink-staining copper granules in hepatocytes.
(Courtesy of Fernando Constantino-Casas, Pathology Department, Department of Veterinary Medicine, University of Cambridge)

- Copper concentrations <350 μg/g DM are normal (qualitative score 0 and 1) and >1000 μg/g DM (qualitative scores 3, 4 and 5) are definitely abnormal
- If copper is >350 but <2000 μg/g DM and there are structural changes, it is significant. The dog should be treated with a chelator and a copper-restricted diet
- If copper is >350 but <2000 μg/g DM and there are no structural changes, a copper-restricted diet should be fed. Chelation should not be instituted but a repeat of the biopsy after 6–12 months is indicated. If the copper concentration is then the same or reduced, the diet should be continued; if it has increased, chelation should be considered
- A copper concentration >2000 μg/g DM will cause lysosomes to rupture, resulting in structural liver damage. This is always significant and requires active chelation together with a copper-restricted diet

37.13 Interpretation of quantitative and qualitative hepatic copper levels in dogs and recommendations for treatment. DM = dry matter.

Supportive treatment with antioxidants (SAMe, silymarin and vitamin E) is wise because copper is an oxidizing toxin. Decisions about dietary management and copper chelation depend on the amount of copper in the liver. Copper chelation involves the use of either penicillamine or trientine (2,2,2-tetramine). Neither is licensed for use in dogs, but there are more published studies on penicillamine than trientine, and the latter is currently unavailable. The ACVIM Consensus Group recommends the use of D-penicillamine (Webster *et al.*, 2019). D-penicillamine takes months to effectively decopper the liver. It also has weak antifibrotic and anti-inflammatory properties. The recommended dose is 10–15 mg/kg orally twice a day, 30 minutes before meals. Starting at the lower end of the dose range and increasing the dose after 1 week (or dividing the dose and giving it more frequently) can reduce the common adverse effects of vomiting and anorexia. It has also been reported to cause nephrotic syndrome, leucopenia, and thrombocytopenia in dogs, so blood and urine samples should be monitored regularly during therapy. The recommended dose of trientine in dogs is 10 to 15 mg/kg orally twice a day, 30 minutes before a meal. Reported adverse effects include nausea, gastritis, abdominal pain, melaena and weakness. Neither trientine nor penicillamine should be used in dogs without biopsy confirmation of excess hepatic copper. In dogs treated with D-penicillamine, a decrease in liver copper content of about 900 µg/g dry weight per year can be anticipated.

Copper is an essential metal and necessary in small amounts, and copper deficiency is possible if dogs are overzealously chelated for years. This can result in microcytic anaemia and GI ulceration, stressing the importance of only using chelation when necessary, not continuing it lifelong unless necessary and monitoring the therapy. The efficacy of therapy can be monitored with repeat measurement of liver enzyme activities, although the only really reliable way of deciding when to stop is a repeat liver biopsy for copper measurement.

Chelation should be combined with the use of a low-copper diet, and it is wise to continue to feed a copper-restricted diet for the lifetime of the animal. Commercial therapeutic canine liver diets are low in copper but also have varying amounts of protein, therefore unless the dog is showing signs of protein intolerance (urate urolithiasis or HE), a less protein-reduced commercial therapeutic liver diet should be chosen. Owners should avoid titbits which are high in copper, such as shellfish, liver, kidney, heart, cereals, cocoa and legumes. In addition, if they live in a soft water area, it is advisable to give low copper bottled water rather than tap water because copper concentrations will be high from copper pipes. A rule of thumb is to give bottled water if a dripping tap leaves a blue copper stain in the sink.

Zinc can be added to the food once chelation has finished to block intestinal uptake of copper. It is unwise to add zinc to the diet while chelation is ongoing because the chelator will preferentially chelate the zinc instead of copper.

In severe, acute presentations with haemolysis, treatment should be supportive as detailed in the Acute hepatitis section below. Blood transfusion may be necessary if the haemolysis is severe. In acute cases, consider chelation with trientine (2,2,2-tetramine or 2,3,2-tetramine, if obtainable) because this can chelate rapidly. Penicillamine is not helpful in an acute crisis, as chelation takes weeks to months. On recovery, long-term treatment is continued as outlined above.

Copper storage disease and copper-associated disease in cats

Hepatitis associated with excess copper storage is much less common in cats than dogs but has been reported. The criteria for diagnosis appear to be similar to those in dogs, in that cats with presumed primary copper storage disease have high concentrations of copper that are predominantly centrilobular, whereas cats with copper build-up secondary to other liver diseases, such as cholangitis, have more of a periportal pattern with less copper (Hurwitz *et al.*, 2014). Normal hepatic copper concentrations in cats have been reported to be <180 µg/g DM. In a published study of 11 cats with presumed primary copper storage disease, a cut-off of 700 µg/g DM was chosen for primary disease, although some cats with secondary accumulation also had concentrations higher than this (Hurwitz *et al.*, 2014).

Cats with copper storage disease present clinically, and on clinical pathology and diagnostic imaging, very similarly to cats with chronic cholangitis (see later). Based on a small study (Hurwitz *et al.*, 2014), cats with copper storage disease tended to be younger, with a median age of 2 years. Penicillamine was used to chelate five cats with primary copper storage disease at the same dose as dogs (10–15 mg/kg q12h). Penicillamine should be used with extreme caution in cats, with very careful monitoring, because it is not licensed for use in this species and there is very limited experience of its use. In the published study, one of the five treated cats developed haemolytic anaemia, which resolved on cessation of therapy, so careful monitoring of blood count during therapy would be wise.

Acute hepatitis

Definitions and causes: Acute hepatitis encompasses a spectrum of disease from mild to severe, fulminating and life-threatening. The causes of acute hepatitis are outlined in Figure 37.14. The commonest causes in small animals are infectious, neoplastic or toxic, although many cases remain idiopathic (Lester *et al.*, 2016). Fortunately, most cases of acute hepatitis are focal and patchy. These cases usually do not show clinical signs, except those referable to the underlying cause, so the liver disease is usually unrecognized. Serum liver enzyme activities are often increased on blood samples and this may be the only clue to the clinician that the liver is involved. These animals may go on to complete recovery, but they may also develop CH, although the long-term sequelae of mild and focal acute hepatitis in small animals are poorly understood. By contrast, severe, fulminating acute hepatitis is a serious disease with marked clinical signs and a generally poor prognosis. Some animals go on to complete recovery but they require intensive management. Fortunately, fulminant acute hepatitis is rare in small animals. Dogs suffer more commonly than cats from acute hepatitis, probably because dogs are more likely to ingest toxins than cats.

History and clinical signs: It is very important to try to rule out toxicity when taking the history of an animal with suspected acute hepatitis. The owner should be questioned not only about possible access to toxins in the environment, but also about any nutritional or dietary supplements used. Owners often assume nutraceuticals are completely innocuous and may not mention them, whereas some supplements have been associated with hepatotoxicity. A drug history and any access to the artificial sweetener xylitol should also be ascertained, together

Type of disease	Potential cause

Acute massive hepatocyte necrosis (severe necrosis with signs referable to liver disease)	• Toxic or drug-induced:
	  • Paracetamol (acetaminophen; especially in cats)
	  • Carprofen (especially in Labrador Retrievers)
	  • Diazepam (cats)
	  • Mebendazole (dogs)
	  • Thiacetarsamide (dogs)
	  • Mercury
	  • Potentiated sulphonamides (dogs)
	  • Blue-green algae (dogs)
	  • Xylitol (dogs)
	  • Overdose of glucosamine- and chondroitin-containing joint supplements (dogs)
	• Infectious:
	  • Canine adenovirus type 1
	  • Neonatal canine herpes-virus
	  • Bacterial endotoxaemia
	  • *Salmonella* (dogs)
	• Thermal: heat stroke (uncommon)
	• Metabolic: acute hepatic necrosis in young dogs with copper storage disease

Acute hepatic necrosis: mild to moderate, focal (note that clinical signs are usually referable to primary underlying disease and not to the liver)	• Milder forms of toxic and drug-induced necrosis
	• Hypoxia:
	  • Cardiorespiratory disease
	  • Severe anaemia
	• Cholestasis
	• Septicaemia:
	  • Focal
	  • Diffuse
	• Pancreatitis
	• Chronic enteropathy
	• Infectious causes:
	  • Feline infectious peritonitis
	  • *Salmonella*
	  • *Leptospira*
	  • *Clostridium*
	  • *Ehrlichia*
	  • *Toxoplasma*
	  • Disseminated aspergillosis

Acute loss of hepatocyte function with minimal necrosis (usually marked loss of liver function and signs referable to liver disease)	• Certain toxicities (e.g. aflatoxicosis, especially in dogs)

37.14 Causes of acute hepatitis in dogs and cats.

with vaccination history. Canine adenovirus infection is very unlikely in a vaccinated dog, but infection with atypical leptospiral serovars, which are not covered by vaccination, is possible.

Dogs and cats with acute fulminating hepatitis present with a rapid onset of signs of severe hepatic insufficiency. As noted earlier, acute loss of hepatocytes causes a more profound reduction in liver function than slow chronic loss. The most clinically significant signs are usually acute HE, due to acute loss of hepatic detoxifying function with resultant rapid build-up of blood ammonia and other encephalopathic toxins; acute GI signs, often with melaena and haematemesis; and coagulopathies associated with sudden loss of hepatic function and also triggering of the coagulation cascade and disseminated intravascular coagulation.

Clinical pathology, diagnostic imaging and diagnosis:
Clinical pathology in acute hepatitis typically shows an early, marked increase in hepatocellular enzyme activities (ALT and AST) followed by slightly later increases in ALP, bilirubin and bile acids. Hypoglycaemia is common and

hypokalaemia is not uncommon. Some dogs develop renal failure by both pre-renal and renal mechanisms. Coagulopathies with both prolonged clotting times and reduced platelet counts are not uncommon. Blood ammonia is often increased. The additional presence of azotaemia, thrombocytopenia and glucosuria in the absence of increased blood glucose should increase the index of suspicion for leptospirosis in dogs.

Findings on diagnostic imaging are non-specific. The liver may appear normal or may appear enlarged on radiographs and ultrasonography, with rounded edges and diffusely hypoechoic or hyperechoic.

Definitive diagnosis relies on histology of a liver biopsy sample. However, animals with acute hepatic necrosis are often clinically unstable, with prolonged coagulation times and are poor candidates for general anaesthesia and liver biopsy. A presumptive diagnosis of acute hepatic necrosis might be made on the basis of a suggestive history (e.g. access to a toxin) and classic clinical signs and clinico-pathological findings. Blood and urine polymerase chain reaction tests for leptospirosis are indicated in suspected cases. Treatment is intensive but largely supportive and non-specific, so there is no urgency in obtaining a liver biopsy sample. A biopsy can be considered later, if the animal stabilizes but continues to show evidence of liver disease.

Treatment: Treatment of acute fulminating hepatitis is largely supportive and is outlined in Figure 37.15. Note that steroid therapy is not indicated in these cases – in fact, it potentially worsens the disease. Acute hepatitis results in only temporary and not permanent disruption of hepatic structure and function. Provided the insult is not ongoing, and provided that the limiting plate around the hepatic lobule remains intact and there is not gross destruction of hepatic architecture, there is the potential for complete recovery. The challenge is to support the animal through the acute crisis while awaiting recovery, as it is possible even if 50% of the liver is destroyed. However, there is no effective 'liver dialysis', even in humans, so too great a loss of vital hepatic functions results in death in spite of intensive care. It is difficult to predict the outcome, as some animals start to recover and have an improvement in liver enzyme activities and then deteriorate again. Some animals go on to complete recovery with no permanent histological lesions, whereas others develop CH and fibrosis. It has been suggested that dogs with acute hepatitis

• Treat cause if known – remove drug; give specific antidote (e.g. N-acetylcysteine, cimetidine and SAMe for paracetamol)
• Intravenous fluid support with balanced crystalloids
• Regularly measure serum potassium, phosphate and glucose and supplement as necessary
• Monitor renal output. Do not over-infuse and worsen ascites
• Avoid central line if coagulation times are prolonged
• Treat acute hepatic encephalopathy
• Treat coagulopathy as necessary: consider fresh frozen plasma to replenish clotting factors
• Consider supplementing vitamin K
• Treat GI ulceration if evident: omeprazole and antiemetics
• Treat ascites if evident: spironolactone ± furosemide
• Antibiotic support: use to protect against infectious complications is controversial. Use broad-spectrum agents which are not metabolized by the liver or hepatotoxic. Potentiated amoxicillin is a good choice: can be given intravenously; concentrated in bile and effective against leptospirosis in dogs. If this is a differential, consider a move to doxycycline in the longer term, when liver function has improved

37.15 Summary of supportive treatment of acute fulminating hepatitis in dogs and cats. SAMe = S-Adenosylmethionine.

are less likely to develop chronic lesions if they are fed a single-protein milk or soybean-based diet on recovery than if they are fed ordinary commercial dog food.

Hepatitis caused by drug toxicity

Many drugs can result in hepatotoxicity in dogs and cats by either dose-related or idiosyncratic mechanisms. Most cases of drug toxicity result in acute hepatitis, although this can progress to chronic hepatitis with fibrosis and cirrhosis, particularly when the drug is administered chronically, as for example with anticonvulsants such as phenobarbital. Two important potentially hepatotoxic drugs are outlined below. However, it is important not to assume drug toxicity in every dog or cat with increased liver enzymes. Surveys in humans have shown that drug reactions are over-diagnosed resulting in unnecessary withdrawal of therapeutically important drugs. In cases where there is doubt, a liver biopsy is important in confirming toxicity.

Phenobarbital in dogs

Chronic phenobarbital administration has been associated with an acute hepatic necrosis and also chronic hepatitis and cirrhosis in a small number of dogs. Toxicity is uncommon but hepatic enzyme induction is very common, so the challenge in treated dogs is to differentiate normal enzyme induction from hepatotoxicity. The main differences are outlined in Figure 37.16.

In a normal animal, phenobarbital induces cytochrome P450 enzymes and causes enlargement of hepatocytes by swelling of the endoplasmic reticulum. This in itself is not pathological. The potential for hepatotoxicity may be increased by concurrent medication with other drugs requiring hepatic metabolism, so this should be avoided if at all possible. In addition, the diet fed also appears to affect phenobarbital pharmacokinetics with low protein diets reducing the half-life and increasing the ALP level. It is therefore important to monitor blood concentrations regularly during therapy and adjust dosages according to blood concentrations and not just empirically. Most dogs developing hepatotoxicity with phenobarbital have serum concentrations at, or above, the top end of the therapeutic range and have been on the drug for at least 5 months. If seizures are not adequately controlled at a high blood concentration of phenobarbital it is advisable to add in a second drug which does not require hepatic metabolism,

such as potassium bromide or levetiracetam rather than to increase the dose of phenobarbital yet further. The ideal treatment for phenobarbital toxicity would be to withdraw the drug, but in many cases this is not possible without a recurrence of seizures. In these cases, a reduction in dose rate and combination with another drug as described above is indicated. Reductions in phenobarbital dose of between 25% and 100% have been shown to be sufficient to resolve toxicity in most cases. In addition, S-adenosylmethionine has a particular indication in phenobarbital toxicity where it appears to be hepatoprotective as it is a precursor for antioxidant and detoxifying systems in the liver.

Diazepam in cats

Diazepam has the potential to cause an acute, fulminant hepatic failure in cats with a high mortality. This is uncommon but, because of its seriousness, it is advisable to avoid the use of diazepam in cats as much as possible, particularly chronic use. All reported cases had been receiving diazepam orally for at least 5 days with total daily doses ranging from 1.0–2.5 mg. Unlike phenobarbital, diazepam does not induce hepatic enzymes in normal animals. Therefore, a key finding in affected cats is a sudden dramatic increase in hepatic enzymes, particularly ALT, which is markedly increased. Other clinical and clinicopathological findings are typical of acute hepatic failure. Treatment involves immediate and complete withdrawal of the drug and aggressive intensive support. However, the prognosis is very poor.

Non-inflammatory hepatocellular disease
Feline hepatic lipidosis

Definition and pathophysiology: Feline hepatic lipidosis (FHL) describes a clinical syndrome of acute liver failure associated with marked lipid build-up in hepatocytes. This is recognized as a disease in cats but not in dogs. Both species can develop steatosis where fat accumulates in hepatocytes and there are increased liver enzyme activities, but mild to moderate accumulation does not result in liver failure. Cats have a particular propensity to develop hepatocyte steatosis when they are anorexic for any reason, and this becomes FHL if the cat is clinically ill, with most of the hepatocytes affected with a large amount of lipid accumulation (Figure 37.17)

Parameter	Changes with uncomplicated phenobarbital therapy	Evidence of potential hepatotoxicity
Clinical signs	Sedation, ataxia and polyphagia normal side-effects at high doses	All dogs developing hepatotoxicity initially show sedation and ataxia, followed by signs of acute or chronic hepatitis (not all signs in all cases): anorexia, jaundice, ascites, coagulopathy
Liver size and shape (grossly and on radiography)	Enlarged with smoothly rounded border	Enlarged (acute toxicity) or small (chronic toxicity) often with irregular border
Liver appearance on ultrasonography	As above. No change in echogenicity	As above. May be diffusely increased or normal echogenicity
Hepatic enzyme changes	Typical of enzyme induction: mild to moderate increases in alkaline phosphatase and alanine aminotransferase, transient increase in gamma-glutamyl transferase	Typical, acute or chronic hepatitis: in addition to increase in alkaline phosphatase, alanine aminotransferase and aspartate aminotransferase may become more markedly increased
Hepatic function tests	Normal albumin (may be transiently reduced at start of therapy), normal bilirubin and normal bile acids	Most have low albumin, increases in bilirubin and postprandial ± preprandial bile acids or ammonia

37.16 Clinical, clinicopathological and diagnostic imaging findings, which help to differentiate uncomplicated phenobarbital-induced enzyme induction from hepatotoxicity.

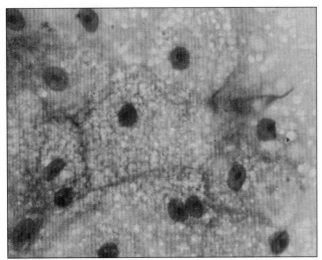

37.17 Cytological appearance of severe hepatic lipidosis in a cat. Note the great accumulation of fat globules in hepatocytes. (Giemsa stain; original magnification X1000.)
(Courtesy of Elizabeth Villiers)

FHL was first reported in the USA in 1977 and it is now increasingly recognized in Europe including the UK, where secondary FHL seems to be more common than the primary idiopathic form. The pathophysiology remains poorly understood. Obesity, anorexia and stress are important predisposing factors. Primary FHL is recognized in overweight cats which have not eaten for a prolonged period with no identified underlying cause. It has been reported with as little as 25–30% weight loss over a few weeks. Cats with secondary FHL have another disease, and are often not as overweight as cats with primary disease. Any other disease can be associated with secondary FHL, but particularly cholangitis, pancreatitis, idiopathic chronic inflammatory enteropathy, neoplasia, diabetes and hyperthyroidism.

The pathogenesis in both forms involves a 'bottleneck' in the liver such that lipids released as a result of peripheral lipolysis cannot be exported rapidly enough. The triglyceride content of the liver increases from the normal 1% to over 40%. The resultant marked fat build-up in hepatocytes causes a form of acute liver failure by interfering with hepatocyte metabolic activity, together with a secondary cholestasis due to compression of small intrahepatic cholangioles. Circulating insulin concentrations in affected cats are normal or reduced, ruling out insulin resistance as the mechanism. The reason why some cats appear to be more susceptible than others is unclear. Concurrent protein, taurine and carnitine deficiency and negative nitrogen balance associated with fasting have been suggested to contribute to the pathogenesis by reducing the ability to metabolize and export fat from the liver, although evidence for these mechanisms is limited.

History and clinical signs: The classic history for FHL is a cat which was previously obese then suffered a period of anorexia, with or without concurrent disease. There is an increased prevalence in young to middle-aged female cats. Idiopathic cases tend to be younger than secondary cases. Clinical signs are typical of acute loss of liver function. In addition to anorexia, cats often show vomiting, weakness and weight loss along with hypersalivation and dullness, which are likely manifestations of HE. In cats with secondary FHL, these clinical signs will be combined with those of the underlying disease. Clinical examination usually reveals lethargy, dehydration, jaundice and hepatomegaly. There is usually evidence of weight loss, with loss of body mass

over the spine but retention of inguinal and abdominal fat, typical of weight loss in cats. The falciform fat pad is typically retained and can be seen on abdominal radiographs.

Diagnosis, clinical pathology and diagnostic imaging: FHL should be suspected in any cat, with or without concurrent disease, which is overweight and then has a period of anorexia or forced starvation. The suspicion is increased by finding typical changes on biochemistry and should be confirmed with cytology or biopsy of the liver.

Blood samples are lipaemic and show increases in circulating triglycerides and also serum beta-hydroxybutyrate, showing there is some ketogenesis in the liver. There are moderate to marked increases in bilirubin, ALP and ALT, whereas classically gamma-glutamyl transferase (GGT) is normal. Therefore, finding a marked increase in ALP with normal or only mildly increased GGT in a cat raises the index of suspicion for FHL rather than biliary tract disease. However, a cat with secondary FHL may also have increased GGT if it has concurrent disease with biliary stasis, such as pancreatitis or cholangitis. Hypokalaemia is common due to prolonged anorexia and vomiting. Hyperglycaemia is reported in 40–50% of cats. It is usually transient, but diabetes mellitus should be carefully ruled out as an important cause of secondary FHL with measurement of serum fructosamine and serial monitoring of blood glucose during treatment (Brown *et al.*, 2000). Coagulation times are prolonged in about half of affected cats. It is advisable to measure serum cobalamin in affected cats because it is low in some cases, presumably reflecting a concurrent enteropathy or, rarely, exocrine pancreatic insufficiency. Parenteral supplementation of cobalamin is recommended if concentrations are subnormal.

Ultrasonography usually shows a diffusely hyperechoic liver, more hyperechoic than the adjacent falciform fat. However, the sensitivity of detection of FHL by ultrasonography is not 100%: obese cats without lipidosis can also have a hyperechoic liver, and in one ultrasonographic study, a correct diagnosis was made based on imaging findings in only 50–71% of cases of FHL depending on the ultrasonographer (Feeney *et al.*, 2008). It is, therefore, important to interpret the ultrasonographic appearance along with clinical and clinicopathological findings. Ultrasonography also allows assessment of other organs for concurrent disease, particularly the pancreas and GI tract.

Definitive diagnosis requires a tissue biopsy. Ideally, an ultrasound-guided Tru-Cut® or wedge biopsy sample should be taken to rule out significant underlying disease. However, taking a biopsy sample requires heavy sedation or general anaesthesia and normal coagulation times, so it is usually not safe in the acute stages of disease. The liver is particularly friable with hepatic lipidosis. Therefore, on initial presentation, a safer, minimally invasive indication of disease can be made using ultrasonographically or digitally guided FNA. Blind aspiration is safe and straightforward if there is palpable hepatomegaly, but should be performed on the left-hand side to avoid accidental puncture of the gall bladder. If cytology is strongly suggestive of FHL, the cat should be treated quickly and a feeding tube placed. If the cat fails to respond as expected, a tissue biopsy sample should be taken after the cat has been stabilized to confirm the diagnosis because fine-needle aspirate cytology has been reported to be unreliable in some cases, and false diagnoses of FHL in cats with hepatic lymphoma or cholangitis have been reported (Willard *et al.*, 1999; Wang *et al.*, 2004). Parenteral vitamin K treatment, as described earlier in this chapter, prior to biopsy together with aggressive treatment of suspected FHL, may normalize coagulation times prior to sample collection.

Treatment: Early aggressive feeding is the single most important factor affecting prognosis in cats with FHL. This always requires some form of tube feeding (Figure 37.18). The mortality in cats with FHL is up to 90% without feeding but reduces to 40% or lower with aggressive dietary management. Rapid institution of tube feeding in one study resulted in a survival rate of six out of seven cats (Biourge *et al.*, 1993). Appetite stimulants do not work in cats with FHL and are not indicated. It is equally important to institute early, aggressive nutritional management in cats with secondary disease, although it is also important to identify and treat, or provide supportive care for, any underlying disease, such as pancreatitis, in these cats.

Fluid and electrolyte imbalances should be addressed within 12 hours of hospitalization and then tube feeding can commence. Serum potassium and phosphate should be measured frequently, particularly after feeding commences, because re-feeding syndrome has been reported in a tube-fed cat with FHL, with a precipitous drop in serum potassium and phosphate resulting in haemolysis (Brenner *et al.*, 2011).

Feeding always requires placement of a feeding tube. Oesophagostomy or gastrostomy tubes are preferred because cats usually need feeding for at least 2 weeks and often longer (Biourge *et al.*, 1993). Naso-oesophageal tube feeding is useful in the short term (the first few days) because it has the advantage of not requiring a general anaesthetic for placement in an unstable cat. A more permanent tube can then be placed once the cat has stabilized. Food should be introduced slowly with initially small volumes (starting with no more than 25% of the calculated resting energy requirement and gradually increasing in 20–25% increments every 24 hours) because there is a significant reduction in stomach volume in cats after prolonged fasting (Armstrong and Blanchard, 2009) and to prevent re-feeding syndrome after prolonged anorexia. The cat should be fed using a high-protein diet, which equates to commercial therapeutic recovery or critical care diets, which are generally also formulated for feline tube feeding. Studies have shown that high-protein diets are the most effective at reducing hepatic lipid in experimentally induced FHL (Biourge *et al.*, 1994). Some authors also recommend adding other nutrients to the tube feed, but there is no evidence that routine addition of extra nutrients to feline critical care diets is necessary, apart from cobalamin, if it has been demonstrated to be deficient (see Chapter 27, the *BSAVA Manual of Rehabilitation, Supportive and Palliative Care* and the *BSAVA Guide to Procedures in Small Animal Practice, 2nd edn.*, for more detail on placing tubes and feeding).

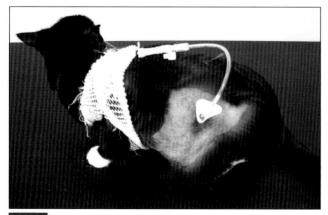

37.18 Cat with hepatic lipidosis with a gastrostomy tube in place.

Some cats with FHL will develop clinically significant HE, most often soon after instituting feeding, while the liver function is still very compromised. However, feeding enough protein is central to the resolution of FHL, so protein restriction as a treatment for HE should be avoided. Instead, HE should be controlled by feeding cats a high quality protein diet. The author recommends ≥ 4.0 g/kg protein to avoid negative nitrogen balance with high fat and low carbohydrate, which would be typically critical care-type diets fed in small, frequent meals, starting at 25–30% calculated resting energy requirement, then gradually building up to 100%. Therapies for concurrent inflammatory disease and electrolyte disturbances should be instituted and cats carefully monitored for hypophosphataemia and hypokalaemia on re-feeding. HE will resolve over a number of days, as the increased protein and calorie intake results in resolution of the severe hepatocyte steatosis and liver function resumes.

Additional therapies which may be used symptomatically in affected cats include antiemetics (maropitant) and prokinetics, such as ranitidine, particularly if there is a delay in gastric emptying after tube feeding, and analgesics (methadone or buprenorphine) if there is pancreatitis. There is evidence that cats with FHL have significant hepatic oxidant injury, so supplementation with antioxidants such as SAMe and vitamin E is recommended (Center *et al.*, 2002).

Vacuolar hepatopathies in dogs

Vacuolar hepatopathies are commonly recognized in dogs and are predominantly secondary to disease in other organs, although some causes are primary; many of the causes are listed in Figure 37.4. In addition, certain lysosomal storage diseases and toxicities can also cause vacuolar hepatopathies. Hepatocytes become vacuolated when they are loaded with fat (steatosis), glycogen or water (hepatocellular swelling or cloudy swelling). Cloudy swelling occurs if hepatocytes are injured and less able to maintain fluid homeostasis. Histological features and special stains can help differentiate the types of vacuolation, but this can be challenging.

There has been a tendency to consider that canine vacuolar hepatopathies are invariably benign and reversible. However, this is not always the case. If hepatocyte swelling is severe and chronic, it can result in hepatocyte cell death, fibrosis and even cirrhosis. Steatosis in humans can also predispose to hepatocellular carcinoma (Takahashi and Fukusato, 2014), and the same appears to be true in the glycogen-like vacuolar hepatopathy of Scottish Terriers.

Glycogen-like vacuolar hepatopathy of the Scottish Terrier: Scottish Terriers can develop a particular form of vacuolar hepatopathy, reported in the USA and France. The condition is characterized by a marked persistent increase in serum ALP with a milder increase in ALT activity and an apparent increase in the risk of hepatocellular carcinoma (Zimmerman *et al.*, 2010; Cortright *et al.*, 2014; Peyron *et al.*, 2015). It is commonest in middle-aged dogs and has no clear male or female predominance. The histological and clinicopathological changes are typical of hyperadrenocorticism and nearly half of the affected dogs show clinical signs suggestive of hyperadrenocorticism (hepatomegaly; pot-bellied appearance; polydipsia and polyuria), but the results of adrenal function testing are variable: there is an inconsistent response of cortisol to adrenocorticotropic hormone (ACTH) stimulation and low dose dexamethasone suppression testing, and in one report five out of seven dogs which had urine cortisol:creatinine ratio testing, showed normal results (Cortright *et al.*, 2014). The most consistent endocrinological abnormalities in affected dogs are increases in progesterone and androstenedione post ACTH stimulation. The adrenal glands are enlarged on ultrasonography in a quarter of cases and gall bladder mucocoele (see below) is reported in 16% of cases (Cortright *et al.*, 2014).

On ultrasonography, the liver usually appears mottled. Hypoechoic nodules may be present, which appear to result from hepatocyte death and collapse (Cortright *et al.*, 2014). Affected dogs respond poorly to traditional treatments for hyperadrenocorticism, with severe side effects reported with mitotane or ketoconazole and lack of efficacy of trilostane. Current treatment recommendations are, therefore, unclear. Antioxidant supplements, particularly SAMe, are recommended because reduced glutathione is reported in other vacuolar hepatopathies in dogs (Center *et al.*, 2002; Center *et al.*, 2005). It is also wise to repeat hepatic ultrasonography regularly to screen for the development of gall bladder mucocoele or hepatocellular masses, which may benefit from surgical intervention.

Canine familial hyperlipidaemia: Familial hyperlipidaemia is another important cause of canine primary hepatic steatosis, particularly in Miniature Schnauzers. It is also recognized in Briards, Rough Collies, Shetland Sheepdogs and a variety of other breeds and crossbreeds. The disease is associated with increases in fasting triglycerides or cholesterol in affected dogs. Familial hypertriglyceridaemia is very common in Miniature Schnauzers and is thought to be caused by delayed clearance of dietary triglycerides by the liver. It is usually not recognized until middle age and there is an increased prevalence with age, due to an interaction between the dog's genetic risk and its environment. As dogs age, the liver becomes less proficient at clearing dietary fat, and if this is superimposed on a hereditary hypertriglyceridaemia, the result is a marked fasting hypertriglyceridaemia and clinical signs. Concurrent diseases associated with increased triglycerides, such as hypothyroidism, also lower the threshold for disease in affected dogs. The condition is diagnosed on the basis of inappropriate increases of triglycerides, and often also cholesterol, in a fasting sample with no other reason identified. The presence of associated diseases also increases the index of suspicion. The most well known disease associated with hypertriglyceridaemia is acute pancreatitis (see Chapter 36). However, vacuolar hepatopathy and gall bladder mucocoele are also common. In one study of Miniature Schnauzers with familial hypertriglyceridaemia, 60% and 45% of affected dogs had increases in serum ALP and ALT activities, respectively, compared with 0% and 9% of Miniature Schnauzers with normal fasting triglycerides.

The disease is strongly suspected to be familial because of the high prevalence in one breed, but the genetics are unknown. It is highly likely that the disease will be polygenic, as it is in humans. Treatment involves long-term feeding of a low-fat diet together with diagnosis and treatment of concurrent disorders, such as hypothyroidism. If a low-fat diet fails to reduce fasting serum triglycerides, then omega-3 fatty acids can be supplemented, as these clear triglycerides from the circulation as a result of a number of proposed mechanisms, including extracellular lipolysis by lipoprotein lipase and enhanced hepatic and skeletal muscle oxidation (Shearer *et al.*, 2012). It is

also wise to repeat hepatic ultrasonography regularly to screen for the development of gall bladder mucocoele or hepatocellular masses, which may benefit from surgical intervention (see below). Symptomatic treatment should be instituted for acute pancreatitis (see Chapter 36).

Superficial necrolytic dermatitis

Pathophysiology: Superficial necrolytic dermatitis, also known as hepatocutaneous syndrome, metabolic epidermal necrosis or necrolytic migratory erythema, is an uncommon canine skin condition associated with a very characteristic hepatopathy, which is assumed to be secondary to an underlying metabolic disorder. Many cases in humans are associated with a glucagon-secreting tumour but this is rare in dogs. One dog reported with the condition had an insulinoma. Superficial necrolytic dermatitis was also reported in 11 dogs being treated with phenobarbitone (March *et al.*, 2004), although the contribution of the drug to the disease was unclear and the response to stopping treatment was not known. However, in most canine cases the cause remains obscure. Superficial necrolytic dermatitis is very rare in cats and has only been reported in five cases, three of which had pancreatic tumours (Kimmel *et al.*, 2003; Asakawa *et al.*, 2013).

Clinical signs and diagnosis: Diagnosis is based on the characteristic histology of skin biopsy samples together with findings on liver ultrasonography and histology. Affected dogs are typically older, small-breed dogs, with a male predominance. They often present because of the skin lesions which are hyperkeratotic, erythematous, crusting lesions, particularly on the extremities: footpads, nose, periorbital and perianal regions, around the genitals and often also on pressure points. Dogs are usually lame because of the footpad lesions. Between a quarter and a half of cases have diabetes mellitus, which usually develops later in the disease process. Dogs rarely present because of clinical signs of liver disease.

Skin biopsy samples demonstrate typical parakeratotic hyperkeratosis, which results in a 'red, white and blue' layered appearance on haematoxylin and eosin-stained sections of skin; the major differential diagnosis is zinc-responsive dermatosis. ALP and ALT activities are usually increased on blood samples, hypoalbuminaemia is common, and hyperglycaemia and glucosuria are recognized in those cases with concurrent diabetes mellitus. Hepatic ultrasonography shows a very characteristic 'Swiss cheese' appearance to the liver with hypoechoic nodules surrounded by hyperechoic borders (Nyland *et al.*, 1996). The nodules correspond histologically to nodular areas of normal hepatocytes surrounded by zones of collapsed parenchyma with vacuolated hepatocytes.

Treatment: Treatment is challenging and the prognosis tends to be poor, with death or euthanasia within 6 months of diagnosis. This likely reflects a lack of understanding of the underlying pathogenesis. Cure is very unusual and has only been reported in one case after successful removal of a pancreatic tumour. In other cases, treatment is supportive and symptomatic. The most important consideration is an ample supply of amino acids because the disease has been associated with amino acid deficiency. For this reason, proprietary hepatic diets are not ideal, and a high-quality, digestible, high-protein diet should be fed. Supplementation with extra zinc and essential fatty acids is often recommended. Some authors use weekly intravenous amino acid infusions, but the efficacy is unproven.

In one case report, a dog was fed a daily egg yolk together with a hepatic support diet, essential fatty acids and colchicine. The skin lesions resolved and the dog was still doing well 22 months after presentation (Hill *et al.*, 2000). Symptomatic treatment of the skin lesions includes appropriate antibiotics for secondary infections, topical shampoos and analgesia. Steroids should be avoided because of the risk of precipitating diabetes mellitus.

Feline hepatic amyloidosis

Pathophysiology: Amyloidosis is caused by accumulation of auto-aggregated beta-pleated sheets of amyloid protein. There are different types of amyloid protein, but the form which accumulates in the liver is serum amyloid A (SAA). This is an acute phase protein made normally by hepatocytes in response to inflammatory cytokines. Together with C-reactive protein, it is the acute phase protein which is produced in the largest amount. An increase in SAA is necessary to develop consequent amyloidosis, but by no means do all individuals with increased SAA go on to develop disease. Amyloidosis due to amyloid light chain, which is monoclonal immunoglobulin G light chain, also occurs in small animals but liver involvement has not been reported.

Amyloidosis can be generalized or localized and can affect different organs. Hepatic amyloidosis, where SAA is largely confined to the liver, is most often reported in cats. The reason why some individuals build up SAA in certain organs and not others is unknown, but it is likely to represent an interaction of genetic susceptibility with environmental triggers. This is supported by breed predispositions in cats: Abyssinian cats usually develop generalized amyloidosis, which presents as renal failure and, although the liver is often involved, it is usually not the reason for clinical presentation or the cause of mortality. In contrast, the amyloidosis recognized in Siamese cats is usually predominantly hepatic. Predominantly hepatic amyloidosis has also been reported in Domestic Shorthaired, Oriental Shorthaired and Devon Rex cats (van der Linde-Sipman *et al.*, 1997; Godfrey and Day, 1998; Beatty *et al.*, 2002; Khoshnegah and Movassaghi, 2010), and the author has diagnosed it in a Persian cat.

Clinical presentation and diagnosis: Affected cats are usually young adults. The commonest reason for presentation is weakness and anaemia as a result of acute intra-abdominal bleeding from the liver capsule: the liver becomes very rigid and friable with amyloidosis, and very susceptible to damage. The haemorrhage can be severe enough to be fatal, or cats may autotransfuse and recover. Other possible causes of acute liver haemorrhage in cats include peliosis and hepatic tumours. Some cats present with jaundice due to hepatic dysfunction. Hepatomegaly is usually obvious on clinical examination. There may also be an obvious concurrent inflammatory disease, such as severe periodontal disease, which is assumed to be driving the production of SAA. On clinical pathology, there is increase of ALT activity and bilirubin, and also usually increased globulins and often anaemia. Cholestatic enzyme activities are rarely increased. Some cats have concurrent azotaemia. Ultrasonography shows a diffusely enlarged, hyperechoic liver with normal biliary tract: important differential diagnoses for this appearance are lymphoma, lipidosis and feline infectious peritonitis (FIP). Definitive diagnosis is made with hepatic biopsy. Fine-needle aspirate cytology is usually misleading, although there is one report of diagnosis of amyloidosis with FNA.

Treatment: There is no effective specific treatment for hepatic amyloidosis in cats. Colchicine treatment has been used in Shar Peis with Shar Pei fever, but this is not reported in cats and colchicine is likely to be toxic in this species. Supportive treatment of the liver disease with a high-quality diet and antioxidants and treating any underlying inflammatory disease can give affected cats a good quality of life, but the owner should be warned of the high risk of sudden death due to hepatic rupture and haemorrhage.

Hepatocellular neoplasia

Pathophysiology: Primary liver tumours are rare in dogs and cats, and much less common than they are in humans. They represent less than 2% of all tumours in dogs and less than 3% of all tumours in cats. This may be because two of the predisposing factors for development of liver tumours (hepatitis virus infection and alpha$_1$-protease inhibitor deficiency) have not been recognized in small animals. However, vacuolar hepatopathy appears to predispose to hepatocellular carcinoma in Scottish Terriers (Cortright *et al.*, 2014) and chronic inflammatory disease may predispose to neoplasia in other dogs and cats. It is interesting to note that cholangiocellular carcinomas are the most common malignant liver tumours seen in cats, which may mirror the high incidence of biliary tract disease in this species. In contrast, hepatocellular carcinomas are the most common primary liver tumours reported in dogs.

In dogs, malignant primary tumours outnumber benign primary tumours, whereas in cats benign primary tumours are much more common and may be incidental findings. The types of primary tumour recognized in the liver in dogs and cats are outlined in Figure 37.19. Canine malignant tumours may be 'massive', which present as a solitary, large mass confined to one lobe; 'diffuse', which describes diffuse involvement of all liver lobes; or 'nodular', in which there is a multifocal disease with involvement of several lobes. The diffuse and nodular forms usually carry a poorer prognosis with a higher metastatic rate than the massive forms.

Secondary tumours are commonly recognized in the liver because of its excellent blood and lymphatic supply and reticuloendothelial function. Metastases have been estimated to be 2.5 times more common than primary tumours, in the liver of dogs. These include particularly haematopoietic tumours, such as lymphoma and, less commonly, leukaemias, histiocytic tumours and mast cell tumours and metastases from other organs, such as pancreas, mammary glands and GI tract. Haemangiosarcomas in the liver may be primary or secondary and sometimes the origin is difficult to ascertain if multiple organs are involved, although the right atrium or spleen are often primary sites.

It is important to note that older dogs and cats can also develop benign nodular hyperplasia (BNH) in the liver, which is clinically insignificant but can be confused with neoplasia. BNH is found at post-mortem examination in at least 70% of dogs 14 years of age or older, and is also reported in cats, although less commonly. The cause is unknown, although nutritional factors including protein restriction are said to play a role in other species. It is most important in that it can be confused on gross appearance, clinical pathology and diagnostic imaging findings with more serious conditions, particularly hepatic neoplasia and also regenerative nodules in cirrhosis.

Type of tumour	Dogs	Cats
• Hepatocellular tumours • Hepatocellular adenoma • Hepatocellular carcinoma (HCC)	Adenoma is usually an incidental finding HCC is the most common primary liver tumour Most are solitary and massive – prognosis is good with full surgical resection. Some are nodular and diffuse – prognosis is poor	Recognized but less common than biliary tumours
• Biliary tract tumours • Cholangiocellular carcinomas (including cystadenocarcinomas) • Cholangiocellular adenomas • Gall bladder tumours	Cholangiocellular carcinomas constitute 22–41% of malignant liver tumours; MR 56–88%	Cholangiocellular carcinomas and adenomas are the most common primary liver tumours in cats
• Neuroendocrine tumour • Hepatic carcinoid	Rare but very aggressive	Rare but very aggressive
• Primary hepatic sarcomas • Haemangiosarcoma • Leiomyosarcoma • Others	Uncommon. Most are locally aggressive and have high MR	Uncommon. Most are locally aggressive and have high MR

37.19 Primary liver tumours in dogs and cats. Note that secondary metastases in the liver are much more common than primary liver tumours and diffuse metastatic disease can present as acute liver failure. In addition, hepatosplenic and hepatocytotropic T-cell lymphomas have been reported in dogs with a rapidly progressive course (Keller *et al.*, 2013). MR = metastatic rate.

Clinical signs and diagnosis: Primary malignant liver tumours are usually seen in older animals (mean age 10–12 years), although they are also sporadically recognized in younger animals. There is no obvious sex predisposition reported, except for canine biliary carcinomas, which were more common in females in several studies.

The presenting clinical signs and laboratory findings of liver tumours are indistinguishable from the findings in any primary liver disease or BNH. About half of affected animals may have palpable hepatomegaly or liver masses on abdominal palpation, and these will be particularly obvious in dogs with massive tumours. However, at least 50% of cats with liver tumours show no clinical signs at all. Most animals present with signs of chronic liver disease, but diffuse hepatic neoplasia, particularly lymphoma, can present as acute liver failure in dogs with a high mortality (Lester *et al.*, 2016).

On clinical pathology, increase in liver enzyme activities and bile acids and a mild anaemia and neutrophilia are common but non-specific findings. Jaundice is uncommon but can occur. Hypoglycaemia is a notable finding, particularly in dogs and particularly with massive tumours. The blood glucose can be low enough to cause clinical signs of weakness and collapse in these cases. BNH also often causes an increase in serum ALP activity, which is usually moderate (2.5–3 times upper end of normal range) but can be as high as 10–14 times normal. This can cause confusion and a fruitless, expensive search for causes of biliary stasis or hyperadrenocorticism in a dog which is in fact healthy, so it is important to be aware of this possibility. Bile acids and bilirubin are usually normal in BNH, but there may be a mild increase in hepatocellular enzyme activities, probably due to cellular regeneration.

Ultrasonography is very helpful in identifying a hepatic mass and also in checking for metastases. However, it is important to remember that BNH can look identical to malignant neoplasia on ultrasonography. Malignant hepatic tumours commonly metastasize to the peritoneum and local lymph nodes and less commonly to the lungs, but it is important to take right and left lateral thoracic radiographs (or perform thoracic CT) in all animals with liver tumours to check for metastases. A thorough abdominal ultrasound examination should be undertaken to check for evidence of metastases.

Hyperplastic nodules are usually macroscopic and multiple and may appear of mixed echogenicity on ultrasonography, mimicking tumours. This underlines the fact that ultrasonography cannot give a histological diagnosis, so it is important on finding a hepatic mass on imaging not to euthanase an animal without biopsy confirmation.

Definitive diagnosis of neoplasia relies on cytology or histopathology. In some cases, fine-needle aspirates may be diagnostic but in others they may be difficult to interpret, particularly with benign hepatocellular tumours, where the cells may look indistinguishable from normal hepatocytes. Ultrasound-guided Tru-Cut® biopsies are usually diagnostic or, alternatively, biopsy samples may be taken at laparoscopy or laparotomy. In the case of an apparently single, massive lesion, the clinician may elect to proceed straight to surgical removal and an 'excisional' biopsy. Coagulation times should be checked prior to any form of biopsy, although it is unusual for these to be prolonged with primary tumours. However, coagulation times can be very significantly and dangerously prolonged in diffuse hepatic infiltration with lymphoma or other diffuse secondary tumours, and biopsies should not be considered in these cases until clotting factors have been supplemented with a plasma transfusion.

Nodular hyperplasia is often difficult to diagnose on a Tru-Cut® biopsy and a wedge biopsy is preferred. A Tru-Cut® biopsy may simply show vacuolar swelling, suggesting an endocrinopathy (causing further confusion in a dog with increased ALP activity), and does not give such a good indication of hepatic architecture, making differentiation from hepatomas difficult.

Treatment: Treatment of primary hepatic tumours relies on surgical removal if they are resectable. This is advisable even with benign tumours, as there is some limited evidence that they may undergo malignant transformation. Resection of hepatocellular carcinomas in dogs carries a good prognosis, if the entire mass can be removed with a lobectomy (Kinsey *et al.*, 2015). Even debulking of large masses can prolong life expectancy if they are slow growing. Treatment of diffuse, nodular and metastasized tumours is difficult. Hepatic tumours generally show a poor response to chemotherapy. It has been suggested that this is because hepatocytes, both normal and transformed, have high expression of the multi-drug resistance membrane-associated P-glycoprotein and also that heptocytes are naturally high in detoxifying enzymes. Radiotherapy is not widely used, as normal liver tissue is very radiosensitive, although it has been reported in a small number of cases. Transarterial catheter chemoembolization has been reported in a small number of animals, but more studies are required to confirm its indications and efficacy. Future therapies may rely more on immunotherapeutics or personalized medicine using cell culture techniques from biopsy samples.

No treatment is required for BNH, as the condition is benign, although it would be worth checking that the animal has a balanced diet, which is not inappropriately protein-restricted.

Biliary tract diseases

Suppurative (neutrophilic) cholangitis and cholecystitis in cats and dogs

Pathophysiology: Suppurative cholangitis and cholecystitis in dogs and cats are believed to be due to bacterial infections. The origin of the infection can be either haematogenous via the portal vein or ascending the bile duct from the small intestine. Suppurative cholangitis and cholecystitis are more commonly reported in cats than dogs, but a recent retrospective case series suggested they are also more common in dogs than previously recognized, representing about 6% of all dogs with hepatitis (Tamborini *et al.*, 2016). It is commonly believed that bile is usually sterile in dogs and cats, and certainly bacteria and inflammatory cells are not seen on cytology of normal bile. The causes and predisposing factors for bacterial infection of the biliary tract are unknown but are suggested from studies to include partial obstruction of bile flow, interference with the function of the sphincter of Oddi, immunosuppressive medication and gall bladder wall abnormalities.

Clinical signs and diagnosis: Suppurative cholangitis/cholecystitis can affect dogs and cats of any age or breed, but is most often seen in young to middle-aged cats and middle-aged dogs. Affected animals usually present acutely, although some dogs have a more chronic history, perhaps because the disease is not recognized initially.

Clinical signs are similar in dogs and cats and reflect biliary stasis with sepsis. However, none of the signs are specific. Affected animals usually show vomiting, lethargy, pyrexia and jaundice. Some dogs show signs of abdominal pain. Not all animals are pyrexic and, in a recent study in dogs, only a third of animals were pyrexic at presentation (Tamborini *et al.*, 2016). A small percentage of affected dogs and cats may present with gall bladder rupture or leakage and, therefore, more severe signs of an 'acute abdomen'. Important differential diagnoses include acute or chronic hepatitis, chronic cholangitis, gall bladder mucocoele and extra-hepatic biliary obstruction with choleliths, neoplasia or pancreatitis.

Blood samples commonly show neutrophilia, increased liver enzyme activities and bilirubin. Clinicopathological findings also show overlap with the other differential diagnoses. On ultrasonography, many affected cats and dogs have abnormalities of the biliary tract, including dilatation of bile ducts and thickening of the gall bladder wall. It is important to look carefully for any evidence of biliary obstruction, including choleliths. If there is any free abdominal fluid, a sample should be taken and analysed cytologically and its bilirubin concentration should be measured: if there is leakage from or rupture of the gall bladder, the bilirubin concentration will be high. This would be an indication for urgent surgical intervention.

A definitive diagnosis of suppurative cholangitis requires bile culture. Culture is also important for antibiotic sensitivity testing since a significant number of infections are

multi-drug resistant. Bile aspirates can be taken safely under ultrasound guidance, provided the animal is heavily sedated or anaesthetized and care is taken. Alternatively, aspirates can be taken under visualization at laparotomy or laparoscopy. Aspirates should not be taken if there is a grossly abnormal gall bladder wall, bile duct obstruction or mucocoele because of the increased risk of bile leakage. Aspirates should be submitted for cytology, which may show bacteria and neutrophils, and culture. It is important to consider taking bile aspirates in any dog or cat which has a laparotomy or laparoscopy for liver biopsy, because bile aspirates or gall bladder wall taken at surgery have a higher yield on bacterial culture than liver biopsy and, therefore, there is a high chance that a biliary tract infection will not be identified if only a liver biopsy sample is taken. The most common organism isolated in cats is *Escherichia coli*, although *Streptococcus* spp., *Clostridium* spp., and even occasionally *Salmonella* spp. may be involved. Bile-tolerant *Helicobacter* organisms have been isolated in a few cats with cholangiohepatitis but also in the bile of cats without liver disease, so their significance is unknown. In dogs, the most common isolates are *E. coli*, *Enterococcus* and *Clostridium* spp. and more than one species is isolated in some individual dogs.

Treatment: Affected animals should be treated with appropriate antibiotics together with supportive care as detailed below. Ideally, antibiotics should be chosen based on culture and sensitivity of the organisms involved: *Escherichia coli* and *Enterococcus* are often resistant to multiple antibiotics and can also alter their resistance patterns during treatment. In the absence of culture, potentiated amoxicillin is a good initial choice as it achieves high concentrations in the bile, is not hepatotoxic or metabolized by the liver and has a broad spectrum of activity. Most specialists recommend 4–6 weeks of treatment in both dogs and cats.

Supportive treatment depends on the severity of the disease. In all cases, the addition of ursodeoxycholic acid and antioxidants is logical and probably helpful, although there are no studies of their efficacy in suppurative cholangitis in dogs and cats. In sick, septic animals and particularly those with biliary tract rupture, early aggressive fluid therapy will be necessary. All affected animals should be fed a high-quality diet: critically ill animals might need tube feeding with critical care diets. There is no need to consider feeding a hepatic diet unless there is concurrent significant parenchymal liver disease. Consideration should also be given to treating any identified underlying cause of the biliary tract infection to reduce the risk of recurrence.

Feline chronic cholangitis

Pathophysiology: Chronic biliary tract disease is common in cats but the causes are very poorly understood. Unlike acute biliary tract disease, most cases are not cured but wax and wane in spite of treatment. The WSAVA Liver Standardization Group suggested standardized nomenclature for feline biliary tract disease (Rothuizen *et al.*, 2006): neutrophilic cholangitis (which is suppurative cholangitis, discussed in the last section), lymphocytic cholangitis and chronic neutrophilic cholangitis. Other terms used in the veterinary literature for lymphocytic cholangitis in the past include lymphocytic cholangiohepatitis, lymphocytic portal hepatitis and non-suppurative cholangitis. Chronic neutrophilic cholangitis, as defined by the WSAVA, may also overlap with lymphocytic cholangitis. Some of the confusion with nomenclature reflects the likelihood that 'chronic' biliary tract disease in cats is not one disease but probably has many aetiologies. The cause of chronic biliary tract disease in cats remains unknown. Lymphocytic cholangitis and small cell lymphoma look very similar histologically and can be difficult to differentiate. There is an association, in some cases, with concurrent pancreatitis and chronic enteropathy (CE), which have similar presenting signs and complicate diagnosis and treatment. The pancreatic and bile ducts join in cats just before entering the duodenum, so blockage of the sphincter of Oddi or reflux of gut contents or bile secondary to CE could explain concurrent disease. It is also possible that all three organs are affected by immune-mediated disease, or that bacteria from the gut settle in the pancreas and/or liver due to increased permeability of the gut wall due to CE.

Clinical signs and diagnosis: Any age or breed of cat can be affected. In some studies, young to middle-aged Persian cats are at higher risk, whereas others include older cats of no particular breed, or a predominance of Norwegian Forest cats. These inconsistencies are likely due to the presence of more than one (unknown) aetiology and geographical variations. Cats tend to show a waxing and waning history of months to years with anorexia, lethargy and jaundice. They may also vomit, but are less often pyrexic than cats with suppurative disease. Presenting signs may be complicated by signs of concurrent pancreatitis or CE. A small proportion of cases present with a high-protein ascites, making differentiation from FIP challenging.

Clinicopathological testing typically shows increases in liver enzyme activities. There is less likely to be a neutrophilia than in neutrophilic (suppurative) cholangitis, but affected cats often show an increase in globulins, again making FIP an important differential diagnosis. Abdominal radiographs show non-specific hepatomegaly in some cats, due to diffuse biliary dilatation. Ultrasonography is more helpful but is not abnormal in all cases: there may be dilatation of the common bile duct and gall bladder, but these may also look normal. It is important to rule out extra-hepatic biliary obstruction wherever possible by following the bile duct ultrasonographically down to the sphincter of Oddi. Since concurrent intestinal or pancreatic disease may occur, assays of serum pancreatic marker enzymes (see Chapter 36) and cobalamin and folate are recommended.

Definitive diagnosis is made on the basis of hepatic histology. Biopsy samples should only be taken after assessment of clotting times and consideration of vitamin K treatment, as discussed earlier. The author routinely treats all cats with suspected chronic cholangitis with parenteral vitamin K for 24–48 hours prior to biopsy.

Treatment: Treatment of affected cats is largely empirical and not evidence-based. Most authors use a combination of immunosuppressive doses of steroids, antibiotics and hepatoprotectants until liver enzyme activities return to normal. Concurrent intestinal or pancreatic disease should also be addressed. However, in many cats, the disease recurs after weeks to months, requiring repeat treatment. A digestible, high-quality diet should be fed and the presence of concurrent CE might prompt the use of a single protein source or hydrolysed diet. There is a logical reason to use ursodeoxycholic acid in all affected cats for its choleretic and hepatoprotective effects, together with antioxidants, although a recent retrospective study of 26 cats with lymphocytic cholangitis, with a preponderance of older male cats and Norwegian Forest cats, suggested

that cats had a longer survival time when given prednisolone alone than when given ursodeoxycholic acid alone (Otte *et al.*, 2012). However, the study was small, biased and did not address the survival time using both drugs together. The author continues to use prednisolone, ursodeoxycholic acid, antibiotics (potentiated amoxicillin) and SAMe in affected cats until there is more understanding about the causes, and potentially infectious cases can be differentiated from potentially autoimmune cases.

Gall bladder mucocoele

Pathophysiology: A gall bladder mucocoele is a cystic mucinous hyperplasia of the gall bladder wall with accumulation of thick mucus (Figure 37.20). A mucocoele can be subclinical and an incidental finding on diagnostic imaging or post-mortem examination. However, many cases grow large enough to cause signs of biliary obstruction and, ultimately, pressure necrosis and rupture of the gall bladder. The causes of mucocoele are poorly understood. They appear to have increased in frequency since they were first reported in dogs in 1995 (Newell *et al.*, 1995) but the reasons for this are not understood. There does appear to be a strong association with hypertriglyceridaemia and hypercholesterolaemia in dogs. They are reported with increased frequency in animals with hypothyroidism, hyperadrenocorticism and idiopathic hypertriglyceridaemia. Other proposed causes are disrupted gall bladder motility, genetic mutations and biliary tract infections. Gall bladder mucocoeles are very rare in cats.

Clinical signs and diagnosis: Affected animals are typically small-breed dogs and there is an overlap with breeds predisposed to familial hyperlipidaemia: Shetland Sheepdogs, Miniature Schnauzers and Cocker Spaniels appear to be over-represented. Border Terriers are over-represented in the UK (Allerton *et al.*, 2018). Clinical signs and clinicopathological findings are very variable: in some dogs, the mucocoele is clinically silent, there are no changes on clinical pathology and these are incidental findings on ultrasound examination. Many mucocoeles are clinically significant and give typical findings of biliary tract obstruction, with anorexia, lethargy, vomiting and jaundice. In these cases, blood samples will show increased liver enzyme activities

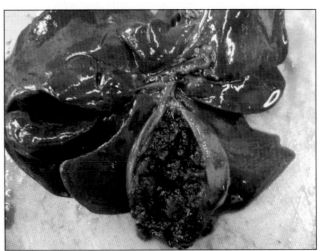

37.20 Gross appearance of a gall bladder mucocoele which was an incidental finding at post-mortem examination in a Cavalier King Charles Spaniel. The gall bladder has been opened to reveal the mucocoele.
(Courtesy of Fernando Constantino-Casas, Pathology Department, Department of Veterinary Medicine, University of Cambridge)

and bilirubin. The gall bladder is well innervated and it is likely that large mucocoeles are painful. It is important also to identify any predisposing factors, such as endocrine disease (hypothyroidism, hyperadrenocorticism or diabetes mellitus) on blood tests if possible. A small number of dogs present acutely as a result of bile peritonitis due to gall bladder rupture.

Treatment: Clinically significant gall bladder mucocoeles should be treated, and most authors recommend surgery for cholecystectomy. The prognosis is reasonable if the gall bladder has not ruptured and if biliary diversion surgery is not necessary. However, there is a real risk of perioperative mortality and bile leakage, and cholecystectomy is generally considered to be a referral procedure. Successful medical management has been reported – particularly when the underlying cause is also identified and treated. Complete resolution has been reported in two hypothyroid dogs after supplementing thyroid hormones together with medical management (Walter *et al.*, 2008). Medical management should only be attempted where there is no evidence of bile leakage or gall bladder wall thinning or necrosis on ultrasonography. The owners should be warned of the potential risk of gall bladder rupture and the mucocoele should be regularly monitored for this with ultrasonography. Medical treatment involves feeding a low-fat diet and giving ursodeoxycholic acid and antioxidants.

It is unknown whether there is any benefit to medically managing asymptomatic mucocoeles. Surgical management would not be advisable in the absence of any clinical or clinicopathological abnormalities because of the risk of perioperative mortality. It is not known if asymptomatic mucocoeles progress nor, if they do, how quickly. It is also unknown whether medical management will delay progression, but the author uses ursodeoxycholic acid routinely in asymptomatic cases and monitors them with repeat ultrasound examinations every 2–4 months.

Extra-hepatic biliary obstruction

Extra-hepatic biliary obstruction (EHBO) is defined as obstruction at the level of the common bile duct or duodenal papilla that impedes bile flow into the duodenum. The causes of EHBO in dogs and cats are listed in Figure 37.21. Most causes are rare except for chronic pancreatitis, which is the most common cause, and for which serum pancreatic markers should be assayed. Animals present with similar clinical and clinicopathological signs to cholangitis and gall bladder mucocoele: typically, jaundice, anorexia, lethargy and vomiting. A particular clinical feature which might raise the suspicion of obstructive disease is marked abdominal pain, particularly in cats. EHBO is only differentiated from non-obstructive biliary tract disease on the basis of diagnostic imaging and, in some cases, surgery. Persistence of abdominal pain in a cat with cholangitis after medical management should prompt consideration of surgical exploration of the biliary tract. There are no pathognomonic findings on clinical pathology: acholic (colourless) faeces are rare and only occur if bile flow has been completely interrupted for several weeks. Most cases in small animals show only partial obstruction. Serum bilirubin is usually very increased in dogs and cats with EHBO but can become normal with chronic obstruction, particularly in cats. The reasons are poorly understood but it is suggested that chronically obstructed cats can reduce the excretion of bile (Figure 37.22). Conversely, cats can develop jaundice with

Extraluminal
• Acute and chronic pancreatitis (D+C – commonest cause)
• Neoplasia in pancreas or liver or other adjacent tissues (D+C)
• Compression by cysts in cystic liver disease (C)
Intraluminal
• Gall bladder mucocoele (D)
• Neoplasia (D+C)
• Choleliths (C+D – more common in cats)
• Stricture post inflammation or surgery (D+C)
• Entrapment in diaphragmatic rupture (C+D)
• Duodenal foreign body (C – rare)
• Liver flukes (not in the UK)
• Heterobilharzia (D)
• Opisthorchis felineus (C)
• Platynosomum (C)
Sphincter of Oddi
• Sphincter of Oddi spasm (C)
• Obstruction by duodenal neoplasia (D+C)
• Obstruction by slow-moving duodenal foreign body (D+C)
Biliary tract rupture
• Traumatic and iatrogenic (D+C)
• Secondary to mucocoele (D)
• Secondary to neoplasia (D+C)

37.21 Causes of extra-hepatic biliary obstruction in dogs (D) and cats (C).

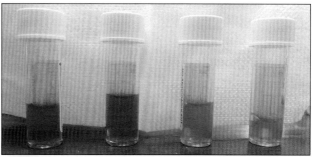

37.22 Samples of urine (two pots on the left) and gall bladder bile (two pots on the right) from a cat with chronic biliary tract obstruction due to a stricture of the common bile duct. Note the grossly abnormal pale appearance of the bile due to reduced excretion of bilirubin into the bile. This is not unusual in cats with chronic biliary obstruction. The serum and urine contained a large amount of bilirubin, so it is assumed that the bilirubin transporters in this case had moved from the luminal surface of the bile ducts to the hepatic side.

inflammatory disease elsewhere, which does not affect the bile duct (e.g. pyothorax), and it is suggested that toxaemia in cats can stimulate the bile transporters to move from the luminal surface of bile duct epithelial cells to the hepatic surface.

Choleliths are uncommon in small animals, but are a more common cause of biliary obstruction in cats than dogs. Canine choleliths are usually composed of calcium bilirubinate, whereas cats usually produce calcium carbonate choleliths, although bilirubin choleliths are reported in cats with pyruvate kinase deficiency. Biliary sludge is also commonly reported in both species and is of unknown clinical significance. Most authors suggest it is incidental (De Monaco *et al.*, 2016), although it is associated with pain in humans. There is some suggestion that biliary sludge in dogs may progress to gall bladder mucocoele in some cases, although this is not proven. It might be wise to monitor dogs with significant amounts of sludge regularly with ultrasonography and to screen for and treat any underlying endocrine disease which may be associated with gall bladder mucocoele (see earlier).

Biliary tract rupture

Rupture of the biliary tract may occur secondary to trauma (such as a kick or bite), as a result of disease of the gall bladder or biliary tract (including mucocoeles and choleliths) or iatrogenically, as a result of careless or inappropriate bile aspiration (e.g. in the presence of EHBO) or surgery. It results in a chemical bile peritonitis as a result of the irritant effect of bile. Early clinical signs are non-specific and similar to those of other diseases of the biliary tract, but these progress as peritonitis develops to vomiting, anorexia, jaundice and signs of shock. There may be a palpable abdominal effusion, and analysis shows an exudate with a high concentration of bilirubin. Treatment is surgical and the prognosis is guarded, but more favourable if the cause is found and can be treated.

Biliary tract neoplasia

Primary neoplasia of the biliary tract is rare but reported in both dogs and cats, although more commonly in cats. Details are given in the previous section and Figure 37.19.

References and further reading

Allerton F, Swinbourne F, Baker L et al. (2018) Gall bladder mucoceles in Border Terriers. Journal of Veterinary Internal Medicine 32, 1618–1628

Andersson M and Sevelius E (1991) Breed, sex and age distribution in dogs with chronic liver disease: a demographic study. Journal of Small Animal Practice 32, 1–5

Armstrong PJ and Blanchard G (2009) Hepatic lipidosis in cats. Veterinary Clinics of North America: Small Animal Practice 39, 599–616

Asakawa MG, Cullen JM and Linder KE (2013) Necrolytic migratory erythema associated with a glucagon-producing primary hepatic neuroendocrine carcinoma in a cat. Veterinary Dermatology 24, 466–469

Azumi N (1982) Copper and liver injury – experimental studies on the dogs with biliary obstruction and copper loading. The Hokkaido Journal of Medical Science 57, 331–349

Bayton WA, Westgarth C, Scase T et al. (2018) Histopathological frequency of feline hepatobiliary disease in the UK. Journal of Small Animal Practice 59, 404–410

Beatty JA, Barrs VR, Martin PA et al. (2002) Spontaneous hepatic rupture in six cats with systemic amyloidosis. Journal of Small Animal Practice 43, 355–363

Bexfield NH, Andre-Abdo C, Scase T et al. (2011) Chronic hepatitis in the English Springer Spaniel: clinical presentation, histological description and outcome. The Veterinary Record 169, 415

Bexfield NH, Buxton RJ, Vicek TJ et al. (2012a) Breed, age and gender distribution of dogs with chronic hepatitis in the United Kingdom. The Veterinary Journal 193, 124–128

Bexfield NH and Lee K (2014) BSAVA Guide to Procedures in Small Animal Practice, 2nd edn. BSAVA Publications, Gloucester

Bexfield NH, Watson PJ, Aguirre-Hernandez J et al. (2012b) DLA class II alleles and haplotypes are associated with risk for and protection from chronic hepatitis in the English Springer Spaniel. PLoS One 7, e42584

Biourge V, Pion P, Lewis J et al. (1993) Spontaneous occurrence of hepatic lipidosis in a group of laboratory cats. Journal of Veterinary Internal Medicine 7, 194–197

Biourge VC, Massat B, Groff J et al. (1994) Effects of protein, lipid, or carbohydrate supplementation on hepatic lipid accumulation during rapid weight loss in obese cats. American Journal of Veterinary Research 55, 1406–1415

Brenner K, KuKanich K and Smee NM (2011) Refeeding syndrome in a cat with hepatic lipidosis. Journal of Feline Medicine and Surgery 13, 614–617

Brown B, Mauldin GE, Armstrong J et al. (2000) Metabolic and hormonal alterations in cats with hepatic lipidosis. Journal of Veterinary Internal Medicine 14, 20–26

Center SA, Warner KL and Erb HN (2002) Liver glutathione concentrations in dogs and cats with naturally occurring liver disease. American Journal of Veterinary Research 63, 1187–1197

Center SA, Warner KL, McCabe J et al. (2005) Evaluation of the influence of S-adenosylmethionine on systemic and hepatic effects of prednisolone in dogs. American Journal of Veterinary Research 66, 330–341

Center SA, McDonough SP and Bogdanovic L (2013) Digital image analysis of rhodanine-stained liver biopsy specimens for calculation of hepatic copper concentrations in dogs. American Journal of Veterinary Research 74, 1474–1480

Coronado VA, Damaraju D, Kohijoki R et al. (2003) New haplotypes in the Bellington Terrier indicate complexity in copper toxicosis. Mammalian Genome 14, 483–491

Cortright CC, Center SA, Randolph JF et al. (2014) Clinical features of progressive vacuolar hepatopathy in Scottish Terriers with and without hepatocellular carcinoma: 114 cases (1980–2013). Journal of the American Veterinary Medical Association 245, 797–808

De Monaco SM, Grant DC, Larson MN et al. (2016) Spontaneous course of biliary sludge over 12 months in dogs with ultrasonographically identified biliary sludge. Journal of Veterinary Internal Medicine 30, 771–778

Dyggve H, Kennedy LJ, Meri S et al. (2010) Association of Doberman hepatitis to canine major histocompatibility complex II. Tissue Antigens 77, 30–35

Dyggve H, Meri S, Spillmann T et al. (2017) Antihistone antibodies in Dobermans with hepatitis. Journal of Veterinary Internal Medicine 31, 1717–1723

Feeney DA, Anderson KL, Ziegler LE et al. (2008) Statistical relevance of ultrasonographic criteria in the assessment of diffuse liver disease in dogs and cats. American Journal of Veterinary Research 69, 212–221

Godfrey DR and Day MJ (1998) Generalised amyloidosis in two Siamese cats: spontaneous liver haemorrhage and chronic renal failure. Journal of Small Animal Practice 39, 442–447

Gomez Selgas A, Bexfield N, Scase TJ et al. (2014) Total serum bilirubin as a negative prognostic factor in idiopathic canine chronic hepatitis. Journal of Veterinary Diagnostic Investigation 26, 246–251

Haywood S (2006) Copper toxicosis in Bedlington Terriers. The Veterinary Record 159, 687

Haywood S, Boursnell M, Loughran M et al. (2016) Copper toxicosis in non-COMMD1 Bedlington Terriers is associated with metal transport gene ABCA12. Journal of Trace Medicine in Medicine and Biology 35, 83–89

Hill PB, Auxilia ST, Munro E et al. (2000) Resolution of skin lesions and long-term survival in a dog with superficial necrolytic dermatitis and liver cirrhosis. Journal of Small Animal Practice 41, 519–523

Hoffmann G, van den Ingh TSGAM, Bode P et al. (2006) Copper-associated chronic hepatitis in Labrador Retrievers. Journal of Veterinary Internal Medicine 20, 856–861

Hurwitz BM, Center SA, Randolph JF et al. (2014) Presumed primary and secondary hepatic copper accumulation in cats. Journal of the American Veterinary Medical Association 244, 68–77

Hyun C and Filippich LJ (2004) Inherited canine copper toxicosis in Australian Bedlington Terriers. Journal of Veterinary Science 5, 19–28

Keller SM, Vernau W, Hodges J et al. (2013) Hepatosplenic T-cell lymphoma: two distinct types of T-cell lymphoma in dogs. Veterinary Pathology 50, 281–290

Khoshnegah J and Movassaghi AR (2010) A very severe case of feline amyloidosis with spontaneous hepatic rupture and chronic renal failure. Comparative Clinical Pathology 19, 519–522

Kimmel SE, Christiansen W and Byrne KP (2003) Clinicopathological, ultrasonographic, and histopathological findings of superficial necrolytic dermatitis with hepatopathy in a cat. Journal of the American Animal Hospital Association 39, 23–27

Kinsey JR, Gilson SD, Hauptman J et al. (2015) Factors associated with long-term survival in dogs undergoing liver lobectomy as treatment for liver tumors. Canadian Veterinary Journal 56, 598-604

Lester C, Cooper J, Peters RM et al. (2016) Retrospective evaluation of acute liver failure in dogs (1995–2012): 49 cases. Journal of Veterinary Emergency and Critical Care 26, 559–567

Lindley S and Watson P (2010) BSAVA Manual of Canine and Feline Rehabilitation, Supportive and Palliative Care, Case Studies in Patient Management. BSAVA Publications, Gloucester

March PA, Hillier A, Weisbrode SE et al. (2004) Superficial necrolytic dermatitis in 11 dogs with a history of phenobarbital administration (1995–2002). Journal of Veterinary Internal Medicine 18, 65–74

McCallum KE, Constantino-Casas F, Cullen JM et al. (2019) Hepatic leptospiral infections in dogs without obvious renal involvement. Journal of Veterinary Internal Medicine 33, 141–150

Newell SM, Selcer BA, Mahaffey MB et al. (1995) Gallbladder mucocele causing biliary obstruction in 2 dogs: ultrasonographic, scintigraphic, and pathological findings. Journal of the American Animal Hospital Association 31, 467–472

Nyland TG, Barthez PY, Ortega TM and Davis CR (1996) Hepatic ultrasonographic and pathologic findings in dogs with canine superficial necrolytic dermatitis. Veterinary Radiology and Ultrasound 37, 200–205

Otte C, Penning L, Rothuizen J et al. (2012) Retrospective comparison of prednisolone and ursodeoxycholic acid for the treatment of feline lymphocytic cholangitis. Veterinary Journal 195, 205–209

Peyron C, Chevallier M, Lecoindre P and Guerret S (2015) Vacuolar hepatopathy in 43 French Scottish Terriers: a morphological study. Revue de Médecine Vétérinaire 166, 176–184

Poldevaart JH, Favier RP, Penning LC et al. (2009) Primary hepatitis in dogs: a retrospective review (2002–2006). Journal of Veterinary Internal Medicine 23, 72–80

Proot S and Rothuizen J (2006) High complication rate of an automatic Tru-Cut biopsy gun device for liver biopsy in cats. Journal of Veterinary Internal Medicine 20, 1327–1333

Raffan E, McCallum A, Scase TJ and Watson PJ (2009) Ascites is a negative prognostic indicator in chronic hepatitis in dogs. Journal of Veterinary Internal Medicine 23, 63–66

Rothuizen J, Bunch SE, Charles JA et al. (2006) WSAVA Standards for Clinical and Histological Diagnosis of Canine and Feline Liver Diseases. Saunders Elsevier, Edinburgh

Shearer GC, Savinova OV and Harris WS (2012) Fish oil – how does it reduce plasma triglycerides? *Biochimica et Biophysica Acta–Molecular and Cell Biology of Lipids* **1821**, 843–851

Takahashi Y and Fukusato T (2014) Histopathology of nonalcoholic fatty liver disease/nonalcoholic steatohepatitis. *World Journal of Gastroenterology* **20**, 15539–15548

Tamborini A, Jahns H, McAllister H (2016) Bacterial cholangitis, cholecystitis, or both in dogs. *Journal of Veterinary Internal Medicine* **30**, 1046–1055

Ullal T, Ambrosini Y, Rao S *et al.* (2019) Retrospective evaluation of cyclosporine in the treatment of presumed idiopathic chronic hepatitis in dogs. *Journal of Veterinary Internal Medicine* DOI: 10.111.Jvim. 15591

van den Ingh TSGAM, Punte PM, Hoogendijk ENLJ and Rothuizen J (2007) Possible nutritionally induced copper-associated chronic hepatitis in two dogs. *Veterinary Record* **161**, 728–729

van der Linde-Sipman JS, Niewold TA, Tooten PCJ *et al.* (1997) Generalized AA-amyloidosis in Siamese and Oriental cats. *Veterinary Immunology and Immunopathology* **56**, 1–10

van de Sluis B, Rothuizen J, Pearson PL *et al.* (2002) Identification of a new copper metabolism gene by positional cloning in a purebred dog population. *Human Molecular Genetics* **11**, 165–173

Villiers E and Ristić J (2016) *BSAVA Manual of Canine and Feline Clinical Pathology, 3rd edn.* BSAVA Publications, Gloucester

Walter R, Dunn M, d'Anjou MA *et al.* (2008) Nonsurgical resolution of gallbladder mucocele in 2 dogs. *Journal of the American Veterinary Medical Association* **232**, 1688–1693

Wang KY, Panciera DL, Al-Rukibat RK and Radi ZA (2004) Accuracy of ultrasound-guided fine-needle aspiration of the liver and cytologic findings in dogs and cats: 97 cases (1990–2000). *Journal of the American Veterinary Medical Association* **224**, 75–78

Watson PJ, Roulois AJA, Scase TJ *et al.* (2010) Prevalence of hepatic lesions at post-mortem examination in dogs and association with pancreatitis. *Journal of Small Animal Practice* **51**, 566–572

Watson PJ (2014) Hepatobiliary and exocrine pancreatic disorders. In: *Small Animal Internal Medicine, 5th edn*, ed. R Nelson and CG Couto, pp. 501–598. Mosby, Missouri

Webb CB, Twedt DC and Meyer DJ (2002) Copper-associated liver disease in Dalmatians: a review of 10 dogs (1998–2001). *Journal of Veterinary Internal Medicine* **16**, 665–668

Webster CRL, Center SA, Cullen JM *et al.* (2019) *ACVIM consensus statement on the diagnosis and treatment of chronic hepatitis in dogs* **33**, 1173–1200

Willard MD, Weeks BR and Johnson M (1999) Fine-needle aspirate cytology suggesting hepatic lipidosis in four cats with infiltrative hepatic disease. *Journal of Feline Medicine and Surgery* **4**, 215–220

Williams JM and Niles JD (2015) *BSAVA Manual of Canine and Feline Abdominal Surgery, 2nd edn.* BSAVA Publications, Gloucester

Zimmerman KL, Panciera DL, Panciera RJ *et al.* (2010) Hyperphosphatasemia and concurrent adrenal gland dysfunction in apparently healthy Scottish Terriers. *Journal of the American Veterinary Medical Association* **237**, 178–186

Liver: vascular disorders

Mickey Tivers

Structure and function

In dogs and cats the liver is divided into distinct lobes: the right lateral and medial, the left lateral and medial, the quadrate and the caudate, which is subdivided into caudate and papillary processes (see Figure 37.1). The hepatic blood supply is unique, with afferent blood delivered by the hepatic artery and hepatic portal vein and efferent blood drained by the hepatic vein.

The portal vein drains the cranial and caudal mesenteric veins, the splenic vein (left gastric vein) and the gastroduodenal vein and, hence, the gastrointestinal (GI) tract, pancreas and spleen. It supplies the liver with approximately 75% of its blood flow and 50% of its oxygen requirements. The right branch supplies the right lateral lobe and caudate process of the caudate lobe (right division). The left branch divides further, with a central branch supplying the right medial and quadrate lobes (central division) and the left branch supplying the left medial and lateral lobes and the papillary process of the caudate lobe (left division). The hepatic artery is responsible for the remaining blood flow and oxygen supply.

Traditionally, the liver is divided into lobules that are roughly hexagonal in cross-section and 1–2 mm wide, made up of sheets of hepatocytes. The lobules are arranged around a central hepatic vein with portal tracts located at the periphery. The hepatic sinusoids are fenestrated capillaries that radiate from around the central vein. In terms of blood flow, the liver can be divided into functional units called acini. The acini are roughly diamond-shaped and are supplied by terminal branches of hepatic portal venules and hepatic arterioles. These venules and arterioles lie within portal tracts, associated with bile ductules. Blood enters the liver lobule via the hepatic portal venules and hepatic arterioles and is transported via the sinusoids to the central vein. Sinusoids are lined with endothelial cells but have a discontinuous basement membrane that facilitates exchange of substances between the blood and the hepatocytes.

Pathophysiology of vascular disease

Normal hepatic blood flow, as outlined above, is crucial for normal liver function. Vascular liver disorders result from derangements in the normal blood flow through the liver,

typically leading to hepatic insufficiency. The precise vascular abnormality depends on the underlying condition (see specific conditions later in this chapter for more detail). However, histopathology of the liver normally shows changes characteristic of portal vein hypoperfusion. As a consequence of reduced portal blood flow, the portal veins in the portal tracts are reduced or absent. Blood flow is increased through hepatic arteries in response to this hypoperfusion, resulting in arteriole hyperplasia. Histopathologically, this results in an increased number of tortuous arterioles in the portal tracts (Figure 37.23). An increased number of bile duct profiles and portal fibrosis are also seen in some animals. Additional changes include hepatocellular degeneration, the presence of lipogranulomas and sinusoidal dilatation.

In a normal animal, the liver metabolises toxic substances, in particular ammonia, absorbed from the GI tract. Animals with vascular liver disorders have reduced liver blood flow and, hence, reduced liver function. Failure of the liver to remove the toxic products of gut metabolism from the portal blood results in hepatic encephalopathy (HE). The pathogenesis of HE is complex (see Chapter 26), although ammonia is recognized as a key factor. In addition, a wide variety of factors have been implicated in animals with HE, including inflammation, aromatic amino

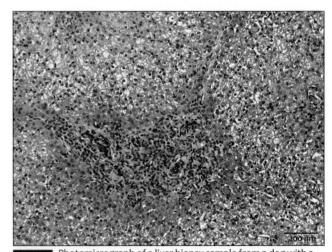

37.23 Photomicrograph of a liver biopsy sample from a dog with a congenital portosystemic shunt, showing an abnormal portal tract with marked arteriole hyperplasia and absent portal veins. The number of aberrant arterioles is dramatically increased. There is also microvesicular vacuolar change affecting the hepatocytes, indicative of hepatocyte degeneration. (Haematoxylin and eosin; original magnification X200.)

BSAVA Manual of Canine and Feline Gastroenterology, third edition. Edited by Edward J. Hall, David A. Williams and Aarti Kathrani. ©BSAVA 2020

acids (phenylalanine, tyrosine and tryptophan), methionine, glutamine, central nervous system inhibitors (gamma-aminobutyric acid (GABA) and GABA receptors), mercaptans and short-chain fatty acids. It is believed that several factors act synergistically in a given animal, and this may partly explain the variation in signs between individuals.

Vascular diseases

Vascular disorders can be congenital or acquired. The most common congenital vascular disorder in dogs and cats is a congenital portosystemic shunt (CPSS). Other, less common, conditions include primary portal vein hypoplasia (PVH) peliosis and hepatic arteriovenous malformation (HAVM). These conditions are discussed in detail below.

Acquired vascular disorders are multiple acquired portosystemic shunts (MAS). MAS develop as a consequence of chronic liver disease resulting in increased portal blood pressure. In response to this increased portal blood pressure (portal hypertension), multiple new vessels develop or pre-existing vessels open up to bypass the liver. Although animals with MAS have blood bypassing the liver, their clinical signs and clinicopathological abnormalities are typically a result of the underlying liver disease.

Congenital portosystemic shunts

CPSS are developmental abnormalities that result in an aberrant vessel that forms a physical and functional communication between the portal vasculature and the systemic circulation. This results in blood from the GI tract bypassing the liver and is associated with hepatic hypoplasia and decreased function. Affected animals have clinical signs associated with hepatic insufficiency, in particular HE.

CPSS have two broad phenotypes: extra-hepatic and intra-hepatic. Extra-hepatic CPSS (EHCPSS) are more common and arise from the portal vein or one of its tributaries outside the liver. EHCPSS typically terminate in the caudal vena cava, azygos vein or phrenic vein and, therefore, have a number of different morphologies. Conversely, intra-hepatic CPSS (IHCPSS) arise from an intra-hepatic portal vein branch and, therefore, lie wholly or partly within the liver parenchyma. IHCPSS can be classified based on the liver lobe they pass through: right divisional (right lateral lobe or caudate process of caudate lobe), central divisional (right medial or quadrate liver lobes) and left divisional (papillary process of caudate lobe, left medial and lateral liver lobes), which is the most common type.

History, physical examination and minimum database

CPSS have been shown to be hereditary in Yorkshire Terriers, Cairn Terriers and Irish Wolfhounds, whilst other breeds are predisposed including West Highland White Terriers, Labrador Retrievers, and Golden Retrievers. In 2001, 0.5% of dogs seen at North American teaching hospitals were diagnosed with CPSS (Tobias and Rohrbach, 2003). In the UK, the prevalence of CPSS in certain breeds of pedigree dogs has been reported as 0.1–2.9% (Asher et al., 2009). Thus, although uncommon, the condition is a significant problem for some dog breeds. CPSS are seen less commonly in cats. The majority of cats with CPSS are Domestic Shorthaired cats (Figure 37.24), although it has been suggested that Persian, Himalayan and Siamese breeds are predisposed.

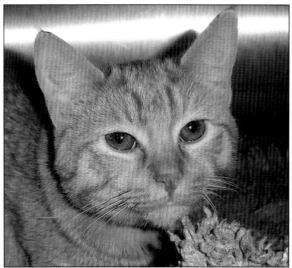

37.24 A cat with a congenital extra-hepatic portosystemic shunt (CPSS). Note the copper-coloured irises that are commonly seen in cats with CPSS.

Animals with CPSS can suffer from a variety of clinical signs, which can affect the neurological, GI and urinary systems (Figure 37.25). Neurological signs are common, particularly in cats, where 93–100% may be affected. Signs are due to HE and vary in frequency and severity. Urinary tract signs result from the formation of ammonium urate stones, which can lead to urinary tract infection or urethral obstruction. Animals typically start to exhibit signs when immature and may be diagnosed as young as 6 weeks of age. Dogs and cats will often have poor growth and weight gain and may appear stunted compared with littermates. However, some animals can initially appear clinically unaffected but demonstrate clinical signs when mature. Some individuals can be presented as emergencies due to severe HE resulting in seizures or coma (Figure 37.26), or due to urethral obstruction secondary to ammonium urate urolithiasis. Occasionally, older animals are diagnosed with CPSS as an incidental finding, and the decision on whether to treat these individuals can be challenging.

System affected	Common clinical signs
Neurological signs (hepatic encephalopathy)	• Reduced mentation • Altered behaviour • Ataxia • Head pressing • Circling • Tremors • Blindness • Seizures • Coma
Gastrointestinal signs	• Vomiting • Diarrhoea • Pica • Gastrointestinal bleeding/melaena
Urinary tract signs – related to ammonium urate urolithiasis	• Haematuria • Dysuria • Stranguria
Miscellaneous	• Polyuria/polydipsia (more common in dogs) • Small stature • Poor body condition • Intolerance to sedatives/anaesthetics • Hypersalivation (cats) • Copper-coloured irises (cats) (see Figure 37.24) • Intermittent pyrexia

37.25 Common clinical signs seen in dogs and cats with congenital portosystemic shunts.

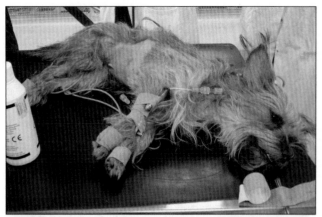

37.26 An 18-month-old female neutered crossbreed dog with severe hepatic encephalopathy (HE) due to a congenital extra-hepatic portosystemic shunt. The dog is collapsed and obtunded. The dog significantly improved with medical management of HE.

Animals with CPSS can have a number of changes on routine haematology, biochemistry and urinalysis, related to impaired liver function (Figure 37.27). Clotting times (activated partial thromboplastin time and prothrombin time) are often increased in dogs with CPSS, although significant coagulopathy is rarely seen.

Parameter	Abnormality	Comment
Haematology	Microcytosis ± anaemia	60–72% dogs 27–54% cats Anaemia less common – 0–15% (cats)
Biochemisty	Hypoalbuminaemia	Less common in cats
	Decreased BUN	
	Hypocholesterolaemia	
	Hypoglycaemia	Less common in cats
	Increased liver enzyme activities (ALP and ALT)	
Urinalysis	Low urine specific gravity	
	Ammonium biurate crystalluria	26–57% dogs 20–43% cats

37.27 Common abnormalities in routine haematology, biochemistry and urinalysis in dogs and cats with CPSS. ALP = alkaline phosphatase; ALT = alanine aminotransferase; BUN = blood urea nitrogen.

Diagnostic imaging

Computed tomography angiography (CTA) is considered the gold standard for preoperative imaging of animals with suspected CPSS, as it provides detailed information on the morphology of the anomaly (Figure 37.28). Abdominal ultrasonography is not as reliable, but is worth doing in some circumstances. Some surgeons also perform intra-operative mesenteric portovenography to gain valuable information regarding the CPSS during surgery (Figure 37.29). The variety of techniques that have been reported for the diagnosis of CPSS in dogs and cats are detailed in Figure 37.30.

Laboratory tests

Assessment of liver function is necessary to further investigate animals with suspected CPSS. Pre- and post-prandial serum bile acid concentrations are considered to be very sensitive (up to 100% for paired samples) for the diagnosis of CPSS (although evaluated alone they do not

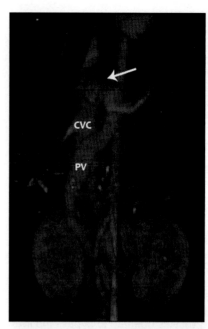

37.28 Reconstructed dorsal plane computed tomography angiography image of a congenital left divisional intra-hepatic portosystemic shunt (arrowed) in a dog. CVC = caudal vena cava; PV = portal vein.

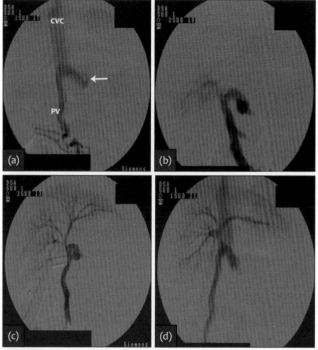

37.29 A series of ventrodorsal intraoperative mesenteric portovenograms from a 19-week-old male entire West Highland White Terrier with an extra-hepatic congenital portosystemic shunt (CPSS). The images are orientated so that cranial is at the top. (a) Intraoperative portovenogram image. Contrast medium has been injected through a jejunal vein under fluoroscopic guidance with digital subtraction. The majority of the contrast medium, and hence blood, flows through the large shunt vessel (arrowed) on the right of the image. The portal vein and intra-hepatic vasculature appear faintly on the left. This is a right gastric vein CPSS entering the post-hepatic caudal vena cava. (b) Repeat portovenogram following temporary occlusion of the shunting vessel. Note the increased opacification of the liver and the lack of contrast medium flow through the abnormal vessel. However, the opacification of the intra-hepatic portal system is poor, and this dog was unable to tolerate a complete attenuation of the shunt. Therefore, a partial suture ligation was performed. (c) Intraoperative portovenogram from the same dog, approximately 3 months after the first surgery. Note the improvement in the intra-hepatic portal blood flow but persistent flow through the CPSS. (d) Repeat portovenogram following temporary occlusion of the shunting vessel. Note the increased opacification of the liver and the lack of contrast medium flow through the abnormal vessel. The dog was able to tolerate a complete ligation of the CPSS at the second surgery. CVC = caudal vena cava; PV = portal vein.

Imaging modality	Advantages	Disadvantages
Radiography	• Readily available • Relatively cheap • Non-invasive	• Non-specific • Cannot provide confirmation of CPSS – can show microhepatica, renomegaly and urolithiasis when present (although, typically, stones are radiolucent and may not be visible unless large or of mixed composition)
Ultrasonography	• Readily available • Relatively cheap • Non-invasive • Sensitivity: 74–95%; specificity: 67–100% • Can provide information on shunt location/morphology • Provides information regarding liver size and presence/absence of urinary calculi • Can be used to assess residual shunt flow following surgery	• Highly operator dependent • Often requires sedation for detailed scan
Scintigraphy (transcolonic)	• Non-invasive • Good accuracy for diagnosis of CPSS • Provides information on degree of shunting • Particularly useful for monitoring response to treatment, i.e. identifying continued shunting postoperatively	• Normally requires sedation or anaesthesia • Not readily available • Use restricted by radiation safety guidelines in the UK • Does not provide information on shunt location/morphology
Computed tomography angiography	• Extremely accurate for diagnosis of CPSS • Provides highly detailed information on shunt morphology and hepatic vasculature • Useful to assess response to treatment in terms of hepatic development/blood flow	• Expensive • Not readily available • Requires sedation or general anaesthesia
Intraoperative mesenteric portovenography	• Allows definitive diagnosis • Provides information on shunt morphology and intra-hepatic vasculature pre-attenuation • Repeat portovenography following attenuation allows confirmation of correct shunt identification and assessment of intra-hepatic vasculature • Allows definitive diagnosis and surgical treatment during one procedure	• Requires intraoperative fluoroscopy – limited availability and increased cost • Increases anaesthesia and surgical time (approximately 15 minutes)

37.30 Comparison of different imaging modalities for the diagnosis of congenital portosystemic shunts (CPSS) in dogs and cats.

differentiate CPSS from other liver diseases). Occasionally, animals may have normal pre- or postprandial values, so a dynamic test is always recommended.

Plasma ammonia concentrations can be measured, but this is not as reliable as dynamic bile acids and false-negatives can be seen (sensitivity 62–88%), unless an ammonia tolerance test is conducted. The availability of ammonia assay is very limited because it is very labile and a specific 'in-house' methodology is required to test samples within 30 minutes or so of collection.

Management of congenital portosystemic shunts

Animals with CPSS can be treated medically or surgically. Medical management is particularly important for stabilising animals with severe HE in the short-term before attempting surgical correction of CPSS. Indeed, there is a suggestion that a period of medical stabilization before surgery decreases the risk of postoperative seizures. However, medical management does not treat the underlying cause of the problem or improve liver function and necessitates lifelong treatment. Individual animals can have a good outcome with long-term medical management. However, surgical treatment is recommended in most instances. It has been shown in dogs that surgical management is associated with a significantly improved survival rate and a lower frequency of ongoing clinical signs compared with medical management (Greenhalgh et al., 2014).

Surgical management: The aim of surgery is to attenuate the CPSS and, hence, restore normal hepatic portal blood flow. A variety of surgical techniques are recommended for the treatment of CPSS in dogs and cats including suture ligation, ameroid constrictors, thin film bands and endovascular coils. Not all animals are able to tolerate complete acute suture ligation of their CPSS due to the development of life-threatening portal hypertension, related to an underdeveloped hepatic portal vasculature. It has been shown that animals that can tolerate a complete ligation have a better long-term outcome than those treated with a partial ligation (Figure 37.31). Ameroid constrictors and thin film bands are gradual attenuation devices, which are intended to slowly occlude the CPSS over a period of weeks (Figure 37.32). These techniques are commonly used to allow complete attenuation ultimately, whilst avoiding the risk of portal hypertension. However, once placed, there is no control over the rate or degree of attenuation that is ultimately achieved. Ameroid constrictors and thin film bands can still result in too rapid attenuation and, hence, the development of MAS. Conversely, the attenuation may not be complete, resulting in persistent shunting. Studies of EHCPSS have shown persistent shunting, in the form of MAS or due to incomplete attenuation, in 24% of dogs treated with ameroid constrictors and 31–37% of dogs treated with thin film banding, as assessed by scintigraphy (Landon et al., 2008; Falls et al., 2013; Matiasovic et al., 2019). An alternative approach for animals that cannot tolerate complete acute ligation is to perform a partial ligation and then a repeat surgery approximately 3 months later to allow complete ligation. Surgical attenuation of IHCPSS is technically more challenging than for EHCPSS as the abnormal vessel is located within the liver. Coil embolization via interventional radiology has been recommended for attenuation of IHCPSS, particularly in dogs, to reduce the morbidity

271

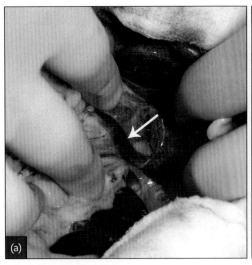

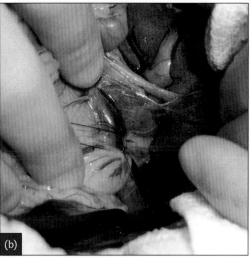

37.31 Intraoperative photographs of an exploratory laparotomy in a cat with a congenital portosystemic shunt. (a) The stomach has been retracted caudoventrally to reveal the shunting vessel in the region of the gastric cardia. This is a left gastric vein CPSS entering the post-hepatic caudal vena cava (arrowed). (b) Forceps have been used to carefully dissect around the shunt vessel. The cat tolerated complete attenuation of the CPSS and, therefore, the vessel has been ligated with polypropylene suture material (Prolene; Ethicon) (the second length of suture will be removed prior to routine abdominal closure).

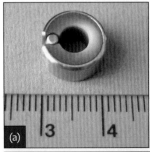

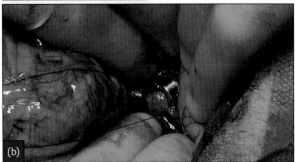

37.32 (a) Ameroid constrictor which consists of a ring of casein with a lumen, surrounded by a stainless steel collar. There is a gap in the ring to allow it to be placed around a vessel and this is closed with a small 'key' of casein. In theory the casein absorbs fluid and expands, and the lumen is gradually occluded over a period of weeks. However, it has been shown experimentally that ameroid constrictors cause vessel occlusion primarily by thrombus formation, that this occlusion may be more rapid than desired, and that recanalization of the vessel is possible. (b) Intraoperative photograph of an exploratory laparotomy in a dog with an extra-hepatic congenital portosystemic shunt. An ameroid constrictor has been placed around a portocaval shunt.

and mortality associated with surgery (Weisse *et al.*, 2014). Overall, there is a lack of good evidence to recommend one technique over another, and all have potential advantages and disadvantages (Tivers *et al.*, 2012; Tivers *et al.*, 2017; Serrano *et al.*, 2019).

CPSS attenuation has been associated with serious complications, including haemorrhage, hypoglycaemia, portal hypertension, post-attenuation neurological signs (PANS) and GI haemorrhage. Life-threatening portal hypertension can occur due to excessive attenuation of the CPSS. The incidence of portal hypertension is reduced by using a gradual attenuation device or by careful intraoperative assessment when using suture ligation. PANS can

vary in severity from mild tremors or ataxia to status epilepticus. Signs can occur up to 72 hours after surgery and can occur with acute or gradual attenuation. The occurrence of PANS is not related to hypoglycaemia or HE. The precise aetiology is unknown, but it is speculated that PANS is related to changes in false neurotransmitters. Despite aggressive treatment with anti-seizure medication, some animals do not recover and die or are euthanased. GI haemorrhage secondary to gastric ulceration is seen as a complication in dogs with IHCPSS and can be severe, resulting in death. The mortality for different treatments varies between studies. The mortality rates for dogs are summarized in Figure 37.33. The reported mortality rate for surgical treatment in cats ranges from 0–22.2%.

Successful surgery results in resolution of clinical signs and improvement in liver function. There are also improvements in liver volume and in the portal vasculature, presumed to be a result of liver regeneration. A good clinical response is normally associated with significant improvements in dynamic bile acids. However, in some animals there remains a mild to moderate increase in bile acids, despite an apparently good outcome. The reason for this is unclear but may be due to subclinical shunting or concurrent PVH. A good to excellent outcome with surgical treatment is reported in 84–94% of EHCPSS in dogs, 50–100% of IHCPSS in dogs and 33.3–80% of CPSS overall in cats. The wide variation in both the method of long-term follow-up and the definition of a 'good' or 'excellent' outcome make direct comparison of the different techniques challenging.

However, despite a good short-term outcome, some animals may experience recurrence of clinical signs in the long term. This can be due to continued shunting, as a result of incomplete attenuation or the development of MAS, presumably due to subclinical portal hypertension.

Technique	Mortality for extra-hepatic CPSS	Mortality for intra-hepatic CPSS
Suture ligation	2–29%	6–23%
Ameroid constrictor	4–7%	0–9%
Thin film band	0–9%	3–27%
Intravascular coil	Only studies with <10 dogs	0–7%

37.33 Reported perioperative mortality of different surgical treatments for congenital portosystemic shunts (CPSS) in dogs.

Medical management of hepatoencephalopathy

The aim of medical management is to control the clinical signs associated with HE, which are detailed in Figure 37.25 and Chapter 26. In animals with a CPSS, medical management is mainly used to stabilise them prior to surgery but can be used for long-term treatment if surgery is not possible or is declined by the owner.

In humans, HE is classified into three types based on aetiology: Type A is caused by acute liver failure in the absence of pre-existing liver disease; Type B by porto-systemic bypass with no intrinsic hepatic disease (i.e. a CPSS); and Type C associated with cirrhosis, portal hypertension and MAS. Thus, primary hepatopathies, such as acute hepatitis, end-stage chronic hepatitis in dogs and cholangitis or hepatic lipidosis in cats, may also manifest with HE, although other signs such as jaundice and/or ascites are often present. The medical management of primary hepatopathies involves many other therapies (see Chapter 37a) but the management of HE is the same as for HE caused by CPSS.

The source of ammonia involved in HE is mainly from the GI tract, although muscle metabolism also produces some ammonia. In the GI tract, ammonia is produced partly by urease-positive gut bacteria metabolizing amino acids derived from dietary protein, and partly as a by-product of enterocyte metabolism of glutamine, which is used in preference to glucose for energy production. The latter mechanism probably explains the rapid postprandial rise in ammonia and worsening signs of HE sometimes seen in animals with CPSS, as most bacterial fermentation is likely to occur in the large intestine hours after eating. However, there is a gastric bacterial population of urease-positive *Helicobacter* in most dogs and cats that may also contribute to ammonia production. The presence of a CPSS (or hepatocellular dysfunction and/or MAS) allows ammonia (and other toxins) generated in the GI tract to enter the systemic circulation and cause HE. Therefore, most of the methods used to manage HE aim to reduce the production and absorption of ammonia from the GI tract.

Medical management treats the clinical signs of HE, primarily by modifying the gut environment to reduce the production and absorption of ammonia and other compounds. However, medical management does not treat the underlying cause of the problem or improve liver function. It is recommended that animals with a CPSS should have a minimum of 2–4 weeks of medical management prior to surgery. Medical management involves treatment with one or more dietary modification, lactulose and antibacterials. It is best practice to start with dietary modification and to add lactulose and then antibacterials to the treatment regimen as needed. In severely affected animals, all three may be necessary prior to reducing treatment once clinical signs are controlled. Medication should be tailored to reach the minimum effective treatment.

A variety of factors have been implicated in worsening HE or precipitating it in a previously stable animal. Dehydration, hypokalaemia and metabolic alkalosis, either because of diarrhoea or overzealous furosemide administration in animals with ascites due to either hypoalbuminaemia in animals with a CPSS, or portal hypertension in animals with chronic liver disease, should be corrected with intravenous fluid therapy and potassium supplementation. If diuresis is necessary, spironolactone should be used in place of furosemide. Other potential risk factors include hypovolaemia, GI haemorrhage, constipation and azotaemia, and these should be addressed when present.

However, a recent study did not show any significant association between these potential triggers and clinical signs of HE (Lidbury *et al.*, 2015).

The exact mechanisms causing HE are not fully understood and involve increased systemic circulation of a variety of chemical mediators including ammonia, as detailed previously. Plasma ammonia concentration is predictive of the presence of HE in dogs with CPSS, although dogs with HE can have normal plasma ammonia concentration (Tivers *et al.*, 2014). Nevertheless, ammonia is the most useful biochemical marker of HE. However, the test is not often available in practice as the sample needs to be collected on ice and analyzed within 30 minutes or false-positive results occur. In-house dry chemistry analyzers are too inaccurate to be recommended (see *BSAVA Manual of Canine and Feline Clinical Pathology*). Before starting medical therapy, the diagnosis of a CPSS, suspected based on clinical signs and dynamic bile acid testing, should be confirmed by imaging (see Figure 37.28)

Diet

Bacterial metabolism of dietary protein, particularly protein in red meats that is rich in aromatic amino acids (e.g. tyrosine, tryptophan, phenylalanine), is a source of ammonia. Therefore, modification of dietary protein content is extremely important in moderating HE. However, severe protein restriction is not recommended as it can lead to malnutrition, reduced serum albumin concentration and a potentially poorer prognosis for medical management (and surgical correction where subsequently attempted).

The ideal diet should be highly digestible to reduce the residue reaching the colonic bacteria, contain protein of high biological value with high levels of branched-chain amino acids and arginine and low levels of aromatic amino acids and methionine, have a highly available carbohydrate as the primary source of calories, contain physiological levels of vitamins and minerals and be highly palatable. Protein modification is not only the most important part of dietary management of HE but potentially the most challenging. Animals with HE are often small and underweight and excessive protein restriction may exacerbate signs of HE due to increased protein oxidation and ammonia production. Protein levels must reach the animal's requirement without being too high. In addition, in young, growing animals there are other important nutrient requirements including calcium and phosphorus, which need to be considered. Therefore, meat proteins are avoided, and vegetable proteins are preferred as they are richer sources of branched-chain (aliphatic) amino acids (e.g. leucine, isoleucine, valine) that produce less ammonia when fermented. Cottage cheese is also a good source of such high-quality protein and a home-cooked diet for HE has historically been cottage cheese and pasta. If a home-cooked diet is recommended, it must be formulated by a board-certified veterinary nutritionist to ensure it is appropriate for liver disease and is complete and balanced for long-term feeding. Soya-based diets may be suitable, especially if they are nutritionally balanced for growth, as CPSS is most commonly diagnosed in young, growing animals. Further, a hydrolysed soya diet balanced for growth (e.g. Purina ProPlan Veterinary Diet HA Canine and Feline Dry) may be preferred, as it is thought to require less glutamine metabolism and cause less ammonia production by enterocytes for its digestion and absorption. Commercial hepatic diets may also be suitable as they are somewhat protein-restricted, although they are of more value in animals with copper hepatotoxicosis due to their high zinc/low copper content and additional antioxidants. The author prefers a hydrolysed soya diet, as it is also suitable for growth.

Lactulose

Successful management of HE often requires the administration of lactulose in addition to dietary modification. However, its mechanism of action and benefit is still debated (Als-Nielsen et al., 2004). Lactulose is an osmotic laxative (see Chapter 28), and therefore may act simply by aiding the evacuation of colonic contents and reducing the substrate available for bacterial fermentation and ammonia production. It is a non-absorbable, synthetic disaccharide (fructose-galactose) that is hydrolysed by colonic bacteria to lactic, acetic and formic acids. These organic acids reduce the pH of the colonic contents trapping free ammonia (NH_3) as ammonium (NH_4^+) ions that cannot be absorbed, increasing faecal ammonia and nitrogen excretion (Beynen et al., 2001).

The effect of lactulose on faecal consistency is quite variable and the recommended initial dose (see table) has to be adjusted empirically until an individual animal is producing two to three soft stools a day. Both too little lactulose, with continued faecal retention, and too much, with consequent diarrhoea, can worsen HE. In animals with severe HE causing stupor or coma, a lactulose retention enema may be given. A retention enema of 20 ml/kg of a warm solution comprising three parts lactulose to seven parts water is instilled per rectum via a Foley catheter for up to 4 hours and repeated as necessary.

Antibacterials

These are used to reduce the urease-positive gut bacteria implicated in the production of ammonia and therefore ameliorate the signs of HE. Ampicillin, amoxycillin, metronidazole and neomycin have all been used successfully in dogs and cats (Figure 37.34). Neomycin may have the advantage in that it is not absorbed from the healthy GI tract. However, the chronic administration of antibacterials is a potential public health risk because of the selection of antibiotic resistance, and their use should be kept to a minimum. Antibacterials are therefore reserved for those animals where dietary modification and lactulose produce inadequate control of signs.

Medical treatment	Recommended dose and frequency
Lactulose	Dogs: 0.5–1.0 ml/kg orally q8–12h (ideally two to three soft stools daily) Cats: 0.5–5 ml orally q8–12h (ideally two to three soft stools daily)
Antibiotics: Ampicillin Co-amoxiclav Metronidazole Neomycin*	10–20 mg/kg orally q8h 12.5 mg/kg orally 12qh 7.5–10 mg/kg orally q12h 20 mg/kg orally q8–12h daily

37.34 Recommended medical management for animals with hepatic encephalopathy. *Contraindicated if concurrent intestinal disease, as may be absorbed and cause nephro- and/or oto-toxicity

Primary portal vein hypoplasia

PVH is a complicated congenital disorder. It has been divided into two subcategories based on the presence or absence of portal hypertension, although it is most likely a spectrum of the same disease.

PVH with no hypertension

PVH with no hypertension was previously known as microvascular dysplasia. It is a microvascular abnormality of the liver vasculature, which may involve shunting at this level. The histopathological findings are consistent with portal hypoperfusion (small intra-hepatic portal vessels, endothelial hyperplasia, portal vein dilatation, random juvenile intralobular blood vessels, central venous hypertrophy and fibrosis) and are similar to those seen with CPSS. These changes seen in the absence of a macroscopic CPSS indicate a diagnosis of PVH. It seems likely that animals with CPSS have a variable degree of PVH, but as the histopathological findings are the same, this is difficult to further categorize.

PVH with portal hypertension

PVH can also occur in combination with portal hypertension (PVH-PH) and this is also known as idiopathic non-cirrhotic portal hypertension or juvenile hepatic fibrosis. Importantly, these animals do not have liver cirrhosis (i.e. no nodular regeneration) but do have portal hypertension, presumably due to the severity of their microvascular abnormality and consequent fibrosis. This results in the development of MAS. Liver histopathology shows changes consistent with portal vein hypoperfusion, similar to PVH without hypertension and CPSS, although there is typically marked fibrosis noted.

History, physical examination and minimum database

PVH: Cairn Terriers have been shown to have hereditary PVH and Yorkshire Terriers are over-represented. Animals with PVH may have similar clinical signs to those with CPSS, including HE and those affecting the GI and urinary tracts. However, these are typically less severe, and some animals may have no overt clinical signs. Animals are diagnosed at an older age than those with CPSS and are typically mature. Routine biochemistry and haematology are typically within normal limits. Increased serum bile acid concentration may be the only biochemical abnormality.

PVH-PH: Animals with PVH-PH are normally purebreed dogs; Dobermanns, Rottweilers and German Shepherd Dogs are over-represented. Most are less than 4 years old and greater than 10 kg in bodyweight. Animals with PVH-PH are more severely affected and show signs of ascites, polyuria/polydipsia, GI abnormalities, HE, stunted growth and weight loss. Routine biochemistry and haematology typically show abnormalities consistent with liver dysfunction including microcytosis, mild anaemia, increased liver enzyme activities, hypoalbuminaemia and decreased urea.

Diagnostic imaging

PVH: Animals with PVH tend to have a normal-sized liver on radiography and ultrasonography. Portovenography and CTA will be normal in animals with PVH and can be used to rule out a macroscopic shunt.

PVH-PH: Ultrasonography is useful to identify reduced liver size, ascites and MAS in dogs with PVH-PH. MAS can be confirmed with portovenography or CTA.

Laboratory tests

PVH: Dynamic bile acids are increased, although typically the magnitude is less than that seen with CPSS.

PVH-PH: Dynamic bile acids and ammonia tolerance test are increased in dogs with PVH-PH.

Treatment

Surgery is not an option for PVH (with or without hypertension). These animals should be treated with medical management of HE (see above) including antibiotics, lactulose and diet.

PVH: Some cases require no treatment and the prognosis is excellent for dogs with PVH managed medically. In one study, 92% of dogs had a good long-term survival or died of unrelated causes (Christiansen *et al.*, 2000).

PVH-PH: The prognosis for dogs with PVH-PH is not as good as that for PVH, although it is still considered favourable. In one study, outcome was available for 19 dogs, of which 13 (68%) had a good outcome, four (21%) were euthanased due to their condition and two (11%) were euthanased for other reasons (Bunch *et al.*, 2001). Duodenal ulceration was the cause of mortality in three of these dogs and, therefore, preventative medication should be considered.

Hepatic arteriovenous malformations

HAVM is a very rare congenital condition that can be seen in dogs and cats. The malformation allows blood flow between the high-pressure hepatic arterial circulation and the low-pressure portal system. Typically, there are multiple vessels connecting a branch of the hepatic artery with the portal vein. This results in hepatofugal (away from the liver) flow in the portal system and, importantly, results in portal hypertension. These malformations are associated with MAS, which form in order to relieve the portal hypertension.

History, physical examination and minimum database

A variety of dog breeds have been reported with HAVM and there is no apparent breed predisposition. Animals with HAVM are typically presented at a young age. Clinical signs can be acute or chronic and typically include GI signs, lethargy and poor growth, with neurological signs of HE less common. A murmur may be audible over the abdomen. Ascites is reported in 75% of dogs due to portal hypertension. This is typically a pure transudate with a protein concentration of <25 g/l.

Diagnostic imaging

HAVM can be readily diagnosed on abdominal ultrasonography with Doppler. CTA and portovenography are used to confirm the diagnosis and, importantly, to obtain more detailed information regarding the nature of the malformation (location and size of the abnormal vasculature) to allow appropriate treatment.

Laboratory tests

Clinicopathological abnormalities are similar to those described in CPSS, including microcytic anaemia, hypoalbuminaemia and increased liver enzyme activities. Dynamic bile acid testing and plasma ammonia are abnormal, consistent with impaired liver function.

Treatment

The majority of HAVM affect a single liver lobe, although a minority of dogs have two lobes affected. Recommended treatments include surgical removal of the affected lobe and/or glue embolization using interventional radiology (Figure 37.35). However, persistent shunting through MAS is common and the majority of dogs (approximately 75%) require ongoing medical and/or dietary management (Chanoit *et al.*, 2007). Glue embolization has been reported to be safer, with a better long-term outcome than surgery (Chanoit *et al.*, 2007). However, this is based on a very small number of dogs.

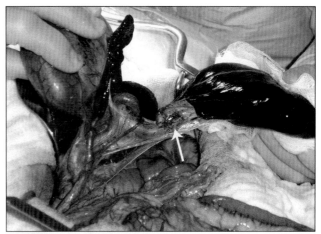

37.35 Exploratory laparotomy in a 6-month-old entire male Labrador Retriever with a hepatic arteriovenous malformation. Note the enlarged hepatic artery supplying the left lateral liver lobe and the dilated portal vein (arrowed).

Peliosis hepatis

Peliosis hepatis is a very uncommon vasculoproliferative disorder in small animals, although it has been reported more frequently in cats compared to dogs. The condition consists of multiple, irregular, cystic blood-filled spaces randomly distributed through the liver. The cysts are typically relatively small (1–5mm) individually but coalesce to cause liver enlargement and mass lesions, and may rupture causing potentially fatal haemorrhage.

The small animal literature is relatively limited, and much of our understanding of this condition has been extrapolated from human beings. The cause of peliosis hepatis remains unknown in most animals with the condition. In people, peliosis hepatis has been associated with a variety of inciting factors, including anabolic androgenic steroids, oestrogenic steroids, HIV and *Bartonella* infection. A single case report suggested an association between peliosis hepatis and *Bartonella henselae* infection in a dog (Kitchell *et al.*, 2000). However, a post-mortem study of the livers of 26 cats with peliosis hepatitis failed to detect evidence of *Bartonella henselae*, suggesting that this is not the underlying cause (Buchmann *et al.*, 2010). Another case report in a dog associated peliosis hepatis with anticoagulant rodenticide (diphacinone) intoxication (Beal *et al.*, 2008).

The exact pathophysiology of peliosis hepatis is unknown although the condition can be divided into two types: parenchymal and phlebectatic (also referred to as telangiectasia). The parenchymal type is due to focal necrosis of hepatocytes as a result of an acute, severe ischaemic lesion. The phlebectatic type develops more slowly as a result of local obstruction of small portal vein branches with associated hepatic atrophy and sinusoidal dilatation. Both types can be seen concurrently in the same individual.

History, physical examination and minimum database

Animals with peliosis hepatis are typically seen with clinical signs relating to abdominal haemorrhage due to rupture of one or more of the cysts (Figure 37.36). In one study 11/16 cats had abdominal haemorrhage identified pre- or post mortem (Brown *et al.*, 1994). Some individuals without haemorrhage, may have signs of liver enlargement or have cystic liver masses identified. However, as some of the animals reported in the literature were diagnosed post mortem it is likely that in some individuals the condition may be an incidental finding or remain unidentified during the animal's lifetime.

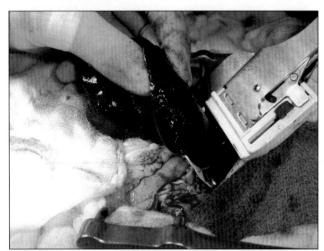

37.36 Intraoperative image of a cat with peliosis hepatis. The left lateral liver lobe is being resected with the aid of a stapling device. Note the blood-filled cystic lesions affecting the lobe.

Diagnostic imaging

Abdominal imaging including ultrasonography or computed tomography will show evidence of liver enlargement with multiple cystic lesions. In animals with haemorrhage, peritoneal effusion will be present.

Laboratory tests

Complete blood count will show evidence of acute and/or chronic haemorrhage in those animals with intra-abdominal bleeding. Sampling of free abdominal fluid, when present, will yield frank blood.

Treatment

There is limited information regarding treatment. Surgery can be performed to remove the affected liver lobe(s) but as the condition can be present in multiple lobes the prognosis is typically guarded due to the potential for ongoing haemorrhage. If an underlying cause such as *Bartonella henselae* or drug toxicity is identified, then treatment of this is likely to be of benefit.

References and further reading

Als-Nielsen B, Gluud LL and Gluud C (2004) Non-absorbable disaccharides for hepatic encephalopathy; systematic review of randomised trials. *British Medical Journal* **328**, 1046–1050

Asher L, Diesel G, Summers JF *et al.* (2009) Inherited defects in pedigree dogs. Part 1: disorders related to breed standards. *Veterinary Journal* **182**, 402–411

Beal MW, Doherty AM and Curcio K (2008) Peliosis hepatis and hemoperitoneum in a dog with diphacinone intoxication. *Journal of Veterinary Emergency and Critical Care* **18**, 388–392

Berent AC and Tobias KM (2009) Portosystemic vascular anomalies. *Veterinary Clinics of North America: Small Animal Practice* **39**, 513–541

Beynen AC, Kappert HJ and Yu S (2001) Dietary lactulose decreases apparent nitrogen absorption and increases apparent calcium and magnesium absorption in healthy dogs. *Journal of Animal Physiology and Animal Nutrition* **85**, 67–72

Brown PJ, Henderson JP, Galloway P *et al.* (1994) Peliosis hepatis and telangiectasis in 18 cats. *Journal of Small Animal Practice* **35**, 73–77

Buchmann AU, Kempf VA, Kershaw O and Gruber AD (2010) Peliosis hepatis in cats is not associated with *Bartonella henselae* infections. *Veterinary Pathology* **47**, 163–166

Bunch SE, Johnson SE and Cullen JM (2001) Idiopathic noncirrhotic portal hypertension in dogs: 33 cases (1982–1998). *Journal of the American Veterinary Medical Association* **218**, 392–399

Chanoit G, Kyles AE, Weisse C and Hardie EM (2007) Surgical and interventional radiographic treatment of dogs with hepatic arteriovenous fistulae. *Veterinary Surgery* **36**, 199–209

Christiansen JS, Hottinger HA, Allen L *et al.* (2000) Hepatic microvascular dysplasia in dogs: a retrospective study of 24 cases (1987–1995). *Journal of the American Animal Hospital Association* **36**, 385–389

Falls EL, Milovancev M, Hunt GB *et al.* (2013) Long-term outcome after surgical ameroid ring constrictor placement for treatment of single extrahepatic portosystemic shunts in dogs. *Veterinary Surgery* **42**, 951–957

Greenhalgh SN, Reeve JA, Johnstone T *et al.* (2014) Long-term survival and quality of life in dogs with clinical signs associated with a congenital portosystemic shunt after surgical or medical treatment. *Journal of the American Veterinary Medical Association* **245**, 527–533

Kitchell BE, Fan TM, Kordick D *et al.* (2000) Peliosis hepatis in a dog infected with *Bartonella henselae*. *Journal of the American Veterinary Medical Association* **216**, 519–523

Landon BP, Abraham LA and Charles JA (2008) Use of transcolonic portal scintigraphy to evaluate efficacy of cellophane banding of congenital extrahepatic portosystemic shunts in 16 dogs. *Australian Veterinary Journal* **86**, 169–179

Lidbury JA, Ivanek R, Suchodolski JS and Steiner JM (2015) Putative precipitating factors for hepatic encephalopathy in dogs: 118 cases (1991–2014). *Journal of the American Veterinary Medical Association* **247**, 176–182

Matiasovic M, Chanoit GPA, Meakin LB and Tivers MS (2019) Outcomes of dogs treated for extrahepatic congenital portosystemic shunts with thin film banding or ameroid ring constrictor. *Veterinary Surgery* DOI: 1111/vsu. 13273

Rothuizen J, Bunch SE, Charles JA *et al.* (2006) *WSAVA Standards for Clinical and Histological Diagnosis of Canine and Feline Liver Disease.* Saunders Elsevier, Edinburgh

Serrano G, Charalambous M, Devriendt N et al. (2019) Treatment of congenital extrahepatic portosystemic shunts in dogs: A systemic review and meta-analysis. *Journal of Veterinary Internal Medicine* DOI: 10.1111/JVIM. 15607

Tivers MS, Hanel I, Gow AG *et al.* (2014) Ammonia and systemic inflammatory response syndrome predicts presence of hepatic encephalopathy in dogs with congenital portosystemic shunts. *PLoS ONE* **9**, e82303. DOI: 10.1371/journal. pone.0082303

Tivers M and Lipscomb V (2011) Congenital portosystemic shunts in cats: investigation, diagnosis and stabilization. *Journal of Feline Medicine and Surgery* **13**, 173–184

Tivers M and Lipscomb V (2011) Congenital portosystemic shunts in cats: surgical management and prognosis. *Journal of Feline Medicine and Surgery* **13**, 185–194

Tivers MS, Lipscomb VJ and Brockman DJ (2017) Treatment of intrahepatic congenital portosystemic shunts in dogs: a systematic review. *Journal of Small Animal Practice* **58**, 485–494

Tivers MS, Upjohn MM, House AK *et al.* (2012) Treatment of extrahepatic congenital portosystemic shunts in dogs – what is the evidence base? *Journal of Small Animal Practice* **53**, 3–11

Tobias KM and Rohrbach BW (2003) Association of breed with the diagnosis of congenital portosystemic shunts in dogs: 2,400 cases (1980–2002). *Journal of the American Veterinary Medical Association* **223**, 1636–1639

Villiers E and Ristić J (2016) *BSAVA Manual of Canine and Feline Clinical Pathology, 3rd edn.* BSAVA Publications, Gloucester

Weisse C, Berent AC, Todd K *et al.* (2014) Endovascular evaluation and treatment of intrahepatic portosystemic shunts in dogs: 100 cases (2001–2011). *Journal of the American Veterinary Medical Association* **244**, 78–94

Index

Note: Page numbers in *italics* refer to figures

Hyperbilirubinaemia *114, 115*, 121
Hypercoagulability secondary to PLE 120
Hypertriglyceridaemia 233
Hypertrophic gastritis 181, 189–90
Hypoadrenocorticism (Addison's disease)
    acute diarrhoea *84*, 85
    haematemesis 94
Hypoalbuminaemia 120
    fluid therapy 125
Hypocalcaemia 120
Hypoglycaemia 120
Hypokalaemia 120
Hyponatraemia 120
Hyporexia *see* Anorexia/hyporexia

Icterus *see* Jaundice
Idiopathic chronic colitis (ICC) 228
Idiopathic chronic gastritis 188–90
Idiopathic gastric motility disorders 194
Idiopathic non-inflammatory gastropathies 190
Imaging
    acute diarrhoea 86
    diagnostic approach 3
    GI tract 12–19, 184–6
    intestinal obstruction 210–11
    liver 19–22
    pancreas 22–4
    (*see also individual techniques*)
Immune system, gastrointestinal 199
Immune-mediated haemolytic anaemia *114, 115, 247*
Immune-mediated disease
    and drooling 57
    haemolytic anaemia *114, 115, 247*
    oropharynx 154–5
Immunoglobulin A, faecal biomarker 5
Immunohistochemistry 43
Immunosuppressive/anti-inflammatory agents 138–9
    (*see also individual drugs*)
Infectious diarrhoea 84
Infectious chronic gastritis 187–8
Infectious colitis 226–8
Infectious enteritis 205–10
Inflammatory hepatocellular disease 251–7
Insulinoma 37–8
Intestinal obstruction 210–12
Intestine *see* Colon and rectum; Gastrointestinal biopsy;
    Gastrointestinal surgery; Small intestine
Intussusception *84*, 85, 210, *211*, 230
Irish Setters
    breed-specific diseases *3*
    gluten-sensitive enteropathy (GSE) 218
Irritable bowel syndrome (IBS) 222, 230
Isospora see Cystoisospora
Itraconazole 188

Jaundice *78*
    bilirubin metabolism *114*
    classification 114
        hepatic 115–16
        post-hepatic 116
        pre-hepatic 115
    diagnostic algorithm *117*
    diagnostic tests 117
    differential diagnosis 118
    history 116
    non-hepatic hyperbilirubinaemia *114*
    physical examination 116–17
    treatment 118

Kaolin 135
Kernicterus *see* Bilirubin encephalopathy

Lactoferrin, faecal biomarker 6
Lactulose 137, 274
Large intestine *see* Colon and rectum
Laxatives and cathartics 136–7
Leucopenia 122
Liver
    biliary tract diseases 263–6
    diagnostic imaging 19–22
    differences between cats and dogs *245*
    hepatobillary diseases
        classification 250–1
        diagnosis 247–50
        hepatitis *250*, 251–3, 255–7, 257
        inflammatory 251–7
        non-inflammatory 257–63
        pathophysiology 245–7
    structure and function 244–5, 268
    vascular disorders
        congenital portosystemic shunt (CPSS) 269–72
        pathophysiology 268–9
        hepatic arteriovenous malformation (HAVM) 275
        hepatic encephalopathy (HE) 119, 268–70, *269*, 273–4
        peliosis hepatis 275–6
        portal vein hypoplasia (PVH) 274–5
        (*see also* Biliary tract diseases; Hepatic; Hepatitis;
        Hepatobiliary disease)
Loperamide 136
Low-fat/GI diets 127
Lymphangiectasia *3*, 18, *47, 90*, 110, *112*, 127, 138, *201, 216*, 218, 220–2
Lymphoma 194, 220, 229
Lymphoplasmacytic gastritis 188–9

Macroglossia 152
Macrolides 143
Malabsorption 201–2
Maropitant 130–1, 204, 207
Masticatory muscle myositis (MMM) 157–8
Megaoesophagus
    acquired 167–8
    aetiology 166
    congenital 166–7
    diagnosis 166–8
    prognosis 169
    treatment 168–9
Melaena
    diagnostic algorithm *97*
    diagnostic tests 96–7
    differential diagnoses 98
    history 96
    physical examination 96
    primary and secondary GI diseases *2*
    small intestine 202
Ménétrier's disease-like gastritis 181, *182*
Menrath's ulcer 157
Mesalazine 138
Mesenchymal tumours 182
Methadone 207
Metoclopramide *123*, 131, 132, 195, 204, 207
Metronidazole *123*, 143, 213, 219, *274*
Microbiome, small intestine 199
Microbiota *see* Gut microbiota
Miniature Schnauzer, breed-specific diseases *3*
Mirtazapine 139

pathophysiology 232–3
prognosis 236
treatment *140*, 141
medical 234–6
surgical 38–9
(*see also* Exocrine pancreas; Exocrine pancreatic
insufficiency)
Pantoprazole 135, 207
Paraffin 137
Paraneoplastic effects, sign of GI disease 121
Parasites 84
antigen detection 7, *10*
ascarids (roundworms) *9*, 84, 145, 209, 214
cestodes (tapeworms) *7, 8*, 145, 209, 214–15
colon 226
culture *7–10*
egg size *7*
faecal concentration methods 6–7, *8–9*
faecal examination 6
gastric *180*
hookworms *9*, 145, 209, 214
immunodetection 7
nematodes *145*, 226
pancreas 242–3
polymerase chain reaction 10
small intestine 209–10, 213–15
treatment 145–7
trematodes 226
whipworms *7, 9, 145*, 209
zoonotic considerations 214–15
Parasitic gastritis 188
Parasiticides 145–7
Pectin 135
Peliosis hepatis 275–6
D-penicillamine 255
Periodontitis *153*
Pharyngeal dysphagia 64–5
Pharyngitis 154
Phenobarbital 131, 257
Phenothiazines 131
Physalopteria spp. *180*
Phytochemicals, oropharynx 156
Poloxamers 137
Polymerase chain reaction 10, 11
Polyphagia 46–8
diagnostic algorithm *46*
diagnostic tests 47–8
differential diagnoses *47*
and exocrine pancreatic insufficiency (EPI) *48*
history 46–7
physical examination 47
primary and secondary GI diseases *2*
Polyps
colon 229
non-neoplastic 190
rectal *107*
Polyuria/polydipsia, sign of GI disease 120
Portal hypertension 246
Portal vein hypoplasia (PVH) 274–5
Portosystemic shunts 269–72
Postural (elevated) feeding 126
Prebiotics 128
Prednisolone 138, 217, 222, 236
Probiotics 128–9
Processionary moth caterpillars, oropharynx 156
Prochlorperazine 131
Prokinetics 132–3
Prostaglandins 133

Protein-losing enteropathy (PLE)
ascites 110
clinical presentation 221
complications 222
diagnosis 221
diseases causing 220–1
and hypercoagulability 120
Norwegian Lundehund 218
and pulmonary thromboembolism 122
small intestine 202
Soft Coated Wheaten Terrier 218
treatment 222
Yorkshire Terrier 218
Proton pump inhibitors (PPIs) 134–5, 165, 192
and haematemesis 94
Prototheca zopfi 228
Protozoa
and acute diarrhoea 84
faecal examination 6, *8*
infectious colitis 227
infectious enteritis 209–10
small intestine 213–14
treatment 145–7
Ptyalism/pseudoptyalism *see* Drooling
Pulmonary thromboembolism 122
Pyloric stenosis 194
Pyogranulomatous stomatitis 154

Rabies
drooling *57*, 58, 59
zoonotic considerations 59
Radiography
dental 62
dysphagia 67
GI tract 12–13, 13–16, 184–5
intestinal obstruction 210–11
liver 19–20
pancreas 22–3
Ranitidine 134, 192, 204
Regurgitation 121
diagnostic algorithm *69*
diagnostic tests 69–70
differential diagnoses *68*
history 68–9
physical examination 69
primary and secondary GI diseases *2*
signalment 68
treatment 70
Renal/urinary signs of GI disease 120–1
Respiratory signs of GI disease 121–2
Resting energy requirement (RER) 126
Rickettsia 143
Ronidazole 123
Rottweiler, breed-specific diseases *3*
Roundworms (ascarids) *9*, 84, 145, 209, 214
Rupture of the biliary tract 266

Saline purgatives 137
Salivary glands 148, *149*, 150, 160–1
(*see also* Oral cavity; Oropharynx)
Salmonella spp. 10, *140, 141*, 227
Scottish Terrier, glycogen-like vacuolar hepatopathy
259–60
Shar Pei, breed-specific diseases *3*
Sialadenitis 161
Sialadenosis 160
Sialocoeles 160

BSAVA Manuals

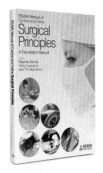 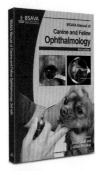 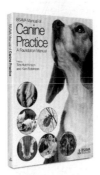 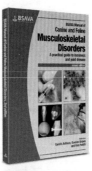 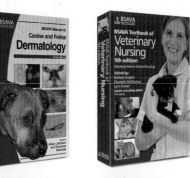

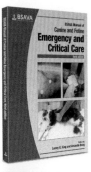 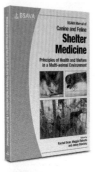 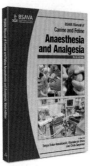 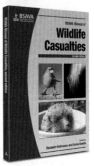 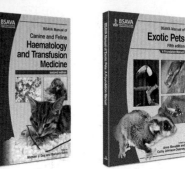

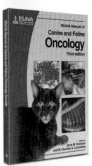 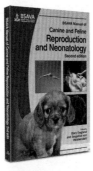 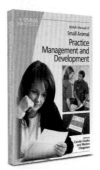 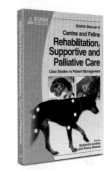 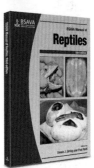 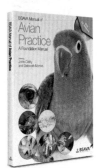

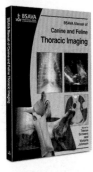 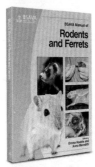 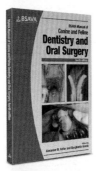 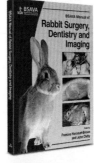 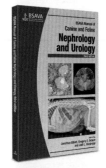 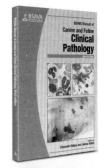

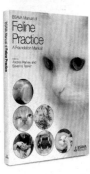 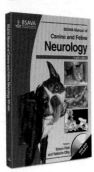 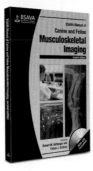 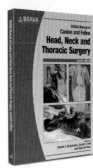 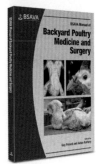 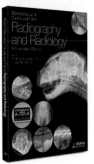